DATE DUE

AG 3 '00			
MR 3 0 '01			
AP1 8 '01			
JE 4 '06			
DE 1 0 '03			

DEMCO 38-296

SPORTS AND EXERCISE FOR CHILDREN WITH CHRONIC HEALTH CONDITIONS

Barry Goldberg, MD
Yale University School of Medicine

Editor

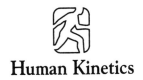

Human Kinetics

Library of Congress Cataloging-in-Publication Data

...th chronic health conditions /
[edited by] Barry Goldberg.
     p.   cm.
    Includes bibliographical references and index.
    ISBN 0-87322-873-1
    1. Sports for the handicapped. 2. Chronically ill children.
3. Sports for children. 4. Exercise for children. I. Goldberg,
Barry, 1943-   .
GV709.3.S646   1995
796'.0196--dc20   95-30663
                                     CIP

ISBN: 0-87322-873-1

Copyright © 1995 by Human Kinetics Publishers, Inc.

Permission notices for material reprinted in this book from other sources can be found on page 374.

Developmental Editor: Christine Drews
Assistant Editors: Karen Bojda, John Wentworth, and Ann Greenseth
Editorial Assistant: Andrew T. Starr
Copyeditor: Kirsten Kite
Proofreader: Karen Bojda
Indexer: Joan Griffitts
Typesetting and Text Layout: Sandra Meier and Yvonne Winsor
Layout Artist: Tara Welsch
Text Designer: Keith Blomberg
Photo Editor: Boyd LaFoon
Cover Designer: Keith Blomberg
Medical Illustrator: Beth Young
Illustrators: Dianna Porter, Studio 2D, and Craig Ronto
Printer: Braun-Brumfield

Printed in the United States of America

10 9 8 7 6 5 4 3 2 1

Human Kinetics
P.O. Box 5076, Champaign, IL 61825-5076
1-800-747-4457

Canada: Human Kinetics, Box 24040, Windsor, ON N8Y 4Y9
1-800-465-7301 (in Canada only)

Europe: Human Kinetics, P.O. Box IW14, Leeds LS16 6TR, United Kingdom
(44) 1132 781708

Australia: Human Kinetics, 2 Ingrid Street, Clapham 5062, South Australia
(08) 371 3755

New Zealand: Human Kinetics, P.O. Box 105-231, Auckland 1
(09) 523 3462

This book is dedicated to my wife, Betty;
my children, Mickey, Rachel, Daniel;
and my parents, Harry and Elsie,
whose support carried me through frustrating periods
and whose understanding tolerated the closed door to my study.
It is also dedicated to the courage and perseverance of children
with chronic health conditions who endure and relentlessly battle.

Contents

Preface

Over 2 million children in the United States suffer from a chronic medical disease. Physical symptoms and recurrent, sometimes traumatic, medical therapy are a regular part of many of their lives. When restrictions on a child's physical activity are required, quality of life is further hampered. Sports and exercise are popular among children and important to them, and exclusion adds to the feelings of social isolation and personal vulnerability. The child with a chronic health condition is also deprived of the potential health promotion of exercise, both generally so and specific to the disease process. Physicians and educators are appropriately conservative in dealing with the physical activity of children with chronic health conditions, but often decisions must be intuitive, because appropriate activity guidelines are not readily available.

Sports and Exercise for Children With Chronic Health Conditions was written so these decisions would not need to be intuitive. This is the first-ever comprehensive set of guidelines for how children with chronic health conditions can participate in sports and exercise. Now the decisions about participation can be based on the recommendations of physicians who have a wealth of experience in diagnosing and treating these conditions as well as in helping their patients find activities that are enjoyable and safe—and even beneficial—to participate in. This book brings together clinical diagnoses and participation guidelines, so physicians can judge where their individual patients may be on the participation continuum—from not being able to participate in most physical activities to being able to participate fully in many activities.

The contributors have concentrated on how physical activity can affect the child's quality of life. They have looked at the total child to see that children with chronic health conditions deserve to be able to achieve all that they can within acceptable safety limits.

Physicians, educators, health and fitness professionals, and parents will find the four chapters in Part I helpful in understanding the general issues affecting the child with a chronic health condition and physical activity participation.

Chapter 1 discusses general problems for children with chronic health conditions, such as possibly impaired psychosocial and physical development. By understanding these more global problems, the physician can effectively plan preventive and therapeutic interventions. The benefits of physical activity participation are discussed in chapter 2, as are the potential adverse effects of sports and exercise, such as sudden death, injury, and the pressures for successful performance.

Chapter 3 deals with general principles for selecting sports and exercise activities: preparatory conditioning, understanding the various demands of sports, and establishing programs that respond to and prevent potentially adverse responses. Sports are categorized by specific demands. Legal ramifications regarding the inclusion or exclusion of children in sports and exercise activities are discussed in chapter 4, along with the uncomfortable liabilities assumed by physicians and educators should activity recommendations yield some adverse result. Mechanisms to minimize this exposure are reviewed.

Physicians and educators will derive practical benefit from the specific recommendations given in Part II. Physicians can couple the guidelines given in these chapters with their knowledge of their patients to create appropriate physical activity recommendations for individual patients. Educators may be able to enter into discussion with parents and physicians if some children are being more limited in participation than what these guidelines suggest.

Each of the chapters in Part II deals with a specific chronic disease. The chapters include a brief description of the pathophysiology, presentation, assessment, and natural history of the condition. The intent is not to be all-inclusive, because other sources are readily available, but rather to review the disease so the later references to sports and exercise are understandable. The chapters deal directly with the interface of the disease entity with sport and exercise. A discussion of the effect of the condition on exercise tolerance and a description of potential adverse effects are provided. Preventive measures to avoid adverse consequences are reviewed, and the appropriate immediate response to an emergency in a school or recreational environment is outlined. The important potential benefits of sport and exercise are discussed, both specific to the disease process and more generally concerning the child's development.

Each chapter includes specific and practical recommendations, including appropriate conditioning activities and recommended sports. You will learn which activities can be permitted as well as those that should be avoided. The issue of level of competition, from recreational to organized team, is also addressed. With these guidelines, physicians and educators can plan the most appropriate program for the child with a chronic health condition, a program that will avoid the potential adverse effects of sport and exercise while permitting the health and psychosocial benefits.

The chronic conditions chosen for discussion certainly do not include all of the entities that afflict children, and the exclusion of such handicapping conditions as mental retardation, paraplegia, blindness, and deafness does not in any way minimize their importance. Much has been written concerning these conditions, and a single chapter would not do justice to the available literature. The illnesses included were selected either because information is not readily available to physicians and educators or because no true literature exists. Where there is no literature, authors were chosen for their broad clinical experience and their commitment to carefully matching children to appropriate sport experiences.

Sports and Exercise for Children With Chronic Health Conditions has been developed through the diligence of its many contributors, who are committed to optimizing quality of life for children with chronic health conditions. The medical care of the underlying disease is the appropriate primary concern of the physician, and protecting the child from adverse environmental situations must be an objective of educators, but concern for psychosocial development, physical fitness, and quality of life is significant. The contributors hope that this book will provide the information and generate the confidence physicians and educators need to recommend activities that will let children with chronic health conditions maximize their life's experiences and their personal potential.

Acknowledgments

The development of a text of this dimension requires the efforts of a great many individuals. First, the American Academy of Pediatrics and its Committee on Sports Medicine and Fitness deserve recognition for understanding the need for this book and encouraging its development. The academy's committee also participated in the early planning of the book. The authors of each chapter must also be commended for their willingness to take the time to write and for the excellent manuscripts they developed. For many, their chapter required not only a review of the literature but also a survey of their colleagues to form a consensus. The national status of our authors reflects their true commitment to the concept of expanding the activities and improving the quality of life for children with chronic health conditions; time may be limited for many of these children. Finally, our reviewers of each article deserve special commendation as we picked only individuals with national reputations. Their reviews were carefully performed, often provoked interesting dialogue, and created a forum for discussion and recommendation in an area poorly researched. I believe many interesting research projects will result from the issues raised by this text.

A book cannot be completed without the assistance of a committed publisher. Human Kinetics has supported this book from its inception, and Christine Drews, the developmental editor, has been diligent in corresponding with the authors and reviewing chapters. Finally, thanks to my assistant and right hand, Stephanie Muzyka, who performed her role brilliantly. Without her dedication, loyalty, and perseverance, this book would not be possible.

PART I

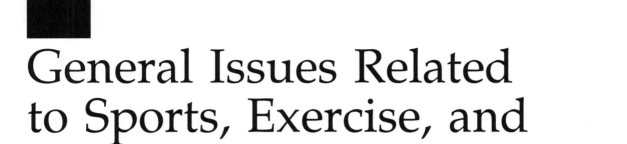

General Issues Related to Sports, Exercise, and Chronic Health Conditions

CHAPTER 1

Impact of Chronic Health Conditions in Childhood

Nancy E. Lanphear
Genesee Developmental Unit, Rochester, NY

Gregory S. Liptak
University of Rochester School of Medicine and Dentistry

Michael Weitzman
University of Rochester School of Medicine and Dentistry

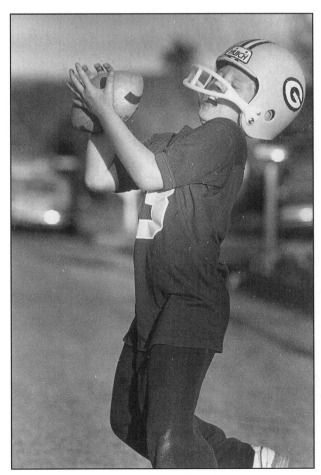

© Mary Langenfeld

Children are generally believed to be the healthiest segment of the American population; their health care needs are usually thought to be preventive or acute and the cost of their care modest. For a significant proportion of children, however, this picture is inaccurate. Chronic health conditions affect approxmiately 1 in 10 children between the ages of 4 and 17 years in the United States (8), although estimates of affected children vary widely because no universal definition of a chronic health condition exists. Some restrict this term only to conditions in which physical limitations occur, others broaden it to encompass conditions that limit any aspect of functioning, and still others argue that any condition that lasts at least three months in a given year should be included (12, 22, 23). The distinction between chronic and self-limited conditions is important because chronic health conditions are much more likely to have far-reaching developmental and psychosocial implications (13).

For purposes of this discussion, chronic health conditions in children may be said to include physical impairments, sensory (visual and auditory) impairments, and cognitive impairments (e.g., specific learning disabilities, attention deficit hyperactivity disorder, or mental retardation). Some conditions, such as congenital heart disease, isolated renal disease, and asthma, are limited to a specific organ or system; others affect multiple organs or systems, as is the case with spina bifida, cerebral palsy, and many syndromes and congenital anomalies. Conditions can also occur in combination: for example, sensory deficits and cognitive impairments may be isolated difficulties or may accompany other conditions.

Although the incidence of most chronic conditions has remained stable, the actual number of children with many of these disorders has increased. For conditions such as congenital heart disease, childhood cancers, and spina bifida, improved technology and treatment have resulted in longer life expectancy (7). The improved survival rates of very low-birth-weight babies also has led to increased numbers of children with physical or neurocognitive problems such as speech and language disorders, attention deficits, mental retardation, and visual and hearing disorders. The natural histories of many other conditions such as congenital hypo-thyroidism and phenylketonuria have also been altered dramatically owing to early identification and the implementation of appropriate therapy. Even for many conditions that are ultimately fatal, such as cystic fibrosis and childhood HIV infection, life expectancy has been extended and the quality of life vastly improved.

Chronic health conditions of childhood vary widely in terms of severity, progression and prognosis, with only a small minority being fatal. The majority are neither life-threatening nor severely limiting. Many have variable effects on children's health and functioning, and some produce only intermittent signs or symptoms. For example, many children with asthma or sickle-cell disease are free of symptoms most of the time, but occasionally experience acute exacerbations necessitating active intervention. These exacerbations are not always predictable or preventable.

The goals of therapeutic efforts on behalf of children with chronic health conditions are at least twofold:

1. to intervene at the biological level and control disease manifestations or progression to the fullest extent possible with a minimal number of side effects; and
2. to minimize the psychological and social impact of the chronic health condition on the child and family, normalizing their experiences as much as possible.

PSYCHOLOGICAL, EDUCATIONAL, AND SOCIAL ISSUES

The prevention of psychological, social, and educational difficulties and the minimization of the functional impact of chronic health conditions are well recognized as central to the care provided to children with chronic health conditions (21). One area of importance is the functional status of the child as indicated by, for example, school attendance and performance, activities of daily living such as personal hygiene and household chores, the maintenance of peer relationships, and play. Also important is the psychological well-being of the child and family, including the development of self-esteem, a sense of competence, social integration, and the maintenance of appropriate expectations. A further consideration is the impact of the condition on family finances and functioning.

Psychological Issues

Although specific health conditions require specific and often highly specialized medical or surgical interventions, many of the altered psychological and social experiences encountered by children with chronic conditions and their families are not disease-specific and are likely to be encountered irrespective of the particular medical aspects of the condition. Thus, even children with rare conditions frequently share experiences similar to those of children with more common conditions. Many of these common experiences are listed in Table 1.1. The perspective that children and families with various health conditions share common issues has been termed a noncategorical approach (28, 29) and has improved our insight into the dynamics of adaptation in the child and the family.

Psychological and behavioral problems are somewhat more common in children with chronic health conditions than in their healthy

Table 1.1   Common Issues for Childen and Families With Chronic Health Conditions

Unpredictable and chronic course of the condition

Pain and embarrassment of treatments

Isolation from peers

Frequent school absenteeism

Increased risk for psychological and behavioral problems

Potential for growth and development to deviate from the norm

Strained family relationships

High cost of care (in time and money)

Frequent health care visits and hospitalizations

Substantial amount of daily care needed by affected individual

Potential conflicts between care providers

Conflicts between home life and therapies

Restricted access to buildings and activities

Ever-changing health reimbursement systems

Lost opportunities for families and children in day-to-day experiences

Restrictions on friends and activities

peers (23). However, except in children with neurological conditions, neither the prevalence, type, nor severity of these secondary problems is disease specific. In other words, a child with a given health condition is not at risk for any particular social or psychological adjustment difficulty (24, 25). Rather, children with chronic conditions are subject to alterations in social experiences, expectations, self-esteem, and interactions, and to some degree of activity restriction (11). These alterations and the attendant psychosocial problems are sometimes more disabling or handicapping than the health conditions themselves.

It may be difficult to predict which children are more likely to develop these secondary problems. In a study of children with juvenile arthritis, for example, all children with arthritis were more likely to have emotional problems than were children in the control group, but the children with only minor disability were at higher risk for these problems than were children with severely disabling arthritis (14). An epidemiological survey of children from 4 to 16 years of age with chronic health conditions found that children both with and without physical disability were at greater risk for mental health difficulties such as overanxious disorder, depression, obsessive-compulsive disorder, conduct disorder, and attention deficit hyperactivity disorder. In another study, however, an increased risk for social adjustment problems was seen only in children with a physical disability; problems included isolation, difficulty interacting with peers, low participation and competence in outside-the-home activities, and school difficulties (2). It is also important to remember in both the child's and parents' viewpoints the possible social stigma that is felt from appearing different.

Primary prevention of psychosocial difficulties is an important component of care in any child who has a chronic health condition, and the primary care physician is in an ideal position to monitor and intervene if evidence of psychosocial difficulties occurs (10, 15, 18). Unfortunately, community and school resources are often underutilized in the prevention and remediation of mental health and social adjustment difficulties (24).

Family Issues

Family stress is frequently heightened in a family with a member who has a chronic health condition. One area of difficulty is economic: medical care in many cases is both expensive and time-consuming (24). Many parents miss work because of the child's illness, medical appointments, or hospitalizations. Added stress occurs from the rising cost of health care and the inadequacies of many health insurance packages, which may require a portion of the cost to be paid by the family or which may not cover needed supplies and equipment. Other non-reimbursable expenses may include transportation, housing, and food connected with health-related visits. Adequate respite care is not only difficult to find, but costly. This added financial burden may in turn limit the family's ability to provide opportunities such as vacations and outside-the-home activities for the entire family (31).

Not all of the stress experienced by families of children with chronic health conditions is economic, however (26). The daily burden of care for a child with a chronic health condition may be substantial and time-consuming, and this can strain both parental and sibling relationships. Unaffected sisters or brothers may feel that they are in competition with their sibling; they may also feel guilty about their sibling's illness, excessively vulnerable themselves, or resentful of altered expectations or parental availability.

The family's perception of a child's well-being can be shaped by events that occur quite early in the child's life. This is certainly true of illnesses, especially those from which the child is not expected to survive; attitudes are further influenced by information that physicians communicate or withhold. Altered perceptions of the child's well-being may adversely affect the parent-child relationship and disturb the child's psychosocial development, which may lead to difficulties with separation, expectations, educational achievement, and independence. Parents may perceive that abnormalities occurring in the neonatal period require them to protect their child from normal day-to-day developmental experiences, and the limit setting necessary for the eventual development of independence may not be provided. This distorted perception has been called the vulnerable child syndrome (3, 6, 9).

Developmental Issues

Parents face challenges from all children during the different stages of development. However, there are also certain developmental issues that are unique to children with chronic health conditions.

Infancy

As Erik Erikson has proposed in his theories of child development, infancy is a time when the child establishes a sense of trust (5). During the infancy of a child with a chronic health condition, however, the environment may be disrupted and unpredictable, and the time and space necessary for optimal bonding of the infant and parents may be difficult to achieve. Physical abnormalities or restrictions may alter the infant's perception of the world and affect his or her ability to move freely in the environment. This can delay the acquisition of developmental milestones and affect the toddler when exploration of the environment is essential to the attainment of autonomy (20).

Preschool

During the toddler and preschool years, gains in cognitive skills rely on the language and fine motor activities that children attempt and eventually master. The child with a chronic health condition may not be exposed to preschool settings, peer activities, or environments that foster development at these stages. In some instances, parents may actively avoid social situations that are perceived as risky, and overly restrict the child's environment and his or her active exploration of it.

School-Age Years

The social activities of school-age children increasingly involve their peers and are more often located outside the home. Critical issues during this time include family separation, acquisition of social skills and competence, adjustment to a work setting, and the development of a sense of personal accomplishment or industry (5). School is the avenue by which children experience early societal successes and failures, refine social niceties and etiquette, interact with adults and peers outside the home, and learn academic skills and personal work habits. These necessary lessons can be difficult for all children to master, but they may be especially difficult for children with chronic health conditions (30).

Emotional behaviors and patterns are developed by a child's day-to-day interactions with family and others. The experiences and environment of a child with a chronic health condition may have both positive and negative affects on emotional functioning. Research on the emotional characteristics of children with chronic health conditions has suggested that these children tend to have significantly higher levels of empathy and emotional responsiveness, but also of depression, and in some instances, poor self-concept (19). Some of these characteristics place the child at risk for the psychosocial difficulties already described.

One of the challenges facing children with chronic health conditions and their families is to avoid frequent absences from school, as such absences may lead to significant educational disadvantages. These absences may be occasioned by visits to health professionals, inappropriate health beliefs and perceptions of excessive vulnerability, exacerbations of symptoms, or hospitalizations. Daily routines may be further disrupted by frequent changes in diets, therapies, surgeries, or medications. Social experiences may therefore be altered, and the acquisition and maintenance of friendships may be more difficult. Children with chronic conditions may also be set apart from their peers because of restrictions on physical activities or diet, or because of the need to administer medications in school. Many medications also have noticeable side effects. In addition, some children with chronic conditions have visible physical or cognitive differences, which may make them or their peers anxious or uncomfortable.

Adolescence

Because of restrictions on activities, peer interactions, and physical and social enviornments, adolescents with chronic health conditions may have increased difficulty making a successful transition to adulthood. Diminished expectations of performance and future goals may also affect choices and the pursuit of educational opportunities on both the child's and parents' part. This need not be the case, however: at least one study of adolescents with chronic health conditions demonstrated that their transition to early adulthood was generally similar to that of their unaffected peers in terms of self-esteem, marriage, and educational attainment. On the other hand, the study included few adolescents with severely limiting chronic health conditions, and it is quite possible that performance in these areas may be more compromised among more severely affected youth (6).

EVALUATION FOR PARTICIPATION IN PHYSICAL ACTIVITIES

Children with chronic health conditions have a wide range of abilities and possibilities for participation in sport. Some children who are severely limited in their ability to perform in sport events may nonetheless enjoy being team manager or supervisor. Very few children cannot physically perform in any sport. It is therefore important to prevent overprotection and to devise creative or collaborative strategies that enable children with all sorts of chronic health conditions to participate in physical activity. Not all sport needs to be organized or competitive, and many of the fundamentals of peer relations can be learned in the neighborhood pickup game.

When devising a prescription of recommended physical activities for an individual with a specific chronic health condition, an overly cautious approach may result in a more limited scope of physical activities than is medically necessary. It is also important to ascertain that the diagnosis is appropriate and is understood by the child and parents. In a classic study, Bergman and Stamm evaluated children who had a history of "heart disease" recorded on school records. Evaluation of school and medical records, followed by cardiology evaluation, found that 80% of children originally reported in school records to have heart disease had no medical findings. Of these children, 30% had already been restricted in their physical activities (1).

Subsequent chapters in this book review issues related to sport and physical activity for a host of specific conditions. However, no matter what the chronic condition, children should be evaluated with the following criteria before

Table 1.2 Evaluation Criteria for Children With Chronic Health Conditions for Participation in Sports

---

What are the child's cognitive abilities?

What are the child's social skills?

Are any effects of condition or treatments anticipated on stamina skills?

Will specific activities post substantial risk?

Will interventions or modifications in preparation be necessary?

How can activities or rules be modified to allow participation?

What level of participation is best for the child?

---

health professionals make recommendations regarding their participation (see also Table 1.2):

- What are their cognitive abilities (e.g., can they follow rules)?
- What are their social skills (e.g., can they interact with team members or do they require additional structure)?
- What effect does their condition or treatment have on their stamina and skills (e.g., can a child with cyanotic heart disease play badminton for 10 minutes)?
- Will specific sports activities pose a substantial risk to health and well-being (e.g., can a child with shunted hydrocephalus safely play football)?
- Will specific interventions or modifications in conditioning or preparation be required (e.g., will a child with asthma need inhaled beta-agonists or cromolyn before an event or activity)?
- How could an activity be modified to allow a child to obtain maximal benefit (e.g., will changing the rules in wrestling allow a child with paraplegia to compete)?
- What level of activity would be best for this particular child (e.g., will an obese child need more consistent aerobic activity)?

Physical Assessment

It is important that the physical health of every child with a chronic health condition be considered prior to participation. This assessment should include cardiovascular status, muscle strength, motor skills and deficits, and any other system that could be affected by the chronic condition. Assessment information is critical not only to determine appropriate activities, but also to determine the training needed to allow a child to participate at the optimal level of activity.

Nutritional Assessment

The nutritional status of a child with a chronic health condition also may be an important area for intervention. Some children with chronic health conditions may be underweight or overweight due to their specific condition, and appropriate dietary counseling to allow the child to perform optimally may be imperative. For example, children with diabetes will need to appropriately alter caloric intake and insulin with any significant modification in their activities. Athletic food fads such as carbohydrate loading or restrictive dieting and medications such as androgenic steroids are questionable and potentially dangerous in all children, but may pose an especially significant risk in a child with a chronic health condition.

Clearing a child from medical concerns is as important as appropriately restricting activities and experiences. Restriction of activities can be a radical and often unnecessary component of care in children with chronic health conditions. Failure of a primary care physician or subspecialist (11) to discuss these issues clearly with the family and to assure understanding may lead to poor knowledge of the true limitations of a condition and an overly restrictive environment.

ENCOURAGING PARTICIPATION IN PHYSICAL ACTIVITIES

Socialization in childhood includes many activities such as free play, learning to play cooperatively with other children, and the experience of nonthreatening competition. These fundamental social skills begin early in childhood and are redefined as new challenges are met. Sport activities for children provide social experiences that can be sources of great enjoyment and enhance the mastery of physical skills. Involvement in sport has traditionally been a way in which children gain self-esteem, pride in abilities, and physical pleasure. Sport also can provide a venue to learn conflict resolution. It is not absolutely necessary that a child be involved in organized or competitive team activities, but the social skills learned in these activities are necessary for the achievement of independent adulthood.

On the other hand, no child should be forced to compete in activities that will be upsetting or demeaning. Activities need to be offered in a nonthreatening manner, and participation needs to be encouraged by the family, school, and health care providers. The influence of parents and coaches is extremely important in the positive experience of sport. Unrealistic parental expectations and pressure to excel can also elevate the stress experienced by a child and decrease personal enjoyment. Parents and coaches can increase the child's enjoyment by expressing satisfaction in the child's performance and acting as supportive and positive influences (27).

Because a chronic condition can impair the development of social skills, parents, teachers, and coaches may have to make special efforts to provide children with chronic health conditions the opportunities to engage in peer and physical activities. For example, parents may have to take the initiative to invite other children to their home to allow their child to play. This is especially true if there is not a neighborhood peer group or if the child attends a school outside the neighborhood.

It is important to remember that most children with chronic health conditions will attend school in a regular setting and should be expected to participate in many usual childhood and school-related activities. Accurate knowledge of the specific aspects of a particular child's condition, gained from information obtained from the parent, teacher, physician, and the child, can lead to the identification of physical activities that are not only safe, but also beneficial. Physical activities initiated during early childhood may promote the maintenance of physical fitness for a lifetime. Long-term benefits include weight control, increased flexibility, and improved cardiovascular status.

Adolescence may be particularly difficult for an individual with a chronic health condition. If the condition is visible, the child will need to face not only the physical changes of puberty but also the social stigma of looking different. The child may refuse to participate in physical education classes or in social situations that require body awareness or changing clothes in a public place. Reluctance to disrobe is natural in childhood, but may be exaggerated in a child with a disability. Providing privacy and other accommodations may increase the adolescent's participation in these activities.

Appropriate role models are critical for the development of children and adolescents. However, it may be difficult for a child with a chronic health condition to locate and contact a successful adult who has a similar condition. Television and movies all too often mark achievement by physical prowess or beauty; they fail to demonstrate positive images of persons with chronic health conditions, and do not adequately show the richness of life possible for such individuals.

THE OPTIMAL PROGRAM

Devising an optimal physical exercise curriculum for a child with a chronic health condition requires certain components. The program needs to be devised with the child's interests, skills, and weaknesses in mind, and should encourage growth in these areas. It must remain flexible to changes in the child's health status and adapt performance expectations as necessary while maintaining the child's motivation and interest. Arranging a safe but boring program of repetitive activities will only serve to further teach the child that enjoyable physical activities are not available.

A physical conditioning program is beneficial for any child undertaking new physical activities, and it may be essential for a child with a chronic health problem. Previous experience may be limited, and the child may be less able to define appropriate limits, particularly if an attempt is made to compete with children without disabilties. The conditioning program should accomplish a slow buildup of physical stamina without added health risk. Once the child's activity program begins, it is important to periodically monitor physical and emotional status and to provide important feedback to the child and family. This process needs to be a creative collaboration with the child, family, and, if these are school-related activities, the coach or school nurse. The physician and nurse practitioner should act as consultants in the decision-making process and give appropriate feedback on the child's health condition.

A successful program will be consistent with activities that exist for children without chronic health conditions, such as dance, team sports, skiing, or swimming. If possible, a child with a chronic health condition should be allowed to participate alongside children without chronic conditions; except in the case of the most competitive teams this should be possible at all ages. For a few activities, children with chronic conditions may prefer to participate only with children who have similar physical limitations, for example, in wheelchair races or wheelchair basketball. Another avenue of segregated participation is the Special Olympics, which have given many children a chance to participate and win in physically challenging situations.

To be successful, physical activities for children with chronic health conditions need to address children's relationships to their families, schools, and communities. Too often these activities are planned in isolation, with little input from the family or child. Ideally, however, the physical education teacher who will be involved with the child gathers input from parents, therapists, and teachers in the context of an Individualized Education Plan meeting (see chapter 4). The physician involved in this child's care could be invited, and if unable to attend could transmit any important information and restrictions. The physical education teacher should also accept input from the child in devising a tentative program. In this manner, the child has additional time to build a relationship of trust with his or her "coach." Periodic evaluations aid in the further evolution of the program and of plans for future programs.

CURRENT STATUS OF PROGRAMMING

Assessment of past physical education programming has revealed somewhat discouraging findings. For example, a study conducted in the 1980s indicated that physical education teachers were usually not involved in the placement process for children with chronic health conditions, lacked knowledge of the legal requirements of Public Law 94-142, had little experience in conducting physical assessments of children with health conditions, and tended to have little interest in working with these students. Teachers also stated that they would exclude students from planned activities on the basis of health conditions and specific abilities (17).

Clearly, much work needs to be done to improve organized athletic opportunities for children with chronic conditions. Education of physical education teachers and college instruction concerning chronic health conditions is essential if the full potential of school-based physical education programs is to be reached. Effective programs have been piloted but are still rare (16).

On a positive note, the theories behind physical education teaching have been changing. In the traditional, formal method of instruction, an activity is demonstrated and the student replicates that activity. However, recent publications support the use of a combination of different instruction approaches, including formal, learner-centered or indirect, and game-oriented methodologies (4). These fundamental changes could add flexibility to the teaching of sports education, thereby opening the door to the individualization and adaptation of many traditional activities.

Programs outside the school are often difficult to find and may need to be invented by parents and children. It may be helpful to contact local parent associations, athletes who have chronic health conditions, and health care facilities which serve children and adults with chronic health conditions. Ingenuity and an exhaustive search of community resources should make it possible to locate programs that can be utilized by every child.

CONCLUSION

Most children with chronic health conditions do not require limitations on their activities. Unnecessary restrictions may indeed have greater negative effects on children's psychosocial and physical development than the chronic conditions themselves. When restrictions are unavoidable it behooves health care providers, teachers, and families to devise creative alternatives so that all children can experience the positive rewards of exercise and live as normal a life as is possible.

Children with chronic conditions may have problems that can affect their psychological well-being and activity levels. Furthermore, the visible reminders of certain conditions may affect the child's body image and hinder the development of adequate self-esteem. Thus, it is vital that children with chronic health conditions have advocates who will foster the least restrictive environment for home, school, work, and recreation. An advocate may be a parent, a teacher, a family member, a friend, or a health care professional. Ideally, all of these people, and most importantly the child, will work together to find positive activities which will become a source of enjoyment for a lifetime. All children should be encouraged to perform to their best ability and to experience all which is within their power. Finally, children with chronic conditions should be encouraged in their dreams for the future and taught realistic expectations of the limitations that their conditions have on their activities.

REFERENCES

1. Bergman, A.B.; Stamm, S.J. The morbidity of cardiac nondisease in school children. New England Journal of Medicine 276:1008-1013; 1967.
2. Cadman, D.; Boyle, M.; Szatmari, P.; Offord, D.R. Chronic illness, disability and mental and social well-being: findings of the Ontario child health study. Pediatrics 79:805-813; 1987.
3. Costanza, M.; Lipsitch, I.; Charney, E. The vulnerable children revisited: a follow-up study of children three to six years after acute illness in infancy. Clinical Pediatrics 7:680-683; 1968.
4. Emmanouel, C.; Zervas, Y.; Vagenas, G. Effects of four physical education teaching methods on development of motor skill, self-concept, and social attitudes of fifth-grade children. Perceptual and Motor Skills 74:1151-1167; 1992.
5. Erikson, E. Childhood and society. New York: Norton; 1964.
6. Gortmaker, S.L.; Perrin, J.M.; Weitzman, M.; Sobol, A.M. An unexpected success story: transition to adulthood in youth with chronic physical health conditions. Journal of Research in Adolescence; in press.
7. Gortmaker, S.L.; Sappenfield, W. Chronic childhood disorders: prevalence and impact. Pediatric Clinics of North America 31:3-18; 1984.
8. Gortmaker, S.L.; Walker, D.K.; Weitzman, M.; Sobol, A.M. Chronic conditions, socio-economic risks, and behavioral problems in children and adolescents. Pediatrics 85:267-276; 1990.
9. Green, M.; Solnit, A.J. Reactions to the threatened loss of a child: a vulnerable child syndrome. Pediatrics 58-67; 1964.
10. Kanthor, H.; Pless, B.; Satterwhite, B.; Myers, G. Areas of responsiblity in the health care of multiply handicapped children. Pediatrics 54:779-785; 1974.
11. Leventhal, J.M. Psychosocial assessment of children with chronic physical disease. Pediatric Clinics of North America 31:71-87; 1984.
12. Mattsson, A. Long-term physical illness in childhood: a challenge to psychosocial adaptation. Pediatrics 50:801-811; 1972.
13. Mattsson, A.; Weisberg, I. Behavioral reactions to minor illness in preschool children. Pediatrics 46:604; 1970.
14. McAnarney, E.R.; Pless, I.B.; Satterwhite, B.; Friedman, S.B. Psychological problems of children with chronic juvenile arthritis. Pediatrics 53:523-528; 1974.
15. McInerny, T. The role of the general pediatrician in coordinating the care of children with chronic illness. Pediatric Clinics of North America 31:199-209; 1984.
16. Melograno, V.J.; Loovis, E.M. Effects of field-based training on teachers' knowledge and attitudes and the motor proficiency of their handicapped students. Perceptual and Motor Skills 72:1211-1214; 1991a.
17. Melograno, V.J.; Loovis; E.M. Status of physical education for handicapped students: a comprehensive analysis of teachers in 1980 and 1988. Adapted Physical Activity Quarterly 8:28-42; 1991b.
18. Merkens, M.J.; Perrin, E.C.; Perrin, J.M.; Gerrity, P.S. The awareness of primary physicians of the psychosocial adjustments of children with a chronic illness. Developmental Pediatrics 10:1-6; 1989.
19. Nelms, B.C. Emotional behaviors in chronically ill children. Journal of Abnormal Child Psychology 17:657-668; 1989.

20. Perrin, E.C.; Gerrity, P.S. Development of children with a chronic illness. Pediatric Clinics of North America 31:19; 1984.

21. Perrin, J.M.; MacLean, W.E. Children with chronic illness: the prevention of dysfunction. Pediatric Clinics of North America 35:1325-1337; 1988.

22. Pless, I.B.; Pinkerton, P. Chronic childhood disorder: promoting patterns of adjustment. London: Henry Kingston Publishers; 1975.

23. Pless, I.B.; Power, C.; Peckham, C.S. Long-term psychosocial sequelae of chronic physical disorders in childhood. Pediatrics 91: 1131-1136; 1993.

24. Pless, I.B.; Roghmann, K.; Haggerty, R.J. Chronic illness, family functioning and psychological adjustment: a model for the allocation of preventive mental health services. International Journal of Epidemiology 1:271-277; 1972.

25. Revell, G.M.; Liptak, G.S. Understanding the child with special health care needs: a developmental perspective. Journal of Pediatric Nursing 6:258-268; 1991.

26. Sabbeth, B. Understanding the impact of chronic childhood illness on families. Pediatric Clinics of North America 31:47-57; 1984.

27. Scanlan, T.K.; Lewthwaite, R. From stress to enjoyment: parental and coach influences on young participants. In: Brown, E.W.; Branta, C.F., eds. Competitive sports for children and youth, 1988: 41-48.

28. Stein, R.E.K.; Jessop, D. A non-categorical approach to chronic childhood illness. Public Health Rep. 97:351-362; 1982.

29. Stein, R.E.K.; Jones-Jessop, D. General issues in the care of children with chronic physical conditions. Pediatric Clinics of North America 31:189-197; 1984.

30. Weitzman, M. School and peer relations. Pediatric Clinics of North America 31:59-69; 1984.

31. Worley, G.; Rosenfeld, L.R.; Lipscomb, J. Financial counseling for families of children with chronic disabilities. Developmental Medicine and Child Neurology 33:679-689; 1991.

CHAPTER 2

The Benefits and Risks of Sports and Exercise for Children With Chronic Health Conditions

Michael A. Nelson
University of New Mexico School of Medicine

Sally S. Harris
Palo Alto Medical Clinic

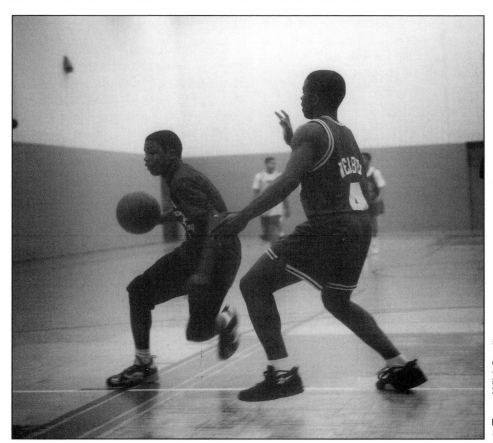

Physical activity is considered essential for optimal health, development, socialization, and well-being of children. However, children with chronic diseases are often restricted from participation in exercise programs or sport activities because of real or perceived limitations imposed by their disease. In addition, coaches, parents, and physicians are often concerned about potential dangers of exercise. As a result, children with chronic diseases are among the least active children and are at additional risk for a variety of health conditions associated with a sedentary lifestyle. Growing attention is being placed on the need to integrate physical activity into the lives of children with chronic diseases, whatever their physical or mental limitations, and to do so in a way that is both safe and beneficial.

Most of the research on the beneficial effects of exercise has been done on populations of healthy children. Much less is known about the potential benefits of physical activity for children with chronic disease. However, children with chronic diseases can attain the same general benefits of exercise as healthy children, including enhanced physical fitness, preventive health benefits, and improved psychosocial well-being. In addition, for certain chronic diseases exercise may carry disease-specific benefits. This chapter reviews the general and specific benefits of exercise for the physical and psychosocial health of children with chronic disease.

GENERAL PHYSICAL FITNESS BENEFITS OF EXERCISE

Physical fitness encompasses a diverse set of traits. Some components of physical fitness include balance, coordination, speed, and power. Improvement in these factors can contribute to motor development, skill mastery, feelings of competence and achievement, and athletic success for all children. Other components of physical fitness, while also contributing to athletic success, are of additional importance for health maintenance and disease prevention. Health-related components of physical fitness include cardiopulmonary endurance, body composition, muscle strength and endurance, and flexibility (see Table 2.1). Improvement in these areas is associated with reductions in risk factors associated with various disease states. Enhanced

Table 2.1   Health Benefits of Physical Fitness

Fitness component	Health benefit
Cardiopulmonary endurance	Improved aerobic exercise capacity Increased caridac output Increased ventilatory capacity
Body composition	Decreased obesity Decreased body fatness Increased lean body mass
Muscle strength and endurance	Improved musculoskeletal function Prevention of muscle atrophy and injury Increased strength Increased oxidative capacity
Flexibility	Improved musculoskeletal function Prevention of joint contractures and injury

physical fitness may be particularly important for children with chronic diseases because it may improve their ability to tolerate physical activities.

Cardiopulmonary Endurance

Cardiopulmonary endurance reflects aerobic capacity—the ability of the heart and lungs to meet the oxygen demands of exercising muscle and the ability of the muscles to use the discharged oxygen to perform sustained physical activity. Maximal oxygen uptake ($\dot{V}O_2$max), defined as the body's maximum capacity to consume oxygen over a fixed period of time, is the variable most often used to measure aerobic capacity in the laboratory setting. It is a measure of the greatest amount of oxygen that can be taken in and utilized by the body during a maximal exercise challenge. It reflects the three components of the oxygen delivery system.

1. Oxygen inhaled and transferred to blood by the respiratory system
2. Oxygen delivered to exercising muscles by the cardiovascular system
3. Oxygen processed by muscle metabolic system (mitochondria)

Low values of $\dot{V}O_2$max indicate low levels of aerobic capacity and poor cardiopulmonary endurance.

All children can improve cardiopulmonary endurance as a result of appropriate physical conditioning. Research shows that when training programs meet adult standards (in terms of the intensity, frequency, and duration of the training stimulus), children demonstrate a similar magnitude of improvement in $\dot{V}O_2max$ (7–26%) as seen in adults (74). Usual recommendations for an appropriate conditioning program to improve cardiopulmonary endurance would include aerobic activity (sustained rhythmic movement of large muscle groups resulting in an increase in heart rate and respiratory rate) performed at a frequency of 3–5 times per week, intensity of 60–85% $\dot{V}O_2max$, and duration of at least 15 minutes, for a minimum of 6 weeks (8). The necessary conditioning stimulus depends on an individual's baseline fitness level. Thus, individuals with low levels of baseline fitness, such as many children with chronic disease, can make appreciable improvements in cardiopulmonary fitness with significantly lower levels of physical conditioning. In many children with chronic disease significant improvements in aerobic fitness can be achieved with very modest physical conditioning programs that would not be intense enough to elicit improvement in healthy children.

Positive physiological effects of aerobic exercise include

- cardiovascular,
- pulmonary, and
- muscle metabolic responses.

Cardiovascular Effects

The cardiovascular response primarily involves increased cardiac output, which a conditioning program can improve by 10–50% (5). This increase in cardiac output during maximal exercise is achieved primarily by an increase in stroke volume and to a lesser extent by an increase in heart rate. Cardiac output is usually the limiting factor in determining exercise tolerance in healthy children and most children with chronic disease, except those with severe lung disease. Children with some forms of heart disease experience more marked limitations of cardiac output. However, many of these children can improve cardiopulmonary endurance with physical conditioning (33).

Pulmonary Effects

Like the heart, the lungs also respond to acute exercise demands by increasing output in volume (tidal volume) and frequency (respiratory rate). Tidal volume can increase to 50% of vital capacity, and respiratory rate can reach a maximum frequency of 50–70 beats per minute, resulting in an increase in minute ventilation during exhaustive exercise of 10–15 times resting values (5). Ventilatory capacity is unlikely to be a limiting factor in determining exercise tolerance in children with healthy lungs, since the limits of cardiac output are reached during exercise long before maximal ventilation occurs. For example, during a maximal exercise challenge, minute ventilation rarely surpasses 50–70% of a child's maximal voluntary ventilation capacity at rest (35). Because significant ventilatory reserve exists during exercise, most children with mild to moderate chronic lung diseases should be able to withstand the demands of moderate physical activity without exceeding their ventilatory capability. Children with severe forms of lung disease, in whom ventilatory insufficiency limits exercise tolerance, may benefit from the potential conditioning effect of exercise on respiratory function. For example, children with cystic fibrosis experience improvements in exercise tolerance and specifically in respiratory muscle endurance as a result of physical conditioning (47, 65).

Metabolic Effects

The third component of the oxygen delivery chain contributing to aerobic fitness is the oxidative capacity of muscle, that is, the ability of exercising muscle to process the oxygen delivered in the bloodstream into usable energy in the form of ATP. This conversion occurs in the mitochondria, which make up the metabolic machinery of muscles. Physical conditioning can increase the density of mitochondria in muscle, thereby increasing oxidative capacity. Children with and without chronic diseases who engage in aerobic conditioning will show improvements in muscle oxidative capacity, which can contribute to improved aerobic fitness.

Body Composition

Both aerobic conditioning and strength training can lead to increased lean body mass and decreased body fat. Mechanisms include energy expenditure (burning calories), utilization of fat stores, and muscle development. Exercise may be particularly important for weight management in children with chronic diseases, in whom underactivity rather than excessive caloric intake may be the main contributory factor to the development of obesity. Favorable changes in body composition are associated with decreased risk of a variety of health conditions associated with obesity.

Muscle Strength and Endurance

Muscle strength and endurance are important in promoting optimal physical function. Traditional dogma held that prepubertal children were incapable of improving muscle strength. This belief was based on the myth that improvement in strength is dependent on the presence of androgens and their ability to increase muscle mass. However, significant strength gains can occur in children and women, not by increase in muscle mass but by alteration in neurological factors. These include increased neural drive, synchronization of motor unit fibers, and improved motor skill coordination. For example, studies of weight training in children show that both boys and girls demonstrate significant strength gains, equivalent to those observed in adolescent males and adults (79). Strength training is safe for children when closely supervised and appropriately designed. The emphasis should be on multiple sets of low resistance, high repetition exercises of large muscle groups, and proper technique; maximal lifts should be avoided. In addition to strength gains, strength training programs can lead to small improvements in aerobic fitness and body composition. Concerns that strength training might create muscle-bound children with decreased flexibility appear unwarranted (73, 78, 79). For children with chronic diseases characterized by physical disabilities, strength training may increase strength, prevent disuse atrophy of muscles, and improve physical work capacity. As in the geriatric population, these changes are important to maximize the ability to perform tasks of daily living and participate in recreational activities, thereby enhancing self-reliance, independence, and overall quality of life.

Flexibility

Flexibility, like muscle strength, is important for optimal musculoskeletal function. Flexibility can be maintained and improved by regular stretching programs emphasizing sustained rather than jerky stretching techniques. Poor flexibility is thought to contribute to injuries in active children, particularly during the adolescent growth spurt, during which the rapid growth of bones may cause decreases in flexibility of surrounding muscles, tendons, and ligaments. This may lead to increased risk of acute injury in the form of strains, sprains, or overuse injuries. Extreme forms of inflexibility can restrict physical movement at joints, lead to joint contractures, and interfere with the ability to perform activities of daily living. Optimal flexibility is particularly important for children with chronic diseases who may already have restricted motion. A regular stretching program can maintain and perhaps improve flexibility, and promote optimal musculoskeletal function.

PREVENTIVE HEALTH BENEFITS

The potential health benefits of exercise are many. Epidemiological studies in adults suggest that regular physical activity contributes to longevity and decreases the risk of death from a variety of causes (Table 2.2; 18, 52, 67). Physical activity is associated most strongly with the prevention and control of

- coronary artery disease (CAD),
- hypertension (HTN),
- non-insulin-dependent diabetes mellitus (NIDDM),
- osteoporosis,
- obesity, and
- psychological disorders (40, 49, 80).

The mechanisms by which physical activity leads to improvements in health are not well understood, but it appears that different mechanisms and different forms of physical activity may be involved, depending on the desired health effect. Traditionally, health benefits of exercise were thought to stem primarily from improvements in the health-related components of physical fitness, such as cardiopulmonary endurance, body composition, muscle strength

Table 2.2   Preventive Health Benefits of Physical Activity

Health concern	Effect of physical activity
Coronary artery disease	Improved cardiac function Decreased thrombus formation Improved lipoprotein profile Reduction of other CAD risk factors
Hypertension	Decreased systolic and diastolic blood pressure
Obesity	Increased lean body mass Decreased percent body fat Increased caloric expenditure Increased basal metabolic rate Suppression of appetite
Osteoporosis	Increased bone density
Diabetes mellitus	Improved glucose clearance Increased insulin sensitivity
Psychological disorders	Reduction in anxiety Improved mood and sense of well-being Improved self-esteem

and endurance, and flexibility. However, significant health benefits are also associated with physical activity that does not improve fitness levels. These effects may be particularly important for many children with chronic disease whose ability to exercise at levels required to improve physical fitness is impaired. There is increasing evidence to suggest that physical activity, as opposed to physical fitness, may play a greater role in disease prevention than was previously thought, particularly for those who are most sedentary. It appears that many forms of exercise can serve to improve health, and involve a diverse range of biochemical, physical, physiological, anatomical, and psychological adaptations.

Although there is little doubt that physical activity exerts a protective effect on health in adults, the benefits with regard to disease prevention in children are less clear. However, many of the adult diseases related to physical inactivity have their origins during childhood. Modification of risk factors associated with these diseases during childhood may forestall the development of later adult disease. This strategy is based on the assumption that such risk factors can be modified by physical activity during childhood and will lead to a sustained improved risk profile as the child enters adulthood. These concepts will be discussed with regard to prevention of CAD, HTN, obesity, NIDDM, and osteoporosis.

Coronary Artery Disease

CAD is the leading cause of morbidity and mortality in the United States; it is estimated that an average of one in five persons will acquire CAD by age 60. Physically inactive adults are twice as likely to develop CAD as persons who are regularly physically active (70). It is well recognized that the atherosclerotic process begins during childhood. Autopsy studies have shown the presence of fatty streaks and fibrous plaques in children and adolescents (43), and the presence of these atherosclerotic precursors correlates with childhood levels of CAD risk factors such as systolic blood pressure and serum cholesterol levels (14). Indeed, it is estimated that 40% of children by the age of 12 have at least one major risk factor for heart disease (34). Some children, moreover, exhibit multiple CAD risk factors, particularly obesity, hypercholesterolemia, and hypertension (97); children with certain chronic diseases such as diabetes and renal disease may be at particularly increased risk of this clustering phenomenon. Finally, risk factors present during childhood track to some extent into adulthood (96, 98). Thus, physical activity during childhood may reduce risk of CAD later in life by early modification of the disease process or by reduction of associated risk factors.

Physical activity may modulate the development of CAD by directly influencing cardiac function or by modifying factors associated with CAD risk. Aerobic exercise leading to improved cardiopulmonary fitness will cause direct improvement in cardiac function, as evidenced by increased cardiac output, stroke volume, collateral circulation, capillary density, and myocardial contractile performance (19). However, beneficial changes in CAD risk factors such as blood pressure, body composition, insulin sensitivity, thrombus formation, and high-density lipoprotein levels may occur at all physical activity levels, including weight training, independent of improvement in components of physical fitness (41, 45, 51).

Specific evidence in children confirms a correlation between physical activity level and CAD risk factor status. For instance, cross-sectional studies show that active children have more favorable lipoprotein profiles (elevated HDL-C) than sedentary children (53). However, intervention studies of physical conditioning in populations of healthy children have not shown a consistent effect of modifying lipoprotein profiles. Studies in adults suggest that favorable changes in lipoprotein profiles are observed more consistently in those with greater baseline abnormalities before training (92). This may be particularly relevant for some children with chronic diseases who may be at increased risk for hypercholesterolemia due to physical inactivity, obesity, or disease-specific risk (i.e., diabetes mellitus and renal disease).

Hypertension

Cohort studies in adults suggest that physically inactive persons have a 35–52% greater risk of developing HTN than physically active persons. The protective effect of physical activity on hypertension appears to be even stronger among those at high risk due to obesity (17, 68). Intervention studies in adults indicate that physical conditioning utilizing aerobic activity can reduce Hg by 5–25 mm in resting systolic blood pressure and by 3–15 mm in diastolic pressure (90). Some studies in children also show an inverse relationship between physical activity level and prevalence of HTN: usually, training studies in children with baseline mild or moderate HTN show a decrease in blood pressure with aerobic conditioning (39), although few changes are seen in normotensive children (59). It is not known whether regular exercise during childhood will suppress the progressive risk in blood pressure seen with increasing age. The implications of elevated blood pressure during childhood and later risk of hypertensive complication as adults are also unknown. Blood pressure values during childhood do show limited tracking into adulthood, and track more consistently for adolescents than for younger children (55). Those children most likely to sustain elevation in blood pressure are those with concurrent obesity, for whom physical activity intervention could be particularly effective.

Obesity

Obesity is associated with physical inactivity during infancy, childhood, and adulthood. While it is unclear whether inactivity causes obesity or whether extra body weight leads to reduced activity, obese children often have lower caloric intake than their lean peers, which would suggest that inadequate physical activity rather than overeating is the major contributing factor (88). Epidemiological evidence, including randomized intervention trials, has consistently shown that physical activity is efficacious for weight control (29), the predominant mechanism being increased energy expenditure. However, other potential mechanisms may include appetite suppression, increase in basal metabolic rate, effects on the growth of adipocytes, and modification of the thermogenic effect of food (88, 93). Besides reduction in body weight, physical conditioning interventions in obese children and adolescents have led to favorable changes in body composition, blood pressure, and blood lipid profiles, which may then reduce the risk of development of medical conditions associated with obesity in adulthood such as CAD, HTN, and NIDDM.

From a behavioral standpoint obesity should ideally be controlled before adulthood, because 75% of obese adolescents will go on to become obese adults (1). In addition to the long-term medical risks, obesity can affect the psychological health of children during critical phases of their emotional development. Physical conditioning programs for obese children have resulted in improvements in mood, self-esteem, body image, and socialization with peers.

Non-Insulin-Dependent Diabetes Mellitus

NIDDM is a metabolic disease of adulthood typically characterized by insulin resistance leading to hyperinsulinemia and hyperglycemia. This form of diabetes has a strong hereditary component and is closely associated with obesity. It is distinct from the childhood form of diabetes, insulin-dependent diabetes mellitus (IDDM), which is caused by insulin deficiency.

Exercise is a cornerstone in the treatment of NIDDM because of its value in controlling obesity and because of its specific effects on glucose regulation. The acute effect of exercise is an increase in glucose utilization as a result of energy expenditure. The chronic effects of exercise conditioning include increased insulin sensitivity and improved glucose clearance (71, 82). These effects are seen in nondiabetic persons as well and may have implications for primary prevention of NIDDM. Some studies suggest that differences in physical activity level may account for differences in the prevalence of NIDDM found in certain populations (86, 89). A recent epidemiological study in adults found that leisure-time physical activity level was inversely related to risk of developing NIDDM (42). Risk from physical inactivity appeared strongest for those at greatest risk for NIDDM, such as those with obesity, HTN, or parental history of diabetes. No studies have addressed the issue of whether physical activity during childhood plays a role in prevention of subsequent NIDDM.

Osteoporosis

Physical activity is one of several factors that promote bone deposition. Physical stress on bones produced by weight-bearing activity is important in maintaining bone mass. Patients confined to bed and astronauts under weightless conditions lose up to 1% of trabecular bone mass per week; however, normal bone density is restored upon resumption of weight-bearing activity (57). Significant loss of bone mass also occurs with immobilization, such as for treatment of fractures. The detrimental effects of bed rest or immobilization on bone mass are of particular relevance for some children with chronic diseases; however, the beneficial effect of physical activity on bone deposition may also be important for all children for achievement of maximal bone mass during the first several decades of life. Failure to achieve peak bone mass during this time may have implications for future risk of osteoporosis.

A variety of evidence links physical activity to improvements in bone mass. Cross-sectional studies indicate athletes have greater bone density than nonathletes (26, 61). Studies in young women have found associations between bone mass and level of physical activity and muscle strength (72, 81). Intervention studies in both young adults and postmenopausal women have shown that weight-bearing physical activity and strength training activities can improve bone mass at a variety of body sites (24). Both mechanical and dynamic loading appear to produce improvements in bone mass that appear specific to the sites of skeletal stress. Moreover, it appears that the greatest improvement in bone mass results from small increments in physical activity among the most sedentary groups (72). This is particularly encouraging for children with chronic disease who may not be able to participate in physical activity at high levels.

PSYCHOSOCIAL BENEFITS

The benefits attributable to exercise are not limited to physical health. The value of regular exercise in promoting both a healthy body and healthy mind has been recognized from the time of the ancient Greeks. In addition to its effects on psychological health, sport and other physical activity is thought to play an important role in the cognitive, social, and moral development of children.

Children with chronic diseases face particularly difficult issues in psychosocial adjustment. Often they are faced with having a disease of unknown cause, with poor long-term prognosis and limited treatment options. At a stage in life where fitting in and peer acceptance seems crucial, children with chronic disease often feel that they are unacceptably different or isolated. Exercise programs provide children with chronic diseases the same opportunity for enjoyment and social interaction as healthy children, and may promote feelings of normality. Apart from any specific effects of exercise on mental health, exercise programs simply help children to feel good about themselves; exercise and participation in sport often produces a general sense of well-being. The mechanism is unclear but may involve biochemical changes in levels of neurotransmitters such as beta-endorphins. In addition, skill mastery may lead to improvement in self-concept, self-esteem, and self-confidence, as well as a sense of competence and achievement. Evidence supports a consistent association between physical activity and self-esteem in school-age children (37). This relationship is seen in healthy children but particularly in children who are emotionally, mentally, or physically handicapped.

A variety of specific beneficial effects of exercise on mental health have been documented (22, 31, 44). The acute psychological response to exercise is a reduction in anxiety and muscle tension, presumably brought about by a relaxation effect. These effects have been seen in children as young as four years old (23). In addition, single exercise sessions are also associated with improved mood. Chronic effects include improved mood, self-confidence, self-esteem, and self-concept. These changes are associated primarily with participation in aerobic exercise programs, although they are not necessarily associated with improvement in measures of aerobic fitness such as $\dot{V}O_2$max (20, 48). The beneficial effects of exercise on psychological well-being are most apparent and well documented for high-risk individuals who at baseline experience increased anxiety or depressive mood. In particular, exercise is helpful for the management of depression in adolescents, and its effect is comparable to other forms of therapy for treating moderate depression in adults (28). Objectively measurable changes in indicators of psychological well-being are less apparent for individuals who are psychologically normal at the outset of a training program. For this reason, physical activity programs are likely to be most beneficial for those in greatest need and may be particularly important for children with chronic diseases. Although specific studies of the psychological benefits of physical activity in children with chronic disease are lacking, there is much anecdotal evidence for them, primarily derived from surveys conducted at special summer camps.

DISEASE-SPECIFIC BENEFITS

The general benefits of exercise on physical fitness, health, and psychosocial well-being that accrue to all children are especially important for children with chronic disease. These children often experience the greatest limitations to functional fitness and face the greatest health risks and challenges of psychosocial adjustment. In addition, the physiological adaptations that occur with exercise may be beneficial with regard to the disease process itself. While exercise is unlikely to alter the disease process per se, a variety of disease-specific benefits of exercise

for children with chronic diseases have been documented. While the following chapters of this text will address this subject in detail, the disease-specific benefits for some of the most common conditions are summarized in Table 2.3, and will be briefly reviewed here.

Cardiac Disorders

Most chronic heart disease in children is due to congenital structural defects. The extent to which exercise tolerance is impaired depends on the type and severity of the defect. Despite the potential for these disorders to result in cardiac inefficiency and thereby limit exercise capacity, only a minority of children with congenital heart disease actually have clinically significant limitations of exercise capacity. Low

Table 2.3 Disease-Specific Benefits of Exercise

Disease	Benefits
Cardiac disorders	Improved cardiac function and aerobic capacity
Asthma	Possible reduced severity of EIB
Cystic Fibrosis	Improved respiratory muscle endurance Improved clearance of airway mucus
Insulin-dependent diabetes mellitus	Increased insulin sensitivity Increased glucose utilization Prevention of obesity Reduction in associated CAD risk factors
Muscular dystrophy	Maintain muscle strength and endurance Prevention of disuse atrophy Maintain ambulation
Cerebral palsy	Prevent joint contractures Improved ambulation and other motor function Improved aerobic capacity
Arthritis	Preserve range of motion Decreased joint stiffness Prevent disuse muscle atrophy and osteopenia Possible decreased rate of progression of joint disease
Renal disease	Improved blood pressure Improved lipoprotein profiles Improved glucose tolerance

exercise tolerance and depressed levels of fitness in children with congenital heart disease often result from underactivity caused by overprotection rather than by limitations of the disease itself. There is generally a poor correlation between objective measures of exercise tolerance in these children and a family's prediction of their exercise capability (85). Exercise programs for children with a wide variety of cardiac disorders have resulted in direct improvements in cardiac function as well as in noncardiac adaptations. Among these adaptations are enhanced peripheral circulation and aerobic capacity of muscles, with secondary improvement in overall aerobic fitness and exercise tolerance. It appears that children with congenital heart disease can benefit significantly from the conditioning effects of exercise on the cardiovascular system before reaching a point where the underlying cardiac inefficiency becomes a limiting factor. In addition to the improvements in aerobic capacity, children in cardiac rehabilitation programs have shown improvements in social interaction skills, becoming more self-confident and outgoing, and having fewer anxieties surrounding physical activity and reduced fears of death (56, 75, 91).

Asthma

Most children with asthma experience exercise-induced asthma (EIA). Bronchospasm can occur with exercise even when the underlying disease is well controlled. Many children with asthma are excluded from sports because of fears of inducing asthma attacks. Such restriction is usually unnecessary since exercise-induced bronchospasm can be effectively prevented with medication, and exercise activities can be designed to decrease the likelihood of triggering asthma. Physical conditioning programs for children with asthma have the same potential to improve aerobic fitness as they do for nonasthmatic children. Children with well-controlled asthma show no impairment in work capacity, $\dot{V}O_2$max, or pulmonary function during exercise (16). Approximately 10% of U.S. Olympians have exercise-induced asthma, demonstrating that these individuals have normal exercise capacity and can have the potential to excel in sports at a world-class level (69). Some studies suggest that aerobic physical conditioning may reduce the severity of EIA and can lead to reduction in the need for medication. It appears that as aerobic fitness improves, the asthmatic child can achieve a given level of exercise with greater ease and less rapid respirations, thus triggering less EIA at a particular level of exercise than occurred prior to training (12). However, there is no evidence that exercise can improve baseline disease in asthma.

Cystic Fibrosis

Cystic fibrosis (CF) is a disease characterized by excessive production of abnormal mucus secretions and inability to clear this thick mucus from the respiratory tract, leading to airway obstruction, chronic cough, and difficulty breathing. Exercise intolerance is common in children with CF and is proportionate to the severity of pulmonary disease. The limiting factor for exercise tolerance is more likely to be respiratory muscle fatigue secondary to increased work of breathing. Respiratory muscle endurance, like skeletal muscle endurance, can be improved with physical conditioning. This is one of the most important disease-specific benefits of exercise training in children with CF (47, 65). Some studies suggest that exercise also may lead to enhanced clearance of airway mucus and perhaps to decreased need for routine chest physical therapy (9, 58, 66, 99). Studies disagree as to whether exercise can lead to improvements in lung volumes and flows; most show no effect on pulmonary function tests despite improvements in $\dot{V}O_2$max and exercise tolerance. However, improvements in exercise tolerance alone are impressive given the progressive nature of the pulmonary disease.

Insulin-Dependent Diabetes Mellitus (IDDM)

The acute effects of exercise on glucose regulation are decreased blood glucose and increased insulin sensitivity. For this reason exercise is an important part of treatment of diabetes, complementing diet and insulin therapy in managing hyperglycemia on a daily basis. However, it remains controversial whether regular physical activity can improve metabolic control and decrease insulin requirements on a chronic basis.

Some studies have found inverse correlations between physical activity level and glycosuria or insulin requirements on a short-term basis, such as during a summer camp session for diabetic children, but most studies fail to show improvement in long-term markers of glycemic control such as glycosylated hemoglobin (HbA1c). Although it remains unclear whether regular physical activity will improve diabetic control beyond the hypoglycemic effect of acute exercise or reduce the risk of long-term complications of diabetes, there are other nonspecific effects of exercise that are of particular benefit to the diabetic child. For instance, prevention of obesity is important for optimal metabolic control in diabetes. The role of exercise in prevention of CAD and associated risk factors is particularly important for diabetics who have a tendency toward the development of atherosclerosis, hypercholesterolemia, elevated triglycerides, depressed fibrinolytic activity, and subsequent death from CAD and strokes.

Muscular Dystrophy

Inadequate muscle strength, power, and endurance due to deterioration of muscle function are the main factors limiting the physical ability of children with muscular dystrophies. Inactivity may further contribute to loss of muscle function. As a result of inactivity children with muscular dystrophy often become obese, and the burden of excess weight may further contribute to loss of function. Physical activity may aid in preventing obesity and maintaining muscle strength and endurance. Studies in adults with myopathies show that strength training can improve function of skeletal and masticatory muscles (46, 58). In addition, adults with myopathies show rates of improvement in aerobic fitness similar to those seen in healthy adults (30, 38). Strength training studies of children with muscular dystrophy show only small if any improvements in muscular strength (2, 27, 76, 95). However, maintenance of existing muscle strength is important for children in whom the natural course of the disease is progressive deterioration in muscle function.

Cerebral Palsy

Children with cerebral palsy have diminished exercise tolerance proportionate to the severity of spasticity. Spasticity results in tremendous mechanical inefficiency and, therefore, in markedly increased effort and easy fatiguability with exercise. Improvements in aerobic fitness and muscular strength and endurance would be expected to result in improved exercise tolerance and functional ability. Flexibility exercises may prevent development of joint contractures. Several intervention studies have documented improvements in walking and other motor skills as a result of exercise training (15, 83, 84). Evidence is conflicting about whether training can specifically reduce spasticity.

Arthritis

Range of motion exercises may be important for maintaining flexibility in children with arthritic conditions. In addition, physical activity can reduce muscle atrophy and bone resorption secondary to disuse. Documented effects of exercise training in adults with rheumatoid arthritis include improvements in muscle strength, physical work capacity, and psychological status, as well as reduction in joint stiffness and tenderness, rate of progression of joint disturbance, and need for medication (62, 63).

Renal Disease

Complications of renal dialysis include high blood pressure, glucose intolerance, and unfavorable triglyceride and lipoprotein profiles. Such changes are linked to the development of atherosclerosis and CAD. Exercise may be helpful in reducing the risk of CAD and associated risk factors in these patients. Documented effects of exercise training in adults with dialysis-dependent renal disease include improvement in $\dot{V}O_2$max, glucose tolerance, and lipoprotein profiles (36).

RISKS OF EXERCISE

Relative risk assessment for most chronic diseases is impossible to quantify because of a lack of controlled studies. Individuals must make a decision regarding participation based on theoretical or inferred risk, anecdotes, availability of compensatory safety equipment or procedures, and their own attitude regarding acceptable levels of risk. Fortunately, in the realm of sports and exercise there are relatively few absolute risks to participation.

Death in Sport

Death during sport and exercise participation may be associated with risks inherent in the activity, environmental factors, or the general health of the participant. Fatal injury may occur regardless of the participant's health. However, the inherent risk of death may be increased several times when an individual with a chronic disease participates in sport. For instance, individuals with uncontrolled seizures or with a cardiac pacemaker may be at increased risk because of an inability to protect themselves during a seizure or collision.

Risk of sudden death from the participant's health status is limited almost exclusively to individuals with certain cardiac lesions. Those lesions include

- hypertrophic cardiomyopathy,
- anomalous coronary vessels,
- myocarditis,
- severe aortic stenosis (> 40 mmHg gradient at rest),
- Marfan's syndrome with aortic dilatation, and
- certain arrhythmias (94).

These children may be at risk for fatal outcomes from participation in all strenuous sports and physical activity.

Exercise Intensity

As an isolated risk factor, high exercise intensity rarely if ever directly results in death in healthy children and adolescents. Rather, inadequate attention to environmental conditions and the child's hydration are contributing factors. Nonetheless, some individuals with chronic disease may be at higher risk of dying during high-intensity exercise. Individuals with severe chronic lung disease (i.e., those with forced expiratory volume in 1 second [FEV_1] < 50%) may be at increased risk of oxygen desaturation and hypoxemia. For example, children with cystic fibrosis may experience oxygen desaturation from poor respiratory mechanics during exercise (25). About 15% of patients with sickle-cell

disease, particularly those with a hemoglobin < 8 gm%, have demonstrated ischemic electrocardiogram changes during exercise stress testing (4). However, there was no progressive deterioration in cardiac function over several years (3). High levels of sickle hemoglobin predispose athletes to potentially fatal hemolysis and vaso-occlusive events (77).

Environmental Issues

Extreme environmental conditions place all of those who exercise at risk. The risk of heat-related illness increases with higher environmental temperature and humidity. Children with impaired heat dissipation mechanisms are potentially at greater risk of fatal heat-related illness. Among others, obese children and those with cystic fibrosis are more susceptible to environmental heat stressors. While obesity is clearly associated with decreased heat tolerance, only one obesity-related death during sports participation has been reported (10). Excessive production of hypertonic sweat in children with cystic fibrosis increases the risk of hyponatremic dehydration and associated heat prostration (11). In addition, some children with congenital heart disease sweat excessively (11). Nevertheless, many of these children can continue to participate if proper precautions are taken to compensate for heat dissipation abnormalities.

Other environmental situations that may increase the likelihood of fatal outcomes include those in which an individual would be at risk if temporarily incapacitated. Underwater activities such as scuba diving may increase the risk of fatal injury in children and youth with poorly controlled seizures.

Contact Injuries

A significant inherent risk of trauma exists for sports such as football, hockey, wrestling, and soccer. An equally important risk of inadvertent trauma occurs in other sports such as downhill skiing, bicycling, and gymnastics. Football continues to be the leading organized sport associated with contact injuries, although specific relative risk data for most sports are not available. However, some individuals with chronic conditions such as congenital heart disease or disorders of hemostasis and bone formation may be at greater risk than the normal child in contact/collision and some limited contact/impact sports (6).

Children and youth with congenital heart disease, particularly in the postoperative period, may be at increased risk for dysrhythmias, arrhythmia, and soft tissue damage from blunt trauma. Pacemakers, due to their subcutaneous placement, are particularly susceptible to blunt trauma.

Some bleeding dyscrasias, such as hemophilia A and B and thrombocytopenia, have traditionally precluded participation in contact/collision sports. Traumatic bone, joint, soft tissue, and intracranial bleeding are potential complications of participation in these sports. The potential for recombinant genetic production of clotting factors may reduce the risk of significant injury in the future.

Osteoporosis may be genetically predisposed or associated with poor nutrient intake, end-stage renal disease, or chronic treatment with catabolic steroids. Quantification of osteoporosis is difficult, and radiographic techniques have not been standardized adequately to identify children and adolescents who may be at increased risk of acute fractures (50). Most children with osteogenesis imperfecta (OI) would not be capable of participation in contact/collision sports. However, there are variations (e.g., OI type IV) that may not be recognized until adulthood that would place a child at increased risk for serious fractures (13). Theoretically, individuals with HIV infection and those with hepatitis could pose a risk to other athletes if there is blood exposure during contact/collision sports. However, no proven cases of transmission have been reported. Many organizations, including the American Academy of Pediatrics, have developed guidelines for control of blood-borne pathogens in the sports setting (7).

Overuse Injuries

Overuse injuries occur in children in association with periods of rapid growth, abrupt increase in activity level, abnormal biomechanics, and the use of improper equipment. Individuals with a variety of chronic disorders, particularly those involving the musculoskeletal system, are more likely to have abnormal biomechanics. Cerebral palsy, other myopathic diseases, and various forms of arthritis are commonly associated with limited range of motion and altered biomechanics. Uncompensated deficiencies of joint range of motion as well as increased resting muscle tone and tendon shortening can contribute to an increased incidence of overuse injuries.

The most common contributing factor potentially associated with all chronic disease is a rapid change from a sedentary lifestyle to one of intense physical activity. Avoiding overuse injuries will require a very gradual increase in physical activity for many of these youngsters if they are to include regular exercise programs in their lives.

Adverse Effects on the Disease Process

Adverse effects on the disease process are generally confined to acute problems. A notable exception may be eating disorders, where chronic caloric restriction may be encouraged in some athletic settings. Minimum body fat and intense exercise are an integral part of sports such as gymnastics, dance, and distance running. Restricted diets, intense exercise, amenorrhea, and hypoestrogenemia have all been associated with osteoporosis. It is unclear whether the poor bony matrix formation that occurs with osteoporosis in adolescents is reversible in adult life. The short- and long-term consequences of osteoporosis include serious fractures of the hip and spine (50). At times, the athlete with an eating disorder may remain undiagnosed because of what appears to be socially acceptable behavior associated with a particular sport.

Traditionally, high-intensity exercise has been proscribed for children and adolescents with muscular dystrophy, but research supporting the concept that exercise might accelerate muscle damage in children and adolescents with muscular dystrophy is limited. One study of mice with muscular dystrophy suggests acceleration of muscle degeneration following high-intensity training (87). Conversely, low-intensity, repetitive exercise in dystrophic mice has not been associated with muscle damage (32). Elevated levels of plasma creatinine kinase that occur after prolonged exercise are not clearly indicative of muscle damage, and the prevalence of this response to exercise is uncertain (30). It is very unlikely that low- or moderate-intensity exercise in children and adolescents with muscular dystrophy would result in accelerated muscle degeneration.

Acute adverse events associated with sport and exercise and chronic disease are usually preventable through medical management of the disease process. For example, no long-term adverse effect has been identified for asthma. Acutely, exercise-induced asthma (EIA) may occur at the time of the activity or several hours later (21). Control of EIA is readily achieved with the prophylactic use of inhaled β-2 adrenergic agonists (e.g., albuterol, salbutamol) or cromolyn. Similarly, late onset hypoglycemia several hours after exercise occurs in 16% of patients with diabetes mellitus (54). Both acute and delayed onset hypoglycemia can be managed with proper monitoring and subsequent change of diet, insulin, and exercise. There have been no long-term adverse effects on the clinical course of diabetes mellitus. Recognition of adverse events that may occur as a result of exercise will allow appropriate changes in medical management to prevent sequelae.

Among hypertensive adolescents, maximal exercise testing sometimes results in dramatic elevation of blood pressure greater than normotensive controls (30). Static exercise produces even higher elevations in systolic and diastolic blood pressure. The significance of these elevations is unknown. While cerebral hemorrhage and stroke have occurred during maximal weight lifting, there is no evidence linking hypertension and these adverse events (64). No long-term adverse outcomes on the course of hypertension have been proven as a result of participation in sport and exercise programs.

Adverse Psychosocial Effects

Data from the National Health Interview Survey suggest increasing trends in activity limitation among children with chronic disease (60). Inappropriate restriction from sport and exercise programs is among the many reversible disabilities experienced by children and adolescents with chronic disease. From a psychosocial perspective, studies have consistently documented only beneficial effects from participation of these children in sport and a variety of physical activities (23).

The risk of adverse psychosocial outcomes are generic and not limited to children and adolescents with chronic medical problems. The programs reported in the literature have been designed to meet the needs of the participants. Poor self-esteem may result for any child if program leaders set unreasonable goals or use derogatory methods to elicit better performance. For sport participation and physical activity to result in positive psychosocial outcomes, it is critical that expectations be appropriate for the desires and capabilities of the participant. This responsibility needs to be shared by all involved, including participants, parents, coaches, physical educators, peers, and the local community.

CONCLUSION

In general, the benefits from participation in sport and exercise programs overwhelmingly outweigh potential risks. Individuals working with children and youth who have chronic medical problems should use every approach to allow safe participation. Changes in medical management, use of safety equipment, and variation in the level of participation are considerations for minimizing risk and allowing participation.

REFERENCES

1. Abraham, S.; Nordsieck, M. Relationship of excess weight in children and adults. Pub. Health Rep. 75:263–273; 1960.
2. Abramson, A.S.; Rogoff, J. Physical treatment in muscular dystrophy [abstract]. Proc. 2nd Med. Conf. Musc. Dystrophy Assoc. Am. 123–124; 1952.
3. Alpert, B.S.; Dover, V.; Strong, W.B.; et al. Longitudinal exercise hemodynamics in children with sickle cell anemia. Am. J. Dis. Child 138:1021–1024; 1984.
4. Alpert, B.S.; Gilman, P.R.; Strong, W.B.; et al. Hemodynamic and ECG responses to exercise in children with sickle cell anemia. Am. J. Dis. Child 135:362–366; 1981.
5. American Academy of Pediatrics. Sports medicine: health care for young athletes. Elk Grove Village, IL: Author; 1991.
6. American Academy of Pediatrics Committee on Sports Medicine. Participation in

competitive sports. Pediatrics 81:737–739; 1988.

7. American Academy of Pediatrics Committee on Sports Medicine and Fitness. Human immunodeficiency virus (Acquired Immunodeficiency Syndrome [AIDS] virus) in the athletic setting. Pediatrics 88:640–641; 1991.

8. American College of Sports Medicine. Position statement on the recommended quantity and quality of exercise for developing and maintaining fitness in healthy adults. Med. Sci. Sport. Exerc. 10:vii–x; 1978.

9. Andreasson, B.; Johnson, B.; Kornfaldt, R.; et al. Long-term effects of physical exercise on working capacity and pulmonary function in cystic fibrosis. Acta Paedeatrica Scand. 76:70–75; 1987.

10. Barcenas, C.; Hoeffler, H.P.; Lie, J.T. Obesity, football, dog days and siriasis: a deadly combination. Am. Heart J. 92:237–244; 1976.

11. Bar-Or, O. Pediatric sports medicine for the practitioner. New York: Springer-Verlag, 1983:285–288.

12. Bar-Or, O. Disease-specific benefits of training in the child with a chronic disease: what is the evidence? Ped. Exerc. Sci. 2:384–394; 1990.

13. Behrman, R.E. Nelson textbook of pediatrics. Philadelphia: W.B. Saunders; 1992: 1741–1743.

14. Berenson, G.S. Evolution of cardiovascular risk factors in early life: perspectives on causation. In: Berenson, G.S., ed. Causation of cardiovascular risk factors in children. New York: Raven; 1986:1–26.

15. Berg, K. Adaptation in cerebral palsy of body composition, nutrition and physical working capacity at school age. Acta Paediat. Scand. Suppl. 204; 1970.

16. Bevegard, S.; Eriksson, B.O.; Graff-Lonnevig, V.; et al. Respiratory function, cardiovascular dimensions, and work capacity in boys with bronchial asthma. Acta Paedeatrica Scand. 65:289–296; 1976.

17. Blair, S.N.; Goodyear, N.N.; Gibbons, L.W.; et al. Physical fitness and incidence of hypertension in healthy normotensive men and women. JAMA 252:487–490; 1984.

18. Blair, S.N.; Kohn, H.W.; Paffenbarger, R.S.; et al. Physical fitness and all-cause mortality—a prospective study. JAMA 262:2395–2401; 1989.

19. Blomquist, C.G. Cardiovascular adaptations to physical training. Annu. Rev. Physiol. 45:169–189; 1983.

20. Blumenthal, J.A.; Emery, C.F.; Madden, D.J.; et al. Cardiovascular and behavioral effects of aerobic exercise training in healthy older men and women. J. Geron. 5:M147–157; 1989.

21. Boulet, L.; Legris, C.; Turcotte, H.; et al. Prevalence and characteristics of late asthmatic responses to exercise. J. All. Clin. Imm. 80:655–662; 1987.

22. Brown, D.R.; Wang, Y. The relationships among exercise training, aerobic capacity, and psychological well-being in the general population. Med. Exerc. Nutr. Health 1:125–142; 1992.

23. Brown, R.S. Exercise and mental health in the pediatric population. Clinics in Sports Medicine 1:515–527; 1982.

24. Conroy, B.P.; Kraemer, W.J.; Maresh, C.M.; et al. Adaptive responses of bone to physical activity. Med. Exerc. Nutr. Health. 1:64–74; 1992.

25. Cropp, G.J.A.; Pullano, T.P.; Cerny, F.J.; Nathanson, I.T. Exercise tolerance and cardiorespiratory adjustments at peak work capacity in cystic fibrosis. Am. Rev. Resp. Dis. 126:211–216; 1982.

26. Dalen, N.; Olsson, K.E. Bone mineral content and physical activity. Acta Orthop. Scand. 45:170–174; 1974.

27. De Lateur, B.J.; Giaconi, R.M. Effect on maximal strength of submaximal exercise in Duchenne muscular dystrophy. Amer. J. Phys. Med. 58:26–36; 1979.

28. Dishman, R.K. Mental health. In: Seefeldt, V.S., ed. Physical activity and well-being. Reston, VA: American Alliance for Health, Physical Education, Recreation and Dance; 1986:303–341.

29. Epstein, L.H.; Wing, R.R. Aerobic exercise and weight. Addict. Behav. 5:371–388; 1980.

30. Florence, J.M.; Hagberg, J.M. Effect of training on the exercise responses of neuromuscular disease patients. Med. Sci. Sports Exer. 16:460–465; 1984.

31. Folkins, C.H.; Sime, W.E. Physical fitness training and mental health. Am. Psychol. 36:373–389; 1981.

32. Fowler, W.M.; Abresch, R.T.; Larson, D.B.; et al. High repetitive submaximal treadmill

exercise training: effect on normal and dystrophic mice. Arch. Phys. Med. Rehabil. 71:552–557; 1990.

33. Galioto, F.M., Jr.; Tomassoni, T.L. Cardiac rehabilitation for children with heart disease. Med. Exerc. Nutr. Health 1:272–280; 1992.

34. Gilliam, T.B.; Katch, V.L.; Thorland, W.; et al. Prevalence of coronary heart disease risk factors in active children, 7 to 12 years of age. Med. Sci. Sports Exerc. 9:21–25; 1977.

35. Godfrey, S.; Mearns, M. Pulmonary function and response to exercise in cystic fibrosis. Arch. Dis. Child. 46:144–151; 1971.

36. Goldberg, A.P.; Hagberg, J.M.; Delmez, J.A.; et al. Metabolic effects of exercise training in hemodialysis patients. Kidney Int. 18:754–761; 1980.

37. Gruber, J.J. Physical activity and self-esteem development in children: a meta-analysis. In: Stull, G.A.; Eckert, H.M., eds. The effects of physical activity on children. Champaign, IL: Human Kinetics; 1986:30–48.

38. Hagberg, J.M.; Carroll, J.E.; Brooke, M.H. Endurance exercise training in a patient with central core disease. Neurology 30:1242–1244; 1980.

39. Hagberg, J.M.; Goldring, D.; Ehsami, A.A.; et al. Effect of exercise training on the blood pressure and hemodynamic features of hypertensive adolescents. Am. J. Card. 52:763–768; 1983.

40. Harris, S.S.; Caspersen, C.J.; DeFriese, G.H.; et al. Physical activity counselling for healthy adults as a primary preventive intervention in the clinical setting; report for the US Preventive Services Task Force. JAMA 261:3590–3598; 1989.

41. Haskell, W.L. Physical activity and health: need to define the required stimulus. Am. J. Cardiol. 5:4D–9D; 1985.

42. Helmrich, S.P.; Ragland, D.R.; Leung, R.W.; et al. Physical activity and reduced occurrence of non-insulin-dependent diabetes mellitus. N. Engl. J. Med. 325:147–152; 1991.

43. Holman, R.L.; McGill, H.C.; Strong, J.P.; et al. The natural history of atherosclerosis: the early aortic lesions as seen in New Orleans in the middle of the 20th century. Am. J. Path. 34:209–235; 1958.

44. Hughes, J.R. Psychological effects of habitual aerobic exercise: a critical review. Prev. Med. 13:66–78; 1984.

45. Hurley, B.F.; Kokkinos, F. Effects of weight training on risk factors for coronary artery disease. Sports Med. 4:231–238; 1987.

46. Kawazoe, Y.; Kobayashi, M.; Tasaka, T.; et al. Effects of therapeutic exercise on masticatory function in patients with progressive muscular dystrophy. J. Neurol. Neurosurg. Psychiat. 45:343–347; 1982.

47. Keens, T.G.; Krastins, I.R.B.; Wannamaker, E.M., et al. Ventilatory muscle endurance training in normal subjects and patients with cystic fibrosis. Am. Rev. Resp. Dis. 166:853–860; 1977.

48. King, A.C.; Taylor, C.B.; Haskell, W.L.; et al. Influence of regular aerobic exercise on psychological health: a randomized, controlled trial of healthy middle-aged adults. Health Psychol. 8:305–324; 1989.

49. Kohl, H.W.; LaPorte, R.E.; Blair, S.N. Physical activity and cancer: an epidemiological perspective. Sports Med. 6:222–237; 1988.

50. Kreipe, R.E. Bones of today, bones of tomorrow. Am. J. of Dis. Children 146:22–25; 1992.

51. LaPorte, R.E.; Adams, L.L.; Savage, D.D.; et al. The spectrum of physical activity, cardiovascular disease and health: an epidemiologic perspective. Am. J. Epidemiol. 120:507–517; 1984.

52. Leon, A.S.; Connett, J.; Jacobs, D.R.; et al. Leisure-time physical activity levels and risk of coronary heart disease and death. The Multiple Risk Factor Intervention Trial. JAMA 258:2388–2395; 1987.

53. Linder, C.W.; DuRant, R.H.; Mahoney, O.M. The effect of physical conditioning on serum lipids and lipoproteins in white male adolescents. Med. Sci. Sports Exerc. 15:232–236; 1983.

54. MacDonald, M.J. Post exercise late onset hypoglycemia in insulin dependent diabetic patients. Dia. Care 10:584–588; 1978.

55. Malina, R.M. Growth, exercise, fitness and later outcomes. In: Bouchard, R.J.; Shepard, T.; Stephens, J.R.; Sutton, J.R., McPherson, B.D., eds. Exercise, fitness and health. Champaign, IL: Human Kinetics; 1990:637–653.

56. Mathews, R.A.; Nixon, P.A.; Stephenson, R.J.; et al. An exercise program for pediatric patients with congenital heart disease: organizational and physiologic aspects. J. Card. Rehab. 3:467–475; 1983.

57. Mazess, R.B.; Wheedon, G.D. Immobilization and bone. Calif. Tissue Int. 35:265–267; 1983.

58. McCartney, N.; Moroz, D.; Garner, S.H.; et al. The effects of strength training in patients with selected neuromuscular disorders. Med. Sci. Sports Exer. 20:362–368; 1988.

59. Montoye, H.G. Physical activity, physical fitness, and heart disease risk factors in children. In: Stull, G.A.; Eckert, H.M., eds. The effects of physical activity on children. Champaign, IL: Human Kinetics; 1986: 127–152.

60. Newacheck, P.W.; Budetti, P.P.; Halfon, N. Trends in activity-limiting chronic conditions among children. 76:178–184; 1986.

61. Nilsson, B.E.; Westlin, N.E. Bone density in athletes. Clin. Orthop. 77:179–182; 1971.

62. Nordemar, R.; Edstrom, L.; Ekblom, B. Changes in muscle fibre size and physical performance in patients with rheumatoid arthritis after short-term physical training. Scand. J. Rheumatol. 5:70–76; 1976.

63. Nordemar, R.; Edstrom, L.; Zachrisson, L.; et al. Physical training in rheumatoid arthritis: a controlled long-term study. Scand. J. Rheumatol. 10:17–23; 1981.

64. Nudel, D.B.; Gootman, N.; Bunson, S.C.; et al. Exercise performance of hypertensive adolescents. Pediatrics 65:1073–1078; 1980.

65. Orenstein, D.M.; Franklin, B.A.; Doershuk, C.F. Exercise conditioning and cardiopulmonary fitness in cystic fibrosis: the effects of a three-month supervised running program. Chest 80:392–398; 1981.

66. Orenstein, D.M.; Henke, K.G.; Cerny, F.J. Exercise and cystic fibrosis. Phys. Sportsmed. 11:57–63; 1983.

67. Paffenbarger, R.S., Jr.; Hyde, R.T.; Wing, A.L.; et al. Physical activity, all-cause mortality, and longevity of college alumni. N. Engl. J. Med. 314:605–613; 1986.

68. Paffenbarger, R.S., Jr.; Wing, A.L.; Hyde, R.T.; et al. Physical activity and incidence of hypertension in college alumni. Am. J. Epidemiol. 117:245–256; 1983.

69. Pierson, W.E.; Voy, R.O. Exercise-induced bronchospasm in the XXIII Summer Olympic games. N. Engl. Reg. Allergy Proc. 9(3):209–213; 1988.

70. Powell, K.E.; Thompson, P.D.; Caspersen, C.J.; et al. Physical activity and the incidence of coronary heart disease. Annu. Rev. Public Health 8:253–287; 1987.

71. Rauramaa, R. Relationship of physical activity, glucose tolerance, and weight management. Prev. Med. 13:37–46; 1984.

72. Recker, R.R.; Davies, K.M., Hinders, S.M.; et al. Bone gain in young adult women. JAMA 268:2403–2408; 1992.

73. Rians, C.B.; Weltman, A.; Cahill, B.R.; et al. Strength training for prepubescent males: is it safe? Am. J. Sports Med. 15:483–489; 1987.

74. Rowland, T.W. Aerobic response to endurance training programs in prepubescent children: a critical analysis. Med. Sci. Sports Exerc. 17:493–497; 1985.

75. Ruttenberg, H.D.; Adams, T.D.; Orsmond, G.S.; et al. Effects of exercise training on aerobic fitness in children after open heart surgery. Pediatr. Cardiol. 4:19–24; 1983.

76. Scott, O.M.; Hyde, S.A.; Goddare, C.; et al. Effect of exercise in Duchenne muscular dystrophy. Physiotherapy 67:174–176; 1981.

77. Sergeant, G.R. Sickle cell disease. Oxford: Oxford University Press; 1985.

78. Servidio, F.J.; Bartels, R.L.; Hamlin, R.L.; et al. The effects of weight training using Olympic style lifts on various physiological variables in pre-pubescent boys. Med. Sci. Sports Exerc. 17:288; 1985.

79. Sewall, L.; Micheli, L.J. Strength training for children. J. Pediatr Orthop. 6:143–146; 1986.

80. Siscovick, D.S.; LaPorte, R.E.; Newman, J.M. The disease-specific benefits and risks of physical activity in exercise. Public Health Rep. 100:180–188; 1985.

81. Snow-Harter, C.; Bousxein, M.; Lewis, B.; et al. Muscle strength as a predictor of bone mineral density in young women. J. Bone Miner. Res. 5:589–595; 1990.

82. Soman, V.R.; Koivisto, V.A.; Deibert, D.; et al. Increased insulin sensitivity and insulin binding to monocytes after physical training. N. Engl. J. Med. 301:1200–1204; 1979.

83. Sommer, M. Improvement of motor skills and adaptation of the circulatory system in wheelchair-bound children in cerebral palsy. Lecture No. 11. In: Simon, U., ed. Sports as a means of rehabilitation. Netanya, Israel: Wingate Institute; 1971:1–11.

84. Spira, R.; Bar-Or, O. An investigation of the ambulation problems associated with severe motor paralysis in adolescents. Influence of physical conditioning and adapted sports activities. Final report project no.: 19-P-58065-FO1 Tel Aviv, US Dept HEW, SRS; 1975.

85. Taylor, M.R.H. The response to exercise of children with congenital heart disease.

London: University of London; 1872. Dissertation. Cited in: Godfrey, S. Exercise testing in children. Philadelphia: W.B. Saunders; 1974.

86. Taylor, R.; Ram, P.; Zimmet, L.R.; et al. Physical activity and prevalence of diabetes in Melanesian and Indian men in Fiji. Diabetologia 27:578–582; 1984.

87. Taylor, R.G.; Fowler, W.M.; Doerr, L. Exercise effect on contractile properties of skeletal muscle in mouse muscular dystrophy. Arch. Phys. Med. Rehabil. 57:174–180; 1976.

88. Thompson, J.K.; Jarvie, G.J.; Lahey, B.B.; et al. Exercise and obesity: etiology, physiology, and intervention. Psychological Bulletin 91:55–79; 1982.

89. Thorne, M.C.; Wing, A.L.; Paffenbarger, R.S., Jr. Chronic disease in former college students. VII. Early precursors of nonfatal coronary heart disease. Am. J. Epidemiol. 87:520–529; 1968.

90. Tipton, C.M. Exercise, training, and hypertension. In: Terjung, R.L., ed. Exercise and sports sciences reviews. Lexington, MA: Collamore Press: 245–306; 1984.

91. Tomassoni, T.L.; Galioti, F.M.; Vaccaro, P.; et al. The pediatric cardiac rehabilitation program at Children's Hospital National Medical Center, Washington, D.C. J. Cardiopulm. Rehab. 7:259–262; 1987.

92. Tran, Z.V.; Weltman, A.; Glass, G.V.; et al. The effects of exercise on blood lipids and lipoproteins: a meta-analysis of studies. Med. Sci. Sports Exerc. 15:393–402; 1983.

93. Tremblay, A.; Despres, J.P.; Bouchard, C. The effects of exercise-training on energy balance and adipose tissue morphology and metabolism. Sports Med. 2:223–233; 1985.

94. Tunstall-Pedoe, D. Exercise and sudden death. Br. J. Sports Med. 12:215–219; 1979.

95. Vignos, P.J.; Watkins, M.P. The effect of exercise in muscle dystrophy. JAMA 197:843–848; 1966.

96. Webber, L.S.; Cresanta, J.L.; Croff, J.B.; et al. Transitions of cardiovascular risk from adolescence to young adulthood—the Bogalusa heart study: II. Alterations in anthropometric blood pressure and serum lipoprotein variables. J. Chron. Dis. 39:91–103; 1986.

97. Webber, L.S.; Freedman, D.S. Interrelationships of coronary heart disease risk factors in children. In: Berenson, G.S., ed. Causation of cardiovascular risk factors in children. New York: Raven; 1986:65–81.

98. Webber, L.S.; Freedman, D.S.; Cresanta, J.L. Tracking of cardiovascular risk factor variables in school age children. In: Berenson, G.S., ed. Causation of cardiovascular risk factors in children. New York: Raven; 1986:42–64.

99. Zach, M.S.; Purrer, B.; Oberwalder, B. Effect of swimming on forced expiration and sputum clearance in cystic fibrosis. Lancet 2:102–103.

CHAPTER 3

Considerations for Sports Selection and Preparatory Training

Barry Goldberg
Yale University School of Medicine

Arthur M. Pappas
University of Massachusetts Medical Center

Nancy M. Cummings
University of Massachusetts Medical Center

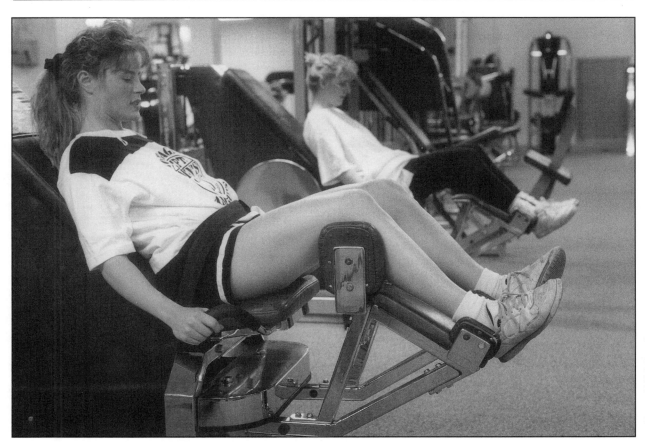

The promotion of moderate to vigorous physical activity is an important preventive health goal for children. As discussed in chapter 2, sport and exercise activities can have positive health outcomes by improving physical fitness and potentially modifying the risks for such chronic diseases as coronary artery disease, hypertension, and obesity. Psychosocial development also can be enhanced in the athletic environment. In appropriately structured programs, an excellent opportunity for excitement and enjoyable social recreation can be provided. Since only 60% of children in the United States engage in adequate levels of aerobic activities (113), physicians have been advised to counsel children and their parents concerning the benefits of exercise and to encourage their participation. Children with chronic illnesses in particular tend to lead sedentary lifestyles either because of limitations imposed by their disease or self-motivated choices (107). These children, who represent the most inactive of the population, could attain significant health benefits from an increase in physical activity while improving the quality of their lives. While physicians caring for a child with a chronic health problem should prioritize attention to the course of the disease process, they should not forget recommendations concerning sport and exercise.

In 1981, over 2 million children, almost 4% of the population up to the age of 16, were restricted in the level of their physical activity by chronic illness (53, 91-93). For 2% of the childhood population these limitations extended to major activities, and it is reasonable to assume that these numbers have remained relatively constant today. Physicians and educators are faced with the challenge of providing activity recommendations to create positive health outcomes, foster a desire for habitual exercise, and provide enjoyment and offer positive psychosocial experiences. This process must occur while avoiding adverse or catastrophic affects on the disease process. To accomplish these goals a preparatory training program may be required, and an understanding of the demands and risks of specific sports is essential. This chapter will address those issues which must be considered when assisting a child with a chronic disease to select appropriate sport and exercise activities.

GENERAL CONSIDERATIONS FOR RECOMMENDING ACTIVITIES

There are many issues that must be taken into consideration before recommending sports and exercise activities for children with chronic health problems. General considerations include understanding what determines a child's desire to participate, assessing physical activity and fitness to make suggestions to optimize success, choosing activities that will have therapeutic benefit, selecting safe activities, and having the child understand the importance of self-limiting activity. The great value of this effort will be the improvement in the child's quality of life.

Determinants of Physical Activity

The factors which determine a child's decision to be physically active or to engage in sport are critical since they represent the issues which will foster a positive experience and motivate the child to continued, lifelong participation. Research has demonstrated that multiple variables correlate with physical activity (122), although direct causal relationships remain to be determined. These variables have been divided into four broad categories, which include

- biological and developmental factors,
- psychological factors,
- social and cultural factors, and
- physical and environmental factors.

Factors within the categories which appear to determine a choice to engage in physical activity include:

- motor skill,
- fitness level (101),
- health status (15),
- knowledge of how to be physically active (54),
- feeling assured in one's ability and intentions to exercise (45, 51, 55),
- higher socioeconomic status (54, 138),
- being of Anglo-American descent (54),
- parental encouragement (68, 83),
- parental and sibling participation in a physically active lifestyle (101, 113, 120, 121),
- good climate conditions (112),
- greater amount of time spent outdoors (67),

- access to exercise and sports facilities and programs (112), and
- possibly, limited television viewing (40, 140).

Surprisingly, issues not associated with activity choices include personality characteristics (28), including independence, achievement motivation, movement satisfaction, and social adequacy and knowledge about the benefits of exercise (96). Time constraints are negatively associated with choosing to be active (139).

Since these studies evaluated healthy children, extrapolation to the child with a chronic health problem must be done with caution. However, the studies do provide the basis for potential interventions (122). It would appear that parents must clearly understand and be supportive of activity recommendations, particularly as it is documented that parents of chronically ill children often discourage physical activity (14). Children should be advised of the importance of exercise and assured of the safety of the recommended activities in the hope they will commit themselves to physical activity decisions. They may have to be assisted in gaining motor skill competence in the sports they choose and may also need specific advice about "how" to be physically active. Such advice can include specific training programs, acceptable sports, and practical modifications in lifestyle which include watching less television and going outdoors when possible. The availability of effective school programs is important, as the school setting represents a location where facilities exist, time is allocated to physical education, and the child is "captured" on the site. Community programs should also be made available for the activities deemed safe.

Studies which have evaluated motivational issues influencing a healthy child to participate in specific sports include three broad factors: intrinsic needs, extrinsic outcomes, and social interaction (50, 78, 98, 124-126, 131, 137, 155). Intrinsic or personal goals appear to be the most significant for all age groups. These include having fun, improving skills, becoming physically fit, engaging in the excitement of competition, achieving success and status, and finding an avenue for the release of energy and the avoidance of boredom. In sport, the child can establish personal goals and attain a sense of fulfillment and confidence through a steady improvement in performance. The importance of these intrinsic goals is reflected in the reasons children withdraw from programs. These include

- not getting a chance to play,
- receiving consistent criticism,
- having no chance for success,
- experiencing constant failure, and
- feeling the stress of expectations beyond their abilities.

Bearing these factors in mind, the child with a chronic illness should be assisted in selecting a sport or activity which provides a reasonable expectation for success as measured by realistic personal standards. Specific programs should be selected based on their ability to provide instruction in sport skills, emphasize participation, and praise improvement. These program characteristics are obviously ideal for all children. However, with the potential existence of underlying problems in ego development, they take on even greater significance for the child with a chronic medical problem.

Issues of social interaction include being with or making friends, becoming a member of a team, and benefiting from the team atmosphere. A chronic illness can make a child feel isolated from his peers, and the sport environment has the potential to permit a feeling of inclusion. Coaches should be aware of the importance of permitting the child to fit into the group. They should avoid behavior which might make the child feel "different" or cause teammates or competitors to interact in a isolating manner. Finally, extrinsic outcomes such as winning awards and games or pleasing parents and coaches are the least important reason children participate in sport. Coaches and programs which overemphasize winning and pay attention only to superior performers should not be recommended.

It is essential to have a full understanding of the motivational factors affecting physical activity and sport participation. Appropriate interventions will promote physical activity, enhance the opportunity for a successful experience, and optimize the development of lifelong exercise habits. Research is needed to further evaluate the specific motivational characteristics of children with chronic medical problems and the interventions which will result in increased activity.

Assessing Baseline Physical Activity and Physical Fitness

Children with chronic disease are frequently inactive. Although hypoactivity can be a direct consequence of the underlying pathology, lifestyle choices are also partially responsible. This conclusion has been documented in such conditions as congenital heart disease (72), asthma (147), diabetes mellitus (76), and obesity (23, 27). Chronically ill, inactive children become physically unfit and are then prone to continue sedentary habits because they are unable to successfully meet the demands of sport and exercise. This cycle of diminished activity deprives children of the positive health outcomes and recreational benefits of sport and exercise. Increasing physical activity and improving fitness is therefore an important goal in the treatment of the child with a chronic health problem, and approprite activity recommendations should be an integral part of medical care.

Physical activity relates to the daily expenditure of energy, while physical fitness represents a composite of neuromuscular, cardiovascular, and body composition characteristics which enhance a child's ability to be physically active (12, 32). Children's physical activity levels have been correlated with physical fitness (101), and physical activity as an independent variable has also been found to have preventive health benefits (51). Lower triglycerides (142), higher HDL cholesterol (145), and low body fat (20) have all been linked with high activity levels, although the relationship to cardiovascular endurance reflects only a weak association (141).

A physician planning activity recommendations must first determine the child's baseline level of activity. All current techniques of measuring physical activity have limitations (46, 71, 82, 119), but a measure of validity can be obtained from questionnaires and diaries provided by both the parent and child. Absolute standards for appropriate levels of physical activity do not exist, but recommedations for healthy children suggest 15-60 minutes of moderate to vigorous physical activity using large muscle groups three to five days per week (54, 111, 136). Specific recommendations for the child with a chronic medical problem might, for example, limit the intensity of the exercise. A sedentary child can also increase total daily activity by lifestyle changes incorporating low-intensity work, such as walking, climbing stairs, or performing household chores.

Physical fitness reflects a capacity to perform vigorous physical activity and can incorporate many attributes. Speed, agility, and coordination represent fitness variables, but although they certainly can affect sport and exercise performance they carry no particular health benefits. In contrast, increases in cardiorespiratory endurance and in neuromuscular and body composition fitness have been associated with decreased risk of hypokinetic diseases (100, 133, 136). These health-related physical fitness parameters can, in a limited way, be assessed in an office setting. Body composition can be measured with relative accuracy by skinfold measurement (75), and flexibility can be assessed by physical examination. Cardiorespiratory endurance and muscle strength can be measured by the assessment of maximal oxygen consumption in a laboratory exercise stress test and with the use of isokinetic or isometric dynamometers in a training facility. However, the measurement of cardiorespiratory endurance by performance tests demonstrates variable validity (63, 117), and the validity of the measurement of muscle strength and endurance by manual muscle tests, pull-ups, flexed arm hang, sit-ups, and push-ups is yet to be determined (12).

Health-related physical fitness parameters should be accurately measured when they are suspected to be significantly abnormal. Obesity or very low aerobic power in a chronically ill child creates a deficiency in fitness that could lead to an adverse health outcome and interfere with daily living. Quantification provides a mechanism to evaluate the magnitude of the deficiencies, to institute specific corrective programs, and to assess the effectiveness of medical intervention. The quantification of fitness parameters can also provide the information for specific training recommendations when a child is committed to successful performance in a demanding activity.

Recommendations for enhancing physical fitness require the provision of specific instructions. Improvements in the level of physical activity can occur simply from general increases in daily energy expenditures. To increase aerobic power an activity must be of adequate intensity in order to improve maximal oxygen consumption (114, 135, 144). This is particularly true for prepubertal children. Resistance exercises are required to improve muscle strength (103, 118, 148, 155), and changes in physical activity and diet can promote weight reduction (99, 143). Optimally, sports and exercise activities should provide the training stimulus to improve fitness. Additionally, a physically fit child is more likely to have a successful sport experience. A later section in this chapter will describe preparatory training programs for the improvement of physical fitness parameters.

Therapeutic Recreation

Sport and exercise can provide therapeutic benefits for specific disease entities. For example, rehabilitative gains in the range of motion of joints, in aerobic endurance, and in muscle strength and endurance can benefit the child with rheumatoid arthritis, diabetes, and cystic fibrosis, respectively. These benefits will be addressed in subsequent chapters which relate to each specific disease. When assisting a child in selecting a sport, desired rehabilitative goals should be incorporated into the performance demands of the sport. Since a broad range of sports will usually achieve the same therapeutic goal, individual activity preferences can be accommodated. If necessary, a supplementary training program can be developed. Thus, recreational rehabiltation is an important consideration in sports selection.

Safety

Sport participation carries a risk of sudden death, physical and psychological injury, and an adverse progression of the underlying disease process. Preventive measures to minimize these risks represent an important component of the sport selection process. Consideration must include

- defining required exclusions,
- establishing periodic reevaluation assessments,
- instituting anticipatory preventive programs, and
- ensuring that the coach, parent, and child understand and will comply with the recommendations provided.

Required exclusions can help to ensure that adverse or catastrophic events do not occur. Factors which must be considered include

- the collision potential of a sport,
- the aerobic demands,
- the dominance of static versus dynamic movements, and
- the dominant motions required.

A classification of sport into these categories will be provided later in this chapter and will be used throughout the text. Unfortunately, classifications are somewhat arbitrary and do not incorporate some important considerations such as the current status of the disease, the competitive level of the chosen program, and the intensity of required training. For example, a child with leukemia who is in remission and on no chemotherapy can be afforded a broader choice of activities than one with active disease. As another example, playing basketball in an interscholastic program associated with intense training places a significantly higher physiological stress than a community program, a nonorganized recreational game, or simply shooting baskets. Sports with high training requirements such as track, crew, and swimming have to be viewed from their total required demand, as well as in terms of the actual competitive event. A broad classification of sports designed for the purpose of decisions of exclusion, such as that of the American Academy of Pediatrics, must be viewed as initial guidelines only; relevant variables should be given appropriate consideration so that individualized recommendations can be made.

Adverse effects from participation in sports must be anticipated. School and community youth leaders as well as medical personnel should be made aware of potential problems. Appropriate plans should be established to prevent and respond to medical complications; specific recommendations will be provided in the future chapters on individual disease entities. Anticipatory and preventive guidance can relieve the anxiety of school and community personnel. Similarly, anticipatory information should also be provided for parents and children. They must be assured that interventional support is available, that the self-limitation of activity is understood by and is acceptable to the coach, and that potential problems can be averted by adherence to specific recommendations.

Compliance with activity recommendations is essential for safe sport partiicpation. The child must adhere to restrictions, follow training directives, and respond to perceived symptoms with self-initiated cessation of activity. It is essential to assess the emotional health and maturity of the child to gauge whether these directives will be followed (7, 44, 56, 97). Children who deny their disesase, act impulsively and immaturely, are depressed with suicidal ideation, or who wish to establish their omnipotence must be regarded as at risk of making inappropriate decisions and will need more supervision. Children who desire stimulation, challenge, and excitement within the context of constructive control of risk variables are more likely to comply with specified recommendations.

Self-Limited Activity

A frequent recommendation made to children and parents is to stop activities when they become stressful. This approach requires that the child be able to recognize both the level of exertion and the appearance of pathological symptoms. Because many parents are concerned that exercise could cause major harm, it is important to discuss self-limited activity and to provide a careful definition of the term. Additionally, it is important to have coaches understand the concept so that the child is free to respond to perceived symptoms without fear of criticism or embarrassment.

Pathological symptoms imply that the abnormalities represented by the underlying disease are creating an abnormal physiological response to the exercise demand. Dyspnea and wheezing in the asthmatic; chest pain, palpitations, and light-headedness in the child with congenital heart disease; sweating, tremors, and light-headedness in the diabetic child; and increasing joint pain in the child with rheumatoid arthritis are representative examples. The more specific we can be about what symptoms are pathological, the easier it is for the child to self-limit activity. A clear and very specific discussion of the potential symptoms provoked by exercise will afford the child the confidence to

stop activity and report symptoms. This decision can prevent a potentially serious event.

Certain children who are permitted to exercise may require limitations on the intensity of exertion allowed. To this end the child may be asked to attend to the peripheral cues of muscle and joint discomfort and to the central signals of ventilation, heart rate, and metabolic change which reflect a high level of effort. A rating of perceived exertion (RPE) has been found to correlate with physiological parameters of effort in adults (21, 31). Although this rating suffers from a lack of specific physiological information (as opposed to, for example, ST changes on an electrocardiogram), it has proven to be a useful clinical tool.

RPE is based on the subjective terms of Borg's 15-point rating (22), which include*

6 No exertion at all
7
8 Extremely light
9 Very light
10
11 Light
12
13 Somewhat hard
14
15 Hard (heavy)
16
17 Very hard
18
19 Extremely hard
20 Maximal exertion

*Reprinted from Borg (1985).

The usefulness of RPE in children requires further study, but restricting activity based on perceived exertion can provide another way of enabling the child to adhere to exercise recommendations. In our experience, this scale, in conjunction with a determination of heart rate by manual palpitation and pulsimetry, has been helpful in maintaining appropriate levels of exercise intensity.

Quality of Life

Chronic health problems can rob childhood of its innocence and fun. Traumatic medical procedures, frequent physician vists, the threat of mortality, and the limitations and isolated feelings are some of the burdens that accompany a chronic disease. Optimizing the quality of a child's life is an important medical consideration and must be considered within the context of total care.

The book entitled "I Will Sing Life" (19) should be read by all medical personnel. In this book, children with life-threatening illnesses express their desire for health and their wish not to feel abnormal because they are sick. They share their wish for fun, challenge, success, and acceptance, as well as for the right to forget their illness for at least part of the day and live in a nonmedical world. Sport is an arena where a child with a chronic health problem can escape and be a "second baseman" rather than a "leukemic." Although sport is not the only avenue of escape it is a popular choice, and these children deserve the effort required to permit sport participation to be a part of their lives.

PREPARATORY TRAINING

A child planning to begin a sport can often benefit from a preparatory training program. This may include exercises to improve aerobic endurance, muscular strength, and body flexibility, as well as advice on optimizing nutrition, body composition, and the capacity to adapt to environmental stresses. Individual instruction in motor skills can also be considered. Programs should be specifically considered in the following circumstances:

- *Sedentary, poorly conditioned children.* A progressive conditioning program can improve physical fitness and facilitate success in a chosen sport activity.
- *Children entering demanding, competitive programs.* A controlled program can enhance fitness and the capacity for successful performance while reducing the potential for overuse injuries, which can arise from sudden changes in repetitive physical stress.
- *Children in need of specific therapeutic rehabilitation.* Specific exercises can be provided to maximize the potential rehabilitative gains from sport participation.
- *Children at risk from the physiological demands of exercise.* A progressive and controlled program can reveal the cardiovascular, pulmonary, metabolic, and musculoskeletal responses to exercise prior to exposure to the less predictable demands of actual sport participation.
- *Older children initially entering a sport.* Skill instruction and general conditioning will facilitate successful performance when competition against more experienced and skilled peers is required.
- *Children who select sports with low aerobic demand.* A training program can improve aerobic fitness which would not otherwise result from participation in the selected sport.

A preparatory training program is an exercise prescription and must be provided with clear instruction, attainable goals, and appropriate safety precautions (74, 77, 115). Time requirements should be reasonable and travel demands limited. Positive reinforcement should be regularly provided by a valued adult and the child should understand the methods, benefits, and goals of the program. These programs need not address all fitness parameters, but rather can be limited to specific desired objectives.

Aerobic Endurance

Cardiorespiratory endurance reflects the capacity of the body to work or exercise at relatively high intensity for a prolonged period of time. Energy must be delivered to the working muscles. This requires the functional integrity of the pulmonary and cardiovascular systems, as well as appropriate perfusion and diffusion and metabolic enzymatic activity (149). One standard measure of cardiorespiratory endurance, $\dot{V}O_2max$ (see chapter 2), increases progressively between the ages of 6 and 12 years in normal children (70). After age 12, boys continue to demonstrate increases while girls display less consistent changes (102). This increase results in gender differences during adolescence. Fourteen-year-old boys have, on average, a 25% higher $\dot{V}O_2max$ than girls. By age 16, the difference can be as much as 50%. These variations appear to be largely related to differences in lean body mass and percentage of body fat, but exercise behavior also seems to play a role. When maximum oxygen consumption is related to body weight, males demonstrate a relatively constant level of approximately 50 ml/kg/min throughout childhood, while females exhibit declining levels throughout the adolescent years. Table 3.1 describes Kranenbuhl, Skinner, and

Table 3.1 The Progression of Maximum Oxygen Consumption in Childhood

Age years (sex)	$\dot{V}O_2max$ – L/min		$\dot{V}O_2max$ ml/kg/min	
	Male	Female	Male	Female
6(M) .... 6(F)	1.1 .... 1.1		53 53	
7(M) .... 7(F)	1.3 .... 1.1		53 51	
8(M) .... 8(F)	1.4 .... 1.2		53 50	
9(M) .... 9(F)	1.7 .... 1.4		53 48	
10(M) .... 10(F)	1.9 .... 1.6		53 47	
11(M) .... 11(F)	2.0 .... 1.7		53 45	
12(M) .... 12(F)	2.4 .... 2.0		53 44	
13(M) .... 13(F)	2.5 .... 2.2		53 43	
14(M) .... 14(F)	2.7 .... 2.3		53 42	
15(M) .... 15(F)	3.0 .... 2.3		53 41	
16(M) .... 16(F)	3.2 .... 2.2		53 40	

Data from Kranenbuhl, Skinner, and Kohrt (1985).

Kohrt's summation of several studies tracking the progression of $\dot{V}O_2max$ throughout childhood (77).

At high levels of work aerobic metabolism becomes unable to meet all required energy demands, and anaerobic metabolism must be called upon to supplement energy production (38, 150, 151, 154). The result of anaerobic metabolism is a rise in blood lactate, metabolic acidosis, and a compensatory ventilatory response. The level of work or oxygen consumption at which anaerobic metabolism becomes prominent is called the anaerobic threshold. This physiological parameter is another measure of cardiovascular endurance. It is usually expressed as a percentage of the maximum oxygen consumption ($\dot{V}O_2$ at anaerobic threshold/$\dot{V}O_2max$). The anaerobic threshold is an important measure of endurance since it reflects a child's ability to use a percentage of his or her aerobic capacity over a period of time without experiencing the fatigue associated with anaerobic metabolism. Studies of the anaerobic threshold of children have revealed varying results, but in general children have higher thresholds than adults, ranging between 60-80% of $\dot{V}O_2max$ (65, 108, 109). There is some evidence that the anaerobic threshold may decrease progressively from prepubescence to adulthood. These findings may explain the relatively good aerobic and poor anaerobic performance of children when compared with adults.

Training can improve cardiorespiratory performance in children. Adolescents have demonstrated 8-20% improvement in maximum oxygen consumption, which is comparable to the results of adult training studies (43, 69, 104, 123, 127). Although trainability of prepubescent children has been debated, reviews of the available literature have generally found that in the presence of an appropriate training stimulus, young children will improve cardiovascular endurance (16, 114, 116, 135, 144). Rowland has recommended that prepubescent training programs utilize large muscle groups for a duration of 15-60 minutes at a frequency of three to five times per week and an intensity that elicits a heart rate of 60-90% of maximum (114).

Chronic illness can impede cardiorespiratory endurance (15). This problem has been confirmed by several studies and will be addressed specifically in future chapters. It is logical that pathological impairment of ventilation, cardiac output, vascular perfusion, muscle function, or fuel metabolism can interfere with aerobic functions. Endurance can also be adversely affected by anemia, malnutrition, mechanical inefficiency, or a sedentary lifestyle. Thus, a child with a chronic health problem can have significantly reduced aerobic power. However, controlled endurance programs can facilitate positive health outcomes and enhance performance both in sport and in activities of daily living.

An optimal aerobic endurance program will employ an effective but safe training stimulus.

Children at risk for adverse or catastrophic responses to high-intensity endurance actitivies require a pretraining cardiopulmonary stress test to evaluate their physiological response to exercise. Simultaneous measurements of work intensity, electrocardiographic response, blood pressure, oxygen saturation, ventilation, and oxygen consumption can detect an abnormal or dangerous response to exercise. Underlying pathology may also dictate the need for a complete evaluation of pulmonary function, a further assessment of cardiac rhythm and an analysis of the metabolic response to exercise.

Children who demonstrate a potentially dangerous response to exercise require either restriction from endurance activity or a training program performed with continuous monitoring under direct physician observation. In our experience (52), children who are at risk but who do not demonstrate abnormalities for a potentially catastrophic cardiac response during exercise testing can be safely trained at home. A program of controlled intensity under parental supervision with regular physician telephone contact is required. A cardiopulmonary progressive exercise test is performed on a bicycle ergometer; alternatively, some laboratories employ treadmill tests. The measurement of maximum oxygen consumption, oxygen consumption at specific work intensities, and the work level and pulse both at the anaerobic threshold

and at maximum heart rate are utilized to establish an appropriate work intensity and to provide baseline information for future evaluations. For training, a work intensity at a pulse 60-70% of maximum and below the anaerobic threshold is selected. The child is provided with a bicycle ergometer, pulse meter, and detailed written instructions. The instructions are reviewed at the initial visit and include a warm-up and cool-down procedure, the requirement for direct observation by an adult, the actions necessary if illness intervenes, and indications for when to stop the program and call for physician advice. These indications include adverse reactions, a heart rate response different from the targeted pulse, or an inability to progress in training. Table 3.2 describes a progressive interval program. The pulse is determined and recorded by manual palpation and pulse meter after each work cycle, and children remain at a specific duration of exercise until they can complete the three intervals. The total time commitment rarely exceeds 30 minutes and children are advised to read, watch television, or listen to music while training. After completion of 12 to 16 weeks of training children return for reevaluation. Based upon their aerobic capacity, specific pathology, and maturity level, as well as their ability to perceive exertion, manually record pulse rate, and recognize adverse symptoms, specific sport and exercise activities are recommended. The ultimate goal is for further aerobic conditioning to arise from recreational activities.

Table 3.2 A Controlled Progressive Exercise Program on a Bicycle Ergometer

Frequency	Intensity	Duration intervals
Performed on alternate days	1. Work intensity at 60-70% maximum heart rate and below the anaerobic threshold	1. Work and rest periods are alternated for three repetitions
	2. Work intensity is increased after the progression in duration is completed	2. Work .... Rest Intervals (minutes)
		3 3
		4 2
		5 2
		5 1/2 2
		6 2
		6 1/2 2
		7 2
		7 1/2 2
		8 2

When there is no risk of adverse reaction to endurance activity but control of training intensity is desired, a Conconi test can be performed (34). The child performs at progressively increasing work intensities (as created, for example, by running or pedaling on a bicycle ergometer), and the pulse rate is recorded at each work level. When the linear relationship of workload to heart rate is deflected such that increments in work exceed increments in heart rate, an indirect measurement of the anaerobic threshold will be determined. This measurement has been shown to be reliable for children (10, 11). Recommendations for aerobic training can be made at a work intensity and/or pulse rate 10-20% lower than that found at the estimated anaerobic threhold. Self-recorded pulse rate can be used as a guide to training intensity. A multitude of training activities can be employed, including swimming, running, or bicycling, as long as criteria for frequency (3-4 times per week) and duration (15-60 minutes) are met while the appropriate intensity is maintained.

Training intensity can be recommended without pretesting by establishing a target heart rate which represents 60-70% of a predicted maximum pulse. Remaining at or below 70% maximum heart rate usually ensures an exercise intensity below the anaerobic threshold (49). The established formula for estimating maximum pulse is 220 minus age in years, although variations exist (57, 58). Endurance programs are not designed to create breathlessness, extreme fatigue, or prolonged weakness after exercise. Children should be advised that the presence of these symptoms indicates that intensity should be reduced and the targeted pulse should not be exceeded.

There are other issues to consider before making training recommendations for children who do not require direct observation. Whenever possible, children with an interest in a sport should train in activities specific to that sport in order to maximize performance. That is, children in running sports should engage in a running program, and swimmers should swim. Variables of intensity and duration should be based on the demands of that choice; for example, sprinters require different programs than distance runners. In addition, when options of training activities exist the child's preferences should always be a priority. Specific goals should always be established as part of the program. These goals should be attainable in a relatively short period of time and the accomplishment should be obvious. A valued adult should be available to provide positive feedback.

Nonspecific recommendations to increase physical activity can result in improved aerobic endurance, but the relationship and the associated variables remain to be established. A correlation between physical activity and cardiovascular endurance certainly exists. However, some issues, such as the minimum required training stimulus and the time required to detect change, need further definition. Adult studies have indicated that low-intensity activities can improve cardiovascular endurance (42, 47, 105, 128). Many children prefer low- to moderate-intensity activities, and if these are proven to be efficacious in improving aerobic capacity in children they will afford another training option.

Muscle Strength

Muscle strength can be defined as the maximum power which a muscle or group of muscles can generate at one time. Prepubescent boys and girls linearly increase muscle strength as they grow (8). At any given height boys are stronger than girls, but the prepubertal rate of gain is similar for both sexes. After puberty, however, the average boy has a more rapid increase in strength compared to the average girl. This is attributed to the presence of circulating androgens. Strength differences are related to the presence of greater muscle mass in males, as strength factored by lean body mass reveals no difference between the sexes.

Children can improve muscle strength by training. Several studies have demonstrated that even prepubescent children can significantly increase muscle strength with low risk of injury when a proper weight training program is employed (110, 132, 156). Necessary ingredients for a proper program include

- close and continuous supervision,
- adequate warm-up and cool-down time,
- uncomplicated training techniques,
- adequate recovery time between sessions, and
- avoidance of maximal or near maximal lifts.

The emphasis should be on how many times a child can correctly lift a weight or perform an exercise, not on how much weight a child can lift. The following prescription for strength training programs is recommended by the American Orthopaedic Society for Sports Medicine (29):

1. Frequency—Two or three times per week.
2. Duration—20 to 30 minutes per session.
3. Intensity—A. In the beginning, no resistance should be used until proper form is achieved.
   B. One set consists of 6 to 15 repetitions.
   C. One to three sets per session.
   D. No maximum lifts.
4. Progressive Resistance—Weight or resistance is increased in 1- to 3-pound increments after the prepubescent can do 15 repetitions in good form.

Any workout involving weight training should include a period of warm-up aimed at maintaining joint flexibility. Special attention should also be directed toward the major muscle groups required for the sport in which the child intends to participate.

The techniques for strength training include isokinetic, isometric, and isotonic exercise. Isokinetic exercise represents the contraction or lengthening of a muscle or muscle group at a constant speed; this requires special equipment and will not be discussed here. Isometric exercise involves the maintenance of a muscle contraction at a constant length (for example, by attempting to extend one's knee against an immovable object). Isotonic exercises involve performing an exercise with constant resistance. Free weights, elastic bands, and tubing are all techniques of creating constant resistance. Progressive Resisted Exercises (PREs), first described by DeLorme (39), are a type of isotonic exercise program. The procedure with PREs is to isolate the exercise to the muscle group that needs to be strengthened, tire that muscle group, and, as strength increases, gradually increase the weight or resistance to the exercise. Maximal repetitions and heavy weights should be avoided as they can result in injury caused by improper form or excess stress on the muscle. Table 3.3 reflects specific exercise programs for general strengthening of the extremities and back. Specific techniques for some of these are described by the following five exercises.

Table 3.3 Strengthening Exercises and Target Muscles

The empty can	Supraspinatus
Prone horizontal abduction	Deltoid, infraspinatus, teres minor
90°/90° external rotation	Teres minor
Side lying external rotation	Infraspinatus, teres minor
Superman	Lower trapezius
Abdominal curls	Rectus abdomini
Quad set	Quadriceps
Straight leg raise	Quadriceps: May perform PRE with more weight on ankle
Knee curls	Hamstrings (PRE) with more weight on ankle
Toe raises/toe walking	Gastrocnemius/soleus
Heel walking	Anterior tibialis

■ "EMPTY CAN"

POSITION: Standing with elbow straight and thumb pointing toward floor; arm adducted 30° toward the midline.

ACTION: Slowly raise arm to eye level and hold for a count of 2 seconds; slowly lower arm.

AMOUNT: Three sets of 10 repetitions.

OPTIONS: A 1/2-pound to 3-pound weight may be added as child gets stronger.

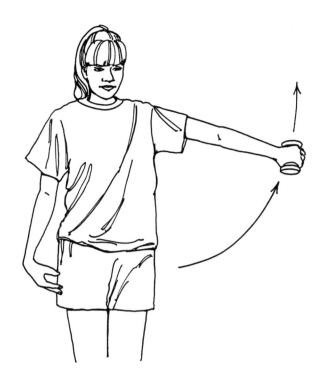

■ PRONE HORIZONTAL ABDUCTION

POSITION: Prone on table with arm hanging straight toward floor.

ACTION: Raise arm (with thumb toward ceiling) out to the side to eye level; hold for a count of 2 seconds and slowly lower.

AMOUNT: Repeat 10 times.

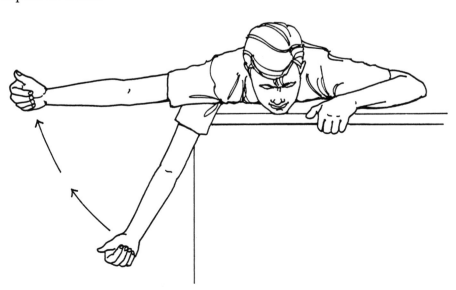

■ 90°/90° EXTERNAL ROTATION

POSITION: Prone on table with shoulder abducted 90° and upper arm supported on table with elbow bent.

ACTION: Keeping shoulder and elbow fixed, raise externally rotated arm 90°; hold for 2 seconds and slowly lower.

AMOUNT: Repeat 10 times.

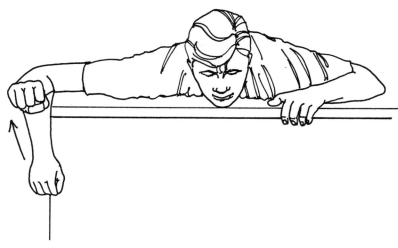

■ SIDE-LYING EXTERNAL ROTATION

POSITION: Lie on opposite side with involved arm at side and elbow bent 90°.

ACTION: Keeping elbow fixed to side, raise arm into external rotation; hold for 2 seconds and slowly lower.

AMOUNT: Repeat 10 times.

OPTIONS: A 1/2-pound to 3-pound weight may be added as child gets stronger.

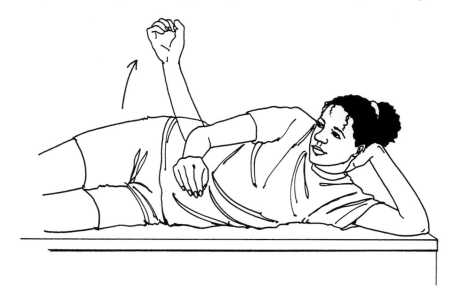

■ "SUPERMAN"

POSITION: Prone with arms outstretched and palms flat on table.

ACTION: With head remaining down, raise arms as high as possible overhead; hold for a count of 3.

AMOUNT: Repeat 10 times.

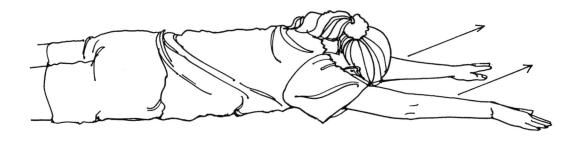

Flexibility

An important parameter in any athletic activity is the ease with which a joint can move through its range of motion. The range of motion of a joint is determined by its bony structure and by the compliance of soft tissue surrounding it. The flexibility of prepubescent children is usually good, but a decrease in flexibility occurs during the adolescent growth spurt. This is attributed to a differential rate of growth in the bones and surrounding soft tissues: the bones increase in length and the ligament and muscles surrounding the bone lengthen secondarily (85). Diminished flexibility can result in increased stress across a joint and may cause injury or diminished performance.

A stretching program should be prescribed if diminished flexibility is identified. The involved area should be slowly stretched until resistance is met, and that position should be held for a period of 10 seconds without bouncing. It is often necessary to stretch the involved area 10 to 25 times per day. Children should be instructed on the correct stretching techniques to enable them to perform stretches over the course of the day.

The following figures show stretches for specific muscle groups.

■ LUMBAR STRETCH

POSITION: Sitting on a stool with hips extended and externally rotated.

ACTION: Gradually bend forward toward floor until a gentle stretch is felt in the lower back; hold for 10 seconds.

AMOUNT: Repeat 10 times.

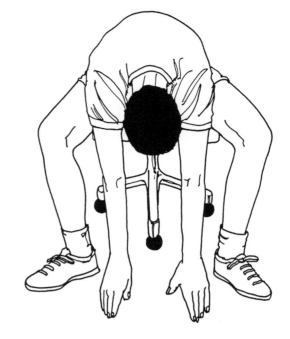

■ HIP ADDUCTORS STRETCH

POSITION: Sitting with back against a wall and soles of feet together.

ACTION: Gently push down on the inside of thighs; hold for count of 30, and then relax.

AMOUNT: Repeat 10 times.

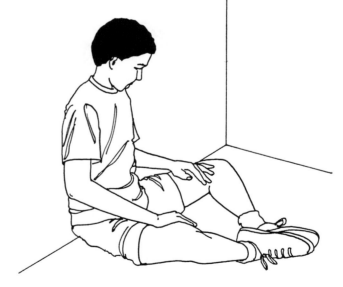

■ HIP FLEXOR STRETCH

POSITION: Supine on table.

ACTION: Bring one knee toward chest while keeping opposite leg straight; gently pull on knee and hold for a count of 30.

AMOUNT: Repeat 10 times each side.

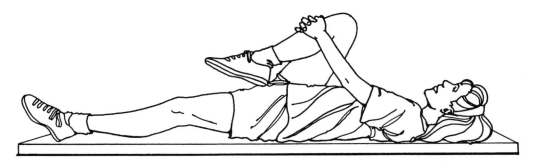

■ QUADRICEPS STRETCH

POSITION: Either standing with ipsilateral arm against wall for support, or in prone position.

ACTION: Grab right foot with left hand and gently pull foot toward buttock. Hold for a count of 10.

AMOUNT: Repeat 20 times alternating legs.

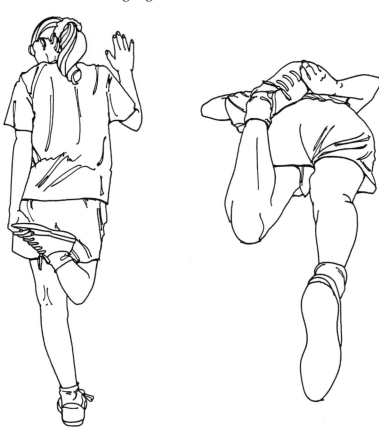

◼ HAMSTRING STRETCH

POSITION: Supine with one leg bent to chest and hands locked behind knee.

ACTION: Slowly straighten knee until gentle stretch is felt; hold for count of 10.

AMOUNT: Three sets of 10 repetitions on each side.

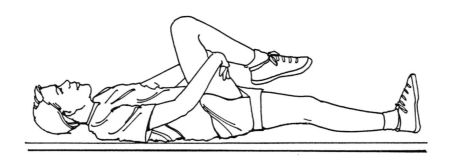

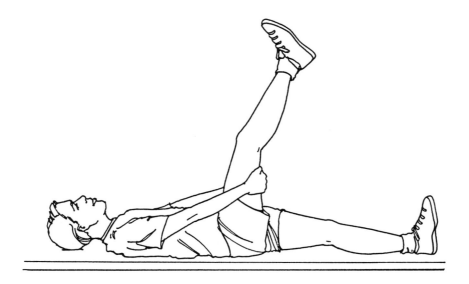

GASTROCNEMIUS/
SOLEUS STRETCH

POSITION: Stand a little distance from wall resting forearms and forehead against wall.

ACTION: Bend one knee while keeping opposite leg straight and foot flat on the floor, until a gentle stretch is felt in calf of straight leg. Hold for a count of 10.

AMOUNT: Three sets of 10 repetitions on each side.

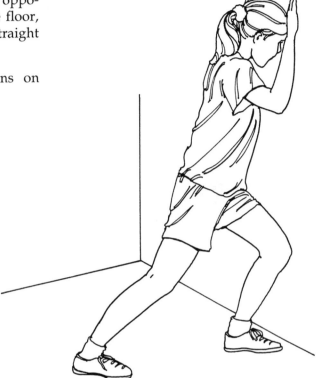

STANDING ABDUCTION/
▮ EXTERNAL ROTATION

POSITION: Sitting with elbows bent 90°.

ACTION: Raise (abduct) arm to shoulder level; pinch shoulder blades together; rotate arms toward ceiling, hold for a count of 5, then slowly reverse movements.

AMOUNT: 25 sets of 5 repetitions.

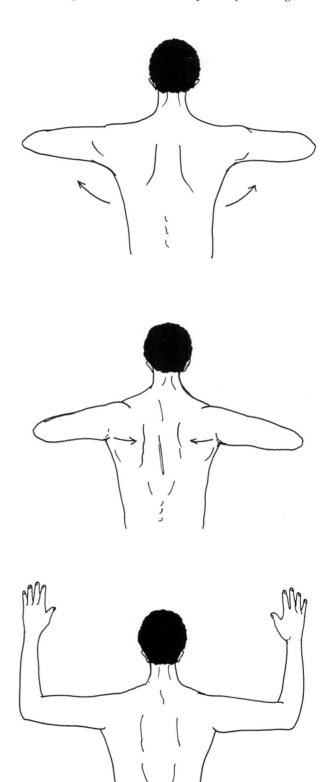

GLENOHUMERAL ADDUCTION STRETCH

POSITION: Supine on table; assistant must stabilize scapula on the thoracic wall.

ACTION: Slowly push arm across chest; hold for a count of 5.

AMOUNT: Repeat 10 times.

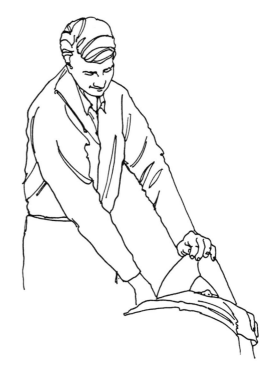

GLENOHUMERAL FLEXION OR FORWARD ELEVATION STRETCH

POSITION: Supine with assistant stabilizing scapula on thoracic wall and arm in neutral rotation.

ACTION: Slowly bring arm up overhead toward table; hold for a count of 5.

AMOUNT: Repeat 10 times.

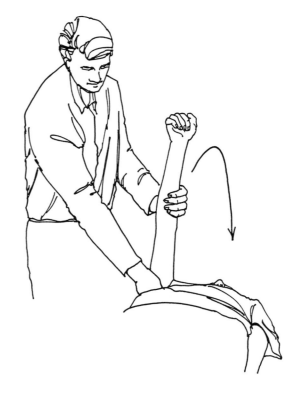

Body Composition and Nutrition

Nutritional disorders are often associated with chronic illness. These disorders may also represent the primary disease entitites of anorexia nervosa or obesity. Nutritional disorders are often accompanied by abnormalities in body composition as reflected by the amount of body fat and lean body mass. Body fat can be measured in the office setting with the use of skinfold calipers (75) and the parameter of body composition is a component of health-related physical fitness. An assessment of body composition and nutrition is thus an important part of the care of the child with a chronic health problem and becomes particularly significant when the demands and benefits of exercise are added to daily living.

Obesity is a common primary chronic disease, and a later chapter is devoted to this subject. Hypoactivity has been directly related to obesity, both as a cause and result, and the chronically ill child who has chosen a sedentary lifestyle is at risk of entering the obesity-hypoactivity cycle (14, 26, 64, 152). Obesity has been associated with reduced maximum oxygen consumption (36) and reduced muscular strength (66). Since the caloric intake of obese children does not appear to be excessive (35, 39), exercise represents an important therapeutic tool. Sport and exercise activities, when combined with caloric control and behavior modification techniques, can promote the loss of body fat (130).

Malnutrition can result from an eating disorder such as anorexia nervosa, or it can be the result of a debilitating neoplasm, chronic malabsorption, anorexia from chemotherapeutic agents, or required nutritional restrictions due to renal insufficiency. If malnutrition results in growth retardation and reduced lean body mass it may limit the capacity to perform physical work (6, 14, 37). Also, poorly nourished children may normally choose to be less active (33). Thus, it is important to establish the nutritional status of chronically ill children before they are encouraged to increase their daily expenditure of calories through involvement in exercise activities.

Exercise results in fluid loss, particularly when the sweat rate is high. Children cannot rely on the thirst mechanism to replenish fluids; typically they will voluntarily consume only two thirds of their fluid replacement requirement (17, 79, 86). Deliberate efforts must be made to correct significant deficiencies in order to avoid hypovolemia and thermoregulatory abnormalities. Electrolyte losses during exercise are usually quite low owing to the hypotonic nature of sweat; however, chronic illness may impose an increased risk of fluid and electrolyte abnormalities. Chronic renal disease, cystic fibrosis, diabetes mellitus, and gastrointestinal disorders can impose either an unusual loss of fluid and electrolytes or an abnormal physiological response to deficits. Careful monitoring of fluid loss (by recording morning and evening body weight) may be required, and specific electrolyte replacement fluids may need to be available. All children should be made aware of the risks associated with persistent excessive fluid loss, including symptoms associated with excessive loss and appropriate interventional responses.

Increased physical activity requires a well-balanced diet, and specific supplementation may have to be added. For example, exercise may increase protein requirements: although specific childhood requirements remain to be determined, adult studies suggest that a 50-100% increase above recommended daily allowances is needed (73). Moreover, disease-related inadequacies in protein intake or absorption may be exacerbated by the addition of exercise activities. The intake of vitamin C and riboflavin may also need to be increased, although these vitamins, as well as thiamine and vitamin E (18, 146), are usually found in adequate amounts in a well-balanced diet. Chronically ill children may need vitamin supplementation if concern for intake or absorption exists. These same considerations should be given to iron intake, particularly if an unusual loss of iron is a conern as with chronic gastrointestinal disease (60).

Motor Skills

The development of motor skills is a complex evolution that begins with the reflex movements of the infant and culminates in the multifaceted motor activities of the athlete (1, 2, 24). It is a progressive process which requires an orderly maturation of the neuromuscular system facilitated by a nurturing environment. Simple fundamental movements are the first to evolve during the first seven years of life; Seefeldt and Hauberstricker have defined norms for the development of fundamental sports movements (129). Motor skills improve with age, although much individual variability exists in the attainment of a skill and the quality of the movement.

Generally, after the age of six or seven fundamental skills are refined and organized into the more complex motor activities required for sport performance (106). The development of these motor skills appears to be dependent on multiple factors, including

- physical growth,
- strength,
- sensory and motor integration,
- feedback,
- memory, and
- concentration (48).

Environmental factors such as instruction and practice also play a role. While a detailed review of these specific issues is beyond the scope of this text, the recognition that motor skills require an orderly sequence of acquiring and building multiple subunits into a complex whole represents an important consideration for the child with a chronic medical problem or physical limitations.

A child with a chronic disease may be physically limited during the first years of life, and this may impede the natural development of fundamental skills. Restrictions placed on older children may alter the maturation of more complex motor activities. Musculoskeletal, neuromuscular, and other abnormalities may further hinder skill development. A prepatory evaluation should include an assessment of the child's motor proficiency, particularly as it relates to the selected sports activity, to determine the likelihood of success. If necessary, the intervention of individualized instruction or the redirection to another activity can prevent disappointment and frustration.

Environmental Acclimatization

The chemical energy of working muscles produces heat, which must be dissipated for body temperature to remain normal. When intrinsic heat production is combined with extrinsic environmental heat and humidity, a significant physiological burden occurs. Sweating and heat transfer from the skin to the environment by evaporation is the most important physiological thermoregulatory mechanism. Children are particularly at risk for heat illness (13). This problem is due to their large surface area per unit mass, lower sweating rate, and delayed initiation of sweating in response to changes in air temperature as compared with adults. In addition, children acclimate more slowly to heat.

Chronically ill children may have increased sensitivity to heat stress. Malnourished children may have decreased insulation and sweating rates (25). Conversely, some children with congenital heart disease appear to sweat excessively (3, 80). Anorexia nervosa may be associated with an abnormal hypothalamic response to heat (84), while cystic fibrosis is associated with excessive amounts of sodium in the sweat (30). Susceptibility to dehydration may be increased by preexisting fluid and electrolyte deficits from chronic vomiting or diarrhea, or by abnormal urinary losses. Compromises of normal physiological renal function can also present a burden. The potential increased risk of heat illness or dehydration from exercise must be considered when making activity recommendations.

Humidity, radiant heat, and ambient temperature all play a role in physiological heat stress. These variables are incorporated in the wet bulb globe temperature, which is defined by the formula

Wet Bulb Globe Temperature = 0.7 wet bulb + 0.2 black globe + 0.1 dry bulb (87).

Wet bulb temperatures of <25 °C (<77 °F) reflect low-risk conditions. At higher levels, however, a progressive curtailment of activities should occur until wet bulb temperature reaches 29 °C (84 °F), at which point all exercise activities should stop (14, 90). In general, ambient temperatures of less than 80 °F and humidity conditions of less than 70% do not present a significant risk for thermoregulatory stress. As noted earlier, hydrational requirements must be reviewed with children and they should be advised to replace water loss as measured by morning and evening weights. Fluids should also be made available during competition in four- to six-ounce quantities every 20 minutes. Cold water is often the most available and practical replacement fluid. Electrolyte losses can usually be replaced by a well-balanced diet, although Bar-Or recommends an electrolyte replacement solution of 25 g/L of glucose, 10 meq/L of sodium and 4 meq/L of potassium for healthy children (84). Adult recommendations include 10 meq/L sodium and 5 meq/L potassium (5).

All children, but particularly those who are chronically ill and previously sedentary, should be permitted to acclimate to heat before engaging in prolonged exercise. This requires controlled 1-hour exposures for 6 to 8 different days over 1 to 2 weeks (62, 84). They should be encouraged to wear lightweight, absorbent cotton clothing, and hats in sunlight. Children and their parents should also be instructed about the signs of heat illness, including

- weakness,
- faintness,
- dizziness,
- nausea,
- headache,
- disorientation,
- ataxia,
- irritability,
- emotional instability,
- apathy,
- aggressiveness, and
- dry or clammy skin (7, 30).

They must also be advised to stop participation and seek medical attention if these symptoms occur.

Cold can present another environmental stress. Vasoconstriction, increased metabolic rate, and shivering are the thermoregulatory responses (41, 134). Children who exercise are usually protected from cold-related illness by the intrinsic heat production of exercise. However, in extreme conditions, and particularly with high wind, vulnerable areas of the body such as fingers, ears, toes, and the chin should be protected. Swimming at water temperatures below 25 °C presents a problem for children owing to the large surface area per unit mass (61). Children who have abnormally low levels of body fat appear to be at particular risk.

THE CLASSIFICATION OF SPORTS

The final section of this chapter is devoted to the classification of sports by the categories of collision potential, aerobic intensity, static and dynamic demands, dominant motion, and neuromuscular skill demands. These classifications, which admittedly are based on experience and clinical judgment rather than on scientific study, have been developed to assist the physician in recommending sports which can provide a safe and successful experience. Additionally, they provide a listing of activities which can be dangerous and potentially result in sudden death, a life-threatening event, or an adverse affect on the progression of a specific disease

process. Those sports which represent a high risk to the child with a chronic disease should be discouraged. A physician's role is to make recommendations; the final decision to permit a child to participate in a specific sport may involve the consideration of medical, legal, parental, and the child's opinions.

Other variables to be considered include the level of competition, training demands, and the ability to employ appropriate judgment in ceasing activity when adverse symptoms arise. Recommendations may vary, for example, according to whether participation will be in a recreational setting or on an organized, competitive team. The categories do provide a general framework upon which individual recommendations can be made.

Collision-Contact Risk

One category consists of risk of body collision. Levels of risk include contact-collision-impact, limited contact, and noncontact (Table 3.4). These categories are similar to those developed by the Sports Medicine and Fitness Committee of the American Academy of Pediatrics in 1988 (4). In defining collision risk, either between athletes or between an athlete and an inanimate object, consideration has been given to the objectives of the sport, injury statistics available in the literature, the risk should a syncopal episode occur, and the potential for a very dangerous high-impact collision. Chronically ill children who can be dangerously affected by a collision force should be placed in appropriate limited-contact or noncontact activities.

Aerobic Intensity

Sports have also been categorized by the aerobic demands placed on the cardiovascular system (Table 3.5). Levels include high to moderate aerobic intensity, and low aerobic intensity. These categories were developed by the 1984 Bethesda Conference on Cardiovascular Abnormalities in the Athlete (89). The aerobic intensity of any sport will be significantly affected by the level of competition and training demand selected. The classification listed here assumes a competitive level of activity performed by a motivated child. When activities demand an intense aerobic response, children at risk should be directed toward low-intensity aerobic sports.

Table 3.4   Collision—Contact Potential in Sports

Contact/collision/impact

Auto racing	Field hockey	Lacrosse	Skiing—downhill
Basketball	Football	Motorcycling	Skiing—jumping
Bobsledding	Football—flag	Mountain climbing	Soccer
Boxing	Gymnastics	Polo	Water polo
Cycling	Handball—team	Rodeo	Waterskiing
Diving	Hockey—ice	Rope climbing	Wrestling
Equestrian	Karate/Judo	Rugby	

Limited contact

Baseball	Paddleball	Skiing—x-country	Volleyball
Cheerleading	Racquetball	Softball	Weightlifting
Field events	Skating—figure	Squash	
Hockey—floor	Skating—roller	Surfing	
Jai alai	Skating—speed	Ultimate frisbee	

Noncontact

Aerobic dance	Canoeing	Fishing	Running—sprint
Archery	Crew/Rowing	Golf	Running—distance
Badminton	Cricket	Handball	Shuffleboard
Ballet	Croquet	Hiking	Scuba diving
Billiards	Curling	Horseshoes	Swimming
Boccie	Dance	Orienteering	Table tennis
Bowling	Darts	Racewalking	Tennis
Bridge/Chess	Fencing	Riflery	Tetherball
Camping	Field events	Rope jumping	

Table 3.5   Aerobic Intensity of Sports

High and moderate aerobic intensity sports[a]

Aerobic dance	Field events	Polo	Soccer
Auto racing	Field hockey	Race walking	Squash
Badminton	Football	Racquetball	Surfing
Ballet	Football—flag	Rodeo	Swimming
Baseball	Gymnastics	Rope climbing	Table tennis
Basketball	Handball	Rope jumping	Tennis
Bobsledding	Handball—team	Running—sprint	Tetherball
Boxing	Hockey—floor	Running—distance	Ultimate frisbee
Canoeing	Hockey—ice	Rugby	Volleyball
Cheerleading	Jai alai	Scuba diving	Water polo
Crew/Rowing	Karate/Judo	Skating—figure	Waterskiing
Cycling	Lacrosse	Skating—roller	Weightlifting
Dance	Motorcycling	Skating—speed	Wrestling
Diving	Mountain climbing	Skiing—downhill	
Equestrian	Orienteering	Skiing—jumping	
Fencing	Paddleball	Skiing—x-country	

Low aerobic intensity sports[b]

Archery	Camping	Fishing	Sailing
Billiards	Cricket	Golf	Shuffleboard
Boccie	Croquet	Hiking	
Bowling	Curling	Horseshoes	
Bridge	Darts	Riflery	

[a]Includes Bethesda Class IA—High Moderate Intensity

[b]Includes Bethesda Class IB—Low Intensity

Static Dynamic Demands

Dynamic activities involve isotonic muscle contractions in large muscle groups, which result in active movement. Oxygen consumption, cardiac output, and systolic blood pressure usually increase significantly; diastolic blood pressure and mean arterial blood pressure remain constant; and peripheral vascular resistance decreases. Static activities involve isometric contractions usually employing smaller muscle groups and resulting in less movement. Static activities require less oxygen consumption and cardiac output, but are associated with increases in systolic, diastolic, and mean arterial pressure. Peripheral vascular resistance increases slightly. Dynamic exercise, therefore, places a volume demand on the heart while static exercise places a pressure load (4, 9, 81). Specific disease states may be adversely affected by either static or dynamic activity. Thus, sport recommendations should be made to avoid potentially dangerous movements (Table 3.6, a and b).

Table 3.6a   Static and Dynamic Demands of Sports

High dynamic demands

Aerobic dance	Field hockey	Race walking	Soccer
Badminton	Football	Racquetball	Softball
Ballet	Football—flag	Rope jumping	Squash
Baseball	Handball	Rugby	Swimming
Basketball	Handball—team	Running—distance	Table tennis
Boxing	Hockey—floor	Running—sprint	Tennis
Canoeing	Hockey—ice	Scuba diving	Tetherball
Cheerleading	Jai alai	Skating—figure	Ultimate frisbee
Crew/Rowing	Lacrosse	Skating—roller	Volleyball
Cycling	Mountain climbing	Skating—speed	Water polo
Dance	Orienteering	Skiing—downhill	Wrestling
Fencing	Polo	Skiing—x-country	

Low dynamic demands

Archery	Croquet	Hiking	Skiing—jump
Auto racing	Curling	Horseshoes	Surfing
Billiards	Darts	Karate/Judo	Waterskiing
Bobsledding	Diving	Motorcycling	Weightlifting
Boccie	Equestrian	Riflery	
Bowling	Field events	Rodeo	
Bridge	Fishing	Rope climbing	
Camping	Golf	Sailing	
Cricket	Gymnastics	Shuffleboard	

Table 3.6b   Static and Dynamic Demands of Sports

High static demands

Archery	Equestrian	Mountain climbing	Surfing
Auto racing	Fencing	Polo	Ultimate frisbee
Ballet	Field events	Rodeo	Water polo
Bobsledding	Fishing	Rope climbing	Waterskiing
Boccie	Football	Rugby	Weightlifting
Boxing	Football—flag	Running—sprint	Wrestling
Canoeing	Gymnastics	Skating—roller	
Cheerleading	Hockey—floor	Skating—speed	
Crew/Rowing	Hockey—ice	Skiing—downhill	
Cycling	Horseshoes	Skiing—jumping	
Dance	Karate/Judo	Skiing—x-country	
Diving	Motorcycling	Sailing	

Low static demands

Aerobic dance	Curling	Paddleball	Softball
Badminton	Darts	Race walking	Squash
Baseball	Field hockey	Racquetball	Swimming
Basketball	Golf	Riflery	Table tennis
Billiards	Handball	Rope jumping	Tetherball
Bowling	Handball—team	Running—distance	Tennis
Bridge	Hiking	Scuba diving	Volleyball
Camping	Jai alai	Shuffleboard	
Cricket	Lacrosse	Skating—figure	
Croquet	Orienteering	Soccer	

Neuromuscular Skill Demands

Neuromuscular skill is required for all sports. Championship caliber performance in any sport requires a high level of motor proficiency. Based on the classification by Nicholas (94), sports are categorized here by the demands required to attain skills adequate for a successful recreational experience (Table 3.7). Children with poor neuromuscular motor skills can be directed toward activities commensurate with their abilities.

Motion Ratings

Specific sports may place demands on either the upper or lower extremity. In some sports a throwing motion is dominant, while in others running, jumping, and kicking predominate. A classification of sports by dominant motion (95) makes it possible to recommend activities which

will cause the least stress on an existing pathological abnormality in an arm or leg (Table 3.8, a and b).

CONCLUSION

There are many issues to consider when assisting a child with a chronic disease to select sport and exercise activities. One must obviously assess the current status of the disease process, but it is also essential to understand the demands of the activities themselves. Recognizing the nature of the child's motivations and the factors affecting them will help in the selection of a specific sport. Assessing baseline physical activity and fitness defines the need for activity recommendations and preparatory training. Understanding the potential benefits of exercise aids in the selection of sports which can potentially be of therapeutic benefit. An awareness that adverse

Table 3.7   Neuromuscular Skill Demands

High

Auto racing	Diving	Jai alai	Skating—speed
Ballet	Fencing	Polo	Skiing—jumping
Baseball	Football	Rodeo	Surfing
Basketball	Gymnastics	Rugby	
Boxing	Hockey—ice	Skating—figure	

Moderate

Badminton	Football—flag	Paddleball	Squash
Bobsledding	Golf	Racquetball	Tennis
Cheerleading	Handball	Rope jumping	Ultimate frisbee
Crew/Rowing	Handball—team	Running—sprint	Volleyball
Cricket	Hockey—floor	Skating—roller	Water polo
Dance	Karate/Judo	Skiing—downhill	Waterskiing
Equestrian	Lacrosse	Skiing—x-country	
Field events	Motorcycling	Soccer	
Field hockey	Mountain climbing	Softball	

Low

Aerobic dance	Canoeing	Horseshoes	Scuba diving
Archery	Croquet	Orienteering	Shuffleboard
Billiards	Curling	Race walking	Swimming
Boccie	Cycling	Riflery	Table tennis
Bowling	Darts	Rope climbing	Tetherball
Bridge	Fishing	Running—distance	Weightlifting
Camping	Hiking	Sailing	

Table 3.8a   Motion Ratings of Sports—Upper Body

High

Archery	Equestrian	Jai alai	Scuba diving
Auto racing	Fencing	Karate/Judo	Skiing—downhill
Badminton	Field events	Lacrosse	Skiing—x-country
Baseball	Field hockey	Motorcycling	Softball
Basketball	Fishing	Mountain climbing	Squash
Bobsledding	Football	Paddleball	Swimming
Bowling	Football—flag	Polo	Table tennis
Boxing	Hockey—floor	Racquetball	Tennis
Canoeing	Hockey—ice	Riflery	Tetherball
Cheerleading	Golf	Rodeo	Volleyball
Crew/Rowing	Gymmastics	Rope clmibing	Water polo
Cricket	Handball	Rope jumping	Weightlifting
Diving	Handball—team	Rugby	Wrestling

(continued)

Table 3.8a *(continued)*

Moderate

Ballet	Cycling	Skating—figure	Waterskiing
Billiards	Horseshoes	Soccer	
Boccie	Orienteering	Surfing	
Curling	Sailing	Ultimate frisbee	

Low

Aerobic dance	Dance	Running—sprint	Skating—speed
Bridge	Darts	Running—distance	Skiing—jumping
Camping	Hiking	Shuffleboard	
Croquet	Race walking	Skating—roller	

Table 3.8b   Motion Ratings of Sports—Lower Body

High

Aerobic dance	Handball—team	Running—distance	Surfing
Ballet	Hockey—floor	Running—sprint	Tennis
Basketball	Hockey—ice	Rugby	Ultimate frisbee
Cheerleading	Jai alai	Skating—figure	Volleyball
Cycling	Lacrosse	Skating—roller	Weightlifting
Dance	Mountain climbing	Skating—speed	Wrestling
Field hockey	Paddleball	Skiing—downhill	
Football	Race walking	Skiing—jumping	
Football—flag	Racquetball	Skiing—x-country	
Gymnastics	Rope climbing	Soccer	
Handball	Rope jumping	Squash	

Moderate

Auto racing	Diving	Motorcycling	Swimming
Badminton	Equestrian	Orienteering	Table tennis
Baseball	Fencing	Polo	Tetherball
Boxing	Field events	Rodeo	Water polo
Crew/Rowing	Hiking	Scuba diving	
Cricket	Karate/Judo	Softball	

Low

Archery	Bridge	Darts	Sailing
Billiards	Camping	Fishing	Shuffleboard
Bobsledding	Canoeing	Golf	
Boccie	Croquet	Horseshoes	
Bowling	Curling	Riflery	

results can occur allows for preventive intervention and careful instruction in the self-limitation of activity.

Sports recommendations often require a preparticipation assessment of the physiological response to exercise and the physical fitness of the child. This may include an evaluation of aerobic endurance, muscle strength, flexibility, and body composition. When indicated, specific preparatory training programs can be provided that improve underlying deficiencies and optimize safety and the potential for a successful experience. Motor skills can also be evaluated and the child directed toward either individual instruction or a sport which requires less neuromuscular demand. The preparticipation assessment also provides an opportunity to discuss precautions for nutrition, fluid requirements, heat and cold stress and precautions, and also response to specific symptoms caused by exercise-induced problems.

Individual sport selection in these areas requires not only a consideration of the factors enumerated above but an awareness of the demands and risks of each sport. To assist the physician and child, sports have been classified by collision/contact potential, neuromuscular skill demands, dominance of upper- and lower-body motions, aerobic requirements, and static and dynamic motions. These classifications should assist in selecting sports which are safe and which provide an opportunity for a successful experience. Assisting a child with a chronic disease to select sport and exercise activities can be challenging, but the effort can have a major impact on the child's quality of life, health, and psychosocial development.

REFERENCES

1. Adams, J.A. Historical review and appraisal on research as the learning, retention and transfer of human motor skills. Psychol. Bull. 101:41-44; 1987.
2. Adams, J.A. The changing face of motor learning. Hum. Movement Sci. 9:209-220; 1990.
3. Alter, B.P.; Czapek, E.E.; Rowe, R.D. Sweating in congenital heart disease. Pediatrics 41:123-129; 1968.
4. American Academy of Pediatrics. Recommendations for participation in competitive sports. Pediatrics 81:737-739; 1982.
5. American College of Sports Medicine. Position statement on the prevention of heat injuries during distance running. Med. Sci. Sports 7:7-8; 1975.
6. Areskog, N.H.; Selinus, R.; Vahlquest, B. Physical work capacity and nutritional status in Ethiopian male children and young adults. Am. J. Clin. Nutr. 22:471-479; 1969.
7. Armstrong, L.E.; Hubbard, R.W.; Kraemer, W.J.; et al. Signs and symptoms of heat exhaustion during strenuous exercise. Ann. Sports Medicine 3:182-189; 1987.
8. Asmussen, E. Growth and muscle strength and power. In: Physical activity human growth and development. New York: Academic Press; 1973:60-79.
9. Asmussen, E. Similarities and dissimilarities between static and dynamic exercise. Cir. Res. 48:3-10; 1981.
10. Ballatein, E.; Borsetto, C.; Cellini, M.; Patracchini, M.; et al. Adaptation of the "Conconi Test" to children and adolescents. Int. J. Sports Med. 10:334-338; 1989.
11. Baraldi, E.; Zanconato, S.; Santus, P.A.; Zacchello, F. A comparison of two non-invasive methods in the determination of the anaerobic threshold in children. Int. J. Sports Med. 10:132-134; 1990.
12. Baranowski, T.; Bouchard, C.; Bar-Or, O.; Bricker, T.; et al. Assessment prevalence and cardiovascular benefits of physical activity and fitness in youth. Med. Sci. Sports Exerc. 24:S237-S247; 1992.
13. Bar-Or, O. Climate and the exercising child—a review. Int. J. Sports Medicine 1:53-65; 1980.
14. Bar-Or, O. Pediatric sports medicine for the practitioner. New York: Springer-Verlag; 1983.
15. Bar-Or, O. Pathophysiological factors which limit the exercise capacity of the sick child. Med. Sci. Sports Exerc. 18:276-282; 1986.
16. Bar-Or, O. Trainability of the prepubescent child. Phys. Sportsmed. 17:65-82; 1989.
17. Bar-Or, O.; Dotan, R.; Inbar, O.; et al. Voluntary hypohydration in 10- to 12-year-old boys. J. Appl. Physiol: Respir. Environ. Exercise Physiol. 48:104-108; 1980.

18. Belko, A. Vitamins and exercise—an update. Med. Sci. Sports Exerc. 19:S191-S196; 1987.

19. Berger, L.; Lithwick, D. I will sing life. Boston, MA: Little, Brown and Company; 1992.

20. Berkowitz, R.I.; Agras, W.S.; Korner, A.F.; Kraemer, H.C.; Zeanch, C.H. Physical activity and adiposity: a longitudinal study from birth to childhood. J. Pediatr. 106:734-739; 1985.

21. Birk, T.J.; Birk, C.A. Use of ratings of perceived exertion for exercise prescription. Sports Medicine 4:1-8; 1987.

22. Borg, G.N.A. An introduction to Borg's RPE-scale (1985). Ithaca, NY: Mouvement Publications.

23. Bradfield, R.B.; Paulos, J.; Grossman, L. Energy expenditure and heart rate of obese high school girls. Am. J. Clin. Nutr. 24:1482-1488; 1971.

24. Branta, C.; Haubenstricker, J.; Seefeldt, V. Age changes in motor skills during childhood and adolescence. Exerc. Sport Sci. Rev. 12:467-520; 1984.

25. Brooke, O.G. Response of malnourished babies to heat. Arch. Dis. Child 49:123-127; 1974.

26. Bruch, H. Obesity in childhood. IV. Energy expenditure of obese children. Am. J. Dis. Child 60:1082-1109; 1940.

27. Bullen, B.A.; Reed, R.B.; Mayer, J. Physical activity of obese and nonobese adolescent girls appraised by motion picture sampling. Am. J. Clin. Nutr. 4:211-223; 1964.

28. Butcher, J. Longitudinal analysis of adolescent girls participation in physical activity. Social Sport J. 2:130-143; 1985.

29. Cahill, B.R., ed. Proceedings of the conference on strength training and the prepubescent. Chicago: American Orthopaedic Society for Sports Medicine 10; 1988.

30. Canny, G.J.; Levison, H. Exercise reponse and rehabilitation in cystic fibrosis. Sports Medicine 4:143-152; 1987.

31. Carton, R.L.; Rhodes, E.C. A critical review of the literature on ratings scales of perceived exertion. Sports Medicine 2:198-222, 1985.

32. Casperson, C.J.; Powell, K.E.; Christiansen, G.M. Public Health Rep. 100:126-131; 1985.

33. Chavez, A.; Martinez, C.; Bourges, H. Nutrition and development of infants from poor rural areas. Nutritional level and physical activity. Nutr. Rep. Int. 5:134-144; 1972.

34. Conconi, F.; Ferrari, M.; Ziglio, P.; Droghetti, P.; et al. Determination of the anaerobic threshold by a noninvasive field test in runners. J. Appl. Physiol. 52:869-873; 1982.

35. Corbin, C.B.; Pletcher, P. Diet and physical activity patterns of obese and nonobese elementary school children. Q. Assoc. Health Phys. Educ. 39:922-928; 1968.

36. Davies, C.T.; Godfrey, S.; Light, M.; et al. Cardiopulmonary responses to exercise in obese girls and young women. J. Appl. Physiol. 38:373-376; 1975.

37. Davies, C.T.M. Physiological responses to exercise in East African children. The effects of schistosomias, anaemia and malnutrition. Environ. Child Health 19:115-119; 1973.

38. Davis, J.A. Anaerobic threshold: review of the concept and directions for future research. Med. Sci. Sports Exerc. 17:6-21; 1985.

39. DeLorme, T.L. Restoration of muscle power by heavy resistance exercises. J. Bone Joint Surg. 27:645-652; 1945.

40. Dietz, W.H.; Gortmaker, S.L. Do we fatten our children at the television set? Obesity and television viewing in our children and adolescents. Pediatrics 75:807-812; 1985.

41. Doubt, T.J. Physiology of exercise in the cold. Sports Medicine 11:367-381; 1991.

42. Edwards, M.A. The effects of training at predetermined heart rate for sedentary college women. Med. Sci. Sports. 6:14-19; 1974.

43. Ekblom, B. Effect of physical training in adolescent boys. J. Appl. Physiol. 27:350-355; 1969.

44. Farley, F. The big T in personality. Psychology Today 20:44-52; 1986.

45. Ferguson, K.V.; Yesalis, C.E.; Pomrehn, R.R.; Kirkpatrick, M.B. Attitudes, knowledge and beliefs as predictors of exercise intent and behavior in school children. J. Sch. Health 59:112-115; 1989.

46. Freedson, P.S. Electronic motion sensors and heart rate as measures of physical activity in chidren. J. Sch. Health 61:220-223; 1991.

47. Gaesser, G.A.; Rich, R.G. Effects of high and low intensity exercise training on aerobic capacity and blood lipids. Med. Sci. Sports Exerc. 16:269-274; 1984.
48. Gentile, A.M. A working model of skill acquisition with application to teaching. Quest 17:3-23; 1972.
49. Gibbons, E. The significance of the anaerobic threshold in exercise prescription. J. Sports Med. 27:357-361; 1987.
50. Gil, D.L.; Gross, J.B.; Huddleston, J. Participation motivation in youth sports. Intern. J. Sports Psychol. 14:1-14; 1983.
51. Godin, G.; Shephard, R. Psychosocial factors in influencing intentions to exercise of young students from grades 7 to 9. Res. Q. Exerc. Sport 57:41-52; 1986.
52. Goldberg, B.; Fripp, A.E.; Lister, G.; Loke, J.; et al. Effect of physical training on exercise performance of children following surgical repair of congenital heart disease. Pediatrics 68:691-699; 1981.
53. Gortmaker, S.; Sappenfield, W. Chronic childhood disorders. Prevalence and impact. Ped. Clin. North America 31:3-18; 1984.
54. Gottlieb, N.; Chen, M. Sociocultural correlates of childhood sporting activities: their implications for heart health. Soc. Sci. Med. 21:533-539; 1985.
55. Greenockle, K.M.; Lee, A.A.; Lomax, R. The relationship between selected student characteristics and activity patterns in a required high school education class. Res. Q. Exerc. Sport 52:301-310; 1990.
56. Groves, D. Why do some athletes choose high risk sports? Phys. Sportsmed. 15:186-194; 1987.
57. Hammond, H.K.; Froelicker, V.F. Exercise testing for cardiorespiratory fitness. Sports Med. 1:234-239; 1984.
58. Hammond, H.K.; Kelly, T.L.; Froelicker, V.F. Radionuclide imaging correlation of heart rate impairment during maximal exercise testing. J. Amer. Col. Cardiol. 2:826-833; 1983.
59. Haskell, W.L.; Montoye, H.J.; Orenstein, D. Physical activity and exercise to achieve health-related physical fitness components. Public Health Rep. 100:202-212; 1985.
60. Haymes, E.M. Nutritional concerns: need for iron. Med. Sci. Sports Exerc. 19:S197-S200; 1987.
61. Horvath, S.M. Exercise in a cold environment. Exerc. Sport Sci. Rev. 9:221-263; 1981.
62. Inbar, O.; Bar-Or, O.; Dotan, R.; Gutin, B. Conditioning versus exercise in heat as methods for acclimatizing 8 to 10 year old boys to dry heat. J. Appl. Physiol. Respir. Environ. Exercise Physiol. 50:406-411; 1981.
63. Jackson, A.S.; Coleman, A.E. Validation of distance run test for elementary school aged children. Res. Q. 47:86-94; 1976.
64. Johnson, M.L.; Burke, B.S.; Mayer, J. The relative importance of inactivity and overeating in the energy balance of obese high school girls. Am. J. Clin. Nutr. 4:37-44; 1956.
65. Kanaley, J.A.; Boileau, R.A. The onset of the anaerobic threshold at three stages of physical maturity. J. Sports Med. Phys. Fit. 28:367-374; 1988.
66. Kitagowa, K.; Miyashita, M. Muscle strength in relation to fat storage rate in young men. Eur. J. Appl. Physiol. 38:189-196; 1978.
67. Klesges, R.L.; Eck, L.H.; Hanson, C.L.; Haddock, C.K.; Klesges, L.M. Effects of obesity, social interactions and physical environment on physical activity in preschoolers. Health Psychol. 9:435-449; 1990.
68. Klesges, R.C.; Malott, J.M.; Boschee, P.F.; Weber, J.M. The effects of parental influences on children's food intake, physical activity, and relative weight. Int. J. Eating Disord. 5:335-346; 1986.
69. Kobayashi, K.; Kitanura, K.; Miura, M.; Sodeyama, H.; et al. Aerobic power as related to body growth and training in Japanese boys: a longitudinal study. J. Appl. Physiol. 4:666-672; 1978.
70. Krahenbuhl, G.S.; Skinner, J.S.; Kohrt, W.M. Developmental aspects of maximal aerobic power in children. Exerc. Sports Sci. Rev. 13:503-538; 1985.
71. Lamb, K.L.; Brodie, D.A. The assessment of physical activity by leisure-time physical activity questionnaires. Sports Medicine 10:159-180; 1990.
72. Lambert, J.; Ferguson, R.J.; Gervais, A.; Gilbert, G. Exercise capacity, residual abnormalities and activity habits following total correction for tetralogy of Fallot. Cardiology 66:120-131; 1980.
73. Lemon, P.W. Protein and exercise. Med. Sci. Sports Exerc. 19:S179-S190; 1987.

74. Locke, E.A.; Latham, G.P. The application of goal setting to sports. Sports Psychology Today 7:205-222; 1983.

75. Lohman, T.G. Applicability of body composition techniques and constants for children and youth. In: Pandolf, K.B., ed. Exercise and sport science reviews. New York: MacMillan; 1987; 14:325-357.

76. Ludvigsson, J. Physical exercise in relation to degree of metabolic control in juvenile diabetics. Acta Paedietr. Scand. (Suppl.) 283:45-49; 1980.

77. Lysens, R.; Auweele, Y.U.; Ostyn, M. The relationship between psychosocial factors and sports injuries. J. Sports Med. 26:77-84; 1986.

78. Martens, R. The uniqueness of the young athlete: psychologic considerations. Amer. J. Sports Med. 8:382-385; 1980.

79. Maughan, R.J.; Noakes, T.D. Fluid replacement and exercise stress. Sports Medicine 12:16-31; 1991.

80. McConnell, C.M.; Rostan, S.; Puyau, F.A. Heat dissipation in children with congenital heart disease. South. Med. J. 63:837-841; 1970.

81. McKelvie, R.S.; McCartney, N. Weightlifting training in cardiac patients. Sports Medicine 10:355-364; 1990.

82. McKenzie, T.L. Observational measures of children's physical activity. J. Sch. Health 61:224-227; 1991.

83. McKenzie, T.L.; Sallis, J.F.; Nader, P.R.; et al. BEACHES: an observational system for assessing children's eating and physical activity and associated events. J. Appl. Behav. Anal. 24:141-151; 1991.

84. Meckleburg, S.; Loriaux, L.; Thompson, R.H.; et al. Hypothalamic dysfunction in patients with anorexia nervosa. Medicine 53:147-159; 1974.

85. Micheli, L.J. Overuse injuries in children's sports: the growth factor. Orthop. Clin. North Am. 14:2-16; 1983.

86. Millard-Stafford, M. Fluid replacement during exercise in the heat. Review and recommendations. Sports Medicine 13:223-233; 1992.

87. Minard, D.; O'Brien, R.L. Heat casualties in the Navy and Marine Corps, 1959-1962 with appendices on the field use of the wet-bulb-globe temperature index (Res. Rep. MR005, 01-0001-01). US Naval Med. Res. Inst. Rep. 7:1-15; 1964.

88. Mirwald, R.L.; Bailey, D.A.; Cameron, N.; Rasmussen, R.L. Longitudinal comparison of aerobic power in active and inactive boys aged 7.0 to 17.0 years. Ann. Human Biology 8:405-414; 1981.

89. Mitchell, J.H.; Maron, B.J.; Epstein, S.E. Sixteenth Bethesda Conference: cardiovascular abnormalities in the athlete: recommendations regarding eligibility for competition. J.A.C.C. 6:29-30; 1985.

90. Murphy, R.J. Heat illness in the athlete. Amer. J. Sports Medicine 12:258-261; 1984.

91. National Center for Health Statistics. Vital and health statistics: national health interview survey. Series 10: nos. 61, 63, 96, 115, 130, 141; 1981.

92. Newacheck, P.; Budetti, P.; Halfon, N. Trends in activity limiting chronic conditions among children. Amer. J. Public Health 76:178-184; 1986.

93. Newacheck, P.; Budetti, P.; McManus, P. Trends in childhood disability. Amer. J. Public Health 74:232-236; 1984.

94. Nicholas, J. Risk factors, sports medicine and the orthopedic system: an overview. J. Sports Med. 3:243-259; 1976.

95. Nicholas, J.A.; Grossman, R.B.; Hershman, E.B. The importance of a simplified classification of motion in sports in relation to performance. Orthop. Clin. N. Amer. 8:499-532; 1987.

96. O'Connell, J.K.; Price, J.H.; Roberts, S.M.; Jurs, S.G.; McKinley, R. Utilizing the health belief model to predict dieting and exercising behavior of obese and nonobese adolescents. Health Educ. Q. 12:343-351; 1985.

97. Ogilvie, B.C. The stimulus addicts. Phys. Sportsmed. 1:61-65; 1973.

98. Orlick, T.D. The athletic drop out: a high price for inefficiency. AHPER J. 41:21-27; 1974.

99. Parizhova, J. Physical training in weight reduction of obese adolescents. Am. J. Clin. Res. 34:63-68; 1982.

100. Pate, R. A new definition of youth fitness. Physician Sportsmed 11:77-84; 1983.

101. Pate, R.; Dowda, M.; Ross, J. Associations between physical activity and physical fitness in American children. Am. J. Dis. Child 144:1123-1129; 1990.

102. Pate, R.P.; Kriska, A. Physiological basis of sex difference in cardiorespiratory endurance. Sports Medicine 1:87-98; 1984.

103. Pfeiffer, R.; Francis, R.S. Effects of strength training on muscle development in prepubescent, pubescent and postpubescent males. Phys. Sportsmed. 14:134-143; 1986.

104. Pollock, M. The quantification of endurance training programs. Exerc. Sports Science Rev. 1:155-188; 1973.

105. Porcari, J.P.; Ebbeling, C.B.; Ward, A.; Freedson, P.S.; et al. Walking for exercise testing and training. Sports Medicine 8:189-200; 1992.

106. Rarick, G.L.; Dobbins, D.A. Basic components in the motor performance of children six to nine years of age. Med. Sci. Sports 7:105-110; 1975.

107. Remlow, J.; Kreska, A. Physical activity in the population: the epidemiologic spectrum. Res. Quart. Exerc. Sport 58:111-113; 1987.

108. Reybrouck, T.; Weymans, M.; Ghesquiere, J.; Van Gerven, D.; et al. Ventilatory threshold during treadmill exercise in kindergarten children. Eur. J. Appl. Physiol. 50:79-85; 1982.

109. Reybrouck, J.; Weymans, M.; Stijns, H.; Knops, H.; et al. Ventilatory anaerobic threshold in healthy children. Eur. J. Appl. Physiol. 54:278-284; 1985.

110. Rians, C.B.; Weltman, A.; Cahill, B.R.; et al. Strength training for prepubescent males: is it safe. Am. J. Sport Med. 15:483-487; 1987.

111. Riopel, D.A.; Boerth, R.C.; Coates, T.J.; Hennekens, C.H.; et al. Coronary risk factor modification in children: exercise. Circulation 74:1189A-1191A; 1986.

112. Ross, J.C.; Dotson, C.O.; Gilbert, G.G.; Katz, S.J. After physical education: physical activity outside of school physical education programs. J. Phys. Educ. Recreat. Dance 56:35-39; 1985.

113. Ross, J.; Gilbert; G. The national children and youth fitness study. A summary of findings. J. Phys. Educ. Recreat. Dance 56:45-50; 1985.

114. Rowland, T.W. Aerobic response to endurance training in prepubescent children: a critical analysis. Med. Sci. Sports Exerc. 17:493-498; 1985.

115. Rowland, T.W. Motivational factors in exercise training programs for children. Phys. Sportsmed. 14:122-128; 1986.

116. Sady, S. Cardiorespiratory exercise training in children. Clin. Sports Med. 5:493-514; 1986.

117. Safrit, M.J. The validity and reliability of fitness tests for children: a review. Pediatr. Exerc. Sci. 2:9-28; 1990.

118. Sailors, M.; Berg, K. Comparison of responses to weight training in pubescent boys and men. J. Sports Med. Phys. Fitness 27:30-37; 1987.

119. Sallis, J.F. Self report measures of children's physical activity. J. Sch. Health 61:215-219; 1991.

120. Sallis, J.F.; Patterson, T.L.; Buono, M.J.; Atkins, C.J.; Nader, P.R. Aggregation of physical activity habits in Mexican-American and Angelo families. J. Behav. Med. 11:31-41; 1988.

121. Sallis, J.F.; Patterson, T.L.; McKenzie, T.L.; Nader, P.R. Family variables and physical activity in preschool children. J. Dev. Behav. Pediatri. 9:57-61; 1988.

122. Sallis, J.; Simons-Morton, B.; Stone, H.; et al. Determinants of physical activity and interventions in youth. Med. Sci. Sports Exerc. 24:S248-S257; 1992.

123. Saltin, B. Physiological effects of physical conditioning. Med. Sci. Sport 1:50-56; 1969.

124. Scanlan, T.K.; Lewthwaite, R. Social, psychological aspects of competition for male youth sport participants: predictors of enjoyment. J. Sports Psychol. 8:25-35; 1986.

125. Scanlan, T.K.; Passer, M.W. Factors related to competitive stress among male youth sport participants. Med. Sci. Sports 10:103-108; 1978.

126. Scanlan, T.K.: Passer, M.W. Self serving biases in competitive sport settings: an attributional dilemma. J. Sport Psychol. 2: 124-136; 1980.

127. Scheurer, J.; Tipton, C.M. Cardiovascular adaptations to physical training. Annu. Rev. Physiol. 39:221-243; 1977.

128. Seals, D.R.; Hagberg, J.M.; Hurley, B.F.; Ehsani, A.A. Endurance training in old men and women. Cardiovascular response to exercise. J. Appl. Physiol. 57:1024-1029; 1984.

129. Seefeldt, V.; Haubenstricker, J. Patterns, phases or stages: an analytical model for

the study of developmental movement. In: Kelso, J.A.; Clark, J.E., eds. The development of movement control and coordination. New York: John Wiley and Sons; 1982: 309-318.

130. Seltzer, C.C.; Mayer, J. An effective weight control program in a public school system. Am. J. Public Health 60:679-689; 1970.

131. Simon, J.A.; Martens, R. Children's anxiety in sport and nonsport evaluative activities. J. Sport Psychol. 1:160-169; 1979.

132. Sewell, L.; Micheli, L.J. Strength training for children. J. of Pediatr. Orthop. 6:2-8; 1986.

133. Shephard, R.J. Physical activity and child health. Sports Medicine 1:205-233; 1984.

134. Shephard, R.J. Adaptation to exercise in the cold. Sports Medicine 2:59-71; 1985.

135. Shephard, R.S. Effectiveness for training programs for prepubescent children. Sports Medicine 13:194-213; 1992.

136. Simons-Morton, B.G.; Parcel, G.S.; O'Hara, S.N.; et al. Health related physical fitness in childhood: status and recommendations. Ann. Rev. Public Health 9:403-425; 1988.

137. Smith, R.E.; Zane, N.W.; Small, F.L.; Coppel, D.B. Behavioral assessment in youth sports: coaching behaviors and children's attitudes. Med. Sci. Sports Exer. 15:208-214; 1983.

138. Sunnegardh, J.; Bratteby, L.; Sjolin, S. Physical activity and sports involvement in 8 and 13 year old children in Sweden. Acta. Paediatr. Scand. 74:904-912; 1985.

139. Tappe, M.K.; Duda, J.L.; Ehrnwald, P.M. Perceived barriers to exercise among adolescents. J. Sch. Health 59:153-155; 1989.

140. Taras, H.F.; Sallis, J.F.; Patterson, T.L.; Nader, P.R.; Nelson, J.A. Television's influence on children's diet and physical activity. Dev. Behav. Pediatr. 10:176-180; 1989.

141. Taylor, W.; Baranowski, T. Relationship of physical activity to cardiovascular fitness among preadolescent children in three ethnic groups. Res. Q. Exer. Sport 62:157-163; 1991.

142. Thorland, W.G.; Gilliam, T.B. Comparison of serum lipids between habitually high and low active pre-adolescents. Med. Sci. Sports Exer. 13:316-321; 1981.

143. Trembley, A.; Despres, J.P.; Bouchard, C. The effects of exercise training on energy balance and adipose tissue morphology and metabolism. Sports Med. 2:223-233; 1985.

144. Vaccaro, P.; Mahon, A. Cardiorespiratory response to endurance training in children. Sports Medicine 4:352-363; 1987.

145. Valimaki, I.; Hursti, M.L.; Pihlakoski, L.; Vhkari, J. Exercise performance and serum lipids in relation to physical activity in school children. Int. J. Sports Med. 1:132-136; 1980.

146. van der Beck, E.J. Vitamins and endurance training. Food for running or faddish claims. Sports Medicine 2:175-197; 1985.

147. Verma, S.; Hyde, J.S. Physical education programs and exercise-induced asthma. Clin. Pediatr. 15:697-699; 1976.

148. Vrijens, J. Muscle strength development in the pre- and postpubescent age. Med. Sports (Basel) 11:152-158; 1987.

149. Wagner, P.D. Central and peripheral aspects of oxygen transport and adaptations with exercise. Sports Medicine 11:133-142; 1991.

150. Wasserman, K. The anaerobic threshold measurement to evaluate exercise performance. Am. Rev. Respir. Dis. 129:335-340; 1984.

151. Wasserman, K.; Whipp, B.; Royal, S.; Beaver, W. Anaerobic threshold and respiratory gas exchange during exercise. J. Appl. Phys. 35:236-243; 1973.

152. Waxman, M.; Stunhard, A.J. Caloric intake and expenditure of obese boys. J. Pediatr. 96:187-193; 1980.

153. Weltman, A.; Janney, C.; Rians, C.B.; et al. The effects of hydraulic resistance strength training in pre-pubertal males. Med. Sci. Sports Exerc. 18:629-638; 1986.

154. Weltman, A.; Katch, V.; Sady, S.; Freedson, P. Onset of metabolic acidosis (anaerobic threshold) as a criterion measure of submaximal fitness. Res. Quart. 49:218-227; 1978.

155. Wenkel, L.M.; Kreisel, P.J. Factors underlying enjoyment of youth sports: sport and age group comparisons. Sports Psychol. 7:51-64; 1985.

156. Zaricznyj, B.; Shattuck, L.J.; Mast, T.A.; et al. Sports related injuries in school aged children. Am. J. Sport Med. 8:318-325; 1980.

CHAPTER 4

Legal Issues Regarding Children With Chronic Health Conditions

Leonard Rieser
Education Law Center, Philadelphia, PA

Sarah D. Cohn
Yale-New Haven Hospital

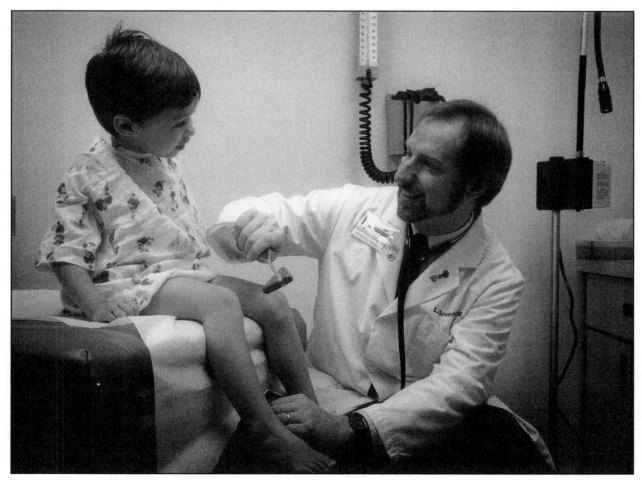

Part A
Legal Rights
of Children With
Chronic Health Conditions

Leonard Rieser

Twenty years ago, the subject of the legal rights of children with chronic health conditions in the area of exercise and sport would hardly have merited a footnote: no such rights existed. Instead, schools, athletic associations, and other organizations were free to include or exclude these children in physical education and sport programs as they saw fit. Often, of course, the decision was to exclude; and even when this decision was based on general assumptions and fears rather than on any specific analysis of the child's condition, there was little or nothing that could be done in response.

In the mid-1970s this legal landscape began to change. First, Section 504 of the Rehabilitation Act of 1973, a federal law often referred to simply as "Section 504," established a prohibition against discrimination on the basis of handicap in federally assisted programs (1). Section 504 began as a single sentence inserted, almost unnoticed, into a set of rules on vocational rehabilitation programs for adults. But through regulation, court decisions, and persistent advocacy, Section 504 was transformed into a broad set of protections for people with disabilities, including children with chronic health conditions.

Section 504 was followed by the Education of All Handicapped Children Act, enacted in 1975 as Public Law 94-142 (2). This statute—recently renamed the "Individuals With Disabilities Education Act," or "IDEA"—created a right to public special education services for children with mental or physical disabilities who need specialized instruction. More recently, in 1990, Congress passed the Americans With Disabilities Act (the "ADA"), a broad bill of rights for people with disabilities—including, under some circumstances, children in private schools (3). Besides these and other federal enactments, moreover, the period from the mid-1970s to the present saw considerable growth in state disability rights laws.

These laws have brought about a drastic change—in some ways, a nearly complete reversal—in the legal status of children with chronic health conditions. At least in the public schools and to some extent in other programs as well, the law now favors inclusion in regular programs, with special modifications and supports as necessary, whenever feasible. When inclusion is not feasible, specialized services and programs tailored to the child's needs must be provided. Decisions on these issues, moreover, must now be made on an individual basis, and the decision-making process, once left entirely in the hands of school officials, is now open to input from medical professionals, parents, and others involved with the child. Finally, when a disagreement arises, procedures, both informal and formal, are available to help resolve the dispute.

This chapter discusses these rights in more detail. Of course, this discussion is only an overview, and a subjective one at that. Some points have not yet been clarified by the courts, and even where the law is clear subtle differences among cases can lead to different results. Thus, sorting out the legal rights of a child in a particular situation will often require specialized expertise. A later section of the chapter notes some sources of legal help.

ELIGIBILITY FOR LEGAL PROTECTION

We begin with the question of which children are protected by the laws discussed in the preceding section. With some exceptions, Section 504, the IDEA, and the ADA do not speak of individuals with "chronic health conditions"; instead, the statutes use the term "disability." Thus, in order to determine whether a child is covered by one of these statutes, one must ask whether his or her condition—taking into account not only the medical diagnosis but also the child's specific combination of needs and abilities—constitutes a disability as that statute defines the term.

The views expressed in this chapter are those of the authors only.

Under Section 504 and the ADA, a person with a disability is defined as one who has a physical or mental impairment that "substantially limits one or more major life activities" (4). "Physical or mental impairment" is broadly defined to include many of the conditions that affect the children discussed in this book (5). Moreover, the phrase "substantially limits one or more major life activities," while obviously intended to exclude conditions that are of only minimal or incidental significance for the individual involved, is also relatively broad in scope (6). In addition, the ADA and Section 504 cover individuals who "have a record of" or are "regarded as having" a disability, whether or not the disability is current or even real. It follows that many children with chronic health conditions will qualify for protection under these statutes.

The eligibility definition under the IDEA is somewhat different. The child must, first, have one or more of several specified disabilities; the list comprises physical as well as mental impairments, and specifically includes

> limited strength, vitality, or alertness, due to chronic or acute health problems such as a heart condition, tuberculosis, rheumatic fever, nephritis, asthma, sickle cell anemia, hemophilia, epilepsy, lead poisoning, leukemia, or diabetes, which adversely affects a child's educational performance.

As the final clause suggests, however, the mere existence of a disability is not enough to bring the child within the scope of the IDEA; rather, the child must also, as a result of the disability, need special education (7). This additional requirement poses no particular problem for many of the children with whom this book is concerned, since their condition does, in fact, result in a need for some special education services (8). On the other hand, the proviso does mean that some children with chronic health conditions are protected by Section 504 and the ADA, but not by the IDEA.

How does a family establish their child's eligibility for rights and services under these statutes? An appropriate first step is a written request, supported by medical and any other relevant documentation, that the child be recognized as having a "disability" (and, if coverage under the IDEA is sought, as requiring special

education). The request should be directed at the agency—for example, a school district—from which protections or services are sought. The IDEA sets out a detailed set of steps that the agency must then take to determine eligibility, including consideration of the child's needs by a multidisciplinary team; Section 504 and the ADA do not set out such elaborate procedures. In any event, however, a response should be forthcoming, and there are legal procedures (discussed later) for challenging either the failure to respond or a response that is adverse.

We turn now to the question of the rights that a child has once he or she has been determined to be eligible for protection under Section 504, the ADA, and/or the IDEA (9).

RIGHTS IN PUBLIC SCHOOLS

Generally, children with chronic health conditions who attend public school have the right to take part in the school's regular physical education and sports program, even if special help or some degree of program modification is required. Moreover, in those instances in which the child cannot participate meaningfully in the regular program even with assistance, the school is still required to provide a specialized program tailored to the child's needs.

The Right to Participate in Regular Physical Education, Sports, and Athletics Programs

Under Section 504, recipients of federal assistance (10) may not deny to a qualified handicapped person the opportunity to participate in any of their services, provide an opportunity unequal to that provided to other persons, or provide services that are less effective than that provided to others. This requirement extends to physical education and athletics. Thus, under Section 504 a child with a chronic health condition has the right to an opportunity to participate in sport and exercise that is fully equal to the opportunity provided to his or her peers (11).

Moreover, the child must generally be permitted to participate in the same programs and services (including not only physical education courses but also "interscholastic, club, or intramural athletics") that are available to his or her peers. This is because the regulations require that, in operating such programs, the school "may not discriminate on the basis of handicap." Indeed, the school is prohibited from providing different or separate services to a student with a disability "unless such action is necessary to provide [the individual] with aid, benefits, or services that are as effective as those provided to others." The school is also required to "ensure that handicapped persons participate with nonhandicapped persons in such activities and services to the maximum extent appropriate to the needs of the handicapped person in question."

These sorts of judgments cannot be made by just any school employee. Rather, decisions concerning placement—presumably including decisions about placement in regular athletics—must be made on the basis of adequate data and by persons "knowledgeable about the child, the meaning of the evaluation data, and the placement options." Therefore, under Section 504, a child with a chronic health condition is entitled to be fully included, with his or her peers, in all school exercise and sports activities, unless an informed review of medical and other data indicates that inclusion would be inappropriate or would fail to provide the child with equal opportunity (12).

For students covered by the IDEA, regulations under that Act reinforce these guarantees. Besides reiterating the "equal opportunity" requirements of Section 504, the IDEA regulations require that each eligible child "be afforded the opportunity to participate in the regular physical education program available to nonhandicapped children unless the child is enrolled full time in a separate facility or . . . needs specially designed physical education." The regulations also require maximum integration of disabled with nondisabled children "to the maximum extent appropriate," and set forth a strong presumption against removal of a child from the regular educational environment. Similar requirements exist for nonacademic and extracurricular programs, including athletics, recreational activities, and the like: a child with disabilities has the right to "participate with non-handicapped children in those services to the maximum extent appropriate to the needs of the [disabled] child." Finally, the IDEA goes beyond Section 504 in requiring that not only qualified experts, but also the child's parents, have the opportunity to participate in decisions concerning the child's participation in regular programs (13).

There are relatively few reported cases applying these provisions in the area of sport and exercise. Those that do exist, however, confirm at least that if the medical evidence shows that participation in the regular program would present no major risk to the student's safety, the student cannot be excluded. For example, in one case decided by the Office for Civil Rights of the United States Department of Education, an eighth-grade student with epilepsy was dropped from the team and made "team manager," apparently out of concern over his safety. The Office for Civil Rights found that the decision, which had been made by the coach and ratified by the school board, had not been arrived at by persons knowledgeable about the student's disability; that, in fact, the student had not suffered any injury during two previous years of playing basketball; and that the available medical evidence indicated that his condition was unlikely to lead to problems on the court. For these reasons, the exclusion was illegal (14).

Similarly, a federal court required a Pennsylvania school district to permit a student with one kidney to play football. Again, the key evidence was medical: a specialist in sports medicine testified that, in view of the protective equipment used by the student, the risk of catastrophic injury to the kidney was minute. (The judge also noted that the student was nearly 18; that he and his parents understood the risks he might be taking; and that football is a dangerous game in any event, with serious perils even for people who have both kidneys!) (15)

In short, then, Section 504 and the IDEA establish that if a child can participate in regular sports without excessive medical risk, he or she has the right to do so. The question of what is excessive is a judgment to be made in each case, based on the circumstances and the views of people with knowledge of the child and his or her medical condition.

A more subtle question arises when the risk involved in including the child in the regular program is excessive but could be reduced to manageable levels through the provision of special assistance or equipment. In this case, the issue concerns whether the school is obligated to make such arrangements. The Section 504 regulations call for the provision of

> regular or special education *and related aids and services* that . . . are designed to meet individual educational needs of handicapped persons as adequately as the needs of nonhandicapped persons are met. (16)

Accordingly, under that Act, the school generally does have the duty to make such modifications and to provide such supports as the child may need in order to participate in the regular program. Thus, for example, a child with motor problems resulting from Niemann-Pick Syndrome was entitled not only to participate in the school swimming program (since the medical evidence was that she could safely do so), but also to the special help that she needed, such as assistance with undressing and getting from the locker room to the pool (17). The IDEA contains similar mandates.

Occasionally, a school system will take the position that the child can be included in the regular program (with or without special supports) only if the family first waives any possible claim of liability against the school. However, if the child is otherwise entitled to participate in the program, the imposition of such "extra" conditions is probably illegal (18).

Taken collectively, these rules obviously add up to a strong legal preference in favor of inclusion. Nevertheless, the school's duty to modify the regular program and to provide extra supports to a child whose condition requires them is not unlimited. The courts have generally held that an individual does not have the right to participate in a program if the modifications and supports that he or she would require are so extreme as to change the fundamental nature of that program. Thus, for example, it might be argued that a school need not permit a non-ambulatory child to play certain key positions on the baseball team, because to do so would require too fundamental a modification of the game. Of course, even if this argument prevailed the child would not lose the right to participate in school sports altogether; rather, as the following section explains, the child would be entitled to a special program appropriate to his or her needs.

Rights to Special Programs and Services

Not all children can manage in regular programs, even with special help. For those who cannot, Section 504 and the IDEA guarantee certain specialized services.

First, as we have noted, regulations under Section 504 entitle children with disabilities to "regular *or* special education and related aids and services that . . . are designed to meet individual educational needs of handicapped persons as adequately as the needs of nonhandicapped persons are met" (19). Since specialized physical education is one form of special education, it must be provided—together with necessary related aids and services—for children who cannot participate in the regular physical education program. Moreover, the specialized program must be "appropriate" to the child's individual needs; that is, it must be based upon a professional, individualized assessment and must be calculated to meet the child's individual needs in the area of physical education as adequately as the needs of nondisabled children are met in that area (20).

The IDEA offers similar but more elaborate protections. Each child covered by this act is entitled to specialized physical education if participation in the regular program would be inappropriate. Moreover, the specialized (or "adapted") instruction to which the child is entitled may address physical and motor fitness, fundamental motor skills, or skills in aquatics, dance, or individual or group games and sports, including "intramural and lifetime sports" (21). Again, moreover, the specific program selected must be "appropriate" to the child's individual needs. Under the IDEA, moreover, this term carries a slightly more extensive meaning than under Section 504. To be appropriate, the program must (among other things) be developed on the basis of a professionally adequate evaluation, including a medical evaluation—at no cost to the family—where necessary; must be reflected in a written "individualized education plan" (IEP), drawn up at a conference in which the family as well as school and evaluation personnel are invited to participate; and must be designed to enable the child to make a reasonable degree of progress (22).

In addition, the IDEA requires the provision of any "related services" that may be needed in order to help a child to benefit from a specialized physical education program. Unlike Section 504, moreover, the IDEA contains a detailed definition of what may constitute related services: they may include (among other things)

- physical and occupational therapy,
- recreation programs,
- assistive devices, and
- school health services (23).

In summary, then, both Section 504 and the IDEA provide that the child who requires specialized physical education services receive them, together with additional services if these are needed in order to benefit from the special program.

RIGHTS IN PRIVATE SCHOOLS

As a general rule, students in private and parochial schools are not protected by Section 504 (24). The IDEA, on the other hand, appears to require states and school districts, at least, to provide special education and related services to private school students requiring them (25); what is less clear is whether all such students are entitled to services, and whether the services provided must be as extensive as those offered to public school students. In general, it appears that a student with a chronic health condition who attends private school but wants some special education services—adaptive physical education, for example—has a right under the IDEA to get them from the public school system.

A broader, but as yet not fully unexplored, set of guarantees is found in the ADA, which applies to private (although not parochial) schools. Specifically, the ADA prohibits "public accommodations," which are defined so as to include most private schools, from discriminating against students with disabilities in the provision of services. "Discrimination" is defined as including, among other things, the use of unnecessary eligibility criteria and the failure to make "reasonable modifications in policies, practices, or procedures" (26). These provisions appear to mean, for example, that even in a private school, a child with a disability must be allowed to participate in regular sports and athletic programs, even if some modifications are required—assuming that those modifications are "reasonable," i.e., that they do not

"fundamentally alter" the program (27). Obviously, there is some line drawing to be done here, but the general idea should be clear. Finally, in some states, state law affords additional rights to private school students.

RIGHTS IN NONSCHOOL PROGRAMS

Finally, we consider the rights of children in nonscholastic organizations such as youth leagues, athletic associations, and the like. If the organization receives federal assistance, even indirectly (28), Section 504 applies and the child probably has the right to participate in the organization's programs, with special modifications and supports as needed, so long as the medical risks are not excessive and the modifications not so extensive as to change the fundamental nature of the organization's program. In addition, the facilities operated by the organization may qualify as a "public accommodation" under the ADA; that category includes "a gymnasium, health spa, bowling alley, golf course, or other place of exercise or recreation" (29). In such event, the child has the right to participate in the program with such reasonable modifications as he or she may require. Finally, state law may provide the child with additional rights.

THE RIGHT TO CONTEST DECISIONS OF SCHOOLS AND OTHER ORGANIZATIONS

All of the federal statutes discussed here, and most state laws as well, provide mechanisms by which a family can obtain resolution of disputes over their child's rights. As we have noted, this is a major change from the situation that existed before the mid-1970s, when decisions of schools and other organizations were, for all practical purposes, unreviewable.

Since there are often several dispute resolution routes available, it is wise to seek advice concerning the most appropriate complaint procedure in any given situation. The endnote lists the available mechanisms, many of which are relatively informal and do not require a court appearance or even a lawyer (30). The important point is that if there is any reason to think that a school or other organization has acted illegally in excluding a child from programs or refusing to adapt its programs to the child's needs, it may well be useful to investigate the possibility of some sort of challenge.

ROLE OF
THE MEDICAL PROFESSIONAL

As this discussion suggests, the medical professional can play a major role in the process of deciding how, and if necessary with what modifications and supports, a child with a chronic health condition should participate in athletic activity. Indeed, a clear report from the physician who best knows the child, describing the child's needs and abilities and spelling out recommendations, will often prove persuasive to those responsible for the child's program. In the smaller number of cases in which a disagreement arises, the professional(s) working with the child can help by contacting school and other officials directly to clarify misunderstandings, address doubts and concerns, and if necessary suggest alternative approaches. Indeed, experience shows that nearly all disagreements can be resolved in this informal fashion—especially if the medical professionals involved find the time to make themselves available for discussion with those on "the other side," and are generally familiar with what the relevant laws require. Finally, in that small minority of cases in which the dispute cannot be resolved and the family resorts to a legal proceeding, a medical professional who knows the child well will very often carry the day in a hearing or in court.

OTHER SOURCES
OF ASSISTANCE

Legal advice and advocacy in this field can, of course, be obtained from many private attorneys and disability law projects. Local and state bar associations can often provide referrals. In addition, for low-income families, civil legal aid offices as well as volunteer and pro bono lawyer programs (which can also be located through bar associations) can be of assistance. Finally, federal law has established a network of state "protection and advocacy" agencies for persons

with developmental disabilities. These offices can sometimes provide direct assistance, and can almost always offer referrals to other agencies. The National Association of Protection and Advocacy Systems, 900 Second Street NE, Suite 211, Washington, DC 20002, telephone (202) 408-9514, can direct families to the protection and advocacy organization for their state.

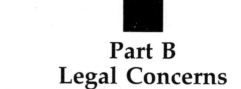

Part B
Legal Concerns
for Health Care Providers
Sarah D. Cohn

Physically and emotionally handicapped children and their parents often desire that the child participate in public or private school recreational activities, community activities such as the Special Olympics, and specialized summer camps. There are some legal concerns associated with persons of differing abilities participating in these activities; while these concerns exist for all participants, there are special concerns for some children with disabilities.

The preceding section discussed the right of the child to participate in at least public school activities; these rights are exercised as against school administrators who may disagree. This section will discuss certain of the legal concerns for physicians and other health care providers.

SCHOOL AND CAMP
PHYSICAL EXAMINATIONS

It is now quite routine for schools to require that students be examined by a health care provider, at least prior to participation in athletics. State law may prescribe some of the content of the examination and its frequency; there may also be a standardized form to use. Some states require that summer camps be licensed, and often, as a condition of licensure, the camp must require that participants undergo a precamp physical examination that is documented and maintained in camp records.

It is important that so-called "physical" examinations of a minor meet professional standards and be well documented. A thorough history should be taken and the child should be examined with the physical and emotional requirements of the proposed activity in mind (31). The professional judgment of the physician should be based on history and physical examination findings that are as objective as possible. The physician then may be guided by professional recommendations made by such groups as the American Academy of Pediatrics, whose Committee on Sports Medicine has published information on such topics as the risks of long-distance running in children (32) and recommendations for participation in competitive sports (33). For example, despite the case law mentioned in the preceding section, the Academy recommends that persons with only one kidney refrain from participation in contact/collision sports such as football.

The physician may determine, based on all of the information available, that there should be no restriction placed on participation, that certain restrictions are prudent, or that the child should be disqualified from participation in some or all of the possible activities. The recommendation and the reasons for them should be documented in the patient's record and in the forms or letters that transmit them.

Regardless of physician recommendations, the child has certain legal rights, some of which were discussed previously. Complicated case law on the legal right of a handicapped child to participate is difficult to summarize, but it would seem to suggest that where protective equipment is available or where reasonably effective safety precautions can be taken, a child will not be prohibited from taking part in an athletic activity. In order to effectively transmit concerns about the child's safety, the physician must document findings, any proposed restrictions, the risks of participation in the activity even with protective equipment, and any discussions the physician has had with parents and with school or camp officials. While the final decision about participation is based at least in part on a physician's recommendation, it is not the physician who makes the final decision about participation.

SPECIALIZED CAMP PROGRAMS

There are now specialized camps for children with cancer, with severe burns, with hematologic disorders, with emotional problems, and with other physical and mental impairments. In addition, there are also general summer camps that accept campers with some disabilities.

Health care providers may volunteer time or be employed by these camps to provide ongoing and emergency health care to the campers (and the staff). The camp is responsible for assuring that these providers are competent, and the providers themselves should have malpractice insurance. Each must be eligible to practice in the relevant state. In some states, licensure will be required; in others, a camp provider may find a special exemption in state law. For example, in Connecticut, a physician licensed in another state but possessing the qualifications for Connecticut licensure may practice without a license as a camp physician for up to 9 weeks (34).

The medical information that accompanies the camper to camp should include the child's medical history and current condition, any medical restrictions and needs, and complete information about medications that may need to be administered.

For any camper, but for these special children in particular, camp personnel should be familiar with

the concept of "the dignity of risk," which maintains that children must be safeguarded but not overly protected. A zero risk of injury is not achievable and this should be understood by all participants. (35)

However, it is also clear that a camp, like a school, will be liable for injuries that occur when camp personnel fail to exercise judgment in determining camp activities.

Agreement to participate forms can be as useful in the camp context as they can in the school. They should be adapted for the special needs of the campers and are discussed later.

HEALTH CARE PROVIDER LIABILITY FOR INJURY

Physicians are clearly vulnerable to suit if a physical examination is improperly conducted, a problem is overlooked, and a child is injured in an activity in which he or she should not have been participating. However, physicians also worry that they may be sued

- if they recommend disqualification from certain activities that are important either to the parent or the child, or
- if they permit participation even in the face of possible injury, and that injury occurs.

There is considerable case law to suggest that the physician will not be liable if the history and physical examination are well conducted and documented, even if the physician recommends limitation or disqualification from certain activities. For example, in *Sitomer v. Half Hollow Hills Central School District* (36), a junior high school student was evaluated for participation in the high school tennis team. New York State law stated that junior high school students could participate on a senior high school team "provided the pupils are placed at levels of competition appropriate to their physiological maturity . . . in accordance with standards established by the commissioner." The physician evaluated the young man according to these standards and found that the student had not reached an appropriate level of physiological maturity to try out for the senior high school team. The student sued for emotional distress and for his lack of ability to further his development as a tennis player. The court found that it would not

substitute its judgment for the judgment of professional educators as to the type of screening devices to be used in determining whether a student should be allowed to participate in an interscholastic athletic program at a level above the grade in which he or she is enrolled.

Further, it found that the physician had an obligation only to administer the screening tests in a proper manner. The court granted summary judgment and dismissed the complaint against both the school district and the physician.

In this case, the physician evaluated the young man based on state screening standards. Where these are not available, the reasons for recommending disqualification from an activity should be made clear in the medical record and in any correspondence on the subject.

Today, total disqualification from all or most activities is unusual. Instead, a health care provider may be asked to judge relative safety and make recommendations. Prior to making a recommendation the physician should inquire of the school, not just of the student or the family, what protective equipment or techniques are available. After recommendations are made it is the responsibility of the school or camp to accept them and see to their implementation. If a school or camp knows of certain limitations and fails adequately to supervise the child, there will be liability for injuries (37).

There is some, but not great, legal risk for a physician who evaluates a child with a disability, determines that participation in certain activities carries increased risk, and nevertheless recommends (or permits) participation with or without protective equipment. This risk can be minimized by the use of certain types of documents designed both to inform and to reduce liability. The first of these is a parental permission form, noting the activity in which the child will participate. If the form contains nothing else, however, it will not serve to limit liability.

A second document is an "agreement to participate." A properly drafted agreement to participate includes

- a description of the activity in which the child will participate;
- a list of potential consequences or injuries that may be incurred during participation;
- a list of expectations for the participants, such as the use of certain protective equipment and an explicit statement that the child will follow the rules and obey the supervisory adults; and
- information about the condition of the participant (may be incorporated by reference to physical forms) (38).

These forms should be signed by the child's parent or guardian. Legally these forms function as a type of "informed consent" for the parent or guardian, and can be used in a legal action to show knowledge on the part of the parent and an "assumption of risk" based on that knowledge.

Although widely used, exculpatory clauses are generally not effective when signed by a parent for a minor. For example, a Florida court considered the following clause signed by a parent:

It is further agreed that reasonable precautions will be taken by the Camp to assure the safety and good health of said boy/girl but that Camp is not to be held liable in the event of injury, illness or death of said boy/girl, and the undersigned, does fully release Camp, and all persons concerned therewith, for any such liability.

The child in question had a psychiatric problem and required the administration of medication on a camping trip. It was alleged that camp personnel did not administer the medication. The court held that the release of liability was contingent on the agreement by the camp to use reasonable care.

Other courts have found exculpatory clauses unenforceable as against public policy. Courts view these clauses with disfavor because they lower the standard of care to gross negligence or willful or wanton misconduct. These clauses may, however, be found valid if they are signed by and for an adult.

CONCLUSION

Physicians, physician's assistants, and nurse practitioners who evaluate children for participation in school and camp activities should be well trained and comfortable making recommendations about participation in the usual activities of childhood. However, each should require that the school or camp provide necessary information so that a focused evaluation can be made, if that is what is required. Detailed information about the child's health condition and any recommended limitations should be transmitted to the parents, and, with their permission, to schools and camps. A copy of this material should be retained for the physician's file; a thorough evaluation and careful documentation are the best protection against any legal risk.

NOTES

1. 29 USC § 794. Regulations of the United States Department of Education implementing Section 504 are found at 34 CFR Part 104. These and the other citations provided here are not comprehensive, but should enable the reader to locate some of the legal provisions on which this chapter is based.

2. 20 USC § 1400 *et seq.* Implementing regulations of the United States Department of Education are at 34 CFR Parts 300 *et seq.*

3. Most of the provisions of the ADA are found at 42 USC § 12101 *et seq.*

4. 29 USC § 706(8)(B); 42 USC 12102(2).

5. For example, regulations under the ADA define "physical or mental impairment" as (i) Any physiological disorder or condition, cosmetic disfigurement, or anatomical loss affecting one or more of the following body systems: neurological; musculoskeletal; special sense organs; respiratory, including speech organs; cardiovascular; reproductive; digestive; genitourinary; hemic and lymphatic; skin; and endocrine; (ii) Any mental or psychological disorder such as mental retardation, organic brain syndrome, emotional or mental illness, and specific learning disabilities; (iii) The phrase physical or mental impairment includes, but is not limited to, such contagious and noncontagious diseases and conditions as orthopedic, visual, speech, and hearing impairments, cerebral palsy, epilepsy, muscular dystrophy, multiple sclerosis, cancer, heart disease, diabetes, mental retardation, emotional illness, specific learning disabilities, HIV disease (whether symptomatic or asymptomatic), tuberculosis, drug addiction, and alcoholism . . . 28 CFR § 36.104.

6. The same regulations define "major life activities" as "functions such as caring for one's self, performing manual tasks, walking, seeing, hearing, speaking, breathing, learning, and working."

7. 20 USC § 1401(a)(1); 34 CFR § 300.5(a), (b)(7)(ii).

8. The IDEA defines "special education" as "specifically designed instruction," without limitation as to type or amount; thus, a child need not require an extensive special program in order to be covered. Moreover, the term "special education" includes special physical education; thus, even a child whose only special need is in that area (defined as including the development of physical fitness, fundamental motor skills, aquatics, dance, and individual and group games and

sports) is covered by the IDEA. 34 CFR § 300.14.

9. As we noted earlier, state laws also provide rights and protections for children with chronic health conditions. Because these laws have widely varying eligibility requirements and substantive provisions, we do not discuss them here; however, they are a crucial part of the legal picture, and practitioners in this field certainly need to be familiar with them.

10. Virtually all public school systems receive federal assistance.

11. 34 CFR § 104.4(b), 204.37(a), (b)(1).

12. 34 CFR § 104.4(b)(iv), 104.34(b), 104.35(c), 104.37(c).

13. 34 CFR § 300.306, 300.307, 300.550, 300.553.

14. Alpena (AR) Public School District (OCR 1984), reprinted at Education of the Handicapped Law Reporter 257:565.

15. *Grube v. Bethlehem Area School District*, 550 F. Supp. 418 (ED PA 1982).

16. 34 CFR § 104.33(b) (emphasis added).

17. Quaker Valley (PA) School District (OCR 1986), reprinted at Education of the Handicapped Law Reporter 352:235.

18. See, e.g., Berlin Brothersvalley (PA) School District, Case No. 03881102 (OCR 1988).

19. Emphasis added.

20. For an example of a decision holding that specialized physical education may be required, see Spokane (WA) School District No. 81 (OCR 1981), reprinted at Education of the Handicapped Law Reporter 257:219. The definition of "appropriate" education is found at 34 CFR § 104.33(b)(1).

21. 34 CFR § 300.307; 300.14(b)(2).

22. See, e.g., *Board of Education of Hendrick Hudson School District v. Rowley*, 458 US 176 (1982).

23. 20 USC § 1401(a)(17), (25)–(26); 34 CFR § 300.308.

24. Exceptions to this general rule include cases in which the private school receives federal assistance, and cases in which a student needing special education is placed in the private school by a public school district at its expense. In these instances, Section 504 will ordinarily apply.

25. 20 USC § 1413(4)(A).

26. 42 USC § 12182.

27. 42 USC § 12182(b)(2)(A)(ii).

28. Indirect assistance is provided, for example, when an organization receives support through a contract with another organization that receives federal assistance.

29. 42 USC § 12181(7)(L).

30. For violations of Section 504, a family can
   • Present an informal complaint to the school or other organization involved.
   • File a formal complaint with the Office for Civil Rights of whatever federal agency provides assistance to the school or other organization involved (often the U.S. Department of Education).
   • Obtain a formal hearing before an impartial official, in matters involving the provision of special education services.
   • File a lawsuit in federal or state court.

   For violations of the IDEA, a family can
   • Present an informal complaint to the school system involved. Frequently, an informal "mediation" program is available.
   • Present a complaint to the state department of education.
   • Obtain a formal hearing before an impartial official and, in some states, an appeal.
   • If the formal hearing and/or appeal results in an adverse decision, take the matter to federal or state court.

   For violations of the ADA, a family can
   • File a complaint with the Attorney General of the United States.
   • File a suit in federal or state court.

   For violations of state law, the family can usually file a complaint with the appropriate board or commission and/or a case in state court.

31. See Committee on School Health, School Health Assessments, American Academy of Pediatrics, *Pediatrics* 88:649 (1991) for a discussion of the recommended content of school health assessments.

32. Committee on Sports Medicine, American Academy of Pediatrics, Risks in Distance Running for Children, *Pediatrics* 86:799 (1990).

33. Committee on Sports Medicine, American Academy of Pediatrics, Recommendations for Participation in Competitive Sports, *Pediatrics* 81:737 (1988).

34. Ct. General Statutes, Section 20-12(d) (1993).

35. Committee on School Health, American Academy of Pediatrics, Medical Guidelines for Day Camps and Residential Camps, *Pediatrics* 87:117 (1991).

36. *Sitomer v. Half Hollow Hills Central School District et al.*, 520 N.Y.S.2d 37 (A.D. 2 Dept. 1087).

37. See *Rodriguez v. Board of Education of the City of New York*, 480 N.Y.S.2d 901 (A.D. 2 Dept. 1984).

38. Van der Smissen, Betty, *Legal Liability and Risk Management for Public and Private Entities* Cincinnati: Anderson Publishing Co., 1990, pp 46–50.

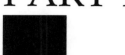

PART II

Sports, Exercise, and Specific Chronic Health Conditions

CHAPTER 5

Spina Bifida

Charles C. Duncan and Eileen M. Ogle
Yale University School of Medicine

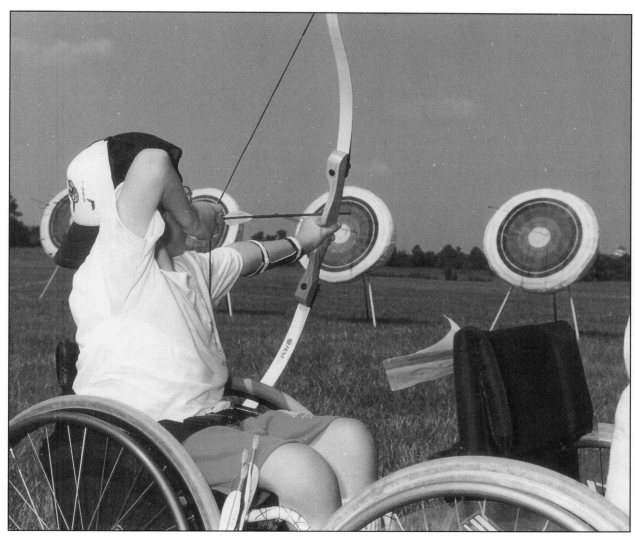

Spina bifida (also known as spina bifida aperta and meningomyelocele) is one of the most complex congenital anomalies compatible with reasonable life expectancy and function. It is a chronic disease that affects the entire central nervous system, with potential for compromise of renal, cardiovascular, and musculoskeletal systems.

Advances in medical technology have afforded this population with an increase in survival. Prior to the advent of antibiotics and cerebrospinal fluid (CSF) shunting devices in the 1950s, the mortality rate was 77% by age 12. It is now estimated to be 15% by the same age (4). As a result, we are now seeing school-age children and young adults with greater medical involvement and disability.

These children vary in clinical presentation but may exhibit cognitive disorders, hydrocephalus, hindbrain dysfunction secondary to an Arnold-Chiari Type II malformation, cerebral dysfunction, musculoskeletal involvement, sensory impairment, and incontinence (Figure 5.1). Not all children will have all of these conditions, so each must be considered separately when evaluating a child for a sport and exercise program. Except for the child with normal motor and cognitive function, most programs will require modification and adaptive measures.

The medical complexity of this illness presents many new challenges to these children and their families, health professionals, school systems, and social administrations. While ongoing physical and occupational therapies are an integral part of these children's lives, the decision to allow for participation in more organized and aggressive sport and exercise programs tends to prompt anxiety from all parties involved. It is hoped that the following discussion of spina bifida and its manifestations will help to alleviate these concerns by imparting an understanding of potential problems and their warning signs.

DESCRIPTION OF THE CONDITION

Spina bifida is a congenital disorder of neural tube development in which there is failure of proper neural tube closure. It occurs in 2-3:1000 live births (3). With spina bifida aperta, or meningomyelocele, the vertebral elements are incompletely formed at the defect site and neural elements are directly visible. The etiology of this defect is unknown, although it is felt to be multifactorial.

The clinical manifestations range from a child with no abnormalities, to a child who is severely mentally retarded and quadriparetic. Children with spina bifida will have one or more of the manifestations in Figure 5.1, each of which will be discussed separately.

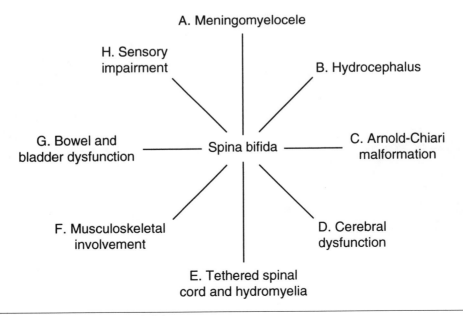

Figure 5.1 The manifestations of spina bifida.

Meningomyelocele

As mentioned above, the meningomyelocele is the spinal defect itself. Not only are the neural elements exposed at birth, but there is an absence of the spinous processes and laminae, an increased interpedicular distance of the vertebral elements, and a reduction in the anterior-posterior size of the vertebral bodies at the site. A kyphotic deformity may also be present. The meningomyelocele is surgically closed within 24 hours after birth.

The surgical closure involves reconstituting a watertight seal around the exposed spinal cord and covering that with several layers of muscle and fascia prior to skin closure. This provides protection to the spinal cord at that site. Very large and kyphotic defects require more complex closures and present a greater risk of injury from trauma. Children with simple closures tend to be well protected from the average falls and skirmishes of sport and play.

Hydrocephalus

Hydrocephalus (excessive fluid within the ventricular system of the brain with increased pressure) occurs in 90% of children with spina bifida, and requires surgical placement of a CSF shunt (4). The shunt diverts CSF from the ventricular system of the brain to an area where the fluid can be reabsorbed. Most frequently the peritoneal cavity is chosen and a ventriculoperitoneal shunt is placed. The diversion of CSF results in a decrease in pressure within the brain, causing the ventricles to decrease in size.

The shunt system is placed under the skin, so it is generally well protected from trauma. The risk of damaging the shunt system in the course of any activity is related to the risk of sustaining a laceration of the scalp or any other location overlying the shunt system. A laceration over the shunt system requires immediate attention by a neurosurgeon.

Shunts may malfunction at any time. A malfunction occurs when the shunt system becomes occluded (usually by infection or mechanical obstruction), and CSF no longer drains properly. As a result, fluid builds up within the ventricular system and the intracranial pressure rises. Children will complain of headaches, double or blurred vision, and photophobia; they may also vomit and be very irritable or somnolent. If this occurs the neurosurgeon should be contacted immediately. Children who have a gradual malfunction, however, may not complain of headaches or visual symptoms, or indeed of any other symptoms. The only signs may be a gradual decline in school performance or memory. If concerns arise that a child's development is slowing down or becoming arrested, medical evaluation is warranted.

Most children with hydrocephalus will have normal IQ scores. However, a significant number will exhibit learning disabilities, processing impairments, perceptual difficulties, and behavioral problems. Even some children with spina bifida but without hydrocephalus exhibit these problems. These cognitive and behavioral parameters must be assessed when selecting activities for these children.

Children with CSF shunts for hydrocephalus are not restricted by the presence of the shunt. Our recommendations for helmet wear are the same as for children without shunts. Helmets should be worn for

- bicycle riding,
- batting in baseball,
- skiing,
- sledding,
- football,*
- hockey,*
- horseback riding, and
- roller blading.
  *Tackle football and competitive ice hockey are contraindicated for children with spina bifida because of the risk of spinal injury.

Arnold-Chiari Malformation

The Arnold-Chiari malformation is a hindbrain malformation in which there is a small posterior fossa, small cerebellum, and downward displacement of the brain stem and cerebellar tonsils through the foramen magnum into the cervical spine. Although imaging studies (MRI and CT scans) indicate that most children with spina bifida have this malformation, not all will be symptomatic.

This malformation with associated hindbrain dysfunction is the major cause of death in infants with meningomyelocele (4). Symptomatic infants clinically present with apnea, cyanosis, vocal cord paralysis, and gastric reflux. Infants who survive this period may have spontaneous remission of these symptoms or remain stable with significant lower cranial nerve deficits and abnormal medullary function. These children are often the most medically involved. Children are now being identified with significantly abnormal sleep patterns involving prolonged periods of hypoventilation, without the normal compensatory response of hyperventilation or hypernea. The long-term effect of this on cardiac function and exercise tolerance is unknown.

Older children and adolescents may exhibit symptoms at any time. Neck pain; changes in motor or sensory function of the face, arms, or legs; the development of swallowing or phonation problems; and respiratory compromise all warrant immediate investigation. Surgical intervention consists of a posterior fossa and upper cervical decompression. Results of this surgery appear promising; however, no published data exist at this time. The results of surgical decompression in infants remains controversial.

The presence of an Arnold-Chiari malformation does contraindicate activities that pose a risk to the cervical spine. These would include football and diving.

Cerebellar Dysfunction

Some children with spina bifida exhibit cerebellar findings of dysmetria, poor fine motor control, tremors, and nystagmus. Cerebellar gait disturbance is difficult to assess since most children have lower extremity motor deficits and utilize a variety of adaptive braces and walkers to maintain stability.

These conditions do not dictate any contraindications, although children may experience difficulties with aim and execution of specific activities such as archery or darts.

Hydromyelia Tethered Spinal Cord

Spinal cord function must be closely monitored in these children. Most children will have either a spastic or flaccid paralysis below the level of their original meningomyelocele, and some children will have upper extremity involvement from hydrocephalus or Arnold-Chiari malformation. However, if changes in muscle tone or strength are noted on physical examination or manual muscle testing, or if scoliosis becomes

rapidly progressive, or if there is a change in bowel or bladder function, the spinal cord should be evaluated for either hydromyelia or tethered spinal cord.

Hydromyelia is a condition in which a fluid cavity develops in the central canal of the spinal cord. It can occur at any time and at any level of the spinal cord. Because of this, children can present with sensory and motor changes in the upper extremity, trunk, and lower extremities, along with scoliosis and bowel and bladder changes. Surgical shunting of the fluid may be required.

Tethering of the spinal cord is a condition in which the terminal portion of the spinal cord is fixed to the surrounding tissues of the spinal canal in a low-lying position (below L1-L2). With growth and movement, traction is placed upon the cord. It is hypothesized that this eventually diminishes oxygen supply to the cord and that neurological changes ensue (5). Children present with rapidly progressive scoliosis, increased lordosis, progressive lower extremity orthopedic deformity, and bowel and bladder changes, as well as with pain at the meningomyelocele closure site. This occurs especially with exercise. Surgery to release the tethered spinal cord is required.

Both of these conditions need to be evaluated and treated as soon as suspected. Their presence requires a termination of sport and exercise until after surgery. Most children will resume activities by 2-4 weeks after surgery; however, it is best to reevaluate the child before determining an appropriate level of sport and activity. The child should be back to normal activities within 2-3 months.

Musculoskeletal Involvement

Children with spina bifida require ongoing follow-up for orthopedic deformity and correction. Motor weakness in the lower extremities is dependent upon the level of the original lesion. Children with lower lumbar lesions may have weakness in the ankles and feet, and some involvement of the knees and hips. Children with higher-level lesions will usually require a wheelchair. Maintenance of proper anatomical alignment for proper bracing is critical to maintaining mobility. Heel cord lengthenings and muscle transfer procedures are frequently necessary.

Hip subluxations and dislocations occur secondary to an imbalance between flexor and extensor muscle groups. Hip dislocations can be painless and, therefore, require regular monitoring by an orthopedic surgeon.

Orthopedic deformity and subsequent intervention are frequently the decisive factors in a child's participation in sport. However, exercise is critical to the maintenance of functional joint alignment with gentle, regular stretching of tight tendons and muscle groups.

Scoliosis is present in most children with meningomyelocele. In children with rapidly progressive scoliosis (where tethered cord and hydromyelia have been ruled out or treated), spinal fusion with placement of either a Harrington rod or Lugue apparatus is performed. This protects sitting posture and prevents the cardiorespiratory compromise associated with untreated scoliosis.

Some children with spina bifida have evidence of upper extremity spasticity. These children may require muscle transfers and tendonotomies. Again, gentle stretching exercises greatly help in the prevention of deformity, along with the use of bracing to maintain functional alignment.

Osteoporosis is frequently seen in children with flaccid paralysis of the lower extremities. Children with this condition are vulnerable to fractures. Fractures will often be painless, and should be suspected when there is erythema, deformity of a limb, and fever. Most children with osteoporosis and secondary fractures are wheelchair users. However, they also can occur in ambulating children with lumbar-level deficits.

All children with spina bifida should seek orthopedic clearance before entering any exercise or sport program.

Bowel and Bladder Dysfunction

The lower sacral roots that supply innervation to the bowel and bladder are almost always involved in children with spina bifida. Aggressive bowel regimens involving diet and scheduled evacuation have successfully helped school-age children to achieve "social continence."

Bladder dysfunction places these children at risk of renal disease because of infection and vesico-ureteral reflux. Incomplete voiding results in frequent urinary tract infections. Renal morbidity has decreased in this population because the use of the Crede Maneuver to empty the bladder has been discouraged (as it promotes greater reflux); other positive developments include the utilization of suppressive antibiotic therapy and the introduction of clean intermittent catheterization programs. Catheterizations done several times daily results in more complete bladder emptying and reduces bacterial growth.

Clean intermittent catheterizations also afford "social continence" in these children. Children who have weak sphincter tone and who tend to "dribble" constantly can achieve continence by taking anticholinergic medication while on a catheterization program. However, children taking such medication may have difficulty producing adequate perspiration in hot weather, and run the risk of heat stroke with too much exertion. Thus, caution is advised.

Adequate fluid intake is to be encouraged, especially with sports involving high levels of exertion. Children with renal impairment should be evaluated and managed as discussed in chapter 18.

Sensory Impairment

All children with meningomyelocele have some degree of sensory loss distal to the level of the lesion. The sacrum and perineum, as well as portions of the lower extremities, will lack sensitivity to temperature and pain. Children and caregivers are instructed to examine these areas for evidence of abrasion, breakdown, or erythema. These can occur very quickly in response to repeated trauma from footwear or poorly fitting orthotic devices. Children in wheelchairs are especially vulnerable to sacral decubiti.

EXERCISE AND SPINA BIFIDA

Children with spina bifida have not been specifically studied with respect to exercise tolerance or to long-term and short-term effects of exercise, and there are few existing data to support specific recommendations for exercise. However, it is becoming increasingly obvious in clinical practice that those children involved in exercise and sports programs have

- higher self-esteem,
- fewer difficulties with obesity, and
- greater social involvement.

There are also growing numbers of handicapped sports programs, and as access to these increase involvement should be encouraged.

Krebs et al. (2) studied a small group of children with spina bifida between the ages of 9 and 12 years. The purpose was to evaluate the effect of active exercise on respiratory and cardiac parameters, as well as on perceptual and cognitive capabilities. Following 6 minutes of active arm exercises there were significant increases in heart and respiratory rate, minute liter volume, and tidal volume. Increases in peripheral vision were also noted. Figure learning trials before and after exercise showed that the number of trials required to learn a given set of figures decreased after exercising.

Although the study was a small one, this improvement in learning ability and peripheral vision is very important in this population, which often experiences learning disabilities and perceptual impairments. The positive effects of this very mild exercise session are felt to result from increased cerebral blood flow secondary to the increased cardiac and respiratory parameters.

Most children with spina bifida will be involved in physical therapy programs from infancy through their school-age years. Most activities performed during these sessions are structured to achieve developmental milestones, to maintain alignment and flexibility of involved muscle groups and joints via stretching exercises, and to maximize the coordination and strength needed to perform activities of daily living. While physical therapy is an integral part of care, sessions are limited and do not constitute a full exercise program.

School-age children have access to physical education within their school systems as a mandatory part of their educational curriculum. Unfortunately, the degree of active participation is often limited by the lack of handicapped-accessible facilities and adaptive equipment, as well as by fear of injury to the child. Although budgetary constraints limit the rapidity with which facilities are made handicap accessible, these changes are being implemented. Likewise, the knowledge and utilization of adaptive equipment is a specialty not available in all school systems. Often the child must independently join a specialty sport group, such as a handicapped skiing or horseback riding group, in order to access the proper equipment.

Fear of injury to the child is a valid concern. For example, children with lumbar meningomyeloceles utilize braces and crutches to ambulate, and will be unstable and fall if involved in a collision with another child. Those children with low sacral meningomyeloceles may have excellent motor function, but may also have cognitive and behavioral impairments, such as impulsivity and inability to comprehend the safety rules of the game, that preclude safe participation in group activities. Children who have higher-level meningomyeloceles will utilize wheelchairs for mobility and are the most stable and at least risk from injury. Wheelchairs have also become lighter, faster, and more maneuverable, and have additional safety features that prevent tipping over during rapid, abrupt moves. The problem for these children is to achieve greater integration into sport activities with the able-bodied.

Children with spina bifida and other disabilities can benefit from being mainstreamed into regular school; however, they may also face difficulties when expected to participate in school physical education programs where most children are able-bodied. Having to avoid collision/contact sports is often perceived as a blow to self-esteem, and may leave such children feeling even more different from their able-bodied peers.

A further consideration is that the time spent in these physical education programs may actually be quite limited, not least because of medical absences. More often than not, the pursuit of physical fitness in this population is dependent upon the motivation of the child and the family to pursue sport programs geared specifically for the handicapped. Physical therapy and school physical education programs provide instruction in proper movement and game rules, but basic fitness needs may more easily be met by supplementary activities.

The Special Olympics programs, National Handicapped Sports, and other specialized activities are available and becoming more utilized by families. In some cases the child's involvement has led parents and siblings to take up the sport as well, thus bringing positive effects on the entire family's physical fitness. With this familial involvement there is a notable decrease in overall family stress, and an increase in independence. The initial fears of injury and failure are replaced with the confidence and inner strength that come from achievement.

EXERCISE AND SPORT PROGRAMS FOR CHILDREN WITH SPINA BIFIDA

Because spina bifida assumes so many forms, there are no global fitness plans. Each child requires individual assessment of motor function, cognitive ability, emotional readiness, and motivation. Indeed, this is also true of children without spina bifida. Each fitness program must be individualized to maximize strengths and minimize weaknesses.

Exercise and Conditioning Programs

Stretching and flexibility routines are a basic element in the exercise regimen. These programs are usually established by a physical therapist and are essential to the daily function and well-being of children with spina bifida. The muscles of the neck, upper extremity, and trunk are often stretched actively; however, lower extremities that are either spastic or flaccid may require passive stretching regimens performed either by the child or with the assistance of a partner. As with the able-bodied, stretching regimens should always precede aerobic or strength training.

Aerobic conditioning should follow stretching. Children who ambulate with braces and crutches utilize a great deal more energy in their mobility than those children with normal motor function or those in wheelchairs. However, the aerobic demand is not sustained over an adequate time period to be beneficial. Many of these children become fatigued and must take frequent rests when walking; thus, walking may not be the best form of training. This must be kept in mind when developing a program for aerobic fitness.

It may prove more beneficial to utilize upper-body activities for a sustained period, for example, by the use of a rowing machine or hand ergometer. Adequate aerobic challenge should be provided by 3 to 5 sessions per week, each lasting 10 to 30 minutes (depending upon the individual's tolerance). National Handicapped Sports has a series of disability-specific videotapes that describe such a program.

Stretching routines and aerobic conditioning exercises should be followed by strength training routines. These routines are critical to the child's later independence. Except for children with sacral-level lesions (and, hence, near-normal motor functioning), spina bifida patients need to develop upper-body strength for mobility and the execution of daily living activities. Free weights may be appropriate for a child with good coordination and upper extremity control; for children with cerebellar involvement, however, stationary resistance training is safer.

Stretching and flexibility routines, aerobic conditioning, and strengthening regimens all require monitoring by a physical therapist or trainer who is experienced in working with handicapped children. These trainers must be able to work with the child in establishing realistic goals—and also make the workouts fun. Pursuing involvement in a handicapped sport program can provide social contact with disabled peers and a chance to apply the coordination and skills learned in the basic program. Success in sport and the satisfaction of peer involvement will help sustain interest in the conditioning portion of the program. An ongoing conditioning program, in turn, is necessary if the child is to remain fit enough to engage safely in sport.

Sports and Spina Bifida

Sport programs for the disabled are growing in number. They include ski clubs, equestrian groups, bowling teams, riflery and archery clubs, wheelchair sports teams, track and field programs, aquatics, tennis clubs, and numerous other activities, many of which offer programs for children. An important feature of such programs is their use of sport-specific adaptive equipment which offers safer and more achievable results (1). Involvement in these programs can open up a whole new world for these children, offering not only local challenges but also national and even international competition. Ultimately, however, the goal of sport programs should be to provide an enjoyable experience for these children so that the habits of exercise become an integral part of their lives.

Children with low-level (sacral) lesions, who can ambulate normally or who wear an ankle-foot orthosis, usually have few limitations in their choice of sport. They can participate in most high collision/impact sports with no more risk of injury than that of an able-bodied child. The activity should be modified, however, if there is coordination, perceptual, or behavioral involvement.

Children with lumbar-level involvement have more limitations in their choices and abilities. These children typically have motor weakness in the feet, knees, and hips, and require the use of higher bracing and crutches. Selecting team sports for these children often involves matching them with other children of similar disabilities. Activities that stress upper-body movement and skill while minimizing rapid lower-extermity response provide a relatively safe choice. Here again, problems with coordination and perception must be taken into consideration, and modifications may need to be made.

Children who utilize wheelchairs for their mobility have many opportunities to participate in wheelchair sport programs. One aspect of these programs involves maneuvering obstacle courses, an activity that requires upper-body strength and control. Other activities include a wide range of track and field events and team sports. These programs foster sportsmanship and individual development, and provide a challenge that is fun for children. They also usually have coaches who have had specialized training and experience with handicapped children.

To list all of the activities that children with spina bifida may participate in would be overly time-consuming. For general considerations the reader may refer to chapter 3; however, there are also certain specific restrictions for this population. These are listed in Table 5.1; for example, while downhill and cross-country skiing are permissible, "jump-skiing" is a specific restriction. Common sense should be the rule when selecting from the many sport activities available.

An example of a specialized program is the annual "teen weekend" for adolescents with

Table 5.1   Contraindications for Children With Spina Bifida

Auto racing	Polo
Bobsledding	Rodeo
Boxing	Rope climbing
Cheerleading (pyramid formation)	Scuba diving
Football	Waterskiing
Jump skiing	

spina bifida in Connecticut. In this 2 1/2-day experience of shared disability, a metamorphosis is observed. The timid, quiet adolescent with poor self-image becomes a formidable defensive player during the basketball game. The young girl embarrassed by her gait and need to catheterize herself hurries to her room to race her roommate in completing the procedure. Comparisons with the able-bodied are pursued as well. During a wheelchair obstacle course the counselors take the chairs to try their skill. Inevitably they find that they have difficulty getting up ramps, and side markers fall left and right—to the delight of the campers who haven't recognized how skillful they really are. The positive effects of such revelations can last a lifetime.

CONCLUSION

We are fortunate to practice health care in a time when infants with disabilities are identified early and enrolled in infant stimulation programs. Physical and occupational therapy regimens are also started early and continue through the school-age years, maintaining flexibility and maximizing strengths. Even severely disabled children can now function better than their predecessors who grew up in the days when therapy did not begin until after the contractures were formed.

The challenge to health care professionals, parents, educators, and therapists is to provide an enjoyable experience for these children so that the habits of exercise stay a part of their adult years. This is most likely to occur if a child is able to attain success in sport, and that requires careful evaluation and matching of skills. A child can develop a highly negative view of these activities if he or she always seems to be last or nearly last, or is pushed to perform beyond physical limitations or preferences.

Children will physically dictate their exercise tolerance levels with fatigue and verbal statements if the activity proves too strenuous; emotional signs that the task is too difficult include despondence and withered determination. If this occurs, the trainer should regress with the child and begin again at an easier level.

Children with spina bifida represent a growing population who are challenging old asumptions about sport and exercise involvement. There are a growing number of agencies that develop, organize, and execute formal competitions for the disabled, and their success and continued expansion into all areas of exercise has been remarkable. Agencies such as Disabled Sports USA, the National Wheelchair Athletic Association, the Special Olympics Organization, and other more sport-specific organizations have been instrumental in increasing opportunities for the disabled to achieve a level of wellness unknown to them in the past.

These organizations and the creativity of dedicated participants, trainers, coaches, kinesiologists, and physical therapists have developed aerobic flexibility programs for specific handicaps (e.g., cerebral palsy, quadriplegia, visual impairment), as well as training programs for the trainers, coaches, and parents themselves. These programs, as well as the development of adaptive equipment, have increased the ease with which the disabled can become involved in sport and exercise, and provide a safer environment for this participation. Information on these programs can be obtained by contacting

Disabled Sports USA
451 Hungerford Drive, Suite 100
Rockville, MD 20850

Participation in sport and exercise programs does of course require a medical evaluation and approval. To make adequate recommendations the health professional must be familiar with the program in which the disabled person will be participating as well as the level of training the supervising coaches have in dealing with neurological problems.

REFERENCES

1. Adams, R.C.; Daniel, A.N.; McCubbin, J.A.; Rullman, L. Games, sports and exercise for the physically handicapped. 3rd ed. Philadelphia: Lea & Febiger; 1982.
2. Krebs, P.; Eickelberg, W.; Krobath, H.; Baruch, I. Effects of physical exercise on peripheral vision and learning in children with Spina Bifida manifestation. Percep. and Motor Skills 68:167-174; 1989.
3. Matson, D.D. Neurosurgery of infancy and childhood. 2nd ed. Springfield, Illinois: Charles C. Thomas; 1969.
4. McLone, D.G.; Naidich, T.P. Myelomeningocele: outcome and late complications. In: McLaurin, R.L.; Schut, L.; Venes, J.L.; Epstein, F., eds. Pediatric neurosurgery. 2nd ed. Philadelphia: W.B. Saunders; 1989:53-70.
5. Yamada, S.; et al. Pathophysiologic mechanisms in the tethered spinal cord syndrome. In: Holtzman, R.; Stein, B.M., eds. The tethered spinal cord. New York: Thieme-Stratton; 1985:29-40.

CHAPTER 6

Epilepsy

Donald R. Bennett
University of Nebraska College of Medicine

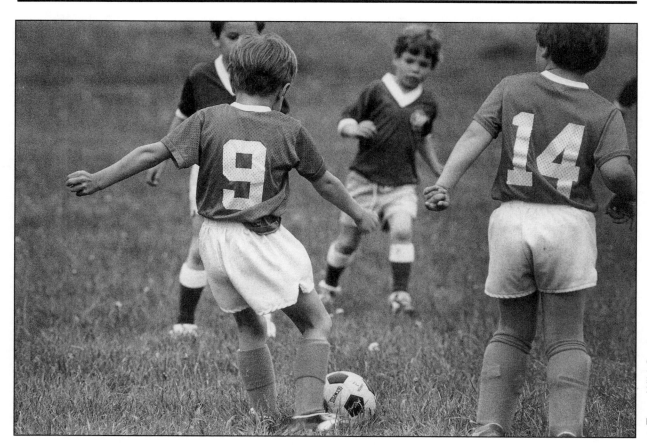

There has been a general reluctance to allow epileptics to participate in physical activity programs and competitive sport. In a recent poll of 760 epileptics between the ages of 7 and 81 (mean age: 36.7 years), 38% listed playing sports as activities limited by their having epilepsy; 32% listed exercising in general (37). Clement and Wallace (10), in a survey of adolescents with epilepsy, found that competitive sports were less popular with them than with controls matched by age and sex. In the early 1980s Bennett (4) conducted a survey of four senior high schools with a total enrollment of 5792 students to determine how many epileptics were playing team sports. School nurses identified 17 epileptics, none of whom participated in high school sports. In another survey of a Division 1 NCAA Conference, only 1 of approximately 3000 student athletes was an epileptic (4). Parental concerns, liability fears, and misconceptions about epilepsy are for the most part responsible for this situation. The attitude is often that the risks far outweigh the benefits.

The critical time for learning the benefits of physical exercise, developing athletic abilities, and experiencing the challenge and excitement of team sports is during the school years. This is also a critical time for developing self-esteem, confidence, and discipline. Participation in physical education programs, whether in gym classes or as a member of a team, can enhance the development of these personal attributes and even may be a valuable adjunct in treating chronic health conditions. Excluding a child with epilepsy from these activities may lead to serious psychosocial problems.

The purpose of this chapter is to provide relevant information on childhood epilepsy so that personal, school, and team physicians, physical education instructors, and school authorities will be better able to make intelligent decisions about sport and exercise programs for epileptic children. While the chapter does not review all facets of childhood and adolescent epilepsy, additional references for health care professionals and teachers can be found on pages 105-106.

BACKGROUND INFORMATION ON CHILDHOOD EPILEPSY

''Convulsive disorders (epilepsy) are states characterized by sudden, brief, repetitive, and stereotyped alterations of behavior, which are presumed to be due to a paroxysmal discharge of cortical or subcortical neurons (32). Before a diagnosis of epilepsy can be made, a person must have more than one seizure. The classification system for epileptic seizures most frequently used today is the one proposed by the International League Against Epilepsy (ILAE) (11) (Table 6.1). A recent proposal for a Revised Classification of Epilepsies and Epileptic Syndromes is currently being studied by the ILAE (12).

Partial Epilepsies

Partial epilepsies are characterized by simple or complex seizures with or without secondary generalization (a progression from a partial seizure to a generalized seizure like a grand mal). In simple partial seizures consciousness is preserved. The clinical manifestations of the seizure depend on the cortical site of the abnormal electrical discharge. For example, if the discharge occurs in the motor area of the frontal lobe, then rhythmical shaking of the extremities on the opposite side will occur. Complex partial seizures are caused by a discharge usually beginning in the mesial temporal lobe or limbic structures. They may be preceded by an aura. For example, the patient may perceive an unpleasant smell (olfactory hallucination). During the attack the patient does not respond to questions and usually has semipurposeful movements, for example, repetitive lip smacking or fumbling with clothes (automatisms). Patients do not remember the events during the seizure (amnesia); frequently they are tired afterward and may wish to sleep. Simple or complex partial seizures may progress into a tonic-clonic convulsion (grand mal). Although there are exceptions (for example, benign Rolandic epilepsy), partial epilepsies are usually caused by a structural brain lesion, such as that caused by damage from head trauma. In addition to seizures the patient may also suffer from mental and physical handicaps. These are related to the location and severity of the brain damage that is responsible for the seizures.

Primary Generalized Epilepsies

These may be convulsive or nonconvulsive. An example of the former is a generalized tonic-clonic seizure. The child, sometimes without

Table 6.1 The International Classification of Epileptic Seizures

I. Partial (focal, local) seizures
    A. Simple partial seizures (consciousness not impaired)
        1. With motor symptoms
        2. With somatosensory or special sensory symptoms
        3. With autonomic symptoms
        4. With psychic symptoms
    B. Complex partial seizures (with impairment of consciousness)
        1. Beginning as simple partial seizures and progressing to impairment of consciousness
           a. With no other features
           b. With features as in I.A.1-I.A.4
           c. With automatisms
        2. With impairment of consciousness at onset
           a. With no other features
           b. With features as in I.A.1-I.A.4
           c. With automatisms
    C. Partial seizures evolving to secondarily generalized seizures
        1. Simple partial seizures evolving to generalized seizures
        2. Complex partial seizures evolving to generalized seizures
        3. Simple partial seizures evolving to complex partial seizures to generalized seizures
II. Generalized seizures (convulsive or nonconvulsive)
    A. Absence seizures
        1. Absence seizures
        2. Atypical absence seizures
    B. Myoclonic seizures
    C. Clonic seizures
    D. Tonic seizures
    E. Tonic-clonic seizures
    F. Atonic seizures (astatic seizures)
III. Unclassified epileptic seizures
    Includes all seizures that cannot be classified because of inadequate or incomplete data and some that defy classification in hitherto described categories. This includes some neonatal seizures, e.g., rhythmic eye movements, chewing, and swimming movements

Reprinted from the Commission on Classification and Terminology of the International League Against Epilepsy (1981).

warning, suddenly emits a shrill cry, the extremities stiffen, and the jaw is tightly clenched. This tonic phase will last about 15-30 seconds, and is followed by rhythmical jerking of the facial muscles and extremities. Tongue biting and urinary and fecal incontinence can also occur. The clonic phase usually lasts 30-60 seconds, but not more than 2-3 minutes unless the seizure becomes continuous (status epilepticus). Following the seizure drowsiness and confusion are present. Children with tonic-clonic generalized seizures may be otherwise neurologically normal, or may have physical and mental handicaps.

Absence seizures (petit mal) are an example of nonconvulsive epilepsy. The child suddenly stops what he or she is doing and stares straight ahead; there may be a few slight jerks of the upper extremities or fluttering of the eyelids, but the child does not lose postural tone. The attack may last several seconds, or as long as 2-3 minutes. Following the episode the patient resumes normal activities and is not fatigued; however, he or she will be amnesic for the events that took place during the attack. Children with uncomplicated absence seizures are otherwise neurologically normal. This type of epilepsy is usually inherited. The other types of generalized seizures, particularly akinetic seizures (sudden drop attacks with or without convulsive movements), occur in severely brain-damaged children.

Epidemiology

One study conducted in two central Oklahoma counties reported the prevalence rate for epilepsies to be 4.71 per 1,000 persons under the age of 20 (13). The prevalence rate was highest in children aged 1-4 years and in blacks. These findings are in general agreement with several other published studies (23, 48, 49). Extrapolating from 1990 United States Census data (8), the number of American children between the ages of 5 and 19 with epilepsy is approximately 265,000. If one accepts a conservative estimate that 60% of these epileptics have excellent to good control over their condition, then approximately 159,000 epileptics in this age group should be able to participate in some type of sporting activity.

Treatment and Prognosis of Childhood Epilepsy

Most childhood epilepsies respond very favorably to treatment with anti-epileptic drugs (AEDs). The drugs used to treat the various seizures, their half-lives, and therapeutic serum levels are listed in Table 6.2. The dose-related and idiosyncratic reactions for each drug are listed in Table 6.3. With the generalized epilepsies, good control can be achieved in 75-85% of patients, particularly in children with absence attacks and generalized tonic-clonic seizures

who are otherwise neurologically normal. Akinetic seizures in severely brain-damaged children are very difficult to control. With the partial epilepsies, seizure control is less optimal (31-80%), with complex partial seizures the most difficult to treat. Patients with complex partial seizures who do not respond to medication may be cured by surgery (temporal lobectomy).

Epilepsy is not always a lifelong illness. Studies have shown that the recurrence rate for children who have been seizure-free for 2-4 years on medication is only about 25-35% when anticonvulsant drugs are withdrawn (16, 20, 26, 27, 50, 53). Most of the relapses occur during the first few months to one year after discontinuing the medicine; the rate of recurrences after more than 3-5 years is quite small. Predictors for recurrence in children are an EEG with epileptic features prior to withdrawal of anticonvulsants, or a history of tonic-clonic or focal motor seizures (41). Less predictive, but probably significant, is the earlier age of onset of the seizure disorder, mental retardation in the patient, and a history of complex partial seizures (42). Also, rapid withdrawal of anticonvulsants can cause a recurrence; thus medications should be withdrawn slowly over a 6-month period.

Table 6.2   Pharmacological Data on Antiepileptic Drugs

	Elimination half-life in adults (hr)	Elimination half-life in children (hr)	Time to reach steady state (days)	Therapeutic range of serum concentrate (µg/ml)	Protein-protein binding (%)
Carbamazepine	14-27	14-27[a] 8-28[b]	3-4	4-12	66-89
Clonazepam	20-40	20-40		0.005-0.070	47
Ethosuximide	20-60	20-60	7-10	40-100	0
Phenobarbital	46-136	37-73[a] 61-173[b]	14-21	15-40	40-60
Phenytoin	10-34	5-14[a] 10-60[b] 10-140[c]	7-28	10-20	69-96
Primidone[d]	6-18	5-11	4-7	5-12	0
Valproic acid	6-15	8-15	1-2	50-140	80-95

[a]Child.

[b]Neonates.

[c]Prematures.

[d]Metabolized to phenobarbital and phenylethylmalonamide; both metabolites have antiepileptic activity.
Reprinted from Penry (1986).

Table 6.3 Dose-Related Toxicities, Non-Dose-Related Side Effects, and Idiosyncratic Reactions to Antiepileptic Drugs Used to Control Generalized Seizures, Listed in Descending Order of Frequency

| Drug | Reactions | | |
	Dose-related	Non-dose related	Idiosyncratic
Carbamazepine	Double vision Blurring of vision Vertigo Cognitive impairment Lethargy Behavioral changes Dyskinesias Cardiac conduction disturbance	Gastrointestinal upset; diarrhea Fluid retention	Granulocyte suppression Allergic dermatitis Stevens-Johnson syndrome Aplastic anemia Hepatic failure Kidney failure
Phenobarbital	Sedation Mental dullness Cognitive impairment Hyperactivity Behavioral changes Ataxia Changes in sleep patterns	Lethargy Decrease in attention span Hyperactivity Changes in sleep patterns Osteopenia	Allergic dermatitis Stevens-Johnson syndrome Serum sickness reaction Hepatic failure Granulocyte suppression
Phenytoin	Nystagmus Cognitive impairment Ataxia Incoordination Dyskinesias Seizure exacerbation	Darkening and increase of body hair Coarsening of facial features Worsening of acne Gingival and other hyperplasias Osteopenia Lymphadenopathy Folate deficiency anemia Neuropathy	Allergic dermatitis Fetal drug effects Hepatic failure Serum sickness reaction Aplastic anemia Granulocyte suppression Lupus erythematosis Hyperglycemia-like reaction
Valproic acid	Gastrointestinal upset[a] Liver enzyme elevations Tremor Hyperammonemia Initial somnolence Behavioral changes	Weight gain Nausea Hair loss and changes in hair texture	Reye-like syndrome Fetal drug effects Hepatic failure Pancreatitis Coma or stupor

[a]May be controlled by giving divalproex sodium.
Reprinted from Penry (1986).

Morbidity and Mortality

Hauser, Annegers, and Elveback have estimated the death rate among epileptics in the United States to be about 1:100,000 persons per year, or about double the expected rate for age-matched controls (22). Wannamaker reports that about 50% of these deaths are directly or indirectly related to the seizure disorder, the major causes being seizures and status epilepticus, accidents, suicide, and sudden unexplained death syndrome (56). Deaths during or soon after a seizure, or status epilepticus, account for an average of 11.6% of the mortality rate (56). Hauser et al. report that accidents are responsible for 7% of deaths (22). However, according to Wannamaker, only 5% are related to injuries suffered during a seizure (57). One study reports that bathtub drownings are responsible for most seizure-related accidental deaths (39) and another states that the risk of drowning during recreational swimming is four times greater for epileptic children than for their peers (45). However, a third study of 274 immersion accidents reports that only 3.3% were actually caused by seizures (44). Suicide accounts for about 7.2% of deaths among epileptics, which is five times higher than the suicide rate in the general United States population (56). The suicide rate for non-institutionalized epileptic children is lower, about 2.2% (7), but still above the national average.

The incidence of sudden unexplained death syndrome (SUDS) in epileptics is about 10-15%, while the risk in the general population has been estimated between 1:525-1:2100 (33). The patients are usually adults (mean age 32 years) with a long history of generalized convulsions. Typically they are found dead at home and have subtherapeutic anticonvulsant serum levels. While it is rare that the deaths are actually observed, mechanisms that have been implicated include seizure with an immediate fatal heart arrhythmia, and seizure with recovery and then delayed secondary respiratory arrest or arrhythmia (15). In addition, it has been well documented that seizures can be associated with cardiac arrhythmias (14, 17). Carbamazepine, a frequently prescribed AED, has also been reported to cause cardiac conduction disturbances (3). SUDS is not common in children and adolescents; in Leestma's (33) study of 124 cases in the Chicago area, only 6% were under the age of 10, and 12% were between 10 and 20 years of age. In another study based in Denver, only 5 cases of 44 involved children between the ages of 3 and 9—a rate of 11%; in contrast to the adult population, only one child had subtherapeutic serum anticonvulsant levels (15). SUDS is not typically associated with exercise: of 19 cases reported by Hirsch and Martin (25), 2 involved sudden collapses after swimming. AEDs were not detected in postmortem drug analyses.

The major complications suffered during seizures are physical injuries, most often during a generalized tonic-clonic spell. Injuries may be related to the intensity of the spell or may result from falls. The most frequent bone injuries include fractures of the humeral neck, femoral trochanter, clavicle, and ankle; dislocations of the shoulder and hip; and vertebral body compressions (35, 46). For adults, at least, there is no evidence that patients on long-term AEDs are predisposed to fractures because of the osteomalacia or secondary hyperparathyroidism which these drugs may produce (2). Brain and spinal cord injuries have also been reported, as well as burns and scalds (1, 47). Foreign matter can also enter the lungs, causing pneumonia. Despite the great physical intensity of generalized tonic-clonic seizures and the confusion and altered states of behavior associated with nonconvulsive seizures, these complications are fortunately not common. Complications from AEDs may constitute another possible cause of morbidity in epileptics (Table 6.3).

SEIZURES AND EXERCISE

The beneficial effects of a regular exercise program in preventing seizures have been suspected since ancient times. Galen (cited in 51, p. 71), in a letter to the father of an epileptic boy, made the following recommendation:

> At the beginning of spring the body ought to be purged and his life ordered as follows: He should rise early, take a moderate walk to the gymnasium where he would meet his master of exercises, who would be charged with the details, but as a general principle the exercises would be calculated to warm up the body in order to expel excess material and should aim at strengthening the head and the cardia.

Galen also mentioned that bowling, bending, and rolling around on the ground were to be avoided, whereas walking, moderate running, and hanging from a bar were to be encouraged.

In this century, Lennox and Lennox (34) wrote:

> Epilepsy prefers to attack when the person is off guard, sleeping, resting, idling. This is easily demonstrable in persons who experience very frequent petits, which may be almost absent during skating, swimming or running and abundant while sewing, eating, or just "sitting." . . . I can remember only a few instances of a person having an attack while running or swimming. (pp. 823-824)

The US Department of Health, Education and Welfare Commission for the Control of Epilepsy and Its Consequences makes the following statement:

Physical activity also appears to play a role in seizure prevention. The need for activity and physical fitness was documented by data collected by the Commission and testimony at the regional hearings. Such activity is important for those with epilepsy since some evidence suggests that activity may, in fact, reduce the likelihood of seizures (54).

In the proceedings of the 19th International Epilepsy Congress (1991), Tettenborn and Krämer (52, p. 530) state that

> common objections such as increased clumsiness, slower performance, fear of accidents or injuries or the assumption that sport increases the frequency or severity of seizures are without foundation, except in refractory patients with associated cerebral impairment.

Despite these testimonials, definite scientific evidence supporting the protective effect of physical activity on seizures is limited. For example, the data supporting the HEW conclusions are not referenced.

Seizures occurring in children and adolescents during or immediately after physical activity are probably uncommon, judging from the paucity of reports in the recent medical literature. Ogunyemi, Gomez, and Klass (43) describe three patients, two of whom were children. One, a 14-year-old boy, reported generalized tonic-clonic seizures only during vigorous physical exercise, usually while running. His baseline EEG, including five minutes of hyperventilation, photic stimulation, and sleep, was normal. However, while the patient was pedaling a stationary bicycle brief bursts of spike-wave activity were noted. These were not accompanied by any clinical manifestations. The second patient, a 7-year-old boy, experienced seizures sometimes while riding a bike, and invariably when swimming. Brief cessation of activity and staring were observed with some of the seizures; during others, he would lose his balance and fall. After 7-1/2 minutes of exercise a spike-wave discharge appeared in the EEG without clinical signs of a seizure, and the baseline EEG also showed diffuse spike-wave paroxysms. Although the case histories do not mention it explicitly, it can be assumed that these two patients were on AEDs. Exercise-induced seizures in

children and teenagers have also been reported by Korczyn (30) and Bennett (4).

A rare form of "seizure" is that induced by a movement, particularly a sudden one. The episodes are usually precipitated by a sudden movement after a period of rest. They are characterized by tonic posturing or writhing movements which frequently only involve one limb. The event is of short duration, rarely longer than 30 seconds. Consciousness is not lost. Patients may respond to treatment with AEDs. Whether the attacks are secondary to an abnormal electrical discharge, as in epilepsy, or are caused by exercise-induced dystonia or chorea-athetosis (24), has not been resolved. Lishman (36) reported seven cases of this interesting paroxysmal disorder. In three patients, the first attack occurred during an athletic event (hockey, track, or cricket).

There is more convincing evidence that exercise-induced seizures in adult epileptics are also uncommon, although most of this evidence is retrospective. Korczyn (30) reported that only 5 of 250 epileptics 10 years and older had ever experienced a seizure while engaged in physical activity. Ninety additional epileptics denied ever having a seizure during physical exertion. Götze, Kubicki, Munter, and Teichmann (21) also reported no seizures in epileptics during intense physical exertion, including swimming, and found fewer abnormal EEG paroxysmal discharges during exercise than at rest or during hyperventilation. Recently, Nakken, Bjørholt, Johannessen, Løyning, and Lind (42) studied the effects of physical training on aerobic capacity and seizure occurrence in 21 uncontrolled adult epileptics. They concluded that "physical activity does not represent an important seizure-inducing factor in general, and that in most people with epilepsy, physical training appears to have a favorable influence" (p. 88). Horyd, Gryziak, Niedzielska, and Zielinski (28) reported a decrease in EEG discharges during exercise but increase in EEG discharges in the immediate postexercise period in 10 of 43 inadequately controlled epileptics. No clinical seizures were recorded. Kuijer, in a personal communication to Fraser and Smith (19), reported that he completed an exercise study on young adults whose epilepsy was active. He compared the effects of continuous versus intermittent exercise on a stationary bicycle. Only one seizure was observed during either type of exercise; however, immediately after exercise, 128 seizures were recorded for the continuous exercise group, as compared to only 27 in those subjects participating in the intermittent exercise program. The number of subjects studied was not mentioned in this communication, and it was unclear whether the events were actual seizures or EEG discharges. An increase in epileptiform EEG discharges during the immediate postexercise period has also been reported in another study by Kuijer (31), as well as by Berney, Osselton, Kolvin, and Day (5). It should be emphasized that the seizures in these subjects were not well controlled. Because of this, it is unlikely that they would have been allowed to participate in competitive sports.

It is still not definitively known why seizures during exercise are uncommon and why physical fitness may improve seizure control. Possible mechanisms include changes in acid-base balance, the release of β-endorphins in brain tissue (β-endorphins tend to inhibit seizure discharges), sensory inhibition, and increased vigilance and attention (55).

Anticonvulsant Drug Metabolism and Exercise

Another possible concern is whether a regular exercise program or a prolonged period of physical activity could adversely affect the pharmacokinetics of anticonvulsant medications. Theoretically, exercise might reduce serum levels because of its hepatic-enzyme-inducing effect. On the other hand, postexercise ketosis may increase serum levels. Studies to date in adults have failed to show that physical training significantly alters serum anticonvulsant levels (6, 9, 40).

Injuries

As previously mentioned, injuries, particularly to the bones joints, can occur during an epileptic seizure, especially tonic-clonic generalized attacks. However, there is no evidence to suggest that seizure-related injuries are increased in epileptics participating in sports (18).

A question that remains unanswered is whether an epileptic is more likely to experience a seizure following blunt head trauma than a nonepileptic child. Livingston and Berman (38),

who cared for over 15,000 epileptic children over a period of 34 years, could not recall a single instance of recurrence of seizures after head trauma in any of their epileptic athletes. In Jennett's study (29) of early posttraumatic epilepsy, 1 of 9 patients with epilepsy experienced a series of generalized seizures immediately after a head injury; however, the patient had no further seizures over the next 10 years. In the remaining 8 patients the frequency of these attacks did not appear to have increased since the accident. Despite this evidence, it remains unclear whether repeated mild head trauma (for example, of the sort incurred by heading a soccer ball) can increase seizure frequency. Further studies are needed.

DECISIONS ON PARTICIPATION IN SPORTS

The major factor in determining whether children and adolescents can participate in individual as well as team sports is seizure frequency type. Other variables that need to be considered are

- a previous history of exercise-precipitated seizures,
- the potential for a serious injury to the athlete or bystanders if a convulsion occurs during the exercise,
- physical skills or handicaps,
- motivation,
- side effects of anticonvulsants that might interfere with performance, and
- environmental, metabolic, and psychological stresses associated with the sport that may activate seizures.

The author recently conducted a survey of six board-certified neurologists, one of whom was a pediatric neurologist, on whether they would allow an epileptic to participate in 62 sports or recreational activities based on seizure control alone. Seizure control was divided into 4 major categories:

I. Excellent—no seizures in the past year.
II. Good control—1-3 convulsions in the past year.
III. Fair control—4-10 seizures in the past year.
IV. Poor control—more than 10 seizures in the past year.

The seizure type was not considered. For each sport or recreational activity they were asked to indicate

- whether the child could participate (P),
- whether the sport was contraindicated (C), or
- whether participation was questionable (Q).

The results for the four categories of seizure control are tabulated in Table 6.4. If there was a majority vote (4 of 6), the sport was listed under P. Sports listed in the questionable category usually had 3 votes for participation, 2 contraindicated, and 1 questionable. Votes of 3 or more against participation placed the sport in the contraindicated category. In Table 6.5 individual sports are listed by seizure frequency according to whether there was a unanimous agreement for or against participation.

As would be expected, the results of this limited survey show that epileptics stand a better chance of being allowed to participate in most activities, even collision and contact sports, if their seizures are well controlled than if they are not. Overall, of 13 major sport categories, the most favorable recommendations were received by the categories of ball, ball plus stick, racquet or paddle, dance (with the exception of gymnastics), outdoor recreational, and track and field. The categories labeled aquatic, combat, snow and ice, horse, and motorbike and roller sports were judged least acceptable. The results of this survey should only be used as guidelines; there are exceptions to the rule.

PREPARATION FOR COMPETITION AND FOLLOW-UP INSTRUCTIONS FOR THE ATHLETE

The following instruction guidelines may be followed once it has been determined that an epileptic can participate in a particular sport.

Notification of Health Care Personnel

School health care personnel, including the team physician, trainer, and school nurse, should be notified that the athlete is epileptic. The athlete (or his or her parents) should also provide information on seizure type and recognition, the dosage and times when AEDs are taken, and whether other mental or physical handicaps are present.

Reporting Seizures or Side Effects From AEDs

The athlete should report immediately any seizures or side effects from AEDs (see discussion in section on instructions for health care personnel).

AEDs

The athlete must be aware of the need for total compliance. AEDs should be taken at the same time every day and not on an empty stomach. They should not be taken immediately before practice or a game. The athlete should inform the team physician when other medications, including over-the-counter drugs, are used to treat other ailments. Certain drugs may alter the pharmacokinetics of AEDs. On overnight trips the athlete should bring a 2-3 day supply of AEDs. The pills should be given to the team physician or other responsible personnel for safekeeping.

Other Health Care Issues

The athlete should follow good nutritional and sleep habits and prevent dehydration. The athlete should abstain from alcohol, stimulant medications, anabolic steroids, and recreational drugs.

Exercise Program

The best procedure is to build stamina with a graded exercise program rather than to attempt too much at the outset. If the athlete feels unusually fatigued even after a graded exercise program, this should be reported to the team physician or school nurse.

INSTRUCTIONS FOR HEALTH CARE PERSONNEL

An increase in seizures may affect an epileptic's ability to continue participation in a particular

Table 6.4   Results of Survey for Participation in Various Sports and Recreational Activities

Sports category	Seizure control		P		Q		C
Aquatic number of sports—8	I	Canoeing Surfing	Crew—rowing Swimming	Diving Waterskiing	Water polo	Scuba diving	Scuba diving
	II	Canoeing Crew—rowing		Surfing	Swimming	Diving Water polo	Scuba diving Waterskiing
	III			Canoeing	Crew—rowing	Diving Scuba diving Surfing	Swimming Water polo Waterskiing
	IV					Canoeing Crew racing Diving Scuba diving	Surfing Swimming Water polo Water skiing
Ball number of sports—7	I	Basketball Bowling Football Handball	Rugby Soccer Volleyball	Football	Rugby		
	II	Basketball Bowling Handball	Soccer Volleyball	Soccer			
	III	Basketball Handball	Bowling Volleyball	Soccer		Football	Rugby
	IV	Basketball Handball	Bowling Volleyball			Football Soccer	Rugby

Ball plus stick, racquet or paddle number of sports—13	I	Badminton Baseball Billiards Cricket Field Hockey Golf Jai alai	Lacrosse Racquetball Softball Squash Table tennis Tennis				
	II	Badminton Baseball Billiards Cricket Golf Jai alai	Lacrosse Racquetball Softball Squash Table tennis Tennis	Field hockey			
	III	Badminton Baseball Billiards Cricket Golf Jai alai	Lacrosse Racquetball Softball Squash Table tennis Tennis	Field hockey			
	IV	Badminton Billiards Golf	Table tennis Tennis	Baseball Cricket Jai alai	Racquetball Softball Squash	Field hockey	Lacrosse
Combat number of sports—3	I	Karate/Judo	Wrestling			Boxing	
	II	Karate/Judo	Wrestling			Boxing	
	III			Karate/Judo	Wrestling	Boxing	
	IV			Karate/Judo		Boxing	Wrestling

(continued)

Table 6.4 (*continued*)

Sports category	Seizure control	P	Q	C
Dance & gymnastics number of sports—4	I	Aerobic dance Ballet Dance Gymnastics		
	II	Aerobic dance Ballet Dance	Gymnastics	
	III	Aerobic dance Ballet Dance		Gymnastics
	IV	Aerobic dance Ballet Dance		Gymnastics
Horse number of sports—3	I	Equestrian	Polo	Rodeo
	II			Equestrian Polo Rodeo
	III			Equestrian Polo Rodeo
	IV			Equestrian Polo Rodeo
Motor, bike & roller number of sports—4	I	Cycling Roller skating		Auto racing Motorcycling
	II	Roller skating	Cycling	Auto racing Motorcycling
	III		Roller skating	Auto racing Motorcycling Cycling

Category	Level						
Motor, bike & roller (continued)	IV			Roller skating		Auto racing, Motorcycling	Cycling
Outdoor-recreational number of sports—4	I	Camping, Fishing	Hiking, Mountaineering				
	II	Camping, Fishing	Hiking			Mountaineering	
	III	Camping, Fishing	Hiking			Mountaineering	
	IV	Camping, Fishing	Hiking			Mountaineering	
Snow & ice sports number of sports—8	I	Curling, Ice hockey, Skating—figure	Skating—speed, Skiing—downhill, Skiing—x-country	Bobsledding		Ski jumping	Ski jumping
	II	Curling, Skating—figure	Skating—speed, Skiing—x-country	Ice hockey	Skiing—downhill	Bobsledding	Ski jumping
	III	Curling	Skiing—x-country	Skating—figure	Skating—speed	Bobsledding, Ice hockey	Skiing—downhill, Ski jumping
	IV	Curling		Skating—figure	Skiing—x-country	Bobsledding, Ice hockey, Skating—speed	Skiing—downhill, Ski jumping
Strength number of sports—1	I	Weightlifting	Weightlifting				
	II			Weightlifting			

(continued)

Table 6.4 *(continued)*

Sports category	Seizure control	P		Q		C
Strength *(continued)*	III					Weightlifting
	IV					Weightlifting
Track and field number of sports—4	I	Field events Race walking	Running—distance Running—sprints			
	II	Field events Race walking	Running—distance Running—sprints			
	III	Field events Race walking	Running—distance Running—sprints			
	IV	Race walking Running—distance	Running—sprints	Field events		
Weapon number of sports—3	I	Archery Fencing	Riflery			
	II	Archery Fencing	Riflery			
	III	Archery		Fencing	Riflery	
	IV			Archery	Fencing	Riflery

Table 6.5   Unanimous Agreement on Sport Participation or Contraindication by Seizure Control

I

Participate

Canoeing	Billiards	Tennis	Figure skating
Crew—rowing	Cricket	Wrestling	Speed skating
Basketball	Golf	Aerobic dance	X-country skiing
Bowling	Jai alai	Ballet	Field events
Handball	Lacrosse	Dance	Racewalking
Soccer	Racquetball	Roller Skating	Running—distance
Volleyball	Softball	Camping	Running—sprint
Badminton	Squash	Fishing	Archery
Baseball	Table tennis	Curling	Fencing

Total = 36/62

Contraindicated

| Boxing | Auto racing |

Total = 2/62

III

Participate

Bowling	Tennis	Handball	Aerobic dance
Badminton	Ballet	Billiards	Dance
Golf	Camping	Table tennis	Racewalking
Softball			

Total = 13/62

Contraindicated

| Scuba diving | Boxing | Auto racing | Cycling |
| Motorcycling | Mountaineering | Bobsledding | |

Total = 7/62

II

Participate

Canoeing	Table tennis	Fishing	Crew—rowing
Racquetball	Curling	Bowling	X-country skiing
Softball	Badminton	Handball	Squash
Field events	Volleyball	Tennis	Racewalking
Aerobic dance	Billiards	Ballet	Running—distance
Running—sprint	Cricket	Dance	Archery
Golf	Camping	Fencing	

Total = 27/62

Contraindicated

| Boxing | Auto racing | Motorcycling | Mountaineering |
| Bobsledding | Ski jumping | | |

Total = 6/62

IV

Participate

| Bowling | Badminton | Billiards | Golf |
| Table tennis | Ballet | | |

Total = 8/62

Contraindicated

| Diving | Scuba diving | Boxing | Rodeo |
| Auto racing | Motorcycling | Mountaineering | Bobsledding |

Total = 8/62

sport or school recreational activity. This is particularly true for athletes with excellent or good seizure control, because the sports that they may be allowed to play, such as collision, combat, aquatic, and ice and snow contests (see Table 6.4) may carry an increased risk of injury not only to the athlete but to others if a seizure occurred during the event. The sports for children whose seizures are less adequately controlled are less of a problem because the risk of injury is not as great.

Seizure Documentation

Seizure documentation can be ascertained from direct and indirect evidence.

Direct

- *School authorities actually witnessing a seizure.* It is beyond the scope of this chapter to provide information on seizure recognition as well as first aid during and after a convulsion. See pages 105-106 for a list of books and periodicals published by the Epilepsy Foundation of America that deal with this subject.
- *Parents.* Parents are a more reliable source of information, and should be instructed to report to school authorities when their child has had a seizure. This is particularly true of those children whose seizures are under excellent or good control. However, the possibility exists that parents who wish their child to excel in a particular sport may not comply.
- *Students.* For reasons of age, relying on the athlete to report when he or she has had a seizure may not be a dependable method of estimating seizure frequency. This also applies to student's peers.

Indirect Evidence

The following events should raise suspicion that the child's seizures may be increasing or that there are side effects from AEDs.

- Unexplained or frequent absenteeism from school
- A decrease in school or athletic performance
- Sleeping in class
- A change in personality

Further investigation is warranted when these problems are identified.

Follow-Up

The following guidelines may be used by the personal physician to follow an athlete whose seizures are under excellent or good control:

- Periodic AED serum levels. The blood should always be obtained at the same time of day, usually in the morning before the first dose. If serum levels are subtherapeutic the athlete should not be allowed to participate until the level is in the therapeutic range.
- Periodic complete blood counts. Other blood studies such as liver function tests may be ordered depending on the toxic side effects of particular AEDs.
- If an athlete or his or her parents report a breakthrough seizure (a seizure that occurs for no apparent reason in a patient with epilepsy under excellent control), or if one is witnessed by school personnel, the personal physician should be consulted. Serum anticonvulsant blood levels should be obtained. If the levels are subtherapeutic or toxic the dose should be adjusted until the levels are in the therapeutic range. This may take several days or as much as 1-2 weeks, depending on the AED. The athlete should not be allowed to participate until blood levels are in the therapeutic range. If the levels are therapeutic the athlete should be observed for one week before resuming practice. To reemphasize, these guidelines are for children and adolescents whose seizures are under excellent to good control.
- If a seizure occurs during competition or practice, particularly during collision or contact sports, the athlete should be taken to the nearest emergency room. The concern in this situation is that the seizure may have been precipitated by an injury, particularly to the head, or by increased body temperature or fluid and electrolyte abnormalities. If causes are not found and serum AED levels are too high or low, follow the recommendations in the preceding paragraph.
- It is difficult to develop guidelines for follow-up of children whose seizures are

under fair or poor control. Clinical judgement must be used in deciding when they can again participate in their activity. The personal physician is the one to make this decision.

First Aid Guidelines

The following first aid guidelines should be followed by the trainer or school health care personnel when caring for a student athlete who is having a generalized or partial seizure.

Generalized Tonic-Clonic Seizure

1. Protect the athlete from self-injury. The head, arms, and legs should be protected but not forcefully restrained.
2. Turn the athlete on one side with head down. This will help in preventing upper airway obstruction and aspiration of vomitus.
3. Do not force objects such as tongue blades between the teeth during a convulsion. Never use your fingers to attempt mouth opening.
4. In the post-ictal period, access the airway and clear any mucus or vomitus from the oral cavity. Check the vital signs.
5. Most generalized tonic-clonic seizures are of short duration, i.e., 1-3 minutes. Therefore, it is not necessary to transport the athlete to the hospital unless there is concern about an injury (particularly head trauma), cardiovascular status, or hyperthermia.
6. The athlete's parents and personal physician should be notified.
7. The athlete should be observed until he or she can be safely escorted home.
8. If the convulsion lasts more than several minutes, or if it is the athlete's first convulsion, paramedics should be called.

Partial Seizures

Simple partial seizures should not present a problem unless they become secondarily generalized. During such seizures the athlete is fully conscious and aware of his or her surroundings. The trainer or health care personnel should

1. Guard against injury;
2. Observe the student over a sufficient period of time to assure complete recovery;
3. Notify parents and personal physician;
4. Forbid continued participation in the sport until cleared by the personal physician;
5. Take the student to an emergency room, if this is the first seizure.

Similar guidelines apply to complex partial seizures. However, as this type of seizure is characterized by abnormal behavior, the trainer should also be careful not to physically restrain the patient since he or she may become combative. Also, the epileptic may be very drowsy after the seizure, and should be allowed to sleep for awhile.

CONCLUSION

Exercise-induced convulsions in epileptics whose seizures are well controlled are uncommon. The injury rate does not appear to be increased in epileptic athletes when compared to their peers. Therefore, the student whose seizures are well controlled should be given the opportunity to participate in most sports available at the grammar and high school levels. However, a safety awareness program should be developed for the athlete as well as for school personnel involved in physical education classes and team sports. Although the number of sports that children and adolescents whose seizures are less adequately controlled may play is somewhat limited, they should be counseled to participate. The epileptic child with mild to moderate physical or mental handicaps should be encouraged to join the Special Olympics programs. A healthy body guards against seizures.

ARTICLES ON EPILEPSY FOR HEALTH CARE PROFESSIONALS

These articles can be obtained by writing:

The Epilepsy Foundation of America
Material Services Department
4351 Garden City Drive
Landover, MD 20785

Current trends in epilepsy: a self study course for physicians. Hauser, W.A. Catalog #137CTS; 1988.

Epilepsy: frequency, causes, and consequences. Hauser, W.A. Catalog #141EPC.

Seizure recognition and first aid. Catalog #031RFA.

Living well with epilepsy. Gumnit, R.J. Demos Publications. Catalog #136LWE; 1990.

Students with seizures: a manual for school nurses. Catalog #148SWS.

Epilepsy and the school-age child. Catalog #065SAC; 1990. The legal rights of persons with epilepsy, 6th edition; Epilepsy Foundation of America; 1992.

REFERENCES

1. Allen, J.W.; Kendall, B.E.; Kocen, R.S.; Milligan, N.M. Acute cervical cord injuries in patients with epilepsy. J. of Neurol., Neurosurg. and Psych. 45:884-892; 1982.

2. Annegers, J.F.; Melton, L.J.; Sun, C-a.; Hauser, W.A. Risk of age-related fractures in patients with unprovoked seizures. Epilepsia 30:348-355; 1989.

3. Benassi, E.; Gian-Paolo, B.; Cocito, L.; Maffini, M.; Loeb, C. Carbamazepine and cardiac conduction blocks. Ann. Neurol. 22:280-281; 1987.

4. Bennett, D.R. Sports and epilepsy: to play or not to play. Seminars in Neurology 1:345-357; 1981.

5. Berney, T.P.; Osselton, J.W.; Kolvin, I.; Day, M.J. Effect of discotheque environment on epileptic children. Br. Med. J. 282:180-182; 1981.

6. Borgà, O.; Juhlin-Dannfeldt, A.; Dahlquist, R. Plasma levels and protein binding of phenytoin during exercise in man: the effect of elevating free fatty acids. Pharmacology 16:37-43; 1978.

7. Bridge, E.M. Epilepsy and convulsive disorders in children. New York: McGraw-Hill; 1949:491-495.

8. Census of Population and Housing. Washington, DC: U.S. Department of Commerce, Bureau of the Census; 1990.

9. Chalmers, R.J.; Johnson, R.H. The effect of diphenylhydantoin on metabolic and growth hormone changes during and after exercise. J. Neurol. Neurosurg. Psychiatry 46:662-665; 1983.

10. Clement, M.T.; Wallace, S.J. A survey of adolescents with epilepsy. Developmental and Child Neurology 32:849-857; 1990.

11. Commission on Classification and Terminology of The International League Against Epilepsy. Proposal for revised clinical and electroencephalographic classification of epileptic seizures. Epilepsia 22:489-501; 1981.

12. Commission on Classification and Terminology of The International League Against Epilepsy. Proposal for classification of epilepsies and epileptic syndromes. Epilepsia 30:389-399; 1989.

13. Cowan, L.D.; Bodensteiner, J.B.; LeViton, A.; Doherty, L. Prevalence of the epilepsies in children and adolescents. Epilepsia 30:94-106; 1989.

14. Dasheiff, R.M.; Dickinson, LaV. J. Sudden unexpected death of an epileptic patient due to cardiac arrhythmia after seizure. Arch. Neurol. 43:194-196; 1986.

15. Earnest, M.P.; Thomas, G.E.; Eden, R.A.; Hossack, K.F. The sudden unexplained death syndrome in epilepsy: demographic, clinical and postmortem features. Epilepsia 33:310-316; 1992.

16. Emerson, R.; D'Souza, B.J.; Vining, E.P.; Holden, K.R.; Mellitis, E.D.; Freeman, J.M. Stopping medication in children with epilepsy. N. Engl. J. Med. 304:1125-1129; 1981.

17. Epstein, M.A.; Sperling, M.R.; O'Connor, M.J. Cardiac rhythm during temporal lobe seizures. Neurology 42:50-53; 1992.

18. Fischer, A.; Daute, K.H. The risk of an accident in sport and at games in epileptic children. Med. Sport (Berlin) 28:93-95; 1988.

19. Fraser, R.T.; Smith, W.R. Adjustment to daily living. In: Sachs, H., ed. Epilepsy: a handbook for the mental health professional. New York: Brunner; 1982:189-221.

20. Gherpelli, J.L.D.; Kok, F.; dal Forno, S.; Elkis, L.C.; Lefevre, B.H.W.; Diament, A.J. Discontinuing medication in epileptic children: a study of risk factors related to recurrence. Epilepsia 33:681-686; 1992.

21. Götze, W.; Kubicki, S.T.; Munter, M.; Teichmann, V. Effect of physical exercise on seizure threshold (investigated by electroencephalographic telemetry). Dis. Nerv. Syst. 28:664-667; 1967.

22. Hauser, W.A.; Annegers, J.F.; Elveback, L.R. Mortality in patients with epilepsy. Epilepsia 21:399-412; 1980.

23. Hauser, W.A.; Annegers, J.F.; Kurland, L.T. Prevalence of epilepsy in Rochester, Minnesota: 1940-1980. Epilepsia 32:429-445; 1991.

24. Hirata, K.; Katayama, S.; Saito, T.; Ichihashi, K.; Mukai, T.; Katayama, M.; Otaka, T. Paroxysmal kinesigenic choreathetosis with abnormal electroencephalogram during attacks. Epilepsia 32:492-494; 1991.

25. Hirsch, C.S.; Martin, D.L. Unexpected death in young epileptics. Neurology 21:682-690; 1971.

26. Holowach, J.; Thurston, D.L.; O'Leary, J. Prognosis in childhood epilepsy: followup study of 148 cases in which therapy had been suspended after prolonged anticonvulsant control. N. Engl. J. Med. 286:169-174; 1972.

27. Holowach-Thurston, J.; Thurston, D.L.; Hixon, B.B.; Keller, A.J. Additional followup of 184 children 15-23 years after withdrawal of anticonvulsant therapy. N. Engl. J. Med. 306:831-836; 1982.

28. Horyd, W.; Gryziak, J., Niedzielska, K.; Zielinski, J.J. Influence of physical exertion on EEG epileptiform abnormalities in epileptics. Neurol. Neurochir. Pol. 15:545-552; 1981.

29. Jennett, B.W. Epilepsy after non-missle head injuries. 2nd ed. London: Heinemann Press, 1975.

30. Korczyn, A.D. Participation of epileptic patients in sports. J. Sports. Med. 19:195-198; 1979.

31. Kuijer, A. Epilepsy and exercise, electroencephalographical and biochemical studies. In: Wada, J.A.; Penry, J.K., eds. Advances in epileptology: the tenth epilepsy international symposium. New York: Raven; 1980:543.

32. Kurland, L.T.; Kurtzke, J.F.; Goldberg, I.D., editor. Epidemiology of neurologic and sense organ disorders. Cambridge, MA: Harvard University Press; 1973.

33. Leestma, J.E. Sudden unexpected death associated with seizures: a pathological review. In: Lathers, C.M.; Schrader, P.L., eds. Epilepsy and sudden death. New York: Marcel Dekker; 1990:61-68.

34. Lennox, W.G.; Lennox, M.A. Epilepsy and related disorders. Boston: Little, Brown & Co.; 1960.

35. Lidgren, L.; Wallöe, A. Incidence of fracture in epileptics. Acta. Orthop. Scand. 48:356-361; 1977.

36. Lishman, W.A.; Symonds, C.P.; Whitty, C.W.M.; Willison, R.G. Seizures induced by movement. Brain 85:51-59; 1963.

37. Living with epilepsy. Report of a Roper poll of patients with epilepsy on quality of life. Carter-Wallace, Inc.; 1992.

38. Livingston, S.; Berman, W. Participation of epileptic patients in sports. JAMA 224:236-238; 1973.

39. Livingston, S.; Pauli, L.L.; Pruce, I. Epilepsy and drowning in children. Br. Med. J. 2:515-516; 1977.

40. Marsh, T.D.; Garnett, W.R.; Poyner, W.J.; Pellock, J.M. Effects of exercise on valproic acid pharmacokinetics. Clin. Pharmacology 2:62-64; 1983.

41. The Medical Research Council Antiepileptic Drug Withdrawal Study Group. A randomised study of antiepileptic drug withdrawal in patients in remission. Lancet 337:1175-1180; 1991.

42. Nakken, K.O.; Bjørholt, P.G.; Johannessen, S.I.; Løyning, T.; Lind, E. Effect of physical training on aerobic capacity, seizure occurrence, and serum level of anti-epileptic drugs in adults with epilepsy. Epilepsia 31:88-94; 1990.

43. Ogunyemi, A.O.; Gomez, M.R.; Klass, D.W. Seizures induced by exercise. Neurology 38:633-634; 1988.

44. Pearn, J.; Bart, R.; Yamaoka, R. Drowning risks to the epileptic: a study from Hawaii. Br. Med. J. 2:1284-1285; 1978.

45. Pearn, J.; Nixon, J.; Wilkey, I. Freshwater drowning and near drowning accidents involving children. Med. J. Aust. 2:942-946; 1976.

46. Pedersen, K.K.; Christiansen, C.; Ahlgren, P.; Lund, M. Incidence of fracture of the vertebral spine in epileptic patients. Acta. Neurol. Scand. 54:200-203; 1976.

47. Richards, E.H. Aspects of epilepsy and burns. Epilepsia 9:127-135: 1968.

48. Rose, S.W.; Penry, J.K.; Markush, R.E.; Radloff, L.A.; Putnam, P.L. Prevalence of epilepsy in children. Epilepsia 14:133-152; 1973.

49. Sangrador, C.O.; Luaces, R.P. Study of the prevalence of epilepsy among school children in Valladolid, Spain. Epilepsia 32:791-797; 1991.

50. Skinner, S.; Vining, E.P.G.; Mellitis, E.D.; D'Souza, B.J.; Holden, K.; Baumgardner, R.A. Discontinuing antiepileptic medication in children with epilepsy after two years without seizures: a prospective study. N. Engl. J. Med. 313:976-980; 1985.

51. Temkin, O. The falling sickness. 1st ed. Baltimore: Johns Hopkins University Press; 1945.

52. Tettenborn, B.; Kramer, G. Total patient care in epilepsy. Epilepsia 33(suppl. 1):528-532; 1992.

53. Todt, H. The late prognosis of epilepsy in children: results of a prospective follow-up study. Epilepsia 25:137-144; 1984.

54. U.S. Department of Health, Education and Welfare. Plan for nationwide action on epilepsy. DHEW Publication NIH 78-276; 1978.

55. van Linschoten, R.; Backx, F.J.G.; Mulder, O.G.M.; Meinardi, H. Epilepsy and sports. Sports Medicine 10:9-19; 1990.

56. Wannamaker, B.B. A perspective on death of persons with epilepsy. In: Lathers, C.M.; Schraeder, P.L., eds. Epilepsy and sudden death. New York: Marcel Dekker; 1990:27-37.

CHAPTER 7

Childhood Progressive Neuromuscular Disease

David D. Kilmer
University of California, Davis, School of Medicine

Craig M. McDonald
University of California, Davis, School of Medicine

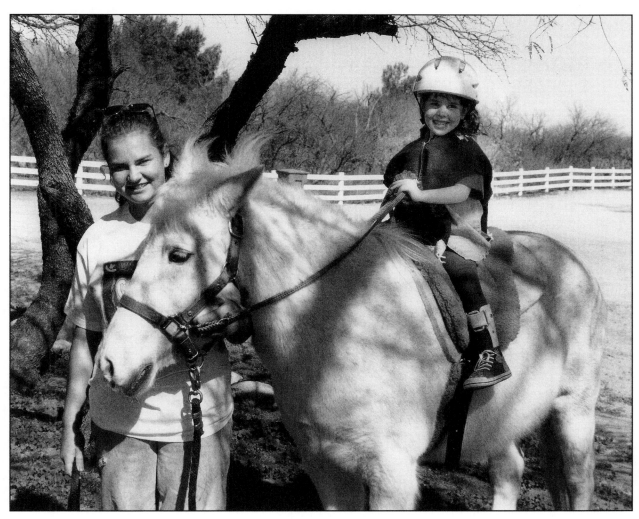

Neuromuscular diseases (NMDs) involve the anterior horn cell, peripheral nerve, or muscle. They are uncommon causes of physical impairment and disability in children. Because of this, many physicians and physical educators have a poor understanding of either the beneficial or detrimental effects of exercise in these children. Excessive caution in the past has too often led to an isolated, sedentary lifestyle. As will be seen, this caution has little scientific support. However, people who deal with children with NMDs need to be aware of functional limitations so that expectations remain appropriate.

The purpose of this chapter is to describe progressive neuromuscular diseases most frequently affecting children, and the role of exercise and sport in treatment of the resultant physical impairment. Very little well-controlled research has been done in this area, so recommendations are based on a critical review of available literature, professsional consensus, and personal experience both in the clinic and exercise physiology laboratory.

COMMON NEUROMUSCULAR DISEASES OF CHILDREN

Diagnosis is based on a clinical pattern of weakness, on family history, and on results of histologic, molecular genetic, and electrophysiological examinations. Many of the slowly progressive NMDs do not cause functional problems until late adolescence or adulthood. However, certain NMDs begin to manifest during childhood and may cause great concern among parents, teachers, and physicians in terms of the amount and type of physical activity to be recommended. Progressive weakness may cause children with these diseases to lose functional abilities as they grow, but preventable secondary complications such as obesity, disuse atrophy, and contractures may be as important as weakness in causing disability.

Duchenne Muscular Dystrophy

Duchenne muscular dystrophy (DMD) is an inherited x-linked recessive disease characterized by a complete absence of the structural protein dystrophin. The disease primarily affects skeletal muscle and the myocardium. Although DMD is usually not clinically apparent until the second or third year of life, histological and laboratory evidence indicates that the disease is active in the neonatal period. This relentlessly progressive dystrophy is universally fatal with death occurring from respiratory or cardiac complications, usually between the ages of 18 and 25. There is currently no known effective cure for DMD. Because current treatment is largely supportive, knowledge of the natural history of DMD is essential for the proper timing of therapeutic interventions.

Early motor developmental delay is rarely noted; however, late walking may occur. Once ambulation is obtained a tendency to fall easily may be noticed. Running and jumping may be particularly difficult, and initially the boys may seem merely clumsy. By 3-5 years of age proximal weakness is usually more obvious, subtle gait changes may be noticed, and the diagnosis is confirmed. The neck flexors are among the weakest muscle groups even at this young age, and boys with DMD may exhibit difficulty lifting their heads against gravity. When arising from the floor the child demonstrates the classic Gower's sign (legs are widely spaced and the child climbs up the lower extremities with hands), owing primarily to proximal weakness involving the hip extensors.

Between the time of diagnosis and the age of 5 or 6 boys with DMD may transiently improve in functional motor tasks such as stair climbing, running, and getting up from the floor. However, by the age of 5 or 6 they are increasingly unable to keep up with their peers, and with the realization that they are not normal some become socially withdrawn. Mild intellectual impairment and learning problems are seen in about one-third of cases.

Between the ages of 5 and 14 or 15 loss of strength occurs in a fairly linear fashion, without prolonged periods of plateau or accelerated loss (1). Neck flexors and proximal muscles of the lower extremities (hip extensors, hip abductors, hip flexors, and knee extensors) are the earliest involved, followed by proximal upper extremity

This work was supported by Research and Training Center Grant H133B800016-03 from the National Institute on Disability and Rehabilitation Research (NIDRR), United States Department of Education.

muscles. The least involved muscles are the foot evertors and ankle plantar flexors. In general, upper extremity muscles are relatively stronger than lower extremity muscles at a given point in time (5, 22).

Later in the first decade boys with DMD utilize a number of postural adaptations to conserve energy and maintain upright stance. Trunk and proximal lower extremity weakness leads to a wide-based Trendelenburg gait with anterior pelvic tilt and marked lumbar lordosis. Eventually progressive contractures and the presence of less than antigravity strength at the hip and knee mandate the use of a wheelchair for locomotion. This usually occurs between the ages 9 and 11; although orthopedic surgery and bracing may prolong ambulation for several years in boys motivated to remain upright. However, prolonged ambulation has not been documented to alter the progressive loss of strength, incidence of scoliosis, or patient longevity.

Contractures may be noted as early as 3-4 years of age. They are initially detected in heel cords, iliotibial bands, and hip flexors (5). Coincident with decreasing ambulation some time after the age of eight, patients develop increasing knee flexion, elbow flexion, and wrist flexion contractures. During adolescence progressive spinal deformity occurs very frequently in boys with DMD. Curves can develop quite rapidly and may exceed 100 degrees in some cases. Operative spinal fixation with internal instrumentation appears to be the only effective treatment of progressive spinal deformity in DMD (38).

Restrictive pulmonary disease in DMD is a universal consequence of progressive muscular weakness. This typically becomes a clinically significant issue several years after the boys have begun using a wheelchair. Abdominal weakness leads to limitation in the ability to generate a forceful cough. Diaphragm weakness limits the total amount of air moved during maximal inspiration, resulting in reduced lung volumes. In the late teenage years boys develop progressive difficulty clearing airway secretions and may suffer repeated infections. Widespread microatelectasis with reduced chest wall compliance, ventilation-perfusion abnormalities, chronic hypoxemia, and pulmonary hypertension further complicate the problem. Noninvasive methods of positive pressure ventilatory support through orally or nasally applied

masks is chosen by some patients with DMD as a long-term alternative to ventilation through a tracheostomy, or to early death from respiratory failure. Life may be prolonged for as long as 10 years (2).

Clinical cardiac involvement is primarily due to fibrotic changes in the myocardium leading to intrinsic left ventricular dysfunction and congestive heart failure (16). In DMD, dysrhythmias other than sinus tachycardia are relatively uncommon. Myocardial impairment in DMD remains clinically silent until late in the course of the disease, possibly owing to the absence of exertional dyspnea secondary to lack of physical activity. Cardiac involvement in DMD can be detected before clinical signs and symptoms appear by close cardiac monitoring with electrocardiography (ECG), echocardiography, and, occasionally, radionuclide ventriculographic studies. ECG reveals abnormalities in up to 90% of DMD patients and changes may be seen as early as 4 years of age (34, 41). Findings may include but not be limited to

- resting sinus tachycardia—found in as many as 90 percent of DMD patients (18),
- tall R-waves in V1 with increased R/S ratio, and
- deep narrow Q-waves greater than 4 millimeters in limb and precordial leads (34).

ECG changes may be mistaken for a posterior wall infarct by physicians unaware of their frequent occurrence in DMD patients. Echocardiography may reveal posterior wall hypokinesis, decreased estimated stroke volume and fractional shortening, and other abnormalities. The primary cardiomyopathy will presumably become an increasingly prominent cause of mortality in DMD as noninvasive ventilation is increasingly applied.

Becker Muscular Dystrophy

BMD is a slowly progressive NMD caused by the presence of abnormal molecular weight dystrophin and/or by reduced amounts of normal dystrophin. It is approximately 10 times less frequent than DMD (24). The distribution of muscle weakness is similar to that seen in DMD, with neck flexor, pelvic girdle, and proximal lower extremity weakness preceding the onset of proximal upper extremity weakness. Forearm muscles, hand intrinsics, and ankle plantar flexors remain clinically unaffected until late in the illness. The majority of BMD patients will initially experience difficulties beween the ages of 5 and 15, although the range for age of onset is quite broad. Few BMD patients require a wheelchair before the age of 16 years and many retain ambulation into adulthood.

Unlike in DMD, intellectual impairment is not a prominent feature of BMD. Plantar flexion contractures are common, as is scoliosis; however, these problems are not as severe as in DMD. Restrictive lung disease is rarely clinically significant in patients with BMD. Cardiac involvement, on the other hand, may be commonly seen. ECG abnormalities similar to those seen in DMD are often present in addition to right bundle branch block, left bundle branch block, or total AV block. Echocardiography may show evidence of ventricular free wall and/or intraventricular septal hypokinesis. Early congestive heart failure does occur and the cardiomyopathy can be severe enough to require cardiac transplantation (36).

Childhood Spinal Muscular Atrophy

The spinal muscular atrophies (SMAs) consist of a large group of heterogeneous disorders with selective deterioration of the anterior horn cell, the cell body of the lower motor neuron. The most common mode of inheritance is autosomal recessive, although autosomal dominant forms have been described. Brzustowicz and colleagues have recently localized the genetic abnormality for many of the acute and chronic forms of SMA to chromosome 5q11 (6). Progression may be rapid to very slow. These children are generally of normal intelligence with no underlying cognitive deficits.

Spinal Muscular Atrophy Type I (Infantile Spinal Muscular Atrophy, Werdnig-Hoffmann's Disease)

Onset of SMA Type I is usually prenatally or shortly after birth, and children always present by 3-6 months of age. The baby may be extremely hypotonic with a weak cry. They may develop early respiratory distress and weakness of bulbar muscles, which makes feeding difficult. Death usually occurs by 3-4 years of age.

In a subgroup sometimes known as Chronic Werdnig-Hoffmann's Disease, patients with onset prior to 6 months of age may live well past age 4 and clinically resemble those with SMA Type II.

Spinal Muscular Atrophy Type II (Intermediate Spinal Muscular Atrophy)

This disease is initially manifested between 6 months and 2 to 3 years of age. Inheritance is usually autosomal recessive. Weakness is generalized but involves the proximal muscles of the lower extremities during the earliest stages. Children usually present with delayed gross motor milestones. Many children may be unable to maintain sitting or standing without significant support. Some children with this illness may learn to walk with the aid of long-leg braces. Invariably ambulation is lost and a wheelchair is utilized early in the first decade. Children with the intermediate form of SMA may have fasciculations and wasting of the tongue, but no difficulty with chewing or swallowing. Proximal limb and trunk weakness is more marked with relative sparing distally. Atrophy of proximal musculature can be quite severe. The lower extremities are usually weaker than the upper extremities and progression is usually relatively slow.

Kyphoscoliosis (a spinal deformity with thoracolumbar scoliosis combined with kyphosis) is extremely common in these patients and often more severe than with DMD. This is perhaps because of the early onset of spinal deformity in SMA Type II. Hip and knee flexion contractures are also common, as is hip dislocation. A spinal orthosis is often used during the first decade. Although such an orthosis does not slow the progression of the scoliosis it does allow weaker patients to sit upright. Spinal instrumentation is now utilized with this population in many centers (29, 35).

After the initial progressive weakness the disease may remain stable for years (10, 37). Some believe that a significant amount of disuse atrophy occurs in the first year of life owing to lack of mobility, followed by a more stable course (37). Many children with SMA Type II develop restrictive pulmonary disease due to a combination of diaphragm, intercostal weakness, and severe spinal deformity. Life expectancy is variable with death usually occurring in the second or third decade, although some patients live into their thirties.

Spinal Muscular Atrophy Type III (Late-Onset Juvenile Spinal Muscular Atrophy, Kugelberg-Welander Disease)

Spinal Muscular Atrophy Type III is typically first noted between the ages of 5 and 15. However, it may begin as early as 3 years of age. Pelvic girdle musculature is involved initially, followed by muscles of the shoulder girdle. The slowly progressive loss of strength generally involves the legs more than the arms, and proximal muscles more than distal muscles. Wasting of the involved muscles may be significant. Type III SMA may be mistakenly diagnosed as Becker Muscular Dystrophy or Limb-Girdle Syndrome because of the slowly progressive course, enlarged calves, and pattern of muscle weakness. There is a low incidence of contractures, spinal deformity, restrictive lung disease, and cardiac involvement. Although ambulation may continue for most patients into their fourth decade, some may use a wheelchair by 20 years of age. Most have a normal life span.

Hereditary Motor and Sensory Neuropathy, Types I and II (HMSN I & II, Charcot-Marie-Tooth Disease)

This disease of peripheral nerves often begins in the late childhood, with foot deformity causing the greatest functional difficulties. Orthopedic correction of the foot instability is commonly required by late adolescence. The muscles below the knee are typically involved, and ankle-foot orthoses (AFOs) may be needed to help provide ankle stability and prevent footdrop during gait. If this occurs, running and jumping skills will be compromised by the braces. Weakness of the hands rarely becomes an issue during the school years. The heart is generally not affected, although cardiac conduction defects have been reported in isolated cases (3). Whether this association is coincidental is not known.

Myotonic Muscular Dystrophy (MMD)

Myotonic dystrophy is inherited as an autosomal dominant trait, and is one of the more common NMDs. There is marked variability in severity and age of onset, although it rarely causes impairment before adolescence or early adulthood. The exception is congenital MMD, which is evident at birth and is associated with significant mental retardation. The later-onset form often goes undiagnosed in childhood; only years later does careful questioning reveal a history of being "clumsy" or "slow" in physical education class. MMD is a unique dystrophy for two reasons. First, the patients may develop myotonia, or the inability to quickly relax muscle groups. The child may complain of muscle cramps, stiffness, or the inability to relax the grip. Secondly, distal muscles are generally more affected than proximal musculature. Therefore, AFOs may be needed with the resultant functional limitations. MMD is a systemic disease, with involvement of the eyes (cataracts), smooth muscle (swallowing dysfunction), heart (cardiac conduction defects), and respiratory muscles. However, it is rare for these systemic problems to become a treatment issue during the childhood or adolescent years. Mild intellectual problems may be present, as opposed to the frank mental retardation seen in the congenital form.

Facioscapulohumeral Dystrophy

This autosomal dominant dystrophy typically involves muscles of the face, shoulder, and upper arms, curiously sparing the deltoids. There is marked variability in severity and age of onset, with some evidence pointing to an earlier age of onset being associated with more severe eventual disease (26). However, the onset of symptoms is typically in late childhood or early adolescence. A typical "chicken wings" appearance of the scapulae may be noticed during PE class as the child attempts to perform a push-up or climb a rope. As with most dystrophies, the child will have difficulty performing tasks or handling objects above the shoulder level. Weakness of the hip girdle musculature is generally not a problem until adulthood.

Limb-Girdle Syndrome (LGS)

Rather than a specific NMD, LGS should be considered a heterogeneous group of slowly progressive dystrophies affecting the shoulder and hip musculature without facial weakness. As expected, there is variety in inheritance pattern, age of onset, and rate of progression. However, rarely are problems noticed before adolescence. An exception is autosomal recessive dystrophy of childhood, which is more severe and generally requires wheelchair use between the ages of 15 and 20. In contrast to MMD, systemic manifestions are rare with LGS. Functional problems revolve around the proximal weakness and may include, for example, difficulty with squatting, walking and running up or down inclines, and overhead activities. Orthoses are generally not indicated in these syndromes.

THE EFFECT OF NEUROMUSCULAR DISEASE ON EXERCISE TOLERANCE AND SPORTS PERFORMANCE IN CHILDREN

There is a paucity of literature concerning exercise in children with neuromuscular diseases. The only studies performed have been with Duchenne muscular dystrophy, which has limited relevance to less severe forms of neuromuscular disease. For the slowly progressive disorders it is necessary to extrapolate from investigations of affected adults. Evaluation of previous studies is difficult because normal maturation and age differences naturally produce variations in strength, disease history, degree of weakness of the muscles exercised, preexercise conditioning status, and type of exercise used (42).

The ultimate cause of physical impairment in NMDs is loss of normally functioning muscle fibers. It should be noted that 30-40% of muscle tissue is lost before clinical weakness is appreciated, although exercise performance may be compromised at a lower percentage of loss (39). In the later stages of DMD and SMA, pulmonary and cardiac involvement can become additional factors which may influence exercise performance.

Overwork Weakness

A major concern with exercise in individuals with NMDs is overwork weakness. This topic was recently reviewed by Fowler (14). Over-work weakness was first suggested in DMD by muscle histologic examination demonstrating that most degeneration occurs in muscles typically used during sustained physical activity (4). Muscle enzymes, used as a marker of muscle breakdown, were reduced by bed rest in dystrophic patients and elevated to a greater degree than in normal controls after a vigorous strengthening program (15, 31). Several other anecdotal reports have found asymmetric myopathic weakness in the limb most often used (21), as well as reversal of increased weakness by reducing excessive daily physical activity (44). Thus, the evidence for overwork weakness is circumstantial and based on case reports, leaving a tenuous connection.

Resistance Exercise Performance in NMDs

Traditionally, high resistance exercise has been discouraged in NMDs because of concerns about overworking the weakened muscle. However, several prospective supervised resistance exercise studies have failed to demonstrate this phenomenon. DeLateur and Giaconi studied 4 boys with DMD using a submaximal isokinetic quadriceps strengthening program for 6 months and demonstrated no untoward effects, although 2 boys were actually quite advanced with the disease (8). Vignos included subjects with both slowly progressive and rapidly progressive NMD, and used a high resistance weight-training protocol (43). He found beneficial effects of strength training in the experimental group, with no subjects becoming weaker. Those with slowly progressive NMDs obtained better results than DMD subjects. More recently, adults with slowly progressive NMDs performed weight-lifting programs without detrimental effects, and improvements in isometric and isokinetic strength were reported (28, 30). It seems apparent that stronger muscles are strengthened more than very weak ones. Thus, starting an exercise regimen early in the disease when muscle fiber degeneration and weakness is minimal is generally recommended (17).

The authors have recently completed both a moderate, or submaximal (1) and high, or near-maximal (23) resistance strengthening protocol in adults with slowly progressive NMD. The 12-week moderate-resistance program was well tolerated and provided generally beneficial effects on most parameters of strength. The high-resistance program, although equally well tolerated, demonstrated some evidence of decreased strength in the upper extremities, although only with eccentric (lengthening action) isokinetic testing. Furthermore, the high-resistance program did not provide an incremental benefit over the moderate strengthening program. Additional studies are needed to investigate the differential effects of training using eccentric versus concentric (shortening) contractions.

Aerobic Exercise Performance in NMDs

Measurement of exercise capacity is feasible in children and adolescents with NMDs if they are able to climb stairs with the aid of a railing (7, 40). A study of maximal O_2 uptake in boys with DMD demonstrates the marked reduction in $\dot{V}O_2$max in this population (40). In the absence of significant cardiac involvement, oxygen delivery to the muscles should be intact in NMDs. The limitation appears to be in oxygen uptake at the muscle cell level, proportional to the loss of active muscle tissue (25). There is some clinical evidence to suggest an inverse correlation between functional muscle loss and maximal O_2 uptake (19). There is no evidence for defects in oxidative phosphorylation (32), nor is there abnormal capillary diffusion capacity (33). Likewise, cardiac output seems to increase proportionally to increased O_2 consumption during exercise in muscular dystrophies as occurs in normals (20, 40).

Little work has been done on the response of diseased muscle to endurance exercise. A 12-week cycle ergometry study in 8 slowly progressive or nonprogressive adult NMD subjects demonstrated greater than 20% improvement in $\dot{V}O_2$max without significant change in resting creatine kinase or myoglobin (13). Thus, there is some evidence that the adaptations to endurance exercise in NMDs may not differ from normal individuals.

Respiratory Exercise Training

A program of respiratory exercise training generally consists of incentive spirometry and forced expiration maneuvers with expiratory water bottles. The effect of this on pulmonary function in NMD patients remains unsubstantiated, however. While several studies have indicated that respiratory muscle training either improves or maintains pulmonary function, most of these studies have been uncontrolled with varied training programs (9, 12). One randomized trial of a 2-month respiratory training program in DMD reported significant improvement in respiratory endurance parameters, but no change in vital capacity or maximal static pressures (27). While respiratory exercise training may have an impact on respiratory endurance, there is no evidence that the progressive course of restrictive lung disease in DMD can be delayed with an exercise program. Similar to skeletal muscle training, we would predict less improvement in patients with more advanced NMDs. A cautious approach seems warranted in the later stages of respiratory weakness, since vigorous training may merely add to the work of breathing in patients with limited respiratory reserve.

The Effect of Contractures on Performance

Muscle imbalance leading to contracture may be as important a factor in limiting performance as specific muscle weakness. In the childhood years this is primarily a concern with DMD, although children with early-onset SMA may also have significant contractures. The 2-joint muscles such as the hamstrings, tensor fasciae latae, and gastrocnemius contract the earliest and to the greater extent. Muscle shortened by contracture develops less maximal tension and fatigues more rapidly owing to effects on the normal length-tension relationship of skeletal muscle (39). Contractures may also contribute to the increased metabolic costs of task performance due to activation of muscle groups not usually needed. For example, Eston et al. demonstrated that DMD subjects have a higher heart rate for a given gait speed compared to normal children, with subsequent adjustment of walking speed to maintain the same energy requirement (11).

General Exercise Precautions and Recommendations

Based on available data submaximal strengthening exercises are recommended for postpubertal and adult patients with slowly progressive

NMDs. Because children normally increase the myogenic (protein synthesis/hypertrophy) component of strength more than the neurogenic (improved recruitment of motor units) component, the response of growing diseased muscle to resistance training is unknown. Nevertheless, we feel that children should not focus on formal weight-lifting programs.

Although the incidence and risk of overuse weakness may be overstated, children with NMDs should avoid exercising to the point of exhaustion, and rest periods should be encouraged. As a general rule, if the child feels fatigued or weak on the day following an exercise bout, the workload was probably excessive. Formal exercise treadmill or ergometry testing is generally not necessary before starting an exercise program in these children unless there are specific concerns about cardiac or pulmonary symptoms. Occasionally the most deconditioned children require a supervised exercise program to obtain a fitness level that would allow participation in sports and games. In this situation we follow the general goal of 20-30 minutes of aerobic exercise, 3 days per week. Supervision is required to monitor for excessive fatigue or increased weakness.

If the child can participate in exercise for 10-15 minutes without stopping, we would prefer exercise for enjoyment and socialization rather than in a strictly supervised program. Choice of recreational activity should provide a positive experience, be sufficiently challenging, and offer some opportunity for success. Recommended games and activities at different levels of disability will be discussed subsequently in this chapter.

Potential Benefits of Exercise in Children With NMDs

Although no direct medical benefits of exercise have been scientifically demonstrated in children with NMDs, observation indicates that the value of improved socialization, self-esteem, and independence must not be minimized in these diseases, which often lead to isolation and loneliness. Also, if it can be assumed that weakness and poor endurance stem in part from deconditioning, at least this component of the problem should respond to exercise. Adherence to a stretching program for contractures may help maintain joint range of motion and should be made part of an enjoyable daily routine.

Finally, exercise during childhood and adolescence has been shown to lead to a more active lifestyle as an adult. With appropriate adaptations, the same habits may be instilled in people with slowly progressive NMDs.

EXERCISE AND SPORT PROGRAMS FOR CHILDREN WITH NMDs

The first step in designing and monitoring an exercise program for a child with an NMD is to educate the family and physical educators about the disease. Often the patient and family are fearful and cautious owing to lack of knowledge and the overriding concern of making impaired muscles even weaker. Encouraging discussion of fears while providing guidelines and support is most beneficial in these circumstances. The specific choice of activity may involve discussion among patient, family, physical therapist, occupational therapist, or adaptive physical education teacher.

One psychosocial issue to keep in mind with progressive childhood NMDs is that participation in an activity may be necessarily brief, depending on the rate of disease progression and demands of the activity. For example, horseback riding or roller skating would not likely be continued into adolescence, and the child may feel an additional sense of loss when no longer able to participate in these activities. This should not necessarily preclude a child from participating, but the physician should discuss the natural history of the disease as it pertains to long-term sports involvement with the family, therapists, and teachers. Consideration should be given to the extent to which a sport can be adapted to accommodate increasing impairment.

The recommendations provided here are based on functional levels which take into account the factors of strength, contractures, and pulmonary and cardiac limitations. These levels are summarized in Table 7.1.

Exercise Recommendations Based Upon Functional Level

Known Presence of an NMD But No Overt Sequelae With Routine Activities

These children are less likely to require encouragement to participate in sports but may have

Table 7.1   Functional Levels of Children With Neuromuscular Diseases

Level	Concerns	Examples
I. Known diagnosis no overt sequelae	Low endurance Subpar dynamic strength Possible overwork weakness	HMSN I MMD
II. Ambulatory without aids	Easy fatigue Disuse weakness Reduced endurance Mild contractures Possible overwork weakness	DMD age 5-8 LGS FSH BMD
III. Ambulatory, marked weakness and/or contractures	Limited ambulation Poor endurance Disuse weakness Possible overwork weakness	DMD 8-11 SMA BMD
IV. Functional wheelchair user	Restrictive lung disease Cardiomyopathy Severe contractures Severe weakness	DMD > 11 SMA

Note. DMD = Duchenne Muscular Dystrophy; BMD = Becker Muscular Dystrophy; MMD = Myotonic Muscular Dystrophy; LGS = Limb-Girdle Syndrome; FSH = Facioscapulohumeral Muscular Dystrophy; SMA = Spinal Muscular Atrophy; HMSN I = Hereditary Motor and Sensory Neuropathy, Type I.

difficulty experiencing success and performing at peer level, particularly in activities with high static or dynamic strength or endurance demands. Although there are no obvious limitations exercise capacity may be limited, necessitating frequent rest breaks. Overwork weakness is a potential concern in unsupervised settings, even at this mild level of involvement. For this reason, competitive sports such as football, distance running, sprinting, and wrestling are not encouraged. Rather, these children are more likely to experience success with peers in sports such as golf, swimming, or softball. A goal with this group is to help the child with a slowly progressive NMD to choose a "lifetime sport" which can be performed into adulthood to maintain fitness. Examples would be swimming or cycling.

Children and adolescents with MMD may have little weakness but demonstrate mild grip myotonia, which may often go unnoticed by the patient. This may increase the difficulty of activities requiring fine motor coordination, although exercise warm-up utilizing repetitive hand motion will often reduce the myotonia. Sports using the larger muscle groups should be emphasized.

Ambulatory Without Aids But With Mild Muscular Fatigue, Mild Contractures, or Reduced Endurance

There is often a component of nonmyopathic disuse atrophy in this group because patients have already curtailed activity. This may be caused by fear, familial pressures, or simply the inability to keep up with peers. With encouragement, children may continue physical education which helps maintain social interaction. Competitive sports are generally not possible but recreational ones are definitely appropriate, although patients should avoid exercising to the point of exhaustion and should have frequent rest breaks. Professional supervision is not necessary at all times if the child can be trusted not to do too much. Swimming and water games are ideal sports for providing resistance, endurance, and flexibility training in an enjoyable manner. Golf, hiking, cycling, and table tennis are examples of other activities that may be popular among children with NMDs. Children with reduced endurance may enjoy tandem cycling, canoeing, or rowing with a parent, sibling, or friend. These activities have reasonable neuromuscular skill demands, static and dynamic demands, and upper and lower body motion ratings.

These authors have observed that children often do not adhere to formal stretching programs unless parents are insistent. This may become a control issue and increase stress at home. If the stretching programs can be made part of the warm-up for a game or sport, cooperation may improve.

Ambulatory But Markedly Limited Due to Weakness, Advancing Contractures, Braces, or Poor Endurance

Examples in this category include the late childhood phase of DMD and also some children with SMA. These children often use braces for ambulation, are not functional runners, and demonstrate marked inefficiency with gait because of postural adaptations to compensate for weakness and contractures. Because of the significant weakness, there may be minimal strengthening response seen with conditioning activities. Water sports are ideal for providing freedom of movement and maintaining fitness, as they eliminate the disadvantage of gravity. Support with flotation devices may be necessary. Pool ball games, relay races, tag, and slalom walking in shallow water may be utilized.

In school, adaptive physical education is necessary, with stress on individual sports alongside peers to maintain socialization and goal-oriented skills. Obviously, in the proximal syndromes overhead activities such as throwing and basketball may be quite difficult, and sports with the arms maintained below the shoulders are more appropriate. Unless contractures are severe, three-wheeled cycling may be an enjoyable way for these children to remain active.

Functional Wheelchair Users

This group includes adolescents with DMD and the most severely affected children with SMA. The period of time these children predominantly use a manual wheelchair is usually less than 2-3 years; ultimately, powered mobility is required. Goals of an exercise program in this group include prevention of disuse atrophy and functionally limiting contractures, maintenance of proper posture in the wheelchair, and avoidance of social isolation, which is quite common in

this phase. Restrictive lung disease and cardiomyopathy become concerns, and any exercise program begun in a previously deconditioned child will have to progress at a very slow pace. The few muscle strengthening studies reported demonstrated the least benefit in the weakest subjects (8, 43). Thus, those patients in a wheelchair are not likely to realize significant benefits from a resistive exercise program.

Despite this discouraging data regarding resistive exercises, there are still significant benefits to exercise and recreation in this group, not the least of which include socialization and improved self-concept. A recreational therapist or adaptive physical education teacher can be very helpful in introducing a wheelchair user to a variety of activities. Water activities usually require some combination of flotation devices and one-on-one assistance by a nondisabled partner. The buoyancy of the water provides freedom of movement for the child that can be quite gratifying. Many can still participate in water games such as those involving a lightweight ball. Occasionally, children requiring a wheelchair for mobility have been able to sit ski. This requires fairly preserved upper extremity function and the ability to long-sit (hips flexed and legs extended) in a sled. Sailing, canoeing, and rowing are also popular.

Many activities can be performed from a manual or power wheelchair, including

- wheelchair bowling (with a special wheelchair bowling ramp),
- wheelchair floor hockey (usually played with manual or electric wheelchairs and special stick attachments),
- fishing,
- hiking (at one of the wheelchair-accessible parks),
- wheelchair events and relay races,
- miniature golf, and
- T-ball.

The Muscular Dystrophy Association (MDA) has an extensive summer camp program with more than 90 camps nationwide. These sessions offer a wide variety of activities especially designed for youngsters who have limited mobility or who use wheelchairs. Activities range from outdoor sports such as swimming, boating, baseball, and bowling to less physically demanding programs such as arts and crafts and talent shows. These camps provide an introduction to many adaptive recreational opportunities, as well as an excellent avenue for children to develop friendships, build self-confidence, and improve self-esteem.

CONCLUSION

Clinicians and physical educators are hampered by a lack of information on the benefits and risks of exercise in children with neuromuscular diseases. This has led to prescriptions of excessive caution regarding physical activity and encouragement of a sedentary lifestyle. However, there is increasing awareness that appropriate participation in recreational sports and games is a positive experience for these children who have a wide variety of functional abilities. With some creativity and appropriate adaptations, activities can be enjoyable and promote socialization, and hopefully active participation will encourage this population to develop a lifelong interest in maintaining fitness.

REFERENCES

1. Aitkens, S.G.; McCrory, M.M.; Kilmer, D.D.; Bernauer, E.M. Moderate resistance exercise program: its effect in slowly progressive neuromuscular disease. Arch. Phys. Med. Rehab. 74:711-715; 1993.
2. Bach, J.R.; O'Brien, J.; Krotenberg, R.; Alba, A.S. Management of end stage respiratory failure in Duchenne muscular dystrophy. Muscle Nerve 10:177-182; 1987.
3. Battistella, P.A.; Moreolo, G.S.; Beuetti, E.; Da Dalt, L.; Pellegrino, P.A. Charcot-Marie-Tooth disease and cardiac arrhythmias. Brain Dev. 10:262-263; 1988.
4. Bonsett, C.A. Pseudohypertrophic muscular dystrophy: distribution of degenerative features as revealed by anatomic study. Neurology 13:728-738; 1963.
5. Brooke, M.H.; Fenichel, G.M.; Griggs, R.C.; Mendell, J.R.; Moxley, R.; Miller, J.P.; Province, M.A., CIDD group. Clinical investigation in Duchenne dystrophy: II. Determination of the "power" of therapeutic trials based on the natural history. Muscle Nerve 6:91-103; 1983.
6. Brzustowicz, L.M.; Lehner, T.; Castilla, L.H.; Penchaszodeh, G.K.; Wilhelmsen, K.C.; Daniels, R.; et al. Genetic mapping of chronic childhood-onset spinal muscular atrophy to chromosome. Nature 344:540-541; 1990.
7. Carroll, J.E.; Hagberg, J.M.; Brooke, M.H.; Shumate, J.B. Bicycle ergometry and gas exchange measurements in neuromuscular disease. Arch. Neurol. 36:457-461; 1979.
8. DeLateur, B.J.; Giaconi, R.M. Effect on maximal strength of submaximal exercise in Duchenne muscular dystrophy. Am. J. Phys. Med. 58:26-36; 1979.
9. DiMarco, A.F.; Kelling, J.S.; DiMarco, M.S.; Jacobs, I.; Shields, R.; Altose, M.D. The effects of inspiratory resistive training on respiratory muscle function in patients with muscular dystrophy. Muscle Nerve 8:284-290; 1985.
10. Eng, G.D.; Binder, H.; Koch, B. Spinal muscular atrophy: experience in diagnosis and rehabilitation management of 60 patients. Arch. Phys. Med. Rehabil. 65:549-553; 1984.
11. Eston, R.G.; Brodie, D.A.; Burnie, J.; Stokes, M.; Griffiths, R.D.; Edwards, R.H.T. Metabolic cost of walking in boys with muscular dystrophy. In: Oseid, S.; Carlsen, K.-H., eds. Children and exercise XIII, intermittent series on sport sciences (vol. 19); Champaign, IL: Human Kinetics; 1989:405-414.
12. Estrup, C.; Lyager, S.; Noeraa, N.; Olsen, C. Effects of respiratory muscle training in patients with neuromuscular diseases and in normals. Respiration 50:36-43; 1986.
13. Florence, J.M.; Hagberg, J.M. Effect of training on the exercise responses of neuromuscular disease patients. Med. Sci. Sports Exerc. 16:460-465; 1984.
14. Fowler, W.M., Jr. Management of musculoskeletal complications in neuromuscular diseases: weakness and the role of exercise. In: Fowler, W.M., Jr., ed. Advances in the rehabilitation of neuromuscular diseases. Philadelphia: Hanley & Belfus; 1988:489-507.
15. Fowler, W.M., Jr.; Gardner, G.W.; Kazerunian, H.H.; Lauvstad, W.A. Effect of exercise on serum enzymes. Arch. Phys. Med. Rehab. 49:554-565; 1968.
16. Fowler, W.M., Jr.; Johnson, E.R.; Yang, C.S. Management of medical complications in neuromuscular diseases. In: Fowler, W.M., Jr., ed. Advances in the rehabilitation of

neuromuscular diseases. Physical Medicine and Rehabilitation: State of the Art Reviews 2(4), Philadelphia: Hanley & Belfus; 1988: 597-615.

17. Fowler, W.M., Jr.; Taylor, M. Rehabilitation management of muscular dystrophy and related disorders: I. The role of exercise. Arch. Phys. Med. Rehab. 63:319-328; 1982.

18. Gilroy, J.; Cahalan, J.; Berman, R.; Newman, M. Cardiac and pulmonary complications in Duchenne's progressive muscular dystrophy. Circulation 27:484-493; 1963.

19. Haller, R.G.; Lewis, S.F. Pathophysiology of exercise performance in muscle disease. Med. Sci. Sports Exerc. 16:456-459; 1984.

20. Haller, R.G.; Lewis, S.F.; Cook, J.D.; Blomquist, C.G. Hyperkinetic circulation during exercise in neuromuscular disease. Neurology 33:1283-1287; 1983.

21. Johnson, E.W.; Braddom, R. Over-work weakness in facioscapulohumeral muscular dystrophy. Arch. Phys. Med. Rehab. 52:333-336; 1971.

22. Kilmer, D.D.; Abresch, R.T.; Fowler, W.M., Jr. Serial manual muscle testing in Duchenne muscular dystrophy. Arch. Phys. Med. Rehabil. 74:1168-1171; 1993.

23. Kilmer, D.D.; Litschert, J.C.; Wright, N.C.; Aitkens, S.G.; Bernauer, E.M. Effect of a high resistance exercise program in slowly progressive neuromuscular disease. Arch. Phys. Med. Rehab. 75:560-563; 1994.

24. Kloepfer, H.W.; Emery, A.E.H. Genetic aspects of neuromuscular disease. In: Walton, J.N., ed. Disorders of voluntary muscle. Edinburgh: Churchill Livingston; 1974:852-885.

25. Lewis, S.F.; Taylor, W.F.; Graham, R.M.; Pettinger, W.A.; Shutte, J.E.; Blomquist, C.G. Cardiovascular responses to exercise as function of absolute and relative work load. J. Appl. Physiol. 54:1314-1323; 1983.

26. Lunt, P.W.; Harper, P.S. Genetic counseling in facioscapulohumeral muscular dystrophy. J. Med. Genet. 28:655-664; 1991.

27. Martin, A.J.; Stern, L.; Yeates, J.; Lepp, D.; Little, J. Respiratory muscle training in Duchenne muscular dystrophy. Dev. Med. Child Neurol. 28:314-318; 1986.

28. McCartney, N.; Moroz, D.; Garner, S.H.; McComas, A.J. The effects of strength training in patients with selected neuromuscular disorders. Med. Sci. Sports Exerc. 20:362-368; 1988.

29. Merlini, L.; Granata, C.; Bonfiglioli, S.; Marini, M.L.; Cervellati, S.; Savini, R. Scoliosis in spinal muscular atrophy: natural history and management. Dev. Med. Child. Neurol. 31:501-508; 1989.

30. Milner-Brown, H.S.; Miller, R.G. Muscle strengthening through high-resistance weight training in patients with neuromuscular disorders. Arch. Phys. Med. Rehab. 60:14-19; 1988.

31. Nakane, K. Change of serum creatine phosphokinase activity after exercise in Duchenne type of progressive muscular dystrophy. Nagoya Med. J. 17:203-216; 1972.

32. Olson, E.; Vignos, P.J.; Woodlock, J.; Perry, T. Oxidative phosphorylation of skeletal muscle in human muscular dystrophy. J. Lab. Clin. Med. 71:220-231; 1968.

33. Paulson, O.B.; Engel, A.G.; Gomez, M.R. Muscle blood flow in Duchenne type muscular dystrophy, limb-girdle dystrophy, polymyositis, and in normal controls. J. Neurol. Neurosurg. Psych. 37:685-690; 1974.

34. Perloff, J.K. Cardiac rhythm and conduction in Duchenne's muscular dystrophy: a prospective study of 20 patients. J. Am. Coll. Cardiol. 3:1263-1268; 1984.

35. Phillips, D.P.; Roye, D.P., Jr.; Farcy, J.C.; Leet, A.; Shelton, Y.A. Surgical treatment of scoliosis in a spinal muscular atrophy population. Spine 15:942-945; 1990.

36. Quinlivan, R.M.; Dubowitz, V. Cardiac transplantation in Becker muscular dystrophy. Neuromusc. Disord. 2:165-167; 1992.

37. Russman, B.S.; Iannacone, S.T.; Buncher, C.R.; Samaha, F.J.; White, M.; Perkins, B.; et al. Spinal muscular atrophy: new thoughts on the pathogenesis and classification schema. J. Child. Neurol. 7:347-353; 1992.

38. Shapiro, F.; Sethna, N.; Colan, S.; Wohl, M.E.; Specht, L. Spinal fusion in Duchenne muscular dystrophy: a multidisciplinary approach. Muscle Nerve 15:604-614; 1992.

39. Siegel, I.M. Muscle and its diseases: an outline primer of basic science and clinical method. Chicago: Year Book Medical Publishers; 1986.

40. Sockolov, R.; Irwin, B.; Dressendorfer, R.H.; Bernauer, E.M. Exercise performance in 6 to 11 year old boys with Duchenne muscular

dystrophy. Arch. Phys. Med. Rehab. 58:195-201; 1977.

41. Tanaka, H.; Nishi, S.; Katanasako, H. Natural course of cardiomyopathy in Duchenne muscular dystrophy. Jpn. Circ. J. 43:974-984; 1979.

42. Vignos, P.G. Exercise in neuromuscular disease: statement of the problem. In: Serratrice, G., ed. Neuromuscular diseases. New York: Raven Press; 1984:565-569.

43. Vignos, P.J.; Watkins, M.P. The effect of exercise in muscular dystrophy. JAMA 197:843-848; 1966.

44. Wagner, M.; Vignos, P.J., Jr.; Fonow, D. Serial isokinetic evaluations used for a patient with scapuloperoneal muscular dystrophy: a case report. Phys. Ther. 66:1110-1113; 1986.

CHAPTER 8

Cerebral Palsy

Carol Adams Mushett
Georgia State University

Duncan O. Wyeth
Michigan Jobs Commission, Lansing, MI

Kenneth J. Richter
Michigan State University

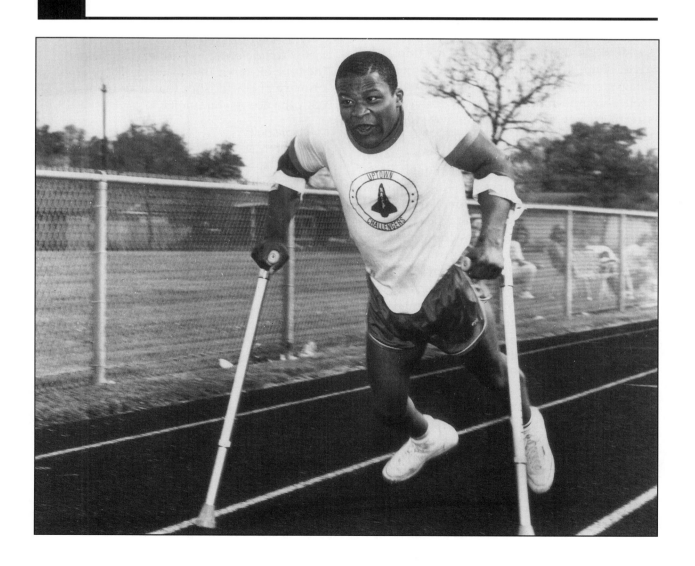

Sporting opportunities for athletes with cerebral palsy, traumatic brain injury, and stroke are organized nationally by the United States Cerebral Palsy Athletic Association (USCPAA), and internationally by the Cerebral Palsy International Sports and Recreation Association (CP-ISRA). The common characteristic linking these athletes is an upper motor neuron lesion of cerebral origin. This chapter will discuss these various conditions and their impact on sport involvement, with specific focus on children with cerebral palsy and like conditions. Cerebral palsy is the neuromuscular orthopedic impairment most commonly found in public schools. There is a reported incidence of approximately 7 per 1000 live births, and a prevalence of 500 cases for every 100,000 persons (27).

The USCPAA provides 16 different sports at the competitive level. Athletes who train for and compete in sport recognize a broad range of benefits. Sport provides persons with disabilities with the opportunity to take risks, to learn team concepts, and to develop personal interactive social skills. Participation in competition also gives children a chance to enhance their self-images and to receive public recognition for their accomplishments. Sport is truly a mainstream activity. Participation allows children to utilize a broad range of community-based facilities and to select their own options—an important part of making independent living choices. Skills learned in sports are also often transferable to other areas of life. For example, an adolescent who uses a power wheelchair and competes in an event such as the slalom can likely apply the same maneuvering skills to everyday living. Sport further provides cross-disability opportunities in which persons with a broad range of physical as well as mental characteristics can come together in a common activity. All of these positive activities can also have an impact on public attitudes, significantly altering the misconceptions of the nondisabled toward the disabled.

Regardless of the extent of their disabilities, participation in competitive sporting events provides young people with an opportunity to better understand their own bodies. Exercise and sport participation can also improve both mental and physical health. For example, athletes who compete and train on a regular basis have a lower incidence of such problems as pressure sores, as well as of other physical and psychological difficulties that often inhibit patients from participating fully in many of life's activities. Individuals who exercise and compete actively in sport increase their strength, flexibility, and stamina for daily living activities.

PATHOPHYSIOLOGY OF CEREBRAL PALSY

To be eligible for participation in the USCPAA or CP-ISRA athletic programs, the athlete must have a condition that results in a non-progressive cerebral motor involvement. Cerebral palsy occurs before, during, or shortly after birth, when the brain is immature (28). Traumatic brain injuries, of course, can occur at any age, and are most commonly caused by motor vehicle accidents. Cerebral vascular accidents, or strokes, tend to be more focal in their involvement of brain function.

Where sporting events are concerned, the key factor for determining athletic participation is the type of motor involvement. There are three primary characteristics that may be associated with the above conditions:

- spasticity,
- athetosis, and
- ataxia.

Spasticity

Spasticity is a hallmark of upper motor neuron lesions (3). In cerebral spasticity there is, of course, weakness, but this is complicated by increased tone and hyperactive stretch reflexes. A good understanding of spasticity and its impact on sport will improve the effectiveness of educators and coaches of athletes with cerebral palsy.

Spasticity is a fluctuating, variable condition which depends upon multiple factors such as the stretch on the muscle, physical and emotional stress, temperature, and fatigue. Spasticity may be significantly increased or decreased. The mediating structure for this condition is a microscopic structure within the muscle, the intrafusal muscle spindle, which is responsive both to static length and to acute or dynamic changes in length. In fact, a key factor is the rate of dynamic stretch: the faster the stretch, the greater the resistance to stretch is developed in the spastic muscle (12).

There comes a point, however, when such tremendous tension is generated in the muscle that the contracting muscle turns off, and the opposing or antagonistic muscle will actually contract. This is the so-called "clasped knife" reflex. Although this is classically described in individuals with spasticity, it is probably present in normal individuals as well. In arm wrestling events, for example, it can be seen that the loser gives way not gradually but suddenly.

In spastic muscles one type of tone tends to predominate within a given muscle group, with the lower extremities tending to be primarily extensor in tone and the upper extremities primarily flexor in tone. This imbalance can lead to major problems such as contractures. Training programs, therefore, need to strive for balance between opposing muscle groups.

Athetosis

Athetosis is a condition that usually arises from involvement of the basal ganglia of the brain (12). Athetosis can be described as an automatic writhing type of movement of the limbs, trunk, and sometimes face. It is often most noticeable when the individual attempts to be stationary or to perform a very slow, controlled movement; it may be much less obvious during a faster, more automatic movement. For example, it is much more observable during walking than during running, and is also clearly evident when performing activities requiring precision. Athetosis can be thought of as the automatic pilot gone awry by failing to turn off when it should.

Ataxia

Ataxia, which originates from involvement of the cerebellum, results in full or partial loss of fine motor control, balance, and equilibrium (12). For example, the patient may have difficulty touching the finger to the nose. Ataxia has also been termed intention tremor, as there is often a significant waver from the normal arc of motion as activities are attempted. Additionally, there is an associated difficulty with the control of rapid alternating movements, which is called dysdiadochokinesia.

Other Characteristics

In addition to the major defining characteristics of spasticity, athetosis, and ataxia, there are other factors associated with cerebral palsy. For example, athletes with these conditions often display primitive reflexes (3). In the asymmetric tonic neck reflex (ATNR) (also called the "fencer's reflex"), when the head is turned to one side the arm on the face side extends and the arm on the back of the head side flexes. The neurologically intact athlete performing a maximal one-handed dumbbell curl displays a remnant of this reflex by turning his or her head away from the weight; however, for athletes with cerebral palsy this reflex may be obligatory. In the symmetrical tonic neck reflex (STNR), neck flexion causes the legs to extend and the arms to flex, while neck extension causes the arms to extend and the legs to flex—a posture that has been likened to that of a cat drinking from a bowl of milk. The tonic labyrinthine reflexes cause flexion in the prone position and extension in the supine position. Familiarity with these reflexes is helpful in coaching: for example, it is very difficult to do the breaststroke if a tonic labyrinthine reflex is keeping one's head under the water. During training one can try to overcome these reflexes, by for example, practicing flexing the arms and neck simultaneously.

Other conditions and characteristics may also be present. Although some authors (2) have associated cerebral palsy with marked levels of mental retardation, in our experience this is less of an issue than has been described. Although there may be some attentional deficits or other cognitive impairment, inappropriate assumptions are sometimes made because of speech difficulties. (Athletes who are truly mentally impaired may be most appropriately placed in Special Olympic activities.) Perceptual deficits may also be present. For example, an individual with hemiparesis may experience loss of the visual field on one side (homonymous hemianopsia). There may also be visual perceptual deficits that can have a significant impact in sporting events. This can sometimes be noted in track events: where the oval lines intersect with the straight lines, the athlete may have difficulty staying in the correct lane.

Seizures can be present in this group of athletes, although they are usually not a significant problem, particularly during aerobic events (8, 18, 20). This is because neurological membranes are more stable in an acidic pH than in an alkaline pH (12), and aerobic events are characterized by a metabolic acidosis that is only partially compensated for by respiration. The decrease in pH thus results in a decreased incidence of seizures. While seizures could potentially be more of a risk in nonaerobic events (particularly if anxiety before the event results in respiratory alkalosis), in our experience this has not been a significant problem. It may be noted, however, that changes in routine (e.g., travel) sometimes cause athletes to neglect to take their seizure medications.

Some medications that are commonly used by this group of athletes affect sport participation. Antiseizure medications such as phenytoin (Dilantin), carbamazepine (Tegretol), and phenobarbital may impair an athlete's attention and concentration. If coaches are aware of this, they can spend more time focusing attention prior to competition. Other medications such as diazepam (Valium) and thorazine hamper heat tolerance. Among the antispasticity medications, diazepam and baclofen (Lioresal) cause sedation, while dantrolene sodium (Dantrium) causes direct muscle weakness by impeding calcium uptake in the sarcoplasmic reticulum, thereby weakening muscle contraction.

CEREBRAL PALSY AND EXERCISE

There is no question that the characteristics associated with cerebral palsy and like conditions give rise to many challenges to performance (23) (Figure 8.1). When it comes to athletic activities, the major problems are twofold. First are the social barriers that reduce opportunities to participate in exercise, recreation, and sport. The other problem is inefficiency and poor economy of movement (26). Both of these factors can be addressed. It is essential to have creative programming which can provide more recreation, exercise, and sport opportunities for individuals with cerebral palsy and related conditions, especially for youth. Issues of economy of motion are more difficult to address, as some of the problems that spasticity, athetosis, and ataxia present are not remediable. Even so, these problems can certainly be minimized through appropriate training and coaching (15). Experience has shown that these athletes are responsive to appropriate aerobic training programs (at least 3 times per week at a pulse rate greater than 65% of the maximum, defined as 220 minus the individual's age).

Strength training is an area of heated controversy in individuals with cerebral palsy and related conditions. Even individuals with diplegia, who only appear to have very minimal involvement in the upper extremities, are affected in upper extremity strength sports. For example, at the 1992 Barcelona Paralimpics, athletes with diplegic cerebral palsy won only 2 out of 30 medals (19). The reasons for this are not completely clear, but may have to do with an inefficiency in the recruitment of motor units in the spastic muscles (21). In fact, some experts argue that resistance training should not be used

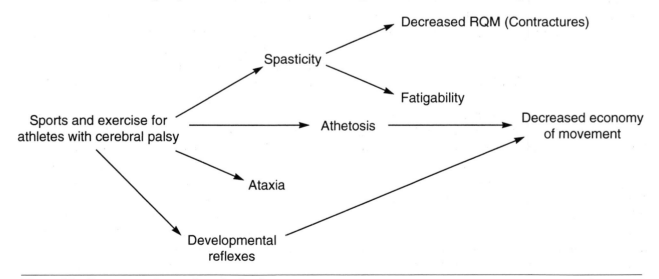

Figure 8.1 Sports, exercise, and cerebral palsy.

in individuals with spasticity of cerebral origin, on the grounds that it could potentially increase spasticity (3). However, this has not been observed to be a problem in the athletes of the USCPAA and CP-ISRA, and research studies have shown that individuals with cerebral palsy and like conditions do indeed benefit from resistance training (13). Certainly it is very important, when constructing a training program for young athletes with cerebral palsy, to be aware of the balance of tone. For example, in the upper extremities flexion often dominates over extension. Therefore, exercise programs should stress strengthening exercises of the extension type, and minimize flexion activities. The athlete should also be monitored constantly to be sure that there is a good balance of tone.

Another important consideration for these athletes is flexibility. Flexibility is a major concern in athletes with spasticity, and to some extent in athletes with athetosis. Many of the key principles of standard stretching are applicable here. For example, in any athlete cold muscles should not be stretched, because they are not as elastic and are more likely to be injured. Thus it is important to start with a warmup period of at least 5 minutes, consisting of an activity such as easy wheeling or running. The stretch itself should occur in a slow, sustained manner so as not to excite the stretch reflex. Stretching should not be painful. The best stretches are prolonged, that is, held for approximately 30 seconds to the point of tightness but not pain. There are also some special considerations for athletes with cerebral palsy. If a coach or fellow athlete is helping in the stretch, hand placement is very important, because tactile stimulation of a muscle with spasticity often causes it to contract. Therefore, when helping an athlete with spasticity stretch flexor muscles, the helper's hand should be on the extensor muscle groups. The contract-relax technique is often helpful in muscles with spasticity. In this technique, the coach or other helper moves the body part to the point of resistance, and the athlete then contracts the muscle isometrically for 10 seconds while the limb is held immobilized. The athlete then relaxes and the coach or helper moves the body part to the new point of resistance. This procedure can be repeated; it should not be painful. For those with special training, proprioceptive neuromuscular facilitation techniques may be useful (17).

Ataxia and coordination deficiencies can also present difficult problems. One way to address them is to train each movement in the simplest fashion. For example, with the body well stabilized, start by only using one arm at a time before the more complex components of the movement are brought in. This is the concept of shaping. Once the activity is established it should be practiced under varying conditions so that the athlete does not fall into stereotypic patterns of control (7).

Visualization of the activity before it is performed may also be helpful. This requires an understanding of neurological involvement. To prevent frustration, the athlete's visualization should reflect his or her individualized sport techniques (7).

Although concern has been expressed that athletes with control disorders such as athetosis may not be able to participate in precision sports, experience has shown that these athletes can successfully and enjoyably participate in precision sports such as boccie. Safety measures are similar to those that should be done with any athlete (16). However, there are a few special considerations of which one should be aware. For example, hydration is very important in an athlete who has difficulty handling oral secretions and who therefore drools. Apart from the fact that a substantial amount of fluid can be lost via drooling, this is often indicative of a swallowing problem, which means the athlete will need even more frequent encouragement and opportunities to drink.

A key concern with cerebral palsy athletes has been the development of overuse disorders (10). Additionally, these athletes, although not at a higher risk for injury, may be at a great risk for more serious injuries and long term residua when they do become injured (10). A possible reason for this is lack of medical intervention. When pain or dysfunction occurs in a cerebral palsy athlete, he or she needs to have prompt and skilled medical assessment and treatment.

One frequently injured site is the shoulder. This tends to arise from a combination of overuse, posture, and spasticity, and occurs most often in wheelchair athletes. Problems can be minimized by proper posture in the chair, as well as by exercise programs that stress stretching of the anterior musculature and strengthening of the scapular stabilizers, humeral depressors, and shoulder external rotators (6).

The benefits of athletic and recreational participation are marked. Psychosocial and self-esteem benefits have been well documented (25). Anecdotal evidence also suggests physical benefits, including improvements in fitness, strength, and range of motion. While some have questioned whether athletes with spasticity of cerebral origin can safely participate in competitive sport (3, 14), these concerns have been unsubstantiated. Studies have shown that there is certainly no increased injury risk (10, 22). In general, the literature indicates that exercise training and sport participation are certainly beneficial (13, 15).

SPECIFIC SPORT AND EXERCISE ACTIVITIES

Because a wide array of neurological characteristics exists in cerebral palsy, there needs to be a wide variety of sports offered to these athletes. A review of the program of the United States Cerebral Palsy Athletic Association gives some idea of the sports available. These include

- archery (see Figure 8.2),
- boccia (also spelled *boccie*),
- bowling,
- track and field sports,
- cross-country events,
- cycling, including tricycling,
- equestrian,
- powerlifting,
- slalom,
- soccer,
- swimming,
- table tennis,
- target shooting,
- wheelchair team handball, and
- winter sports.

Some sports, such as swimming, have the advantage of offering excellent sporting opportunities to a wide range of athletes, from the most severe to those with minimal involvement. Considerable modifications can also be made to adapt these sports to the athletes' needs. Details can be found in the USCPAA and CP-ISRA sports rule manuals. At this time the only true team sports recognized are for wheelchair users, other than soccer.

The classification system for athletes with cerebral motor involvement is based on the three

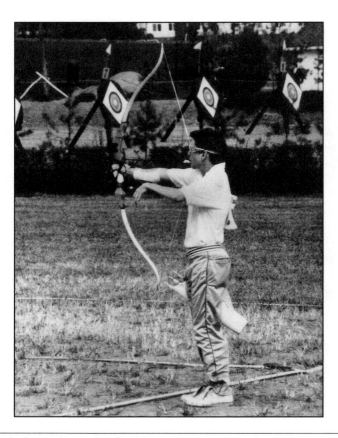

Figure 8.2 A Class VII (ambulatory hemiplegic) athlete competing in archery.

neurological characteristics of spasticity, athetosis, and ataxia. The USCPAA and CP-ISRA share an 8-part classification scheme (Table 8.1). Although it has been called a "functional profile," it is actually an impairment system (that is, it looks at the underlying neurological characteristics). The eight classes include four wheelchair classes and four ambulatory classes. Educators and coaches involved in sport need a solid understanding of this classification system in order to understand the wide range of athletes who can participate in organized sporting events (Table 8.2).

Class I Athletes are those who have severe spastic and/or athetoid involvement with poor functional range of motion. They are unable to functionally propel a manual wheelchair, and must use a motorized wheelchair. However, the mere fact of using a motorized wheelchair does not make a patient eligible for this class; he or she must also meet the neurological profile.

Class II Athletes have severe to moderate spastic or athetoid involvement of all four extremities. They may propel their wheelchair with either their upper or lower extremities. They are able to propel wheelchairs on a level surface and slight inclines. Similarly they may manipulate athletic implements with either their upper or lower extremities.

Class III Athletes are moderately quadriplegic or triplegic, or severely hemiplegic (i.e., with fairly normal functional ability in one upper extremity).

Class IV Athletes are diplegic (i.e., they have primary involvement in the lower extremities). While they have good functional strength in the upper extremities, testing will reveal significant, although subtle, involvement in these extremities as well. This clearly differentiates such patients from spinal cord paraplegic athletes.

Class V Athletes are diplegic, with significant involvement of spasticity in the lower extremities. They participate in sport without the use of a wheelchair.

Class VI Athletes are moderately to severely quadriplegic, spastic, athetoid, or ataxic.

Class VII Athletes are ambulatory hemiplegics.

Class VIII Athletes have very minimal involvement, e.g., minimal hemiplegia or monoplegia. However, they must have a motor involvement significant enough to affect their participation in sport.

Further details on these various classes can be found in the USCPAA and CP-ISRA classification manuals.

Table 8.1 Class Participation in Available Sports

Participation in classes	I	II	III	IV	V	VI	VII	VIII
Archery	x	x	x	x	x	x	x	x
Boccia	x	x						
Cycling	x	x	x	x	x	x	x	x
Equestrian	x	x	x	x	x	x	x	x
Power lifting*				x	x	x	x	x
Track and field	x	x	x	x	x	x	x	x
Slalom	x	x	x	x				
Soccer						x	x	x	x
Wheelchair team handball	x	x	x	x	x	x		

x = appropriate to participate.

*Power lifting based on weight class only—generally Class IV-VIII athletes can participate.

Table 8.2 Topographical Involvement of Cerebral Palsy

Quadriplegia:	All four limbs, head, neck, and trunk
Triplegia:	Primarily three limbs
Diplegia:	Primarily lower limbs, but also some upper limb (different from a spinal cord paraplegic)
Hemiplegia:	One side upper and lower limb, and trunk
Monoplegia:	One limb

Boccia and Cycling

Two sports in particular provide excellent mechanisms for engaging in lifelong recreation. These are boccia, participated in by athletes with rather severe disabilities, and cycling, which most often includes athletes who are ambulatory. In addition to the usefulness of these sports as recreational endeavors, the equipment for both sports is relatively easy to obtain. Unless there are significant problems with balance, most athletes are able to use a standard bicycle and have that bicycle outfitted with basically the same type of equipment used by a nondisabled cyclist (Figure 8.3). Both boccia and cycling can be enjoyed either outdoors or indoors. Boccia is excellent for teaching socialization, strategy, and control. Cycling outdoors can be a leisurely neighborhood activity, or can involve participation in touring clubs, which often undertake extended trips of 50-100 miles or more. Indoors, both bicycles and tricycles can be placed on exercise equipment known as wind trainers, or rollers, which allow individuals to use their own bikes during inclement weather or at night. A wide range of stationary bicycles are also available commercially and can be employed by most people with cerebral palsy. These bicycles may include variations such as arm motion.

Swimming

Swimming has long been recognized for its therapeutic benefits as well as its sport performance opportunities (1). Swimming is appropriate for athletes with a wide range of neurological impairments. As with all swimmers, the development of skills and stroke techniques takes time, energy, practice, and qualified instruction. Far too often athletes, multisport coaches, and parents become discouraged when swim techniques are not mastered in one season. They

may make the inaccurate assessment that the athlete does not have the potential to excel in swimming. Proper instruction by trained swimming professionals experienced in teaching swimmers with disabilities can often make the difference. Once the swimmer has developed basic skills and endurance in the water, then he or she is ready to consider the competitive arena. Further information can be found in *The American Red Cross Adapted Aquatics Manual*.

A few well-trained swimmers appear to be unable to maintain flotation or propulsion without a flotation device. Some coaches promote the use of flotation devices, but their use is controversial (4). Other coaches are of the opinion that if a swimmer initially learns to swim with a flotation device, it may be more difficult to learn to swim without such a device. In elite swimming events, flotation devices are not allowed. On the other hand, a flotation device may enable the beginning swimmer to enjoy success in the water.

The use of shaping techniques, i.e., of working on one isolated skill at a time before introducing the next one, can be very helpful in developing proficiency in swim strokes and kicks. Initially, it is helpful to work with the swimmer's natural strengths; for example, if the swimmer performs the backstroke best, he or she should work on

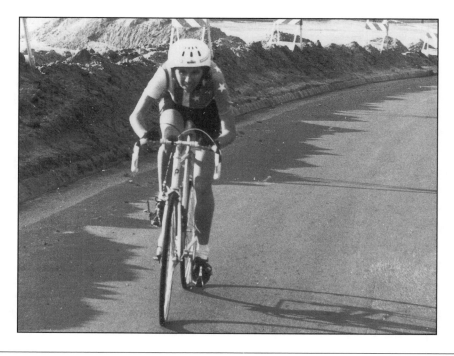

Figure 8.3 A Class VIII athlete competing on a standard bicycle.

that stroke first, developing strength, endurance, breath control, buoyancy control, and skill, before attempting to swim on the front. Strokes may need to be modified according to the swimmer's neurological characteristics, and initial training and movements should be kept slow and simple. If flotation devices are used the coach should monitor the efficiency of the swimmer and change to a different device if the swimmer develops more efficiency in the water. Injuries to swimmers are most often caused by improper transfers into or out of the pool involving undue stress on the arms and shoulders. Proper transfer technique includes primary stabilization of the swimmer by the trunk; pulling on the arms is avoided.

Track and Field Sports

In general, the principles outlined above in the section on neurophysiology must be applied. For ambulatory athletes particular concerns include balance, economy of motion, and technique or skill development and modification. In wheelchair athletes, the most critical factor is positioning. Athletes with cerebral palsy often have spastic involvement of the trunk, with a dominant extensor tone. This tends to extend the hips, put the shoulders backward, and decrease the efficiency of the push. Performance is enhanced when the athlete is positioned in a chair with a "jackknife" seat, that is, a seat that will flex the hips beyond 90 degrees (5). Strapping can also help by bending the knees and keeping the feet on the foot support. Elevating the foot support so that the knees are higher than the hips may also be helpful (Figure 8.4). A strap coming from under the seat across the hips rather than around the waist may help maintain hip flexion and position. Some Class II athletes with cerebral palsy propel their chairs with their feet because of upper extremity limitations; often they use a modified standard lightweight sports chair. Athletes who propel their chairs from a reverse position utilizing a powerful extension thrust benefit from custom-designed racing chairs for control and speed (9).

CONCLUSION

Competitive sport for persons with cerebral palsy allows for a wide range of athlete motivation and rewards. Obviously at the competitive

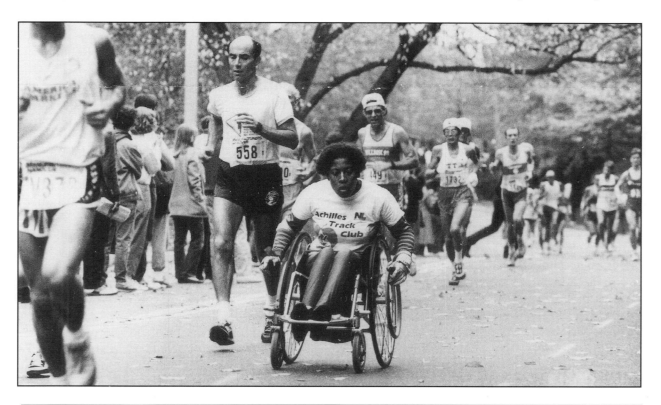

Figure 8.4 A Class III athlete competing in a road race.

level there is a certain degree of intense training and serious competition. At the recreational end of the spectrum the focus is on enjoyment, participation, and gaining a sense of general wellness and fitness. Many activities can be pursued either on an individual basis or in a group setting. The latter allows the person with cerebral palsy to acquire a broad range of interactive social skills in addition to the physical skills associated with the sport or recreational activity.

Whatever the athlete's class or sport, the important thing is to provide opportunities for participation. Studies such as the "Athlete with Disabilities Injury Registry" have shown that athletes with cerebral palsy and other disabilities often fail to meet the minimum American College of Sports Medicine recommendation of 3 days of training per week. Program developers and sports administrators are faced with the challenge of addressing the physical and sociological barriers which limit the quality and quantity of sports opportunities. No matter what a person's neurological characteristics, he or she still has the potential to benefit from, enjoy, and even achieve excellence in physical recreation and sport.

REFERENCES

1. Anderson, L. Swimming to win. In: Jones, J.A., ed. Training guide to cerebral palsy sports. 3d ed. Champaign, IL: Human Kinetics Books; 1988.
2. Bleck, E.E.; Nagel, D.A. Physically handicapped children—a medical atlas for teachers. 2d ed. Orlando, FL: Grune & Straton; 1981.
3. Bobath, B. Motor development: its effect on the general development and application to the treatment of cerebral palsy. Physiotherapy 57:526-532; 1971.
4. Bradley, N.A.; Fuller, J.L.; Pozoa, R.S.; Willmars, L.E. P.F.D.'s. Sports 'N Spokes Minutes p. 23-25; 1981 (May/June).
5. Burd, R.; Grass, K. Strapping to enhance athletic performance of wheelchair competitors with cerebral palsy. Palaestra 3(2):28-32; 1987.
6. Burnham, R.S.; May, L.; Nelson, E.; Steadward, R.; Reid, D.C. Shoulder pain in wheelchair athletes, the role of muscle imbalance. American Journal of Sports Medicine 21(2):238; 1993.
7. Burton, A.W. Assessing the perceptual-motor interaction in the belt mentally disabled and non-handicapped children. Adapted Physical Activity Quarterly 7:325-337; 1990.
8. Cowart, U.S. Should epileptics exercise? Physician Sports Medicine 14(9):183-191; 1986.
9. Davis, R.; Gehlsen, G.; Wilkerson, J. Biomechanical analysis of class II cerebral palsied wheelchair athletes. Adapted Physical Activity Quarterly 1(1):52-61; 1990.
10. Ferrara, M.S. Athlete with disability injury registry study. Miami; 1992.
11. Ferrara, M.S.; Buckley, W.E.; McCann, B.C.; Limbird, T.J.; Powell, J.W.; Robl, R. The injury experience of the competitive athlete with a disability: prevention implications. Medicine and Science in Sports and Exercise 24:184-188; 1992.
12. Guyton, A. Basic human neurophysiology. 3d ed. Philadelphia: W.B. Sanders; 1981.
13. Holland, L.J.; Steadward, R.D. Effects of resistance in flexibility training and strength, spasticity/muscle tone and range of motion of elite athletes with cerebral palsy. Palestra. Summer:27-31; 1990.
14. Hueberman, G. Organized sports activity with cerebral palsy adolescents. Rehabilitation Literature 37:103-106; 1976.
15. Jankowski, L.W.; Sullivan, J. Aerobic and neuromuscular training: an effect of the capacity, efficacy and fatiguability of patients with traumatic brain injuries. Archives of Physical Medicine and Rehabilitation 71:500-504; 1990.
16. Klafs, C.E.; Armheim, D.D. Modern principles of athletic training. 4th ed. St. Louis: C.D. Mosby; 1977.
17. Knot, M.; Voss, D.E. P.N.F.—patterns and techniques. 2d. ed. New York: Harper and Row; 1968.
18. Livingston, S.; Berman, W. Participation of epileptic patients in sports. JAMA 224(2):236-238; 1973.
19. McCubbin, J.; Shasby, G. Effects of isokinetic exercise and adolescents with cerebral palsy. Adapted Physical Activity Quarterly 2:56-64; 1985.
20. Richter, K.J. Seizures in athletes. JOSM 3(4):19-23; 1984.

21. Richter, K.J. Integrated classification: An analysis. Presented at the VISTA 1993 Conference in Alberta, Canada; 1993.

22. Richter, K.J.; Hyman, S.C.; Mushett, C.A.; Ellenberg, M.D.; Ferrara, M.J. Injuries in world class cerebral palsy athletes of the 1988 South Korea Paralympics. Journal of Osteopathic Sports Medicine 5(3):15-18; 1991.

23. Shephard, R. Fitness and special populations. Champaign, IL: Human Kinetics; 1990.

24. Sherrill, C.; Hinson, M.; Gench, B.; Kennedy, S.O.; Low, L. Self-concepts of disabled youth athletes. Perceptual and Motor Skills 70: 1093-1098; 1990.

25. Sherrill, C.; Rainbolt, W. Self-actualization profiles of male able-bodied and cerebral palsied athletes. Adapted Physical Activity Quarterly 5(2):108-119; 1988.

26. Skrotsky, K. Gate analysis in cerebral palsied and non-handicapped children. Archives of Physical Medicine and Rehabilitation 64: 291-295; 1983.

27. Stanley, F.; Blair, E. Postnatal risk factors in the cerebral palsies. In: Stanley, N.F.; Alberman, E., eds. The epidemiology of the cerebral palsies. Philadelphia: J. B. Lippincott; 1984:135-149.

28. Thompson, G.; Rubin, G.; Rubin, I.; Bilenker, R., editors. Comprehensive management of cerebral palsy. New York: Grune & Stratton; 1983.

OTHER RESOURCES

Jones, J.A. editor. Training guide to cerebral palsy sports. 3d ed. Champaign, IL: Human Kinetics Books; 1988.

Sherrill, C. Adapted physical activity, recreation and sport. 4th ed. Dubuque, IA: Brown & Benchmark; 1993.

United States CP Athletic Association (USCPAA)
3810 W. Northwest Hwy.
Dallas, TX 75520
(214) 761-0033

CHAPTER 9

Childhood Arthritis

Shirley A. Scull and Balu H. Athreya
Children's Seashore House
Philadelphia, PA

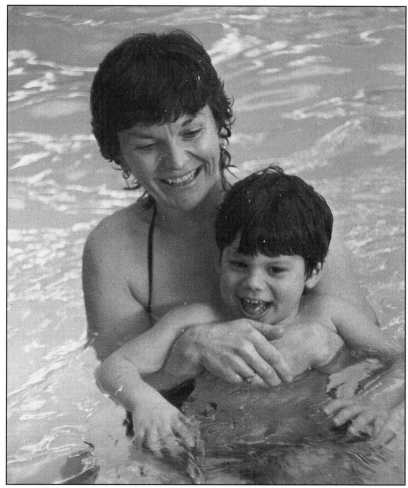

Rheumatic diseases of childhood include a variety of conditions in which inflammation of connective tissues is the primary pathology. Most of these diseases affect multiple organ systems. Juvenile rheumatoid arthritis (JRA) is the most common of these diseases in children in the United States, having replaced rheumatic fever. Other conditions classified as rheumatic diseases include systemic lupus erythematosus (SLE), dermatomyositis (DM), scleroderma (SSC), spondyloarthropathies such as ankylosing spondylitis (AS), polyarteritis nodosa (PAN), and a number of conditions characterized by vasculitis (inflammation of blood vessles), such as Kawasaki disease. Lyme disease can also be considered a rheumatic disorder with a known infectious etiology.

Arthritis is usually a major component of rheumatic diseases. In some diseases it is seen only in the acute stage with no chronic joint disabilities, as in rheumatic fever or Kawasaki disease. In other conditions arthritis may be the major chronic problem leading to deformities, disabilities, and handicaps, as in JRA or AS. Nonrheumatic conditions without inflammation of the joints, such as hemophilia and slipped capital femoral epiphysis, may also cause restricted movement, joint deformities, and serious disabilities.

By definition, *arthritis* means inflammation of the joint. Evidence of joint inflammation must include either swelling of the joint or at least two of the following three features: heat; tenderness or pain on motion; and limited range of motion. One can have an acute arthritis, such as septic arthritis, or chronic arthritis, such as JRA. Children with acute arthritis need joint rest and activity limitation. Children with chronic forms of arthritis need advice on activities and exercises to maintain range of motion, activities of daily living, and a lifestyle as close to age-appropriate normality as possible. The rest of the chapter defines some of these rheumatic diseases and offers advice on appropriate exercise and sport activities.

DESCRIPTION OF JUVENILE RHEUMATOID ARTHRITIS

Juvenile rheumatoid arthritis (JRA) is one of the most common chronic diseases of childhood. Three major subvarieties of JRA exist:

- Systemic
- Polyarticular
- Pauciarticular

Systemic JRA is characterized by high fever, rash, arthritis, enlargement of the liver and spleen, and accumulation of fluid in the pleura and pericardium. Children with this variety are often anemic with high white cell and platelet counts. There are no laboratory tests that are specific for this disease. The diagnosis is based on a pattern of clinical symptoms and is a diagnosis of exclusion. Children with JRA may require hospitalization, particularly in the early stages. They may not be able to take part in any sport activities early in the course of the disease because they often have acute arthritis, general aches and pains, fatigue, and stiffness. If they have pericarditis, activities have to be limited until it is fully controlled. If they have anemia, their energy level is lowered. Although the early course is characterized by fever and systemic features, severe polyarticular disease often develops over a period of months, and the systemic features tend to disappear.

Polyarticular JRA is subdivided into two categories: rheumatoid factor positive (RF+) and rheumatoid factor negative (RF−). Both varieties are characterized by the presence of arthritis involving more than five joints, as well as morning stiffness. However, RF + JRA is more likely to be associated with destructive arthritis, nodules, hip involvement, and systemic vasculitis than is RF − JRA. It is also less likely to enter remission. Almost any joint (including cricoarytenoid of the larynx) may be involved. Knee joints are involved most commonly, but hip disease has greater impact on functional outcome. Involvement of the cervical spine is common, leading to restricted range of motion and subluxation of C1 on C2. Children with arthritis of the cervical spine should not be allowed to do headstands or jump on trampolines. They may have to wear a protective collar during car transport. The RF− variety is likely to enter remission, but the RF+ variety often continues into adulthood.

Pauciarticular JRA is characterized by arthritis affecting four or fewer joints. There are two subtypes: those with the presence of antinuclear antibody in the serum (ANA+), and those without antinuclear antibody (ANA−). The ANA+ variety is usually seen in young females, and the knee is the joint most frequently involved. The major concern in the ANA+ group is the increased incidence of iridocyclitis, or inflammation of the iris and ciliary body, with complications such as cataract, glaucoma and blindness. The eye may be involved even after arthritis enters remission.

The ANA– variety is very similar to the ANA+ variety, except for its more benign prognosis and lower incidence of eye disease. However, when ANA– pauciarticular arthritis occurs in the preadolescent or adolescent age group, it is hard to know whether the condition is pauciarticular JRA or the onset of one of the seronegative spondyloarthropathies. In general, prognosis for remission is better for the pauciarticular group than for the systemic or the polyarticular groups.

The treatment of these diseases is undergoing rapid change with the introduction of many new nonsteroidal anti-inflammatory drugs and methotrexate. Because these are chronic diseases, the focus has to be on helping the whole child and the family grow and develop in spite of the disease.

Pharmacological treatment of JRA includes nonsteroidal anti-inflammatory drugs (NSAIDs) as the first line of therapy. Depending on the type of arthritis and response one may need to modify the regimen, add another drug, or switch to another NSAID. For example, a child with fever (systemic JRA) or severe morning stiffness may do better with indomethacin or small doses of glucocorticoids. In children whose arthritis does not respond to adequate doses of NSAIDs, one may wish to add one of the second-line agents. Examples of this class include intramuscular gold salts, oral gold, d-penicillamine, hydroxychloroquine (Plaquenil), and sulfasalazine (Azulfidine). All of these medications have potential for serious side effects such as bone marrow suppression and kidney disease.

Glucocorticoids are disliked by rheumatologists but must be prescribed for children with severe systemic disease, serositis (pleurisy, pericarditis), rapidly progressive disease, and severe eye disease unresponsive to topical steroid therapy. The adverse effects are numerous. The most relevant to sport and arthritis are

- muscle weakness,
- hypertension,
- osteoporosis, and
- aseptic necrosis of bone.

In spite of adequate treatment, some children do poorly and develop severe deformities. Fortunately, this is a small group (<20%). These children may require surgical intervention, which includes soft tissue releases, synovectomy, fusion, and joint replacement. Mortality is very low (<1%). Amyloidosis, a major cause of mortality in Europe, is rare in the United States.

Ankylosing Spondylitis (AS)

Ankylosing spondylitis belongs to a general category of conditions called seronegative spondyloarthropathies. This category includes

- Reiter syndrome,
- psoriatic arthritis,
- arthritis associated with inflammatory bowel disease, and
- ankylosing spondylitis.

Characteristically, patients have asymmetric arthritis of large and small joints of the extremities. Although the name suggests spondylitis and sacroiliitis as essential features, one may not see these features during the early course of the disease. However, patients with AS may have low back pain, loss of lumbar lordosis, and sacroiliac tenderness. Enthesitis (inflammation at the site of tendon insertion) is very characteristic of this group, especially in the Achilles tendon.

Decrease in chest expansion and spinal mobility are musculoskeletal consequences of these diseases. Aortic regurgitation, cardiac arrhythmia, and acute iridocyclitis are some of the systemic features.

Prognosis for life is good, though there may be long-term morbidity due to involvement of hip joints, spine, aorta, and loss of chest expansion.

Systemic Lupus Erythematosus (SLE)

Systemic lupus erythematosus is a multisystem disease characterized pathologically by vasculitis and serologically by the presence of a variety of circulating autoantibodies such as ANA or antiDNA. Although arthritis is an extremely common manifestation of SLE, it is not usually chronic and is not associated with joint dysfunction and deformity. Bone and joint problems in

SLE are most often associated with glucocorticoids used for treatment. These include aseptic necrosis of bone (e.g., of the femur or humerus), infections, and osteoporosis, which can lead to fractures. Muscle wasting and weakness may be caused by myositis as part of the disease, myopathy caused by glucocorticoid therapy, and inactivity due to fatigue. Cardiac involvement in SLE may produce pericarditis, myocarditis, or valvulitis. Anemia is common and may be caused either by hemolysis, greater need for iron (anemia of chronic disease), or gastrointestinal bleeding (resulting from vasculitis or steroid therapy). Thrombocytopenia may lead to easy bruising or major bleeding into internal organs. Involvement of the central or peripheral nervous system may lead to seizures, coma, stroke, or paralysis of extremities. Behavioral changes may reflect vasculitis of the central nervous system, drug toxicity (steroids), or adaptation to a chronic illness.

The kidney is almost universally involved in SLE. Involvement may be very minor with full remission or very severe, requiring renal transplantation.

Both morbidity and mortality are higher in SLE than in other rheumatic diseases. However, advances in the management of acute problems in intensive care units have contributed to better prognosis for children with SLE. The mainstay of therapy is the use of glucocorticoids. Judicious use of nonsteroidal anti-inflammatory drugs, antimalarials (hydroxychloroquine), and cytotoxic agents (e.g., cyclophosphamide) has made it possible for most of these children to lead a reasonably normal life.

Scleroderma

Scleroderma is characterized primarily by fibrotic changes of the skin and by vaso-occlusive problems. Scleroderma is either localized or systemic. In children, the localized variety is more common than the systemic variety and often involves the extremities. It is characterized initially by linear bands of edema and skin thickening. Atrophic changes may involve deeper tissues and lead to soft tissue contractures, limitation of joint motion, and atrophy.

Systemic scleroderma is also divided into two subtypes. The first, limited form (lSSC), is characterized by calcinosis, Raynaud phenomenon,

esophageal involvement, sclerodactyly, and telangiectasia. The second subtype, diffuse variety (dSSC), is characterized by scleroderma and involvement of the gastrointestinal tract, heart, lungs, and kidneys. Myositis also may occur in combination with scleroderma. Treatment of scleroderma is unsatisfactory. D-Penicillamine and glucocorticoids used early in the course of the disease may be beneficial.

Dermatomyositis

Dermatomyositis is relatively rare and is characterized by skin rash over the face and extensor aspect of the joints, and by severe myositis involving primarily the proximal muscles. During the recovery phase, many children develop calcium deposits under the skin, in muscle, or around the joints. The calcium deposits lead to contractures. Involvement of respiratory muscles and aspiration pneumonia may lead to chronic pulmonary problems.

The mainstay of treatment of dermatomyositis is glucocorticoids. High dose prednisone (pulse steroid) given intravenously and methotrexate have reduced the mortality considerably in this disease. Morbidity is high because of severe contractures, subcutaneous calcification, steroid toxicity, respiratory problems, and gastrointestinal involvement.

Although there are many other arthritis-related conditions, they are less common than those just described. The following sections deal with exercise and sport in childhood arthritis.

EXERCISE AND ARTHRITIS

Benefits and risks exist for children with arthritis who are involved in sport or exercise. The benefits are substantial, and risks can be minimized with appropriate information.

Effect of Arthritis on Exercise Tolerance and Sport Performance

During the acute phase of arthritis, joint effusion may interfere with the force of muscular contraction around the joint. Protective muscle spasm occurs, and agonists and antagonists may fire simultaneously. The joint range of motion is restricted. If this pattern continues even for a few days, muscle mass is lost and the muscles get weaker. Muller, 1970 has shown that muscle atrophies at a rate of approximately 3% per week at rest (14). Biomechanical changes in joint alignment may result, which leads to further pain and effusion and sets up a vicious cycle. This cycle is diagrammed in Figure 9.1.

Myositis, which accompanies many of the rheumatic diseases, may also contribute to muscle weakness. Glucocorticoids used to treat many of the rheumatic diseases are known to cause myopathy. Anemia of chronic disease adds to the problem of general fatigue and weakness. All of these factors contribute to generalized inactivity and loss of endurance.

As shown in Figure 9.2, in the presence of chronic arthritis, contracture of soft tissues around the joints and destructive changes within the joints lead to limited range of motion. Muscle mass and strength are lost because of disuse. Because the growth plates are still open in the immature skeleton, deformities such as leg length discrepancy, scoliosis, or genu valgus (knock knees) may occur. Deformities become accentuated from continued use of the joint in an unnatural position. Limited joint range of motion, muscle weakness, and deformities lead to abnormal gait patterns and impairment of other activities of daily living.

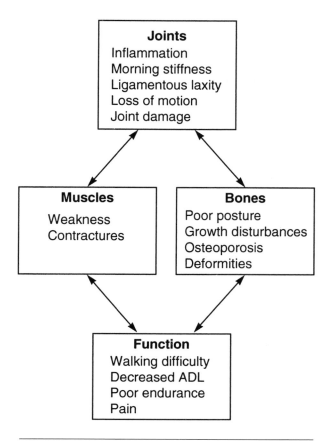

Figure 9.2 Musculoskeletal problems in chronic arthritis.

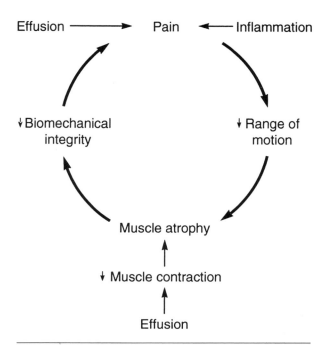

Figure 9.1 The vicious cycle of musculoskeletal impairments, which can lead to disability.
Reprinted from Hicks (1990).

Children with chronic arthritis have reduced cardiopulmonary reserve. Giannini & Protas (8) studied cardiopulmonary capacity in 30 subjects having JRA and controls matched for age, sex, and body surface area. The researchers used cycle ergometry to test $\dot{V}O_2$max, highest workload completed, exercise duration, and peak heart rate. They concluded that all parameters were significantly less for the JRA population than for their matched controls, but that the decreased aerobic capacity did not correlate with the severity of articular disease. To prevent deconditioning, the authors recommend early exercise programs for patients with arthritis.

Klepper, Darbee, Effgen, and Singsen (12) used the Health Related Physical Fitness Test (HRPFT) to compare 20 children with polyarticular JRA with matched controls. They also compared the scores with published normative values. Children with JRA had significantly poorer scores on the 9-minute walk-run and sit-ups. They scored in the 24th percentile on the sit-and-reach test, but this did not reach significance when compared with controls. There was no difference in skinfold thickness and no correlation between severity of disease and fitness scores. Therefore, it appears that children with chronic arthritis are deconditioned in comparison to their peers, regardless of the severity of their disease.

Potential Benefits of Exercise on Arthritis

Exercise has the following beneficial effects for children with arthritis:

- Maintains maximum joint flexibility
- Maintains normal muscle strength
- Prevents deconditioning of the cardiopulmony system
- Maintains normal bone density
- Improves self-esteem

Limited research describing the effects of exercise on children with arthritis is available. For example, can children with chronic arthritis such as JRA continue to be active in games, physical education, and sports if they want to? Do children with arthritis who continue to be active develop flares of arthritis more often or develop degenerative disease earlier than those who are more sedentary? There are very few studies on which to base recommendations.

Recently, one controlled study on adults with osteoarthritis of the knee showed that exercise three times a week for over 12 weeks did not lead to increased cartilage breakdown (3). In another study, voluntary aerobic exercise two times a week by patients with rheumatoid arthritis was not associated with radiological progression of the disease over a period of 4 years (21).

In the absence of solid evidence about the effects of exercise on children with arthritis, recommendations are based on the following two realities:

1. It is hard to keep children inactive when they feel well—unlike adults!
2. Activity is clearly better for the emotional well-being of a child.

In chronic diseases, it is important to plan for the child's whole future, not just for the disease category. Therefore, the authors encourage children to be as active as possible, with precautions taken for specific conditions such as cervical spine instability or for potential risks such as contact sport.

Potential Adverse Effects of Exercise on Arthritis

Exercise or sport activities done in excess have the potential to exacerbate the disease. If after an activity the child experiences pain, fatigue, weakness, decreased ROM, or swelling for more than an hour, it can be assumed that the child has gone beyond the safety threshold. Wear and tear on cartilaginous defects can occur, especially with activities that load additional weight onto the joints, such as jogging. Joints not protected properly by normal muscle strength are at greater risk for ligamentous injuries, such as those that might occur with a valgus stress to the knee joint. Joints without full range of motion and with underlying osteoporosis are also at greater risk for fracture when external forces are applied. Therefore, contact sports such as hockey, football, and wrestling are generally contraindicated for patients with arthritis. Other restrictions include:

- gymnastics that place weight on the upper extremity joints, such as occurs when using the parallel bars, rings, or pommel horse; also, push-ups, handstands, cartwheels
- excessive collision of the unprotected wrist with outside forces, such as in volleyball and perhaps basketball
- extreme neck motions or weight-bearing on the cervical spine, such as with forward and backward rolls, headstands, and the like
- repeated jarring of the lower extremities, such as occurs with jogging and high-impact aerobics.

Precautions to Prevent Adverse Effects

Children should be encouraged to participate in physical education class to their tolerance. Floor exercises emphasizing flexibility and strengthening are beneficial. Sometimes activities can be modified by using lighter-weight equipment such as foam balls, or wiffle balls and plastic bats, to decrease the forces on the wrist and allow participation in the sport. Sometimes orthotics are worn to protect an involved joint such as the knee, ankle, or wrist. Some children may require an individualized adaptive physical education program or even physical therapy treatments in school (22). Children with severe disease might also become involved in wheelchair sports or may participate in sport activities as the trainer.

Depending on the number of joints involved, children may be able to participate in carefully selected sports with proper coaching and protective gear. Table 9.1 outlines suggestions regarding sport selection. As already noted, children with arthritis should avoid contact sports such as football, hockey, and boxing because of the potential for joint injury. Students may attempt sports requiring high neuromuscular skill, but may not be successful. Ability to use the upper

Table 9.1 Sport Selection for Patients With JRA

Recommended: Most individuals with JRA can participate safely.

Badminton	Darts	Swimming
Billiards	Fishing	Table tennis
Croquet	Horseshoes	Walking/hiking
Cycling	Shuffleboard	Wiffle ball

Self-limiting: Reasonable activities in which students may try to participate to the best of their ability. The risk/benefit ratio should be evaluated for each individual.

Baseball (not pitcher/ catcher)	Cross-country skiing	Ice skating
	Dance	Roller skating
Basketball	Golf	Rowing
Canoeing	Horseback riding (supervised)	Softball
Cheerleading		Tennis

Contraindicated: Sports for which the risk of joint damage outweighs the benefits.

Ballet (on pointe)	Gymnastics	Track
Bowling	Hockey	Trampoline
Boxing	Lacrosse	Tumbling
Diving (if C spine involved)	Martial arts	Volleyball
	Skateboarding	Weightlifting
Downhill skiing	Soccer	Wrestling
Football	Speed skating	

Note. Those general guidelines should assist in planning sporting activities for the student with JRA. However, specific recommendations for each child should be developed jointly with the physician or physical therapist since children with rheumatic disease exhibit a wide range of disabilities.

body or the lower body will depend on each student's particular joint involvement. Obviously, a student with pauciarticular JRA involving one ankle and wrist may succeed at a racket sport using the uninvolved upper extremity. Lower-body sports are generally more difficult because of the need to run or maneuver in some way. An exception to this is cycling, which avoids joint trauma because it is non-weight-bearing. Activities classified as low-dynamic, such as croquet, will be easier than highly dynamic or mobile sports, and highly static sports should be easiest. Aerobic precautions should be related to the cardiopulmonary status of the student, and aerobic activity should be encouraged if precautions do not exist.

Coaches must be mindful that JRA has a fluctuating course, causing children with the diseases to have good and bad days. Joint conservation and daily pacing are important principles. Exercise is not the cure for arthritis, and when children with JRA request a break they should be given one. Indeed, they should not be scheduled for as much playing time as their peers. Coaches should have a clear understanding of the child's problems and should know whether they involve joint inflammation, muscle weakness, ligamentous laxity, reduced flexibility, or a combination of these. Joints should be moved through their available range of motion, allowing muscles around the joints adequate time to warm up prior to play.

Consideration of joint pathology should be given when deciding the position a child will play on a team. For example, children trying to begin Little League should not be trained as pitchers or catchers because of the potential for overuse injuries to the elbow during throwing or to the knees during squatting. Children who cannot participate physically may be involved as scorekeeper or trainer, and may benefit from learning the rules of the game and socializing with peers.

Sometimes a sport orthotic such as a knee cage or wrist splint can be used during the game to protect a joint that is at risk for injury. The orthotic should be individually prescribed and fitted with input based on a thorough musculoskeletal evaluation. To protect the knee joint, adequate medial and lateral uprights must be present to prevent valgus and varus forces. The pull-on type of elastic sleeve has no place as a sport orthotic. At the ankle, airsplints may be used to reduce varus and valgus stresses. Properly fitting sneakers are essential, and cushioned orthotic insoles may be needed to redistribute the weight-bearing forces onto the foot surfaces that can tolerate them. In the upper extremity, the wrist may require stablization from a splint in about 20 degrees of extension. Wrist splints may be worn during racket sports.

Appropriate Responses to Adverse Effects

Rest, ice, compression, and elevation (RICE) is the appropriate first-aid protocol for an injured child with arthritis. After an injury, the player should not return to the game for a minimum of 24 hours. Treatment in the locker room may involve whirlpool and range-of-motion exercises to decrease pain and maintain flexibility. Active range-of-motion exercises in a non-weight-bearing position (e.g., ankle pumps) may be useful for reducing swelling. Some players may require an assistive device such as crutches if an involved knee is severely aggravated by the sport. This is actually just another form of rest for lower extremity joints. Crutches may not be useful if the player also has significant elbow or wrist involvement.

EXERCISE AND SPORT PROGRAMS FOR CHILDREN WITH ARTHRITIS

The exercise program for a child with arthritis should progress in a slow and logically graded manner (see Figure 9.3). The foundation of the exercise prescription should consist of active and active-assisted range-of-motion exercises to promote flexibility. Isometric and/or isotonic exercises can be added to improve strength. The next level of difficulty consists of aerobic exercises. Patients with sufficient flexibilty, strength, and aerobic conditioning may be considered for recreational exercises appropriate for their disease (11). Depending on the severity of disease, the exercise program may be integrated with regular physical education, or conducted by a physical therapist.

Flexibility exercises that move each joint of the body through their available range of motion

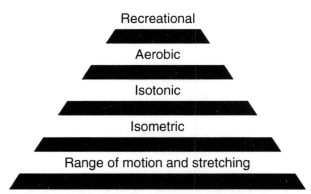

Children with arthritis should begin with range-of-motion exercises. They may progress upward on the pyramid as their disease regresses or is controlled medically.

Figure 9.3 Pyramid of graded progress in an exercise program.
Reprinted from Hicks (1990).

are the foundation of the exercise prescription. Slow, rhythmic movements that involve several joints are recommended. Students must be observed to ensure that they do not substitute movements through the trunk, for example, when shoulder or hip joints are restricted. Exercises must also be planned to stretch the muscles that cross two joints, such as the hamstrings or gastrocnemius (19). Figure 9.4 illustrates several flexibility exercises. Generally, active exercises done by students themselves are preferred to stretching or passive exercises. Exercises should be done in positions that allow gravity to assist in the direction of the movement.

Positioning is also used to maintain flexibility. Stretching out prone or supine, as opposed to sitting all day, helps overcome the tendency for flexion contractures to develop in the hips and knees for the student with severe arthritis (18).

Students may be most stiff in the morning, causing difficulty walking and poor school attendance. Stiffness may also occur after periods of prolonged sitting. It is generally recommended that students get up and walk about the room at least every hour to avoid inactivity stiffness (2).

Strengthening exercises should be done for all major antigravity muscle groups and for those muscles that are antagonistic to contractures (7). In the lower extremities these include the hip extensors and abductors, knee extensors, and ankle muscles.

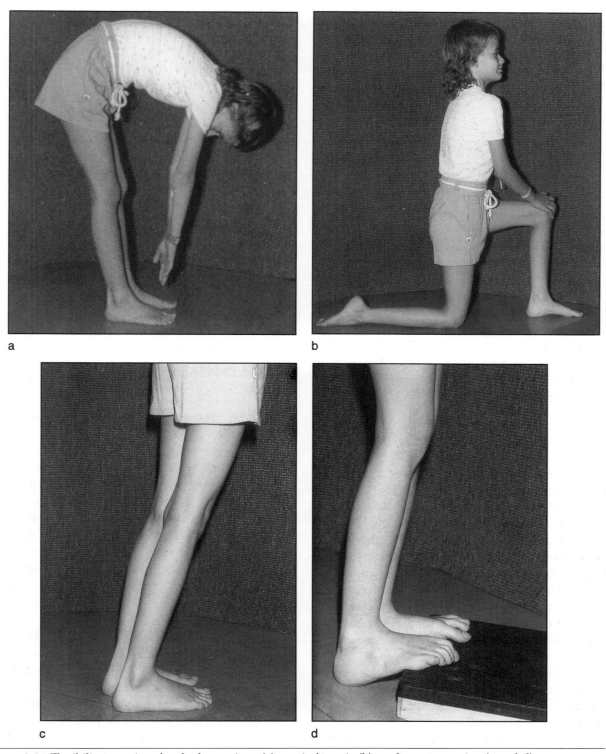

Figure 9.4   Flexibility exercises for the hamstrings (a), rectis femoris (b), and gastrocnemius (c and d).

Strengthening exercises can be either *isometric*, involving no motion, or *isotonic*, involving motion as muscles shorten or lengthen. Isometric exercises are ideal for joints with acute arthritis because there is no joint surface movement. Children should hold contractions for 3 to 6 seconds to increase muscle strength. Isotonic exercises (especially concentric, or shortening, contractions) are done using a program of low weights with repetitions just to the point of muscle fatigue. Resistance is increased when students are strong enough to complete 20 repetitions actively without fatigue, but should always be less than 1 kilogram. *Eccentric* exercises are those in which the muscle lengthens instead of shortening; an example for quadriceps would be squatting.

The same exercise principles apply to the upper extremities. Wands may be used in the upper extremity to encourage using both arms overhead. Special emphasis should be placed on the rotator cuff and the deltoid, which stabilizes the glenohumeral joint. The triceps and wrist extensors should be strengthened to oppose typical flexion contracture at the elbow and wrist. Grip may be strengthened with a variety of materials such as putty or elastic bands.

Aerobic exercises should be considered to prevent deconditioning. To have a conditioning effect, exercises must be performed for at least 20 minutes, three times per week. Aerobic exercises can be safely planned at about 60% of maximum heart rate (which is calculated using the formula 220 – the individual's age × 60%) (16).

Aquatic Exercise

Aquatic exercise is one of the best therapeutic modalities for patients with arthritis (4, 13, 20). Total-body exercise can be accomplished with minimal stress or strain on the joints because the buoyancy of the water supports the weight of the limbs and protects the joints from bearing weight. A warm pool also provides muscle relaxation and reduces pain. The upper body and lower body are involved in total movement patterns during aquatic programs. The Arthritis Foundation sponsors therapeutic aquatics programs across the country, although many are geared toward adults rather than children.

Specific aquatic exercise programs can be designed to improve flexibility and strength. Depending on the patient's position, the water may assist the movement when moving toward the surface, resist the movement when moving toward the bottom, or simply eliminate gravity when moving horizontally. Exercises should be done slowly, and rhythmically, without stopping. The faster the speed of the exercise, the greater the resistance of the water against the limb. The patient can also perform postural exercises such as pelvic tilts against the side of the pool wall. Diaphragmatic breathing can improve chest expansion, promote relaxation, and increase buoyancy.

An aerobic exercise program may also include non-weight-bearing exercise in deep water or jogging in water. Rhodes (17) conducted a pilot study of 7 subjects, aged 4 to 18, who underwent 20 minutes of aerobic training in the pool three times per week for 12 weeks. The subjects showed a lower resting heart rate and had no exacerbation of their disease, even though $\dot{V}O_2$max did not change significantly. Swimming or walking laps in the pool can also improve cardiovascular endurance. The amount of time spent in each session may be increased as the patient's endurance improves.

Walking laps forward, backward, and sideways may be done in deep water. If the instructor cuts a path in the water by walking ahead of the student, the activity will be easier because of less water turbulence. Braiding sideways, also known as the grapevine, is an exercise involving cross steps alternating in front and in back of each other. Some patients who are unable to walk on land are able to walk comfortably in deep water.

Pool water should ideally be heated to a temperature bewteen 88° and 92 °F (31° to 33 °C) for the patient with arthritis. Because this temperature may be difficult to find at community pools, students may swim in cooler water and evaluate the effect on stiffness and pain. Cardiovascular responses will need to be monitored more closely as the pool temperature increases. Aerobic programs are performed most safely in a pool temperature between 82° and 86 °F (27° to 30 °C).

Each participant should be evaluated for swimming ability and the need for flotation devices. Young children or older nonswimmers may benefit from a personal flotation device, while others may be assisted by inflatable water wings worn on the upper arms, flotation belts around the waist, or bar floats that are grasped during activities. Sometimes one-on-one assistance is necessary in the water until a student feels comfortable. Safety issues such as the ratio of students to instructors must also be considered when deciding on flotation equipment.

Other special devices for increasing resistance include water mitts or hand paddles for arm exercise, and flipper fins for the feet. Snorkels may allow some children with restricted cervical spine motion to enjoy the water in a face-down position. Preschoolers may use various water toys such as boats, containers, or waterwheels; older children may be involved with a variety of aquatic games such as floating volleyball or basketball.

Water depth is extremely important. The student should be able to stand holding onto the side in some area of the pool. Shallow water exercises may be done in the sitting and prone positions if water depth is 1 to 2 feet. The amount of weight-bearing on the lower extremities may be controlled by varying the water depth (20), which can be especially important following an injury or an orthopedic procedure where the physician orders limited weight-bearing for a period of time. A movable pool floor such as those available from AFW of Olean, New York, allows full barrier-free access to the pool as well as selection of any depth desired (see Figure 9.5).

Patients with severe arthritis who walk with an assistive device or who use a wheelchair will require a barrier-free locker room with accessible showers and toilets. The entrance and exit to the pool should have ramps or be outfitted with a special chairlift. Instructors should plan ahead to know that students have a safe method of entering and exiting the pool. Care must also be taken on the deck and locker room floor to avoid falls on slippery surfaces.

The student with mild impairment may be able to progress to swimming. Swimming is the best activity for patients with arthritis to improve flexibility, strength, and endurance. Teaching the student a variety of strokes such as the crawl, the sidestroke, and the breaststroke assures a workout for all muscle groups. Stroke choice may also need to be based on the pattern of joint involvement. Recreational swimming is usually best for this population, but individuals may choose to compete either individually or on a team if their skills warrant this. Atlantoaxial stability should be cleared prior to allowing diving starts, the butterfly, or the breaststroke (6).

Cycling

Cycling, whether on a tricycle, bicycle, or exercise ergometer, is an ideal form of exercise for most children with arthritis (15). It can improve lower-extremity strength, flexibility, and cardiovascular endurance. Upper-body cycle ergometers are also available. Cycling can be done year round by children over age 3, indoors or outdoors, individually or in groups. It is easy to learn and the equipment is simple and inexpensive, although some minor modifications may be necessary to accommodate students' specific limitations. Cycling is generally noncontact and provides reduced loads on the lower-extremity joints as compared with walking or jogging. It may also be considered a functional means of mobility for younger children by allowing a child with limited ability to play on the playground at recess or to get to and from the cafeteria or library, for example.

The bicycle is extremely energy-efficient and causes no trauma to the joints. The torso weight is supported by the seat, reducing the compressive forces at the knee to 1.2 times body weight, as compared to walking, which places 2 to 4 times body weight on the knee (15). Because of the seat support, even patients who are obese can exercise comfortably. Bicycling strengthens the large muscle groups of the lower extremities, especially the quadriceps (vastus medialislateralis), gluteals, and gastrocnemius. With the addition of toe clips, the hamstrings may also be given a workout.

As an aerobic exercise, cycling has been shown to increase $\dot{V}O_2max$ to levels reached while running. Harkcom, Lampman, Banwell, and Caster showed that a minimum of 15 minutes of cycling three times per week improved aerobic capacity, decreased joint counts, improved daily living activities, and decreased pain and fatigue in adult women with arthritis (9).

The bicycle should be lightweight with at least 10 gears and a comfortable foam or gel-padded seat. An all-terrain bike (ATB) or mountain bike has a broad wheelbase, fatter tires, and upright handlebars with the brakes and shifting equipment mounted on them. Riders with arthritis will be most comfortable in an upright posture because this decreases the need to bear weight on the wrists or hands and decreases the lumbar kyphosis that may aggravate back pain. A girl's frame (called a *mixte frame*) will be easier to mount and dismount.

A bicycle helmet is a requirement for preventing head injury. Padded gloves can decrease the road shock transmitted to the upper extremities.

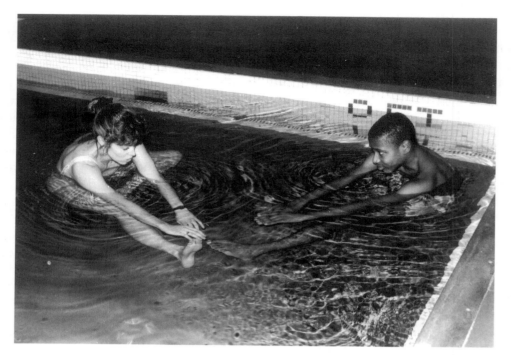

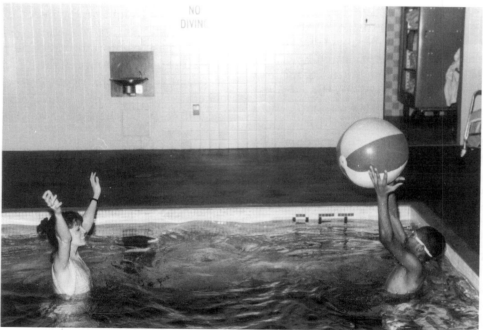

Figure 9.5   Aquatic exercises can be planned for both shallow and deep water if the pool is equipped with a movable floor.

A mirror to view approaching traffic is added for safety. Elbow and knee protectors can be slipped on to add protection from falls. Toe clips or sandals with straps allow new riders to learn to ride more easily and allow experienced riders to use their flexors as well as their extensors. Hand brake extensions can increase the ease of gripping the brake. It is essential that riders be able to operate the braking mechanism easily and independently.

For indoor bicycling, a special stand that raises the rear wheel off the floor can be purchased to convert a standard bike to an exercise bike. Patients with limited knee range of motion can purchase a range limiter that shortens the distance from the shaft to the pedal.

The bicycle must be fitted to the correct size. The seat height should be set with the foot at the apex of the downstroke, with the knee in 10° to 15° of flexion. If the seat height is set much higher, riders will shift weight from side to side while riding. The handlebars should be raised to allow upright posture and prevent excessive weight-bearing through the arms.

The ideal cycling program should allow 2 to 5 minutes of warm-up, 20 minutes of riding at 70 to 90 rpm, and 5 minutes of cooldown. Patients with moderate to severe joint disease or with poor endurance may need to build up to this level. Exercise should be done at least 3 times per week in order to obtain a training effect. Cadences of less than 70 rpm as well as a seat height that is too low increases the patella-femoral forces at the knee. Outdoor riders should be taught to shift to lower gears when hills are encountered.

Some children with arthritis have never learned to ride a two-wheeled bike because their disease has interfered with the usual developmental schedule for introducing this activity. Most children learn to balance by taking a few falls when their training wheels are removed. Letting the child with knee involvement fall may not be advisable, but extra pads may be added to the knees and elbows and training wheels can be left on. Alternatives include a large chain-driven tricycle, a tandem bike, or an indoor exercise bike.

Dance

Dance is not as safe a form of exercise as swimming or cycling, but may be undertaken by some students with certain guidelines and an interested teacher. There are various types of dance, including classical ballet, jazz, tap, ballroom, square dance, aerobic dance, and others. Gymnastics is also included in the curriculum of many dance classes. A typical dance class for a young school-age child might include ballet work at the barre, ballet floor exercises, gymnastics, and tap for a total of 1 hour. Private lessons are usually more focused, and may be scheduled for half an hour.

Students with joint disease will find it easier to perform the barre exercises than to perform floor work. Many of the basic postures in classical ballet require 90 degrees of external rotation of the hip; teachers must ensure that students toe out from the hip joint and do not substitute with tibial torsion. Extension postures of the hip will also be difficult, and students may substitute with lumbar lordosis. Teachers must be aware of normal postural alignment and ensure that students are completing the maneuver with the appropriate joint range of motion rather than substituting. Dance activity should not be undertaken if it increases joint pain.

Ballet using pointe technique in toe shoes (shoes with blocked toes) should be avoided for children with lower extremity joint disease because this places unnatural forces on the metatarsal-phalangeal joints, the arch, and the ankle. Instead, it is preferable to encourage jazz, modern, or character dance performed in flat slippers on the ball of the foot.

Tap can be undertaken if ankle and foot involvement is not severe. Some tap steps that require a hop may be modified to decrease the compressive forces. Certain steps or routines will be harder than others.

Gymnastics should generally be avoided because almost all postures involve weight-bearing on the upper extremities (e.g., back-bends) or cervical spine.

Aerobics may be low-impact or high-impact. The low-impact variety of aerobic dance may be undertaken if there are no cardiopulmonary precautions. Variety in the routine helps to avoid muscle fatigue. Weight shifting and knee flexing may substitute for running maneuvers.

Several dance routines have been designed specifically for patients with arthritis. Teenagers and adults can perform the "Range-of-Motion Dance" (10) or "People with Arthritis Can Exercise (PACE)" (1) that can be done from a sitting position or a wheelchair. Younger children may enjoy a range-of-motion video called "Where Are the Indians?" that includes eight different dances to music with varying levels of difficulty (5). Each dance focuses on joints in different parts of the body.

Certainly one of the appeals of dance is that exercise is set to music. The patterns generally involve total body movement, and can often be done to the best of the learners' ability while still being enjoyable. They may be done individually or in groups, and are part of the normal activities undertaken by their peers.

CONCLUSION

This chapter reviewed the common rheumatic diseases of childhood and discussed appropriate exercise and sport activities, as well as those that may be harmful. Specific recommendations for each child are best formulated by interacting directly with the medical team responsible for the child's care. Children with rheumatoid disease exhibit a wide range of disabilities, and each child must have an individualized plan. An understanding and caring teacher or coach should help the child lead as active a life as is safely possible.

REFERENCES

1. Arthritis Foundation. People with arthritis can exercise (PACE). Atlanta: Arthritis Foundation; 1987.
2. Arthritis Foundation. When your student has arthritis: a guide for teachers. Atlanta: Arthritis Foundation; 1992.
3. Bautch, J.C.; Malone, D.G.; Vailas, A.C. Osteoarthritis of the knee: effects on articular cartilage. Arthritis Care and Res. 5:S20; 1992 (abstract no. 62).
4. Campion, M.R. Hydrotherapy in paediatrics. 2nd ed. Oxford: Butterworth-Heinemann Ltd.; 1991.
5. Carmen, D. Where are the Indians? An exercise video for children. Dallas: Texas Scottish Rite Hospital for Children; 1991.
6. Committee on Sports Medicine. Recommendations for participation in competitive sports. Pediatrics 81:737-739; 1988.
7. Emery, H.M.; Bowyer, S.L. Physical modalities of therapy in pediatric rheumatic diseases. Rheum. Dis. Clin. of North Amer. 17:1001-1014; 1991.
8. Giannini, M.J.; Protas, E.J. Exercise response in children with and without juvenile rheumatoid arthritis: a case-comparison study. Physical Therapy 72:365-372; 1992.
9. Harkcom, T.M.; Lampman, R.M.; Banwell, B.F.; Caster, C.W. Therapeutic value of graded aerobic exercise training in rheumatoid arthritis. Arthritis Rheum. 28:32-39; 1985.
10. Harlowe, D.; Yu, T. The ROM dance. Madison, WI: New Ventures of Wisconsin; 1984.
11. Hicks, J.E. Exercises in patients with inflammatory arthritis. Rheumatic Disease Clinics of North America 16:845-870; 1990.
12. Klepper, S.E.; Darbee, J.; Effgen, S.K.; Singsen, B.H. Physical fitness levels in children with polyarticular juvenile rheumatoid arthritis. Arthritis Care & Research 5:93-100; 1992.
13. McNeal, R.L. Aquatic therapy for patients with rheumatic disease. Rheumatic Disease Clinics of North America 16:915-929; 1990.
14. Muller, E.A. Influence of training and inactivity on muscle strength. Arch. Phys. Med. Rehabil. 57:449-462; 1970.
15. Namey, T.C. Adaptive bicycling. Rheumatic Disease Clinics of North America 16:871-886; 1990.
16. Pollock, M.L.; Wilmore, J.H.; Fox, S.M. Exercise in health and disease: evaluation and prescription for prevention and rehabilitation. Philadelphia: W.B. Saunders Co.; 1984.
17. Rhodes, V.J. Physical therapy management of patients with juvenile rheumatoid arthritis. Phys. Ther. 71:910-919; 1991.
18. Scull, S. Juvenile rheumatoid arthritis. In: Tecklin, J.S., ed. Pediatric physical therapy. Philadephia: J.B. Lippincott Co.; 1994.
19. Scull, S.A.; Dow, M.B.; Athreya, B.H. Physical and occupational therapy for children with rheumatic diseases. Pediatric Clinics of North America 22:1053-1077; 1986.
20. Skinner, A.T.; Thomson, A.M., eds. Duffield's exercise in water. 3rd ed. Philadelphia: Bailliere Tindall; 1986.
21. Stenstrom, C.H. Does voluntary aerobic exercise frequency influence radiological progression in rheumatoid arthritis? Arthritis Care and Res. 5:S20; 1992 (abstract no. 61).
22. Whitehouse, R.; Shoppe, J.T.; Sullivan, D.B.; Kulik, C.L. Children with juvenile rheumatoid arthritis at school. Clinical Pediatrics 28:509-514; 1989.

CHAPTER 10

Exercise-Induced Asthma

David Cypcar
Regional Allergy and Asthma Consultants
Asheville, North Carolina

Robert F. Lemanske, Jr.
University of Wisconsin Medical School

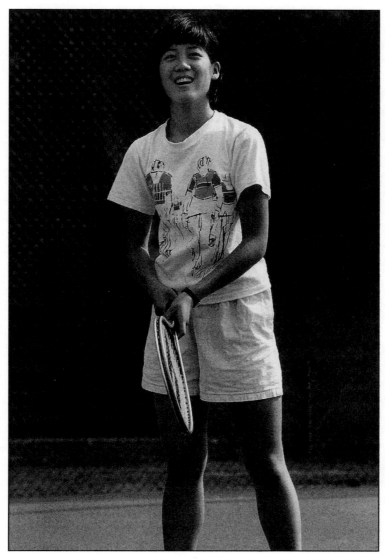

Exercise-induced asthma is lower airway obstruction that develops during or following exercise. Symptoms of lower airway obstruction include wheezing, coughing, and shortness of breath. Although exercise is only one potential triggering factor for asthma, it is a common one; in many patients, it may be the only one. This chapter will first review the basic pathophysiology of asthma in general, and then specifically focus on the mechanisms by which exercise may precipitate episodes of lower airway obstruction. Finally, treatment approaches to attenuate or abrogate exercise-induced asthma will be discussed.

BRIEF DESCRIPTION OF ASTHMA

Asthma is a heterogeneous disease or syndrome which can be triggered by a number of factors, including allergens, irritants, viral infections, and exercise. Pathologically, it is characterized by bronchial smooth muscle contraction, mucus secretion, airway wall edema, and inflammation. Clinically, it is characterized by episodic wheezing, coughing, and shortness of breath that can range in severity from mild to life-threatening. It is the leading cause of chronic illness and the most common chronic respiratory disorder in children through the age of 17 years (22). Despite improved modalities of treatment, for unknown reasons the overall incidence, prevalence, morbidity, and mortality due to asthma are increasing; these trends are particularly evident in poor minority children 5-14 years of age (53).

Pathophysiology

Until recently, asthma was regarded mainly as a "bronchospastic" disease, and most therapies focused on attempting to relieve bronchoconstriction. Recent insights into the pathogenesis of asthma, however, have revealed that even patients with mild and otherwise well-controlled disease have a moderate degree of airway inflammation (26). The National Heart, Lung and Blood Institute (32) has recently defined asthma as a lung disease characterized by:

- airway obstruction;
- complete or partial reversibility, either spontaneous or with treatment;
- airway inflammation; and
- increased airway responsiveness to a variety of stimuli.

In children these stimuli (or "triggers") include viral upper respiratory tract infections, allergens, irritants (such as cigarette smoke), and exercise. It may be that differential exposure to relevant triggers dictates not only the heterogeneity but also the day-to-day variability of the disease.

Airway obstruction is responsible for the clinical manifestations of asthma and is the result of multiple interrelated factors, including airway smooth muscle constriction, mucosal edema, mucus secretion, airway inflammation, and abnormalities in neural control of airway tone. Today, the inflammatory component of asthma is considered to play a central role in the pathogenesis of the disease and is often the prime target in therapy. The inflammatory infiltrate is multicellular, but with a predominance of T-lymphocytes and eosinophils (26).

The pathogenesis of exercise-induced asthma (EIA) may differ from that of other triggering factors in that it is unclear whether exercise alone as a stimulus is capable of producing airway inflammation. In fact, bronchoalveolar lavage performed after exercise has not convincingly demonstrated that either mediator release (8) or cellular infiltration (21) is involved in the airway obstruction that follows exercise. Hence, EIA is often referred to as exercise-induced bronchoconstriction (EIB), reflecting this pathophysiological difference.

The major variables that determine the magnitude of EIA include minute ventilation and the temperature and humidity of inspired air during and following exercise (3). For a given set of air conditions, increased levels of minute ventilation produce more obstruction than do low levels. Likewise, for a fixed ventilatory rate, warming and humidifying inspired air reduces the severity of obstruction, whereas cooling and drying inspired air exacerbates obstruction (9). Therefore, most of the differences in asthmogenicity among various sports are due to the inherent minute ventilation, climatic conditions, and

This work was supported by grant numbers AI34891, AI00995, and HL51843 from the National Institutes of Health.

levels of allergen and pollutants in the air that are associated with that particular sport.

There are several theories regarding the precise stimulus that induces acute EIA (Table 10.1). Normally, the nasal airway conditions inspired air so that alveolar air is close to body temperature and fully saturated with water. With exercise, metablic demands stimulate increased minute ventilation, leading to mouth breathing. Loss of nasal airway conditioning results in the inspiration of cooler and drier air, in turn causing the loss of water (42) and heat (30). This creates a hyperosmolar and dry microenvironment which directly (or possibly through basophil and mast cell degranulation) causes bronchospasm. A second theory is that heat loss during exercise creates a thermal "gradient" across bronchial epithelium; prompt reduction of this gradient (or rapid rewarming) following the cessation of exercise induces vasodilation and increased capillary permeability, physically compromising airway caliber and resulting in EIA (30). Another hypothesis suggests that exercise directly induces mast cell mediator release through the formation of hyperosmolar conditions in the airway resulting from water loss. Supporting evidence for this theory is that other physical stimuli can directly induce mast cell mediator release (51), and that medications that work, in part, by preventing mediator release (13) are effective in preventing EIA. However, the expected rise in mast cell mediators (such as histamine and neutrophil chemotactic factor of anaphylaxis) following exercise is not consistent (31) and, in fact, such rises in plasma levels have also been identified in patients who do not develop bronchospasm following exercise (25). Further, as mentioned previously, mast cell mediators are not found in bronchoalveolar lavage fluid following EIA (8). Thus, the precise contribution of mast cell mediator release remains unknown.

Table 10.1   Proposed Mechanisms Contributing to EIA

1. Hyperosmolar microenvironment due to respiratory heat and water loss
2. Rapid rewarming
3. Mast cell mediator release
4. Inadequate catecholamine response

Finally, there are some data to suggest that patients with asthma have an inadequate or subnormal endogenous catecholamine response to exercise (50).

Physical Symptoms and Clinical Signs

The most common clinical symptoms of asthma are intermittent wheezing, cough, dyspnea, and "chest tightness," characteristically related to exposure to a known environmental trigger, and often more pronounced at night. Patients with chronic asthma, however, may experience acute exacerbations without any known precipitant. Young athletes with asthma are often reluctant to admit to such symptoms for fear of "being different," and may present with exercise intolerance or an inability to keep up with peers when otherwise apparently well-conditioned. This is an especially important feature of EIA that is often overlooked by patients, trainers, and physicians who tend to attribute breathlessness to poor physical conditioning. Thus, it is possible that some individuals experience asthmatic symptoms only when they exercise, while others experience daily symptoms related to a number of triggering factors, including exercise.

The signs of asthma reflect the degree of airway obstruction. Inspiratory and expiratory wheezes with a prolonged expiratory phase are common. Most severe degrees of obstruction are manifest by the use of accessory muscles of respiration, nasal flaring, sweating, and mucous membrane cyanosis. However, it should be noted that EIA is usually self-limited and rarely results in obstruction severe enough to warrant hospitalization.

Clinical and Laboratory Assessment

To make the diagnosis of asthma, the documentation of clinical or pulmonary function data consistent with airflow obstruction, reversibility, and hyperresponsiveness are needed. This is most easily performed by the serial monitoring of peak expiratory flow rate (PEFR) readings before and following bronchodilator use. The patient should be instructed to follow these steps to use the peak flow meter (Figure 10.1):

1. Stand up.
2. Place the indicator at the base of the numbered scale.
3. Take a deep breath and place the meter in your mouth, sealing your lips around the mouthpiece.
4. Blow out as hard and as fast as possible.
5. Repeat the process two more times, and record the highest of the three numbers achieved.

A baseline reading <80% of predicted (based on sex, race, and height) with >15% improvement following the use of a bronchodilator is consistent with asthma. More detailed physiological data can be obtained using spirometry, in which forced expiratory volume in one second (FEV_1), forced vital capacity (FVC), and forced expiratory flow rate between 25% and 75% of FVC (FEF_{25-75}) can be calculated. A decreased FEV_1, FEV_1/FVC, and FEF_{25-75} are all indicators of airflow obstruction and are consistent with asthma. Response to bronchodilator medications can also be assessed using these spirometric values.

Bronchial hyperresponsiveness (BHR) is somewhat more difficult to document. BHR ("twitchy airways") can be demonstrated in many lung diseases, including cystic fibrosis, bronchitis, and emphysema; it can even occur in normal individuals following a viral upper respiratory tract infection (27). However, the severity of BHR tends to be the greatest in asthma. A variation of more than 20% in the best morning and evening PEFR readings is consistent with BHR. Alternatively, either chemical or physical stimuli may be administered in an attempt to provoke bronchoconstriction in susceptible individuals. The chemical stimuli, histamine and methacholine, are more sensitive bronchoprovocation agents than exercise in detecting BHR (40); exercise, however, is far more specific for BHR related to asthma.

To standardize exercise intensity, the stimulus must be of sufficient intensity to increase the patient's heart rate to 80% of maximum (maximum heart rate = 220 minus age in years) for 6-8 minutes. This is most commonly performed on an exercise treadmill or bicycle ergometer. Serial measurements of PEFR or FEV_1 are recorded prior to exercise and every 5 minutes for 30 minutes after the cessation of exercise. A positive response is denoted by a 15% or greater decrement in PEFR or FEV_1, usually occurring 5-10 minutes after exercise. Decreases in either parameter between 10-14% are suggestive of EIA. Bronchoprovocation maneuvers should not be performed with individuals who have baseline airway obstruction, cardiac disease, or upper respiratory infections (which enhance airway reactivity). Exercise testing should be performed with continuous electrocardiographic and heart rate monitoring; appropriate emergency equipment should also be readily available.

One of the most useful purposes of exercise testing is to objectively demonstrate bronchospasm in a patient who subjectively experiences "breathlessness" with exercise. A negative challenge in the routine patient does not invariably exclude the diagnosis of asthma. Indeed, it should be noted that well-conditioned athletes may not experience EIA under the heart rate and oxygen consumption constraints of the test, but may do so under more strenuous conditions. Exercise testing can also be an important tool for evaluating the efficacy of therapy. In addition to bronchoprovocation tests, many clinicians feel that in the typical case of EIA the diagnosis can be confirmed by a therapeutic trial of preexercise albuterol, cromolyn, or nedocromil.

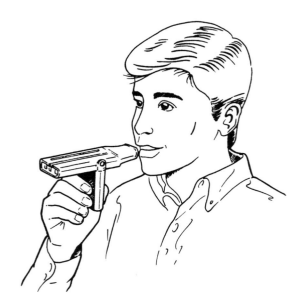

Figure 10.1 Correct use of a peak flow meter.
Reprinted with permission of HealthScan Products Inc., Cedar Grove, NJ 07009.

Natural History

It was once felt that some patients with asthma were more apt to "outgrow" their illness than others. However, it has been well documented that clinically asymptomatic individuals with a previous history of asthma have continued evidence of BHR, and that many of these individuals redevelop the clinical features of asthma later in life. It is therefore preferable to use the term *remission* to describe an asymptomatic time period that may occur in individuals with a previous history of symptomatic asthma.

Prospective studies have indicated that the risk factors (not causes) associated with the development of asthma include male sex, maternal cigarette smoking (19), atopy, and onset of the first episode of wheezing after the age of 2 (43). Risk factors associated with a decreased likelihood of remission include atopy (and for unknown reasons, especially atopic dermatitis), male sex, and onset of the first episode of wheezing before the age of 1. With the exception of age, it thus appears that many of the factors associated with the development of asthma are also associated with its continuation.

Therapeutic Intervention

A comprehensive review of the therapeutic options available for children with varying degrees of asthma is beyond the scope of this discussion. In view of the recent pathophysiologic evidence that the inflammatory component plays a primary role in the development and continuation of the disease (even in patients with mild and otherwise well-controlled symptoms), the therapeutic focus has shifted from relief of acute and episodic bronchoconstriction to prevention of inflammation. Hence, most of the medications used to treat asthma may be broadly classified either as bronchodilators or as anti-inflammatory agents (see Table 10.2). Although the treatment plan needs to be tailored to the individual needs of the patient, it is now generally felt that a patient who develops symptoms more than a few times per week, has acute exacerbations lasting several days, and requires occasional emergency treatment should be maintained on prophylactic anti-inflammatory medications (32). The specific medications available to treat EIA and chronic asthma will be reviewed subsequently.

Table 10.2   Treatment Modalities for EIA

Nonpharmacological
Induction of refractory period
Appropriate climatic conditions
Scarf/mask in cold air

Pharmacological
First line
   β_2-adrenergic agonists—inhaled (metered dose inhaler or nebulizer)
   Cromolyn sodium—inhaled (metered dose inhaler or nebulizer)
Adjunctive
   Theophylline—oral
   Corticosteroids—inhaled (metered dose inhaler)

Morbidity and Mortality

The overall mortality from asthma increased 31% between 1980 and 1987 (10). Risk factors for fatal asthma include age (infants and elderly), African-American or Hispanic ethnicity, previous history of respiratory failure requiring intubation, hospitalization for asthma within the previous year, underestimation of disease severity by the patient or physician, lack of access to medical care, and the concurrent presence of psychological or psychosocial problems, especially depression (32). Athletes with one or more of these risk factors should be identified and appropriately counseled.

EXERCISE AND ASTHMA

The philosophy several decades ago was to limit or even exclude patients with asthma from participating in athletic events. However, thanks to a better understanding of the pathogenesis of the disease and the development of newer and improved medications, even athletes with moderate to severe asthma can participate in competitive athletics. In fact, 11.2% (67/597) of 1984 US Olympic team members demonstrated EIA, but nevertheless 38 of them went on to win 41 medals (15 gold, 21 silver, and 5 bronze) (36).

Effects of Asthma on Exercise Tolerance and Sport Performance

Exercise is a known trigger of acute asthma, and if untreated, will limit the young athlete's tolerance for even mild levels of physical activity. Not only will the patient be less likely to exercise, but may also develop the inaccurate belief that the primary disease process is limiting in this regard. This leads to a sedentary and physically unconditioned person. With appropriate preventive treatment, however, most patients with asthma can participate in competitive athletics without inducing an acute episode of EIA. Knowing that they are able to exert some control over their asthma, patients will be more likely to follow through with an exercise program. Although most studies have failed to identify any significant change in the degree of bronchial responsiveness with various aerobic conditioning programs, the potential benefits are nonetheless valuable and include improved fitness, decreased frequency and severity of acute attacks, decreased medication usage, decreased school absenteeism, and improved self-image (Figure 10.2).

In 40-50% of patients with EIA, induction of a mild attack of asthma will attenuate subsequent asthma responses to identical exercise tasks performed within the next 2 hours. This is known as the refractory period. The mechanism for this response is not fully known, although various theories have been proposed including mast cell mediator depletion, increases in circulating levels of catecholamines, and possibly endogenous

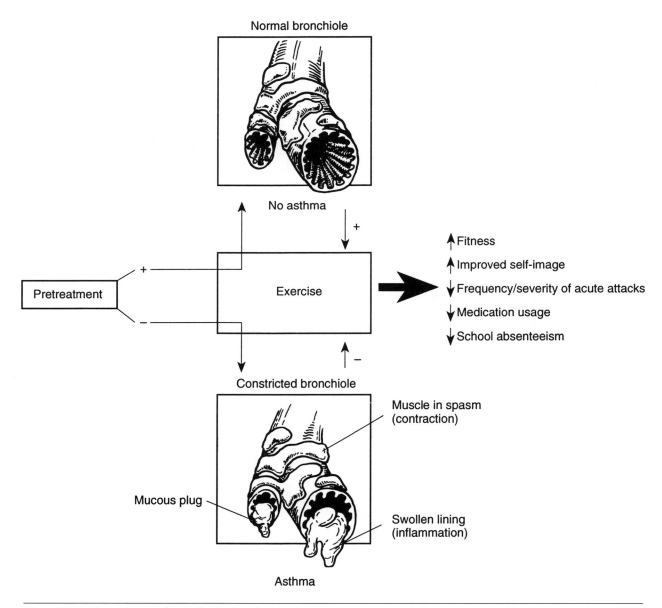

Figure 10.2 Interaction of exercise and asthma.

production of an inhibitory prostaglandin (34). How the young athlete can use this response to his or her advantage will be discussed in greater detail below.

Potential Adverse Effects of Sport and Exercise

As noted already, exercise is a recognized trigger of acute asthma. The symptom complex occasionally develops during exercise, but most commonly occurs 5-10 minutes after the cessation of exercise (see Figure 10.3). In fact, bronchodilation is the initial response to exercise in both normal individuals and patients with asthma, and is felt to be mediated by the release of endogenous catecholamines (29). This response is fairly transient, peaks mid-exercise, and returns to baseline levels by the end of the exercise period. Progressive bronchoconstriction then ensues, with maximal obstruction occurring 5 to 10 minutes after the cessation of exercise. Bronchoconstriction begins to spontaneously and gradually remit, such that pulmonary functions are completely normal by 60 minutes. Some (7), but not all (37) investigators have noted that 20-25% of patients may experience a recurrence of symptoms 4-8 hours after exercise without exposure to a second exercise stimulus. This is known as a late phase response, and may be more likely to occur if the early phase reaction was either severe or prolonged (24). Recent data suggest that this reaction may represent a previously unappreciated diurnal variation in pulmonary function (37).

EIA is more apt to occur following short periods of intense exercise (e.g., windsprints); however, exercise-induced symptoms have been known to occur following exercise durations of up to 30 minutes. Although this is not recommended, some athletes can run through their symptoms. That is, despite continued exercise in the presence of acute EIA, gradual spontaneous resolution of airway obstruction occurs, giving such individuals a second wind. Finally, it is important to appreciate that several factors are important in determining an asthmatic athlete's response to exercise, and include concomitant allergen exposure, ambient temperature and humidity, and baseline airway reactivity.

Precautions to Prevent Adverse Effects

Several therapeutic strategies are available to prevent EIA in susceptible individuals. Although the specific preventive measures are the same for patients with chronic asthma as for patients with EIA alone, it is unlikely that any therapeutic intervention will be successful if the patient's baseline obstructed lung function is not treated first. A practical approach to treatment is depicted in Figure 10.4.

If the patient has a history of cough, wheezing, dyspnea, or chest tightness which develops with exercise or when exposed to known environmental triggers, baseline spirometry or serial monitoring of PEFR should be measured. If the initial parameters are consistent with airflow

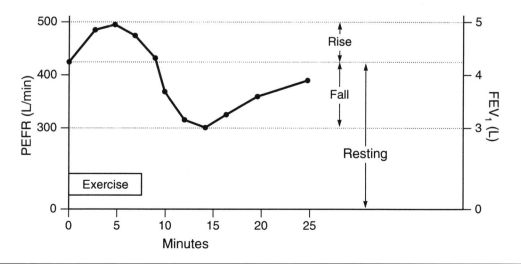

Figure 10.3 Effect of exercise on asthma.
Adapted from Anderson, Seale, Ferris, Schoeffel, and Lindsay (1979).

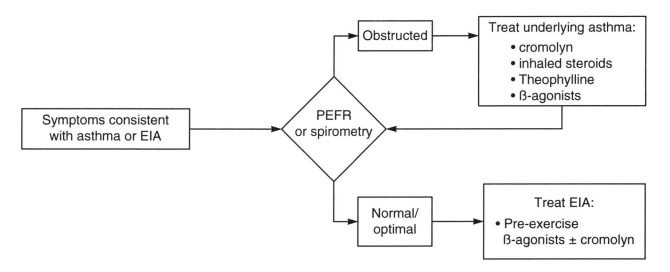

Figure 10.4   Approach to the patient with symptoms suggestive of asthma or exercise-induced broncho-constriction (EIB).

obstruction (FEV_1/FVC, FEV_1, or PEFR <80% predicted; or FEF_{25-75} <70% predicted), or bronchial hyperresponsiveness (>20% variation in diurnal PEFR), the patient's underlying asthma should be treated first. Once pulmonary function is normal (or is felt to represent the patient's optimal baseline), nonpharmacological and pharmacological treatment modalities for EIA (as detailed in Table 10.2) should be instituted.

Nonpharmacological Modalities

The preventive treatment of EIA can be broadly divided into two primary categories, pharmacological and nonpharmacological (Table 10.2). The nonpharmacological measures include the induction of a refractory period and the appropriate choice of climatic conditions less likely to provoke EIA.

As stated previously, 40-50% of patients with asthma will experience a refractory period up to two hours following an acute attack of EIA. Those patients who do develop a refractory period may use this response to their advantage by inducing the refractory state 45-60 minutes prior to the EIA-inducing event. Unfortunately, there are no clinical or laboratory parameters that effectively predict which athletes will experience a refractory period and which athletes will not; empiric induction is therefore recommended for all athletes with asthma and EIA. A universal warm-up prescription that will consistently induce the refractory state has not been

established. Since EIA is more likely to occur following brief intense periods of exercise, many sports medicine physicians recommend a series of half a dozen 50–100-yard sprints. From a practical standpoint, however, exercises related to the EIA-inducing event may be equally effective. Because EIA usually remits within 10-20 minutes and the refractory period lasts up to 2 hours, these exercises are best performed 45-60 minutes prior to the EIA-inducing event. This time frame also permits the use of a β-agonist inhaler between the initial exercises and the EIA-inducing event, either as a rescue agent (if needed), or as a premedication.

Exercising under appropriate climatic conditions cannot be overemphasized. With the knowledge that cool dry air is one of the two major variables that determine the magnitude of EIA, reasonable precautions should be taken to minimize this exposure. Indoor athletics are preferable to the same event played outdoors, for sports where this may be an option (e.g., tennis, basketball, running, volleyball). Likewise, the use of a face mask or scarf may help warm and humidify the cool dry air that would otherwise be inspired during outdoor winter athletics (snow skiing, ice skating, hockey).

Pharmacological Modalities

Several medications have been shown to be effective in the prevention and treatment of asthma and EIA. Most of these medications are not banned by the International Olympic Committee (IOC) or the United States Olympic Committee (USOC). However, many patients with asthma have concurrent allergic rhinitis, treated with combination antihistamine/decongestant medications or access to narcotic antitussives, both of which are banned by the IOC and the USOC. Furthermore, a few approved asthma medications are marketed in combination with banned medications. Thus, there is high potential for an athlete with asthma unknowingly to receive an IOC-banned medication. Before taking any medication prior to competition, athletes should have it verified by the appropriate senior physician or knowledgeable USOC medical staff member. Table 10.3 lists medications likely to be used by patients with allergic rhinitis and asthma and which are currently banned in international competition by the 1992 USOC (49).

β-Adrenergic Agonists. Beta-adrenergic agonists are the most potent bronchodilators available today and are effective in the prevention of EIA in 90% of patients. In addition, they may be used for the treatment of acute bronchospasm and are therefore considered the drug of choice for EIA. By stimulating β2 receptors on bronchial smooth muscle, β-adrenergic agonists induce increases in intracellular cAMP (cyclic adenosine

Table 10.3 Medications Commonly Used by People With Asthma and Allergic Rhinitis

---

Medications Banned in International Competition

1. Sympathomimetic amines/stimulants: ephedrine, pseudoephedrine, epinephrine, phenylephrine, phenylpropanolamine, isoetharine, isoproterenol

2. Oral β-agonists: metaproterenol, albuterol, terbutaline

3. Narcotic antitussives: codeine, hydrocodone, oxycodone

4. Enteral (oral) and parenteral (IM, IV) corticosteroids

Medications Approved in International Competition

1. Antihistamines (caution: classic antihistamines may diminish alertness and cause drowsiness)

2. Topical oxymetazoline and xylometazoline

3. Inhaled and aerosolized formulations

4. Dextromethorphan and expectorants

5. Inhaled and intranasal formulations

Data from United States Olympic Committee (1992).

monophosphate) with consequent smooth muscle relaxation. Their onset of action occurs within 5 minutes, peaks at 15-60 minutes, and dissipates after 4-6 hours; they are therefore best administered 15 minutes prior to exercise. Beta-agonists are available in several formulations; the inhaled and nebulized preparations are of greater efficacy and cause less systemic side effects (tremor, tachycardia) than the oral formulations. Furthermore, the inhaled and nebulized preparations are USOC-approved whereas oral formulations are USOC-banned. Most patients require two puffs of a metered dose inhaler (MDI) to prevent EIA; the dose may be increased to four puffs as needed. Figure 10.5 illustrates the proper use of an MDI. The patient should be instructed to follow these steps:

1. If uncertain, check how much medicine is in the canister: place the canister (but not the mouthpiece) in a cup of water. If the canister sinks to the bottom, it is full; if the canister floats sideways on the surface, it is empty.

2. Remove the cap and shake the inhaler.

3. Tilt your head back slightly and completely exhale.

4. Position the inhaler in one of the following ways (A is optimal, but B is acceptable for those who have difficulty with A. Spacer devices [C] may improve the coordination of canister activation and inspiration in patients unable to do technique A or B effectively.)

5. Activate the inhaler once to release the medication as you start to inhale slowly (i.e., over 3-5 seconds).

6. Hold your breath for 10 seconds after complete inspiration.

7. Wait one minute, and repeat as necessary.

Albuterol (salbutamol), terbutaline, and pirbuterol are the most β2-selective medications; metaproterenol has less β2 specificity and a shorter duration of protection against EIA compared to albuterol (39). The bronchodilating effect of β-agonists and their efficacy in preventing EIA are independent of one another (41). These drugs should therefore not be abandoned as a rescue agent if they fail to prevent EIA.

Cromolyn and Nedocromil Sodium. Cromolyn sodium is less effective than the β-agonists in the prevention of EIA. Forty percent of patients

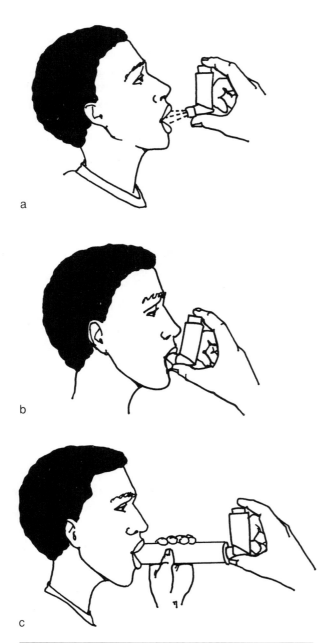

Figure 10.5   Correct use of a metered-dose inhaler:
(a) open mouth with inhaler 1-2 inches away;
(b) place in the mouth; (c) use spacer (recommended especially for young children).
Modified from National Asthma Education Program (1991).

will demonstrate complete prevention of EIA with the use of cromolyn, and an additional group will demonstrate partial efficacy (decrement in PEFR less than one-half that of placebo) (17). For reasons that are unclear, cromolyn tends to be more effective in patients who are capable of inducing a refractory period or patients who have late responses following exercise (5). The precise mechanism of action of cromolyn is unknown. However, it has been shown

to inhibit mediator release, phosphodiesterase activity, and reflex bronchospasm; it may also modify heat flux in the airway (14). Some of these effects may be due to the ability of cromolyn to modulate calcium influx across cellular membranes. Cromolyn's peak effect occurs within 15-30 minutes, and lasts up to 2 hours. It is available in either an MDI (800 mcg/puff) or solution for nebulization (20 mg/2 mL vial), both USOC-approved. Since cromolyn is an ineffective rescue medication, β-agonist drugs are usually prescribed first. However, cromolyn can be added to the patient's therapeutic regimen when it is clear that he or she is not responding sufficiently to β-agonists alone (23). The starting dose is 2 puffs of an MDI 15 minutes prior to exercise, preceded by the β-agonist MDI. Unique to cromolyn's therapeutic profile is its virtual lack of systemic side effects. Nedocromil sodium, a structurally unique compound with a therapeutic and safety profile similar in many respects to that of cromolyn, was recently approved by the FDA for the treatment of EIA.

Theophylline.   Short acting forms of theophylline should not be used in patients with EIA, as they are less effective bronchodilators than the β-agonists as a group and need to be administered about 2 hours before exercise. In addition, intermittent theophylline administration increases the potential for adverse effects (e.g., central nervous system stimulation, headache, nausea and vomiting, or tachycardia). Mechanisms of action include phosphodiesterase inhibition, adenosine receptor antagonism, adenyl cyclase stimulation, and decrease in the release of intracellular calcium, among others (6). Sustained-release theophylline preparations are frequently prescribed in moderate to severe chronic asthma and, when used in this manner, can be helpful in attenuating any bronchospastic response to exercise. Theophylline blood levels between 5-15 µg/mL are currently considered to be therapeutic.

Cholinergic Antagonists.   Cholinergic antagonists treat the component of bronchoconstriction due to vagal efferent activity. As cholinergic mechanisms have little (if any) role in the pathogenesis of EIA, the role of cholinergic antagonists in the prevention and treatment of EIA is not fully established. In comparison to β-agonists, they have a slower onset and somewhat longer duration of action. The only available formulation approved for inhaled use in the USA is ipratropium bromide. Because this is poorly absorbed, the incidence of systemic anticholinergic side effects is low. In contrast to cromolyn, ipratropium does not augment the effects of β-agonists, if used in combination prior to exercise (38). Ipratropium might be of value for the rare athlete with asthma who develops bronchoconstriction while taking β-blockers. Ipratropium is approved by the USOC.

Corticosteroids. Inhaled corticosteroids are being used more frequently for children with moderate to severe asthma who are incompletely responsive to cromolyn sodium or nedocromil sodium. The regular use of inhaled steroids for chronic asthma may reduce the propensity to EIA by decreasing airway responsiveness. Although recommended doses of inhaled corticosteroids are generally considered safe, recent data have demonstrated that short-term (i.e., 18-day) use of high-dose inhaled steroids may affect growth rates in asthmatic children (52). Thus, while corticosteroids are the most effective agents currently available for reducing asthmatic symptoms and improving pulmonary function, they should still be prescribed judiciously in children. Inhaled corticosteroids are approved by the USOC; parenteral (IV, IM) and oral corticosteroids are banned.

The Difficult-to-Manage Patient. The majority of patients with EIA will respond to the use of albuterol or cromolyn prior to exercise, in conjunction with treatment of any baseline lung obstruction. If a lack of response is seen with either drug alone, the two in combination may result in effective blockade of EIA. Patients continuing to manifest exercise intolerance should be tested under their usual therapeutic regimen to determine the basis for their problem (e.g., poor physical fitness, improper use of medications [poor inhaler technique], unresponsiveness to medications, muscular weakness, and so forth). From a practical standpoint, this may be done by treadmill testing (discussed previously) and/or PEFR monitoring before exercise and with the onset of symptoms.

Some patients with severe asthma require daily or alternate-day oral corticosteroids in order to maintain asthma control, and hence are referred to as *steroid-dependent*. Despite maximal treatment for chronic asthma and preventive treatment for EIA, some of these patients may become symptomatic with even mild levels of physical activity. These patients should be referred to a qualified physician and physical therapist capable of determining fitness levels, appropriate level of exercise, rate of buildup, and expected achievable goals. Depending on the severity of asthma, the prescribed exercise program may therefore differ substantially from physical education designed for children with lesser degrees of (or no) asthma. It is desirable for the physician and physical therapist to work with the patient and physical education instructor in order to determine activities that not only meet the patient's exercise needs, but are enjoyable to the patient, utilizing available facilities and personnel.

Appropriate Response to Adverse Effects in the School and Recreational Environment

It is especially important that all patients with EIA follow the therapeutic plan prescribed by their physicians, whether this involves the regular use of medications or medications only prior to exercise. Because of the potential for the development of progressive life-threatening symptoms if treatment of acute exacerbations of asthma is delayed, an expert panel from the American Academy of Allergy and Immunology recommends that children with asthma who have sufficient maturity to control the use of inhaled medications be permitted to carry their β-agonist inhalers with them at school and use them as needed (1).

Very rarely will airflow obstruction be so severe that initial treatment by the inhaled route is ineffective. Under these circumstances, the administration of subcutaneous autoinjectable epinephrine by the patient or a knowledgeable person is indicated. This situation almost invariably reflects advanced unattended disease in a patient with severe chronic asthma. Children with this type of clinical history should have a written action plan that details specific intervention strategies. This plan should be provided by the child's physician in conjunction with input from the parents and school personnel.

As stated above, airflow obstruction severe enough to warrant hospitalization or to cause death from exercise alone is exceedingly rare. With this knowledge, parents and teachers should not discourage children with asthma from participating in athletic activities. Physicians should likewise not unnecessarily exclude patients with asthma from participating in various sports.

Potential Benefits From Exercise

Several studies have demonstrated that patients with asthma are physically unfit (11, 28, 47). As noted earlier, it is a common misconception that the disease process per se is limiting in this regard. Two recent independent studies have challenged this notion, however. One study correlated the physical fitness of asthmatic children with several medical and psychological variables and found that the measure of the child's psychological adjustment correlated better with fitness than with all of the medical variables combined (46). Although the relationships between poor fitness and phychological adjustment was not defined, it is likely that the voluntary withdrawal from physical education programs exacerbates the "distance from normality" that these individuals already perceive, leading to poor self-image and low self-esteem. A more recent study found that physical fitness did not correlate with objective measures of disease severity (namely bronchial responsiveness and FEV_1), but rather with the degree of physical activity (16). These investigators postulate that patients with inadequately treated lung disease experience breathlessness at lower levels of activity than individuals without asthma. To avoid this sensation, the patient reduces his or her level of activity, creating a vicious cycle which results in a sedentary and physically unconditioned person. They further found that with appropriate preventive treatment, objective measures of exercise performance were not significantly different from, and often higher than, predicted norms. One-half of these patients nevertheless subjectively experienced wheezing and dyspnea, suggesting that the normal sensation of breathlessness with exercise was subjectively equated with asthma.

To date, several studies have evaluated the potential benefits of exercise on the overall cause and management of asthma. Most well-controlled, prospective studies have failed to identify any significant change in the degree of bronchial responsiveness following various aerobic conditioning programs (12, 15, 33, 35). Some studies, however, have found an attenuation in the exercise-induced decrease in FEV_1 or PEFR, following such exercise programs (4, 18, 20). This may be attributable to improved fitness, insofar as the fit person will have decreased minute ventilation for a given work load, which in turn will decrease the coincident respiratory heat and water loss with exercise, thereby attenuating the stimulus for EIA. Other beneficial effects that have been identified include decreased frequency and severity of asthma attacks, decreased use of medications, decreased school absenteeism, and improved self-confidence (48). In addition, an almost universal feature of exercise programs is improved physical fitness.

Patient education is of paramount importance in the successful implementation of an exercise program. Not only does the physician need to convince the patient of the potential benefits of exercise on the overall course and management of his or her disease, but also address the attitude that the underlying disease is limiting in this regard. Even with appropriate premedications, many patients with asthma will interpret the normal sensation of breathlessness with exercise as the beginning of acute asthma. Under these circumstances objective measures of lung function (as measured with a portable peak flow meter) may help to differentiate true bronchospasm from this otherwise normal response. Because acute asthma symptoms will intermittently disrupt the patient's exericse program, it is important not only to continue to reassess and adjust the patient's therapeutic regimen, but also to reinforce attempts to participate in exercise programs despite the occasional development of asthma symptoms.

EXERCISE AND SPORT PROGRAMS FOR CHILDREN WITH ASTHMA

Exercise and Conditioning Activities

Most patients with asthma can exercise enough to maintain fitness levels simply with encouragement and the proper use of medications to prevent EIA. As previously indicated, however, many patients with asthma are not physically fit. It is therefore important to determine fitness levels by standardized tests (treadmill or bicycle ergometer) in patients manifesting exercise intolerance despite the proper use of medications to prevent EIA. Once the level of fitness has been identified a program for physical conditioning can be prescribed, with the level of entry and rate of buildup based on the actual test results. The resources of a physical therapist or exercise physiologist can be helpful in this regard. In addition to one of several forms of aerobic exercise, physical conditioning may also include various breathing and postural exercises (discussed subsequently; see Table 10.4).

The American College of Sports Medicine has established the goal of exercise programs to be performance of either continuous or rhythmic aerobic exercise for 20-30 minutes duration three times per week (2). There are no data to indicate that this recommendation should be altered for patients with asthma. The exercise intensity should be similar to that used in exercise testing, thereby increasing oxygen consumption to 70-80% of maximum, which roughly correlates with 70-80% of maximum heart rate. This exercise period should be preceded by a short warm-up period, and followed by a period of gradual cooling down. Such aerobic exercises include, but are not limited to, swimming, running, aerobic dance, cycling, racquetball, and tennis (see Table 3.5). In prescribing an exercise program, it is important to choose activities that the patient finds enjoyable and meaningful. If the activity does not meet these criteria, there is little likelihood that the patient will incorporate the program into his or her lifestyle.

Table 10.4   Preparatory Training and Conditioning Activities

---

Aerobic exercise
Goal: To $\uparrow$ O_2 consumption (or heart rate) to 70-80% of maximum (maximum heart rate = 220 – age in years)
Duration: 20-30 minutes
Frequency: 3 times per week
Options: See sports classification table in chapter 3; choose enjoyable activities to facilitate incorporation into the patient's lifestyle

Breathing and postural exercises
Goal: To improve posture and increase use of the diaphragm over that of the accessory muscles during normal respiration
Option: See text

Many patients with asthma have what has been described as a "tight posture" characterized by forward slumping of the upper back and flattening of the lumbosacral curvature (45). This posture is associated with underuse of the diaphragm and overuse of the accessory muscles of respiration, which may be further accentuated during acute exacerbations of asthma (44). Breathing and postural retraining exercises have therefore been advocated for patients with asthma. Their benefits, however, are more likely attributable to the added confidence that the patient can maintain some control over breathing during an acute exacerbation, rather than to actual improvements in respiratory muscle function per se (45). The goals of such exercises are to improve posture and increase use of the diaphragm over that of the accessory muscles during normal respiration. One useful maneuver is to have the patient clasp the hands behind the head, allowing an assistant or therapist to pull back at the elbows while concurrently stabilizing the trunk, thereby not only improving posture but also placing the patient in an optimal position to maximize diaphragmatic (over intercostal) breathing. Maximal diaphragm-induced chest expansion is obtained by having the patient take a deep breath while concurrently relaxing the abdominal musculature, followed by active abdominal muscle contraction during expiration.

Sport Programs

Low Asthmogenic Sports

As previously stated, the major variables that determine the magnitude of EIA are minute ventilation and the temperature and humidity of the inspired air. A high level of minute ventilation in cool dry air will induce far greater obstruction than lower levels of minute ventilation in warm, humid environmental conditions. The differences in asthmogenicity between various sports are therefore due to the inherent minute ventilation and climatic conditions associated with each individual sport. It thus follows that the ideal sport program for patients with asthma would entail relatively low levels of minute ventilation and warm and humid environmental conditions (Table 10.5). Most athletic activities

Table 10.5 Low Asthmogenic Sports

Low minute ventilation sports

Tennis	Karate	Football
Handball	Wrestling	Baseball
Racquetball	Boxing	Downhill skiing
Gymnastics	Sprinting	Isometrics
Diving	Golf	

Sports associated with warm and humid climatic conditions
Swimming
Water polo
Diving

characterized by low minute ventilation are associated with brief intermittent bursts of activity. This is a further advantage to the patient capable of inducing a refractory period, as participation may essentially become a series of back-to-back refractory periods. Sport programs inherently associated with a warm and humid environment are primarily water-related.

Highly Asthmogenic Sports

In general, patients with asthma can participate in most physical activities and sports. Patients should be aware, however, that sports with high levels of minute ventilation (high-intensity endurance activities) and/or inherently cool, dry environmental conditions are more likely to provoke EIA than activities with low levels of minute ventilation or warm, humid environmental conditions (as discussed previously). Although not specifically contraindicated for athletes with asthma, these activities will likely require more aggressive medical pretreatment. Sports that require a relatively high level of endurance include those listed in Table 10.6.

Table 10.6 High Asthmogenic Sports

High minute ventilation sports
Long-distance running
Cycling
Basketball
Soccer
Rugby

Sports associated with cool and dry climatic conditions
Ice hockey
Ice skating
Cross-country snow skiing

Special Equipment and Therapeutic Interventions

The successful implementation of a therapeutic program to minimize acute EIA in athletes with asthma depends not only on patient compliance, but also on the willingness of schools to accommodate the individual needs of such patients. It is critical that athletes with EIA have immediate access to their β-agonist inhalers and be able to use them as needed with acute episodes of EIA. For athletes with severe asthma, a coach or trainer should be familiar with the administration of autoinjectable epinephrine. For out-of-town competitions, arrivals should be scheduled so that patients with EIA have adequate time to premedicate and, if needed, to induce a refractory period. (See Table 10.7).

Summary of Recommendations

The nonpharmacological and pharmacological treatment modalities described in Table 10.2 remain the therapeutic foundation for patients with EIA. It is essential that the patient's baseline pulmonary function be determined, as it is unlikely that any therapeutic intervention will be successful if the underlying obstruction is not treated first. Athletes should be cautioned about the use of over-the-counter oral decongestants; physicians should likewise exercise caution in prescribing oral β-agonists, narcotic antitussives, and steroids, as all of these medications are banned in international competition by the USOC.

Table 10.7 Special Equipment and Therapeutic Interventions

1. Pharmacological and nonpharmacological treatment, as outlined in Table 10.2
2. β-agonist MDI readily available
3. Coach or trainer familiar with the administration of autoinjectable epinephrine
4. Appropriate scheduling of events to permit premedication and refractory period induction
5. Participation indoors (vs. outdoors), when an option
6. Face mask or scarf, for outdoor winter athletic events
7. Concurrent treatment of nasal obstruction

In general, self-limited participation is recommended, as most patients with asthma subjectively know when their asthma is acting up, and can take appropriate measures. Patients should not be encouraged to run through their symptoms, but to use their β-agonist MDI with the onset of cough, wheezing, dyspnea, and/or chest tightness. A PEFR reading may help to differentiate the normal sensation of breathlessness with exercise from bronchospasm in patients with asthma who are subjectively uncertain of this clinical distinction.

Coaches and trainers should be aware that the major variables that determine the magnitude of EIA are minute ventilation and the temperature and humidity of inspired air. Intense participation (increased minute ventilation) may therefore provoke EIA in patients with asthma who are otherwise well-controlled at less intense activity levels. Likewise, an event played in cool dry air may induce EIA in a patient with asthma, whereas the same event played under non-polluted, warm and humid climatic conditions is tolerated without complication. Both of these circumstances will require more aggressive therapy. Thus, the therapeutic strategies will differ not only between patients, but also between sports (within an individual patient), depending on the inherent minute ventilation and climatic conditions associated with the particular sport. Physicians should be consulted when the patient continues to experience exercise-induced cough, wheezing, dyspnea, chest tightness, or exercise intolerance despite the use of preventive β-agonists and cromolyn, as exercise testing and/or the evaluation and treatment of concurrent upper respiratory disease may be indicated.

Finally, coaches, trainers, and athletes with asthma should realize that mild to moderate asthma (not requiring daily oral corticosteroids to maintain optimal pulmonary function) should not limit the athlete's ability to participate in various sport programs if appropriately treated. Patients with mild to moderate asthma should therefore not be excluded from participating in athletics, and should, on the contrary, be encouraged to become actively involved in exercise programs and athletic events. Patients with severe asthma (requiring daily oral corticosteroid treatment) should also be encouraged to participate in such events, but will require a multidisciplinary evaluation utilizing the services of the physician, physical therapist, exercise physiologist, and physical education instructor to determine the appropriate degree of participation and expected achievable goals. Because acute asthma symptoms will intermittently disrupt the patient's exercise program, it is likewise important to reassess and adjust the therapeutic regimen as needed, as well as to reinforce the patient's efforts to maintain the prescribed program.

REFERENCES

1. American Academy of Allergy and Immunology. Position statement. The use of inhaled medications in school by students with asthma. J. Allergy Clin. Immunol. 84: 400; 1989.
2. American College of Sports Medicine. Guidelines for graded exercise testing and exercise prescription. 2nd ed. Philadelphia: Lea and Febiger; 1980.
3. Anderson, S.D.; Silverman, M.; Konig, P.; Godfrey, S. Exercise-induced asthma. Br. J. Dis. Chest 69:1-39; 1975.
4. Arborelius, M., Jr.; Svenonius, E. Decrease of exercise-induced asthma after physical training. Eur. J. Respir. Dis. 65(Supplement 136):25-31; 1984.
5. Ben-Dov, I.; Bar-Yishay, E.; Godfrey, S. Heterogeneity in the response of asthmatic patients to pre-exercise treatment with cromolyn sodium. Am. Rev. Respir. Dis. 127:113-116; 1983.
6. Bergstrand, H. Phosphodiesterase inhibition and theophylline. Eur. J. Respir. Dis. 109(Supplement):37-44; 1980.
7. Bierman, C.W.; Spiro, S.G.; Petheram, I. Characterization of the late response in exercise-induced asthma. J. Allergy Clin. Immunol. 74:701-706; 1984.
8. Broide, D.H.; Eisman, S.; Ramsdell, J.W.; Ferguson, P.; Schwartz, L.B.; Wasserman, S.I. Airway levels of mast cell-derived mediators in exercise-induced asthma. Am. Rev. Respir. Dis. 141:563-568; 1990.
9. Bundgaard, A.; Schmidt, A.; Ingemann-Hansen, T.; Halkjaer-Kristensen, J.; Bloch, I. Exercise-induced asthma after swimming and bicycle exercise. Eur. J. Respir. Dis. 63:245-248; 1982.

10. Centers for Disease Control. Asthma— United States, 1980-1987. MMWR 39:493-497; 1990.

11. Clark, C.J.; Cochrane, L.M. Assessment of work performance in asthma for determination of cardiorespiratory fitness and training capacity. Thorax 43:745-749; 1988.

12. Cochrane, L.M.; Clark, C.J. Benefits and problems of a physical training programme for asthmatic patients. Thorax 45:345-351; 1990.

13. Cockcroft, D.W.; Murdock, K.Y. Comparative effects of inhaled salbutamol, sodium cromoglycate, and beclomethasone dipropionate on allergen-induced early asthmatic responses, late asthmatic responses, and increased bronchial responsiveness to histamine. J. Allergy Clin. Immunol. 79:734-740; 1987.

14. Fanta, C.H.; McFadden, E.R., Jr.; Ingram, R.H., Jr. Effects of cromolyn sodium on the response to respiratory heat loss in normal subjects. Am. Rev. Respir. Dis. 123:161-164; 1981.

15. Fitch, K.D.; Blitvich, J.D.; Morton, A.R. The effect of running training on exercise-induced asthma. Ann. Allergy 57:90-94; 1986.

16. Garfinkel, S.K.; Kester, S.; Chapman, K.R.; Rebuck, A.S. Physiologic and nonphysiologic determinants of aerobic fitness in mild to moderate asthma. Am. Rev. Respir. Dis. 145:741-745; 1992.

17. Godfrey, S.; Konig, P. Inhibition of exercise-induced asthma by different pharmacological pathways. Thorax 31:137-140; 1976.

18. Haas, F.; Pineda, H.; Axen, K.; Gaudino, D.; Haas, A. Effects of physical fitness on expiratory airflow in exercising asthmatic people. Med. Sci. Sports Exercise 17:585-592; 1985.

19. Halken, S.; Host, A.; Husby, S.; Hansen, L.G.; Osterballe, O.; Nyboe, J. Recurrent wheezing in relation to environmental risk factors in infancy. A propspective study of 276 infants. Allergy 46:507-514; 1991.

20. Henriksen, J.M.; Nielsen, T.T. Effect of physical training on exercise-induced bronchoconstriction. Acta Paediatrica Scandinavica 72:31-36; 1983.

21. Jarjour, N.N.; Calhoun, W.J. Exercise-induced asthma is not associated with mast cell activation or airway inflammation. J. Allergy Clin. Immunol. 89:60-68; 1992.

22. King, J.T.; Bye, M.R.; Demopoulos, J.T. Exercise programs for asthmatic children. Comprehensive Therapy 10(11):67-71; 1984.

23. Latimer, K.M.; O'Byrne, P.M.; Morris, M.M.; Roberts, R.R.; Hargreave, F.E. Bronchoconstriction stimulated by airway cooling: better protection with combined inhalation of terbutaline sulfate and cromolyn sodium than with either alone. Am. Rev. Respir. Dis. 128:440-443; 1983.

24. Lee, T.H.; Brown, M.J.; Nagy, L.; Causon, R.; Walport, M.J.; Kay, A.B. Exercise-induced release of histamine and neutrophil chemotactic factor in atopic asthmatics. J. Allergy Clin. Immunol. 70:73-81; 1982.

25. Lee, T.H.; Nagakura, T.; Papageorgiou, N.; Iikura, Y.; Kay, A.B. Exercise-induced late asthmatic reactions with neutrophil chemotactic activity. N. Engl. J. Med. 308:1502-1505; 1983.

26. Lemanske, R.F., Jr. Patterns of airway responsiveness. J. Allergy Clin. Immunol. 86:53-56; 1990.

27. Lemanske, R.F., Jr. Mechanisms of airway inflammation. Chest 101:372S-377S; 1992.

28. Ludwick, S.K.; Jones, J.W.; Jones, T.K.; Fukuhara, J.T.; Strunk, R.C. Normalization of cardiopulmonary endurance in severely asthmatic children after bicycle ergometry therapy. J. Pediatr. 109:446-451; 1986.

29. McFadden, E.R., Jr. Exercise performance in the asthmatic. Am. Rev. Respir. Dis. 129:S84-S87; 1984.

30. McFadden, E.R., Jr.; Lenner, A.M.; Strohl, K.P. Postexertional airway rewarming and thermally induced asthma. New insights into pathophysiology and possible pathogenesis. J. Clin. Invest. 78:18-25; 1986.

31. Morgan, D.J.R.; Moodley, I.; Phillips, M.J.; Davies, R.J. Plasma histamine in asthmatic and control subjects following exercise: influence of circulating basophils and different assay techniques. Thorax 38:771-777; 1983.

32. National Asthma Education Program. Guidelines for the diagnosis and management of asthma. Bethesda, MD: National Heart, Lung, and Blood Institute, National Institutes of Health; publication 91-3042; 1991. Also published in J. Allergy Clin. Immunol. 88:425-534; 1991, and in Pediatric Asthma, Allergy and Immunology 5:57-188; 1991.

33. Nickerson, B.G.; Bautista, D.B.; Namey, M.A.; Richards, W.; Keens, T.G. Distance running improves fitness in asthmatic children without pulmonary complications or changes in exercise-induced bronchospasm. Pediatrics 71:147-152; 1983.

34. O'Byrne, P.M.; Jones, G.L. The effect of indomethacin on exercise-induced bronchoconstriction and refractoriness after exercise. Am. Rev. Respir. Dis. 134:69-72; 1986.

35. Orenstein, D.M.; Reed, M.E.; Grogan, F.T.; Crawford, L.V. Exercise conditioning in children with asthma. J. Pediatr. 106:556-560; 1985.

36. Pierson, W.E.; Voy, R.O. Exercise-induced bronchospasm in the XXIII Summer Olympic Games. N. Engl. Reg. Allergy Proc. 9:209-213; 1988.

37. Rubinstein, I.; Levison, H.; Slutsky, A.S.; Hak, H.; Wells, J.; Zamel, N.; Rebuck, A.S. Immediate and delayed bronchoconstriction after exercise in patients with asthma. N. Engl. J. Med. 317:482-485; 1987.

38. Sanguinetti, C.M.; DeLuca, S.; Gasparini, S.; Massei, V. Evaluation of Duovent in the prevention of exercise-induced asthma. Respiration 50(Supplement 2): 181-185; 1986.

39. Schoeffel, R.E.; Anderson, S.D.; Seale, J.P. The protective effect and duration of action of metaproterenol aerosol on exercise-induced asthma. Ann. Allergy 46:273-275; 1981.

40. Shapiro, G.G. Methacholine challenge—relevance for the allergic athlete. J. Allergy Clin. Immunol. 73:670-675; 1984.

41. Sly, R.M. Beta-adrenergic drugs in the management of asthma in athletes. J. Allergy Clin. Immunol. 73:680-685; 1984.

42. Smith, C.M.; Anderson, S.D. Hyperosmolarity as the stimulus to asthma induced by hyperventilation? J. Allergy Clin. Immunol. 77:729-736; 1986.

43. Sporik, R.; Holgate, S.T.; Cogswell, J.J. Natural history of asthma in childhood—a birth cohort study. Arch. Dis. Child 66:1050-1053; 1991.

44. Strick, L. Breathing and physical fitness exercises for asthmatic children. Pediatr. Clin. North Am. 16:31-42; 1969.

45. Strunk, R.C.; Mascia. A.V.; Lipkowitz, M.A.; Wolf, S.I. Rehabilitation of a patient with asthma in the outpatient setting. J. Allergy Clin. Immunol. 87:601-611; 1991.

46. Strunk, R.C.; Mrazek, D.A.; Fukuhara, J.T.; Masterson, J.; Ludwick, S.K.; LaBrecque, J.F. Cardiovascular fitness in children with asthma correlates with psychological functioning of the child. Pediatrics 84:460-464; 1989.

47. Strunk, R.C.; Rubin, D.; Kelly, L.; Sherman, B.; Fukuhara, J. Determination of fitness in children with asthma: use of standardized tests for functional endurance, body fat composition, flexibility, and abdominal strength. Am. J. Dis. Child 142:940-944; 1988.

48. Szentagothai, K.; Gyene, I.; Szocska, M.; Osvath, P. Physical exercise program children with bronchial asthma. Pediatr. Pulmonol. 3:166-172; 1987.

49. United States Olympic Committee, Drug Education Doping Control Program. Guide to banned medications. Colorado Springs: Author; 1992.

50. Warren, J.B.; Keynes, R.J.; Brown, M.J.; Jenner, D.A.; McNicol, M.W. Blunted sympathoadrenal response to exercise in asthmatic subjects. Br. J. Dis. Chest 76:147-151; 1982.

51. Wasserman, S.I.; Soter, N.A.; Center, D.M.; Austen, K.F. Cold urticaria. Recognition and characterization of a neutrophil chemotactic factor which appears in serum during experimental cold challenge. J. Clin. Invest. 60: 189-196; 1977.

52. Wolthers, O.D.; Pederson, J. Growth of asthmatic children during treatment with budesonide: a double-blind trial. Br. Med. J. 303:163-165; 1991.

53. Yunginger, J.W.; Reed, C.E.; O'Connell, E.J.; Melton, J.L., III; O'Fallon, W.M.; Silverstein, M.D. A community-based study of the epidemiology of asthma. Incidence rates, 1964-1983. Am. Rev. Respir. Dis. 146:888-894; 1992.

CHAPTER 11

Cystic Fibrosis

David M. Orenstein
University of Pittsburgh and Children's Hospital of Pittsburgh

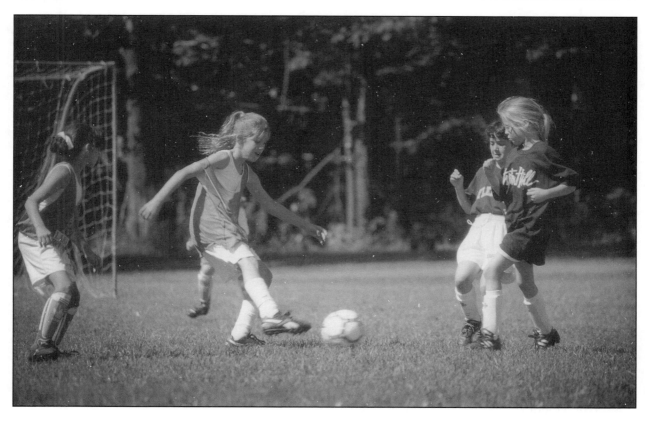

Cystic fibrosis (CF) is the most common life-shortening genetic disease in Caucasian populations (33). It is inherited as an autosomal recessive disorder that occurs in approximately 1 in every 2,500 live births in white American and northern European populations, and in about 1 in every 17,000 births in African-Americans; it is virtually unheard of in Asian populations (26). There are an estimated 30,000 patients with CF in the United States, and some 10 million asymptomatic carriers. The gene for CF apparently alters a protein product, referred to as CFTR (cystic fibrosis transmembrane regulator) (50). Over 400 different mutations at the CF locus have been identified. The natural history of CF is progressive loss of lung function that leads to death; however, with early diagnosis and therapeutic intervention survival into the third and fourth decades is now common.

DESCRIPTION
OF CYSTIC FIBROSIS

Cystic fibrosis can be described according to its pathophysiological characteristics and the signs and symptoms it manifests, including its effects on exercise capacity.

Pathophysiology

Although the signs and symptoms that make up CF have been recognized since 1938 (2), the basic biochemical defect has only recently begun to come to light (28). Cystic fibrosis affects virtually every organ system with epithelial surfaces—most importantly, the lungs, pancreas, intestinal mucous glands, and sweat glands. A common pathogenetic mechanism underlying the involvement of the major target systems is an alteration of ion transport across epithelial surfaces, leading to relative dehydration of luminal secretions (28). These abnormally viscous secretions cause the blockage of ducts and air passages.

Physical Symptoms
and Clinical Signs

Cystic fibrosis can be recognized through signs and symptoms of the gastrointestinal tract, sweat glands, and respiratory tract.

Gastrointestinal Tract and Nutrition

Exocrine pancreatic insufficiency is present in approximately 90% of CF patients (47) and is manifested by maldigestion of fats and protein, with consequent malabsorption and steatorrhea; frequent, smelly, bulky stools; and failure to thrive (47). Malnutrition may be a problem at any age, and is attributable to malabsorption, poor dietary intake, excessive caloric expenditure associated with increased work of breathing and cough, or any combination of these factors. Bowel obstruction may be present in 20–25% of patients (47). Liver abnormalities are common histologically (52); however, hepatic failure or portal hypertension with hypersplenism and bleeding esophageal varices is rare (52).

Sweat Glands

The chloride transport defect seen in all epithelia in CF is expressed clearly in the sweat glands, leading to the characteristic high salt content of CF sweat, and provides the basis for the sweat test, the definitive test for CF. Cystic fibrosis patients lose more salt in the heat than do persons without CF (46), and they may experience heat prostration.

Respiratory Tract

The upper respiratory tract is involved in most CF patients, with apparent sinusitis on X rays. Sinusitis is seldom clinically bothersome to the patient but occasionally is helpful diagnostically. Nasal polyps may be found in as many as 25% of these patients (59).

The lower respiratory tract involvement in CF accounts for over 95% of the morbidity and mortality (33). Although the lungs are histologically normal at birth, obstructive pulmonary disease, beginning in the small airways, eventually is present in almost all patients. Recurrent cough or wheeze, which may be diagnosed as bronchiolitis, asthma, or pneumonia, are often the first indications of pulmonary involvement. As the disease progresses, hyperinflation, crackles, and rhonchi become apparent on physical examination. The rate and intensity of the progression of the lung disease varies tremendously among patients, with some infants having severe disease, and some 30-year olds having normal or nearly normal pulmonary function.

Chronic pulmonary infection with acute exacerbations, often with *Pseudomonas aeruginosa*, is characteristic of CF patients (60). The chain of events begins with bronchiolitis and leads through bronchitis to bronchiectasis, peribronchial fibrosis, and progressive loss of pulmonary function. Low blood oxygen levels result, including during exercise (19). Figure 11.1 shows the cascade of factors leading to bronchial obstruction and destruction in cystic fibrosis: The abnormal gene encodes an abnormal protein that alters the movement of sodium and chloride through epithelial cell membranes, leading to dry mucus that blocks bronchioles and bronchi. With bronchial blockage, infection and inflammation take hold. Both infection and inflammation can cause the release of toxic chemicals that interfere with lung defenses and damage tissues, thus worsening the infection and inflammation. Inflammation also causes swelling of the bronchial wall, thus worsening bronchial blockage. Finally, in some individuals, inflammation may lead to bronchospasm.

Additional Symptoms

Delayed puberty may be seen in either sex as a consequence of chronic illness and poor nutrition. Some adolescents and adults display a unique pattern of diabetes, with hyperglycemia and abnormal glucose tolerance tests, but they almost never have ketoacidosis. Long bones and adjacent joints of patients with severe lung disease may be involved with hypertrophic pulmonary osteoarthropathy, a painful condition responsive to anti-inflammatory drugs or to improvement in the underlying lung condition. Digital clubbing is a nearly universal finding in patients with even mildly abnormal lung function.

Clinical and Laboratory Assessment With Specific Reference to Exercise Capacity

Pulmonary function tests usually show obstructive airways disease, with decreased vital capacity, forced expiratory volume in 1 second (FEV_1)

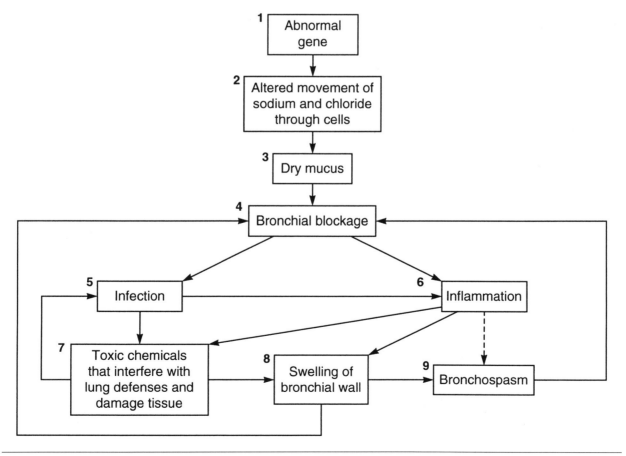

Figure 11.1 Cascade of problems in cystic fibrosis.
Adapted from Orenstein (1991).

and peak expiratory flow, and increased residual volume, which is indicative of air trapping (10). These obstructive changes show varying responses to bronchodilator inhalation; some patients improve, as with asthma, many do not change, and others actually worsen. Also, the response to bronchodilators is not consistent over time (47).

Exercise Testing: Amount of Work Tolerated

CF patients in general perform less well on exercise tests than their healthy peers (5, 11, 18, 39, 44, 52, 61). Patients with normal or nearly normal lung function at rest tend to have normal or nearly normal exercise tolerance, while those with more severe pulmonary function abnormalities fare less well during exercise (11). Despite the high group correlation between pulmonary function and exercise tolerance there is tremendous variation among individuals, making the resting pulmonary function test a poor predictor of exercise tolerance (see Figure 11.2).

Cardiovascular Responses

Heart rate tends to be normal at rest, except in the most severely affected patients, and increases normally with increasing workloads (8). Maximal heart rates, however, do not reach

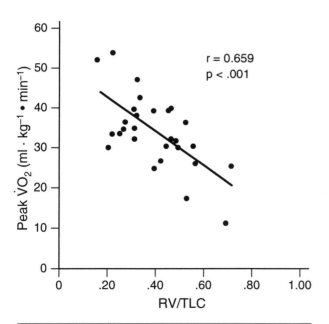

Figure 11.2 Peak oxygen uptake ($\dot{V}O_{2\,peak}$) in ml · kg^{-1} · min^{-1} plotted against residual volume (RV)/total lung capacity (TLC) for 28 patients.
Reprinted from Orenstein and Nixon (1989).

normal, except in those patients with the mildest lung disease (11). This is almost certainly because lung-related factors limit exercise before the heart is pushed to the maximal rates of which it is capable (40). Cardiac output is normal for workload (18, 34, 35), but stroke volume may be reduced (21).

Ventilatory Responses

Ventilation increases with increasing work rate. At peak exercise, minute ventilation is greatest for those with the best pulmonary function and least for those with the most compromised resting pulmonary function, consistent with the amount of work accomplished (42). However, when ventilation is examined in relation to work rates achieved or amount of oxygen consumed, patients with CF require a larger minute ventilation than subjects without lung disease (8), almost certainly in order to compensate for a larger-than-normal dead space (18).

Ventilatory mechanics probably limit exercise tolerance in many patients with CF (18). Many patients employ minute ventilation during exercise that approaches or even exceeds their resting maximum voluntary ventilation (MVV) (18). In healthy children, in contrast, exercise ventilation seldom exceeds 70% of MVV (17). The patient with CF probably has no reserve beyond what is employed to achieve these high levels of minute ventilation.

Gas Exchange

The high minute ventilation used may be inadequate, and some patients may have relative hypoventilation during exercise, with elevated end-tidal carbon dioxide and hypoxemia (8, 11, 19). Most patients do not desaturate during exercise, and some even improve their oxygenation (18, 19). Patients with FEV_1 greater than 50% of forced vital capacity (FVC) are very unlikely to desaturate (19); even those with an FEV_1/FVC ratio of less than 50% are just as likely to maintain their oxyhemoglobin saturation at preexercise levels, or even to increase them, as they are to desaturate (19).

Effect of Desaturation and Oxygen Supplementation on Exercise Tolerance

Despite even profound desaturation in some patients, there is no evidence that oxygenation

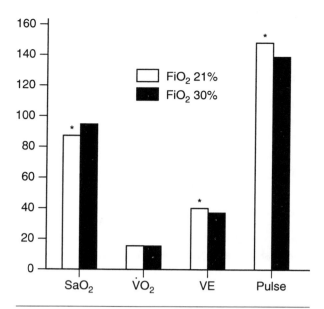

Figure 11.3 Effect of oxygen supplementation on exercise tolerance. SaO₂ in percent, V̇O₂ in ml/kg/min, VE in L/min, pulse in beats/min. Data from Nixon et al. (1990).

limits maximal exercise performance in cystic fibrosis patients; in fact, there is some evidence that it does not. As Figure 11.3 shows, supplemental oxygen given during exercise effectively blocks desaturation in those who desaturate when exercising in room air, and it decreases heart rate and respiratory rate for submaximal work rates. However, it does not increase peak work rate achieved on a progressive test to exhaustion (38).

The pulmonary function and exercise tests are relatively sensitive tools for following progression of disease in the older, cooperative child, adolescent, and adult patient.

Natural History

The natural history of cystic fibrosis includes progressive pulmonary obstruction and infection with progressive loss of lung function, leading to an early death. When the disease was first recognized in the late 1930s, almost all children with cystic fibrosis died before school age. Institution of specialized CF centers and comprehensive, aggressive treatment programs beginning in the 1950s has improved the prognosis tremendously. National median survival was 10.6 years in 1966 and 29.4 years in 1992. Currently, many patients in their 20s and 30s have excellent lung function; at the end of 1992, 32.8% of CF patients in the United States were 18 years old or older (16). Survival probably depends on several factors, including

- inherent severity of the disease, perhaps influenced by genotype (25);
- aggressiveness of the treatment program as prescribed by the physician and carried out by the patient and family; and
- some degree of chance, especially concerning contact with various bacterial and viral pathogens.

Factors with good prognosis include care in a cystic fibrosis center (37), male sex (32), good chest radiograph score (57), good nutrition (30), and high cardiopulmonary fitness (38a). The recent discovery of the gene (24), the uncovering of the basic defect (49), and the very exciting research breakthrough of using gene-transfer techniques to cure the basic defect in CF cells in the test tube (13) have all raised hopes for improved treatments and even the possibility of a cure within the foreseeable future.

Therapeutic Intervention

Cystic fibrosis is a complex disease, and patients require a comprehensive care program. This is usually best carried out in, or at least coordinated from, a specialized cystic fibrosis center where many different specialists are available (37). Therapy has three primary components:

- pulmonary,
- gastrointestinal, and
- psychological.

Pulmonary Therapy

The goal of pulmonary therapy is to prevent or delay progression of the pulmonary lesion, and is accomplished through the relief of airway obstruction and inflammation, as well as control of infection.

Therapy for Obstruction. Chest physical therapy (CPT) with percussion and postural drainage is the effective mainstay of most treatment programs (48). It is recommended that most patients undergo CPT to all pulmonary segments from 1 to 4 times daily, with increased frequency at times of clinical pulmonary exacerbation (48).

Aerosol Therapy. Cystic fibrosis patients who also have asthma respond well to bronchodilator aerosols; in other patients, these aerosols make no difference or may actually reduce airflow (31). Whether long-term use of beta-agonists will be helpful to any or all CF patients is unclear. Antibiotics, especially aminoglycosides and the antipseudomonas penicillin derivatives (60), have been delivered by aerosols, apparently with favorable results.

Several experimental aerosol therapies have been introduced and await definitive study to confirm their safety and efficacy. These include amiloride (27), which may improve epithelial ion transport and make airway luminal contents less viscous; DNase, which can degrade neutrophil-derived DNA and therefore decrease the viscosity of airway secretions (1); and alpha-1 antitrypsin, which may diminish the inflammatory effects of neutrophil-derived proteases (36).

Therapy for Inflammation. Several approaches have been suggested to diminish airway inflammation in CF, including systemic steroids (alternate-day prednisone [4] and ibuprofen [29]). Early studies, particularly with alternate-day prednisone, have had mixed results, with apparent benefits in some patients (4), but unacceptable side effects in others (50).

Therapy for Infection. There is general agreement that antibiotic treatment has probably been the single most important factor in the greatly improved prognosis in CF.

Some CF centers advocate continuous prophylactic antibiotic treatment. Another approach is to restrict the use of antibiotics to times of exacerbation of pulmonary disease, as evidenced by increased symptoms or signs such as cough or sputum production (60), or worsening chest radiograph or pulmonary function test results.

Intravenous antibiotics are indicated when the patient does not respond to outpatient oral administration of antibiotics (60). The important consideration in the decision to hospitalize patients and begin parenteral therapy is whether the patients are sicker than their own baseline, and not whether they seem dreadfully ill. It is clear that a tremendous amount of lung can be lost irreversibly while a child still looks reasonably well. Intravenous antibiotics have traditionally been administered during hospitalization, but in recent years have increasingly been used successfully at home (60).

Aerosol antibiotics may be effective in many patients colonized with pseudomonas (60).

Lung Transplantation. Heart-lung or double-lung transplantation has been successful in a limited number of CF patients with end-stage disease (53). One-year survival ranges from 50% to 80%.

Gastrointestinal Therapy

The main goal of gastrointestinal therapy is to establish good nutrition. With the availability of pancreatic enzyme replacement preparations, and, especially enteric-coated preparations, this once insurmountable problem has become quite manageable (46). Diet need not be especially tailored for the patient whose growth is adequate.

Psychological Considerations

Having a genetic, incurable, progressive, life-shortening, financially draining, and activity-limiting disease places great emotional burdens on patient and family. However, it is remarkable how well the large majority of patients and families adjust; there is a very low incidence of depression (6). Establishing and maintaining a positive, optimistic, yet realistic attitude is extremely important. These goals are attainable, especially if the primary physician shares this attitude and maintains a close, supportive relationship with the patient and family. It is important that the physician encourage an active, normal childhood and adolescence to the extent possible, including participation in sport and recreational activities. Knowledge of the tremendously improved prognosis over the past decades facilitates such an attitude.

Additional Treatment Considerations

Hyperglycemia occurs in a small group of CF patients, who may require insulin therapy (15). Salt loss may be excessive, especially during exertion in warm weather (45). Infants may require small amounts of supplemental salt in warm weather, but older children and adults will regulate their salt intake quite adequately if given free access to the salt shaker. Salt tablets are not necessary and may be harmful.

EXERCISE AND CYSTIC FIBROSIS

Children with CF tolerate exercise well, but those who work with them should be familiar with the potential adverse effects. Figure 11.4 summarizes the impact of CF on sport performance.

Effect of Cystic Fibrosis on Exercise Tolerance and Sport Performance

Single Bouts of Exercise

Just as the severity of airway obstruction varies tremendously among patients with CF, so too does the response to exercise. Some patients are nearly bedridden, while others have completed marathons (54) and Ironman-distance triathlons (swim 2.4 miles, bike 112 miles, run 26.2 miles). In general, studies have shown that exercise tolerance in patients with CF is related to the severity of the underlying lung disease (11, 18, 42, 44) and have suggested that ventilatory mechanics may limit exercise tolerance in these patients. In contrast, in healthy populations the lungs seldom limit exercise. The correlation between lung function and exercise tolerance is highly significant statistically, but nearly useless as a guide to predicting exercise tolerance from the resting pulmonary function. This is not to imply that pulmonary function does not influence exercise tolerance in the individual, but rather that the exact relationship between pulmonary function

testing (PFT) results and exercise tolerance differs from patient to patient. An important study demonstrated what most patients report: A change in pulmonary function changes exercise tolerance in individual patients (7). Seventeen patients with CF were studied at the beginning and end of a 2-week hospitalization for intensive treatment of pulmonary exacerbation. The results are shown in Figure 11.5. The patients achieved much higher work rates, markedly improved peak oxygen consumption, and a lower perception of exertion when their pulmonary function improved (7).

Several different studies have demonstrated that nutritional status correlates significantly with exercise tolerance, separate from the influence of pulmonary function (9, 34, 35). Among patients with comparable disease severity, female patients have lower exercise tolerance than males (42), as is generally true of healthy populations.

Sputum Production. Anecdotes abound associating exercise sessions with improved sputum production (40). A study of 10 hospitalized CF patients measured the volume of sputum expectorated during 15 minutes of cycle ergometer exercise and the ensuing 1.75 hours, and compared it with the expectorated volume during and following a comparable 15-minute session of traditional chest physiotherapy (52). More sputum was expectorated with traditional chest physiotherapy than with cycle exercise, prompting the authors to conclude that "exercise may

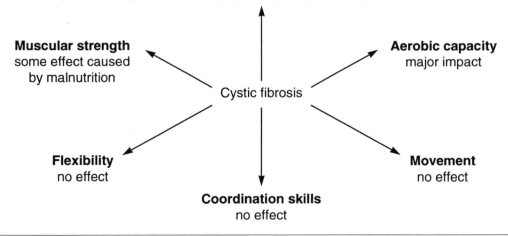

Figure 11.4 The impact of cystic fibrosis on sport performance.

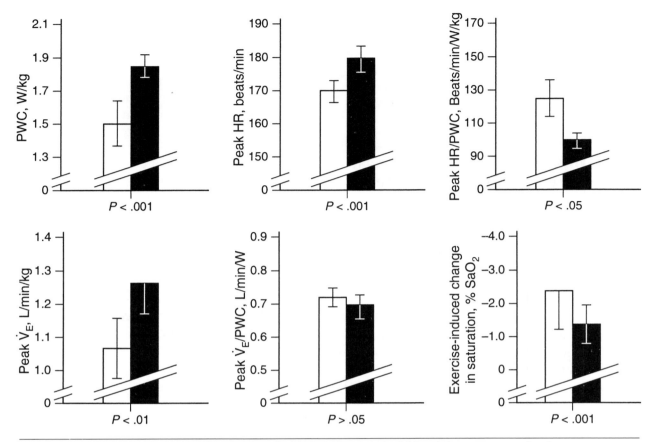

Figure 11.5 Improved exercise tolerance at end of hospitalization (solid bars) for treatment of pulmonary exacerbation after pulmonary function had improved, compared with beginning (open bars). Thus, improved pulmonary function is correlated with improved exercise tolerance. (PWC = peak work capacity; $\dot{V}_E$ = minute ventilation; W = watts.)
Reprinted from Cerny, Cropp, and Bye (1984).

have a role in aiding sputum expectoration in patients with cystic fibrosis but should not be considered as a replacement for physiotherapy" (p. 1006).

Exercise in the Heat. For decades, CF patients have been known to have greater than normal concentrations of sodium and chloride in their sweat (12). In one controlled study, CF patients had normal temperature, heart rate, hormonal (renin, aldosterone), and renal responses, but lost more than normal amounts of sodium and chloride when they exercised for 90 minutes in a heat chamber (100 °F, 38 °C) (46). The sodium and chloride losses were so great that the patients showed decreased concentrations of these ions in serum (45). Another recent study has shown that children with CF underestimate their fluid requirement when they exercise in the heat, a phenomenon that Bar-Or has termed *voluntary hypohydration* (4a). However, once they

have completed the exercise and are out of the heat, CF patients have fully normal homeostatic control: within 24 hours after the 90-minute exercise and heat stress, body weight and serum electrolytes were back to baseline when patients were given a free choice of fluid and food (41).

Repeated Bouts of Exercise (Exercise Programs)

In a number of studies published since the late 1970s, exercise programs have been described for patients with cystic fibrosis. The evidence seems to indicate various benefits from these different programs, and no obvious harmful effects. Table 11.1 summarizes studies published over the past 15 years. The types of exercise intervention can be divided roughly into: ventilatory muscle exercise, jogging and walking, swimming, weightlifting, cycling, and others.

Ventilatory Muscle Exercise. The first published exercise intervention program for cystic fibrosis was by Keens and his colleagues, and focused on the ventilatory muscles (23). This study demonstrated unequivocally that daily exercise directed specifically at the ventilatory muscles could increase the endurance of those most important muscles. (The exercise, which was performed 25 minutes per day, 5 days per week, involved breathing through a tubing system large volumes of air mixed with a small amount of carbon dioxide to keep blood carbon dioxide levels normal.) Similar effects were achieved with less precisely targeted upper body exercise (swimming and canoeing, 90 minutes per day for 4 weeks) (23). Several years later, Asher and colleagues demonstrated that 4 weeks of twice-daily, 15-minute sessions of breathing through an inspiratory resistance brought about increases in both strength and endurance of the ventilatory muscles of patients with cystic fibrosis (3). However, this increased ventilatory muscle performance was not associated with any improvement in overall exercise tolerance (as measured by cycle ergometer testing), suggesting that the ventilatory muscles are not the weak link in the exercise tolerance chain.

Jogging and Walking. The first study to employ general aerobic exercise in cystic fibrosis, instead of exercise targeted specifically at the ventilatory muscles, was of a supervised group who jogged and walked 3 times per week for 3 months (44). They gradually increased the length of time per session devoted to the exercise. Twenty-one CF patients with a wide range of disease severity began with warm-up calisthenics and low-intensity games, and then started jogging and walking at an intensity sufficient to produce heart rates of 70% to 85% of their own maximal heart rates (as determined at the beginning of the program by progressive tests to exhaustion). During the first week of the program, the jogging and walking portion of each session lasted 10 minutes, with 2 minutes added each week; by the 10th week, patients were jogging steadily for 30 minutes. Patients in this study increased their exercise tolerance (as evidenced by higher work rate on a progressive cycle ergometer test to exhaustion) and their cardiorespiratory fitness (as measured by peak oxygen consumption).

In another jogging study, Braggion and colleagues included 10 CF patients with quite mild lung disease for an 8-week (3 times per week) program (5). The intensity of exercise was adjusted "so as to produce a heart rate not exceeding 150 bpm" (p. 147). The length of the exercise sessions was similar to that in the previous study, starting with 10 minutes and gradually increasing to 25 to 30 minutes by the final week. In this study, however, virtually no changes were found in exercise tolerance, cardiorespiratory fitness, or pulmonary function. The authors speculated that the lack of change might have resulted from the relatively mild degree of lung disease and high initial fitness in these patients, or from the low intensity or short duration of the program.

Another study was carried out in Australia by Holzer and coworkers (20). This was a calisthenics and running program with an important difference from the previous studies: it was an at-home, unsupervised study. Compliance was very poor, and no measurable benefits accrued to the patients, forcing the authors to conclude that "there appears limited value in promoting unsupervised home exercise programs for children with CF" (p. 297).

Swimming. Zach and coworkers described a program consisting of 1 hour of swimming 2 to 3 times each week for 7 weeks (63). During the program patients continued their usual chest physical therapy treatments. Exercise tolerance was not measured, but expiratory flow rates were improved at the end of 7 weeks and sputum production was felt to be greater on swimming days than on nonswimming days. However, by 10 weeks after the program, pulmonary function had fallen back to the preexercise baseline. In another study of 12 CF patients, Edlund and colleagues (14) showed a 12-week swimming program to result in improved treadmill endurance but no change in pulmonary function was observed.

Weightlifting. In one study of 9 adults with CF, a 6-month upper-body weight-training program was shown to increase upper-body strength and body weight, and to decrease lung hyperinflation (lower residual volume) (59). It is unclear how this effect on residual volume can be explained, except perhaps by an increase in expiratory muscle strength.

Cycling. A British program prescribed 10 minutes of home exercise on a cycle ergometer 5

Table 11.1   Recent Studies on Exercise Programs for Patients With Cystic Fibrosis

			Exercise program				Study design		
Reference	Frequency	Intensity	Time per session	Type of exercise	Location (supervised)	N start/ N finish (ages)	Disease severity	Controls/ randomization	Length of study
Keens 1977	5 days/wk	Maximal	25 min	Normocapnic hyperpnea	CF summer camp (supervised)	4/4 (16±6)	FEV_1 59 ± 13 % predicted	Non-CF controls Not random	4 wks
Keens 1977	Daily	Intensive	1.5 hr	Swimming & canoeing	CF summer camp (supervised)	7/7 (13 ± 1)	FEV_1 64 ± 8 % predicted	1. Non-CF controls; 2. CF pts vent.musc. trainers not random	4 wks
Orenstein 1981	3/wk	70-85% of pt's own max. heart rate	10 min 1st wk, increase to 30 min by 10th wk	Jogging-walking	Local gymnasia (supervised)	25/21 exercise 10/10 control (10-30)	FEV_1 range 32-81 % of VC	Not random; controls lived far away	3 mos
Zach 1981	2-3/wk		1 hr	Swimming	"Teaching pool" (supervised)	10/10	FEV_1 83 ± 24 % predicted	No controls Not random; pts. lived within 30 km of hospital	7-1/2 wks
Zach 1982	Daily		7.5 hr/day	Swimming, jogging, hiking, gymnastics, soccer, etc.	Paediatric rehab hospital (supervised)	12/10 (2-16)	FEV_1 71 ± 22 % predicted	No controls Not random ("willingness to participate")	17 days
Asher 1982	2/day		15 min	Vent. muscle (breathing through an insp. resist.)	Home (supervised by phone and some home visits)	11/11 (9-24)	Severe FEV_1 < 50% pred.	Pts own controls for 4 wks before or after 4 wks of training	4 wks training; 4 wks control
Holzer 1981	Daily	Graded increase depending on capacity	30 min	Various: Royal Canadian Air Force	Home (unsupervised)	41/? (8-14)	Mild FEV_1 86 ± 19% pred	No controls Not random	3 mos
Blomquist 1986	2/day	HR ≥ 75% of each pt's max	15 min (at least)	Various: skip rope plus: jog, dance, bowl...	Home (unsupervised)	14/12 (13-23)	Mod-mild mean FVC = 77% pred.	Pts own controls Not random	12 mos
Edlund 1986	3/wk	HR 60-75% of pt's max, wk 1-5; then 70-85% of max	5 min 1st wk; increase to 20 min by wk 7	Swimming	University pool (supervised)	12/10 (7-14)	Mild (clin. score 83/ 100); initial VO_2 = 56 ml/kg/min	Controlled Not random (group selection based on proximity to medical center)	12 wk
O'Neill 1987	Daily		11 min	Various: Royal Canadian Air Force Program	Home (unsupervised)	8/7 (17-27)	Mean FEV_1 1.72 ± .97L	No controls Not random	2 mos
Andreasson 1987	Daily	HR 160 or more	30 min	Various: sit-ups, jogging, swimming, ball games, etc.	Home (unsupervised)	7/7 (6-20)	Mild-mod FEV_1 45-106% pred (mean 71%)	No controls Not random	30 mos
Braggion 1989	3/wk	HR 150 or less	10 min 1st wk; increase to 30 min final wk	Jogging (also had warmup and circuit training each session)	? where (supervised by physiotherapists supervised by phys. ed. teacher)	10/10 exercise; 10/10 control (11-15)	Mild FEV_1 43-100% pred (mean 77%)	1. Pts own controls 2. Non-CF control grp. 3. Not random	8 wks
Salh 1989	5/wk	Start at 50% of peak work capacity; increase 5 watts/ wk	10 min	Exercise cycle	Home (not supervised)	19/12 (16-33)	FEV_1 15-94% pred (mean 46%)	No control Not random	2 mos
Cerny 1989	2/day	HR about 1/2 between rest and max.	5-10 min, day 1-3; 15-20 min, day 4-14	Exercise cycle	Hospital (supervised)	9/9 exercise 8/8 control (15.4 ± 4.9)	Moderate-to-severe (study done in pts hosp. for pulm rx)	Randomly assigned to exercise or standard care control	14 days

			Results			
Exercise tolerance	Ventilatory muscle endurance	Peak VO_2	FEV_1	Other PFT	Sputum volume	Comments
No change	Increased 53%	No change	No change	MMEF: No change		Ventilatory muscle endurance incr equally in ventilatory and swim/canoe group. Returned to baseline after program.
No change	Increased 57%	No change	No change	MMEF: No change		(See above)
Improved (exercise group); no change (control group)	Improved (exercise group); no change (control group)	Improved (exercise group); no change (control group)	No change (exercise group); decreased (control group)	No change either group		Exercise group had training bradycardia (lower submax HR) after program. 14 exercise pts who improved began less fit than 7 pts who did not improve.
			Improved (83 > 91% pred.)	FVC, PEFR, FEF_{25-75} all improved	Greater on swimming days (but difference significant in only 2 pts.)	Most pts stopped exercise after program ended; PTFs back to baseline after program ended.
No formal testing, but "a gradual increase in performance & endurance was evident"			Improved (71 > 79% pred.)	FVC, PEFR, FEF_{25-75} all improved	Reached a max between Days 3 & 5, then decreased gradually	Pts stopped regular inhalation and chest physiotherapy for entire 17 days. Authors conclude exercise could replace inhalation-physio for some patients with CF.
No change either maximal or submaximal exercise after program	Increase after ventilatory muscle training; ventilatory muscle strength also increased	No change				Ventilatory muscle training did increase ventilatory muscle strength & endurance, but exercise tolerance did not change.
No change	No change		No change	No change		Very poor compliance. Authors concluded. "There appears limited value in . . . unsupervised home exercise."
No change			No change	Improved PaO_2		No pts did prescribed skipping rope; authors feel self-rx plus exercise is as good as conventional physio.
Increased treadmill time in exercise group; slight decrease in control group		Measured VO_2 no change; predicted VO_2 increase in exercise group	No change	Clinical scores significantly better for exercise groups; no change for controls		Very fit group. Authors concluded: "a swimming program is . . . excellent . . . for improving the clinical status and quality of life in CF"
No change	No change	No change	No change	Decreased RV (1.90 ≥ 1.20L)	"In some cases, a decrease in sputum volume"	Breathlessness significantly reduced on submaximal work, as measured on VAS (visual analog scale).
No change				No change except decreased VTG		After 12 mos, usual chest physio. was eliminated, yet PFTs did not decrease. Conclusion: "conventional chest physio. can be replaced by efficient physical training."
Increased (Wmax: 4.0 > 4.2 W/kg); improved endurance time, faster obstacle course in CF; no change in controls	No change in either group	No change	No change	No change		
Increased (peak work 2.7 > 3.1 watt/kg)		Increased 25.9 > 30.3 ml/gk/min	No change	MVV increased; no change in FVC	Nonsignficant increase in daily sputum volume 24 > 37 gm (with very large std dev.)	In a separate study reported in same paper, compared sputum volume during and after cycle exercise with sputum volume during and after std chest physio: significantly more sputum produced with physio than with exercise.
Increased work load in both groups; no differences between groups			Increased (both exercise and control)	Most PFT's improved in both groups; no differences between groups	No differences between groups in sputum volume	This study was done in hospital, on pts being rx'd for pulm. exac. Exercise group did 2 cycle sessions and 1 physio per day; control did 3 physio sessions per day.

days per week for 2 months for 19 adults with CF (52). Only 12 patients (63%) completed the program, but this group experienced significant increases in peak work capacity and fitness (as measured by maximum oxygen consumption). There was also a nonsignificant increase in daily sputum volume at the end of the exercise program compared with the preexercise baseline. No changes were observed in FVC and FEV_1.

Other Exercise Programs. O'Neill and co-workers (39) prescribed an 8-week at-home program for 8 CF patients based on the Royal Canadian Air Force protocol. Neither pulmonary function nor exercise tolerance changed, but breathlessness during exercise decreased significantly. Zach and colleagues carried out a 17-day program of very intense exercise with 12 children during summer holidays at a pediatric rehabilitation hospital in the mountains of Austria (62). The program included "one hour of swimming and diving twice a day. As the . . . pool was some 2-1/2 km from the paediatric department, the children jogged from one to the other. The children hiked for several hours through the surrounding forests and mountains, collecting firewood, berries, and mushrooms. In addition, all children took part in gymnastics, skipping, and . . . minigolf, soccer, and table tennis" (p. 587). The children did not do their regular chest physiotherapy or inhalation treatments during the 17 days. Daily peak flow measurements increased throughout the program, but fell to baseline by 8 weeks later.

Heat Acclimation. In healthy populations, repeated bouts of exercise in the heat can bring about better tolerance to similar stresses. Patients with cystic fibrosis can also improve their tolerance to exercise and heat stress (41). In one study eight consecutive days of exercise and heat stress enabled CF patients to withstand exercise in the heat with lower heart rates and lower core body temperatures. However, there was no lessening of sweat sodium and chloride concentrations, as was seen in the healthy control subjects.

Potential Adverse Effects of Sport and Exercise

In general, patients with cystic fibrosis, even with severe disease, will tolerate exercise and sport without adverse effects. However, there are several possible adverse effects to be aware of.

Lowered Blood Oxygen Levels

Patients with the most severe lung disease may experience lower oxygen levels in the bloodstream as a result of exercise (19). The dangers from this lower oxygen level are not clear, but most physicians prefer that their patients not experience even brief episodes of low oxygen levels. In most cases, even with profound decreases, blood oxygen levels will be restored within minutes after stopping exercise. Patients who are recognized as being at risk for lowered oxygen during exercise should have been tested by their physician, who will prescribe a level of exercise intensity in terms of a heart rate that should not be exceeded.

Increased Cough

Many patients with cystic fibrosis will cough during exercise. For some patients, and particularly for many bystanders, this may be quite distressing, especially if the patient has a hard coughing spell. It may appear to the naive observer that the patient will not be able to catch his or her breath, and that surely this must be a dangerous problem. In some patients, moreover, these spells may be associated with a profound transient decrease in the blood oxygen level. In fact, however, the spells are not dangerous, and they may even be helpful in clearing mucus from the bronchial tree more effectively than the traditionally prescribed methods of clearing mucus.

Shortness of Breath

With vigorous exertion, some patients with cystic fibrosis may become short of breath, even without cough and with normal oxygen levels. In some cases, this may be due to exercise-induced asthma, as some patients with CF also have asthma. For these youngsters, the approach should be the same as for those patients with asthma who don't have CF (see chapter 10); for example, they should be permitted to use a bronchodilator inhaler before or during practices or competition, and to take short breaks to catch their breath when necessary. If a youngster does not have asthma, a common-sense approach is adequate: that is, the child's own tolerance should dictate the level and timing of exertion. While a few patients not truly limited by their lung capacity may take unfair advantage of this approach, the majority of youngsters with CF will not abuse it and will participate to their full potential.

Salt and Fluid Loss

During sustained exercise in the heat, patients with cystic fibrosis are at risk for greater fluid and salt losses through sweat than their healthy peers.

Preventing Adverse Effects

Preventing Lowered Oxygen Levels

Young athletes with the most severe lung disease from CF (those whose FEV_1 is less than 50% of the FVC) should undergo supervised exercise testing, including monitoring of blood oxygen levels, before engaging in sport. If their oxy-hemoglobin concentration (S_aO_2) falls below 90%, the physician monitoring the test should note the heart rate at which this occurs, and athletes should be advised to keep their heart rate below that level when they exercise during practice or competition.

Preventing Increased Cough and Shortness of Breath

In CF patients who also have asthma, pre-exercise use of a bronchodilator inhaler may help prevent excess coughing and shortness of breath during exercise, and should be encouraged. For most CF patients, no specific measures (other than limiting the intensity of exercise) can or should be taken to prevent exercise-related cough or shortness of breath.

Preventing Fluid and Salt Loss

Cystic fibrosis patients who exercise for more than 30 minutes in the heat should be encouraged to drink water or electrolyte-containing fluid before, during, and after exercise, even if they don't feel particularly thirsty. Cystic

fibrosis patients should also always have free access to the salt shaker and salty foods. Salt tablets are not necessary and may be harmful.

In most cases of adverse effects occurring during exercise in people with CF, little more than allowing the youngster a short break to catch his or her breath is required.

Potential Benefits of Exercise on the Disease Process

Exercise programs in cystic fibrosis have focused on the following different outcome variables, some general, others more specific to CF:

- exercise tolerance and cardiorespiratory fitness,
- ventilatory muscle endurance,
- pulmonary function,
- sputum production, and
- breathlessness.

The influence of exercise programs on the quality of life and its prognosis is also of interest.

Benefits Specific to Cystic Fibrosis

Pulmonary Function. Findings with regard to pulmonary function have been inconsistent, with several studies showing improved pulmonary function and others showing no change, or no difference between an exercise group and a control group. Since cystic fibrosis is characterized by progressive decline in pulmonary function, an intervention that prevented that decline would be a very successful intervention, and a lack of change over time would be a very positive outcome. Unfortunately, few studies have lasted long enough to confirm that the programs have truly delayed or prevented the expected deterioration. For example, Zach's two Austrian studies, one with 7 weeks of swimming (63) and the other with 17 days of very intense, day-long activity (62), both showed improved FEV_1 and FVC during the exercise period, with deterioration back to baseline values after the exercise programs ended.

Sputum Production. Some investigators point to improved sputum production as the main benefit CF patients derive from exercise. However, these studies have been difficult to evaluate. For example, Zach's 7-week swimming program (63) reported that "regular swimming can assist in mucus clearance" (p. 1201), yet the results indicate that only two patients experienced a significant difference between swimming and nonswimming days. In Salh's study (52), daily cycle ergometer exercise brought about a nonsignificant increase in daily sputum weight by the end of the 2-month intervention. The point of several of the exercise studies was to see if an exercise program could substitute for traditional chest physiotherapy. Since the results have been mixed, conservative recommendations would include both exercise and chest percussion and postural drainage.

Breathlessness. One British study evaluated the effects of an exercise program on the amount of dyspnea experienced by patients with CF during exercise. O'Neill and coworkers (39) found that a 2-month program significantly reduced breathlessness for a submaximal exercise task, even though it did not bring about a measurable increase in exercise tolerance on a maximal exercise test.

Prognosis. No studies to date have been long enough or have had sufficient numbers of patients to be able to examine the influence of exercise programs on the prognosis for patients with cystic fibrosis. However, a study by Nixon and her colleagues did demonstrate that fitness was positively correlated with survival in 109 patients with CF (38a) (see Figure 11.6). Patients

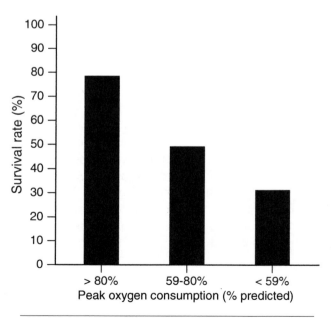

Figure 11.6   The relationship between fitness (peak oxygen consumption) and 8-year survival. Data modified from Nixon et al. (1992).

in this study with peak oxygen consumption under 58% of predicted (corresponding to about 30 ml·kg·min^{-1} were 6.4 times less likely to survive 8 years than those with peak oxygen consumption over 82% of predicted (roughly 38 ml·kg·min^{-1}). Resting pulmonary function tests played a much smaller role in predicting survival than the exercise tests. Several years before, it had been shown that it was possible to increase aerobic fitness in patients with CF (44). Taken together, these two observations suggest that an aerobic exercise program might have the potential actually to improve longevity for patients with CF.

Physical Fitness

Most of the exercise programs studied have brought about an increase in physical fitness and exercise tolerance, which might be the most important outcome for an exercise program. Programs that have been shown to increase exercise tolerance include 3 months of supervised jogging (44) or swimming (14), 3 times a week, and 8 weeks of daily trampoline exercise (55) (see Table 11.1 for further details).

Psychosocial Development and Quality of Life

Although the effects of exercise on psychosocial development have not been studied rigorously in CF, there are suggestions of beneficial effects, particularly on patients' self-concept and self-image (14, 56). In one study of 44 patients with cystic fibrosis, a general scale measuring the quality of well-being (the Quality of Well-Being Scale) was found to correlate significantly with exercise test results (43).

EXERCISE AND SPORT PROGRAMS FOR CHILDREN WITH CYSTIC FIBROSIS

Specific exercise programs and sports can be recommended for youngsters with CF, and none are absolutely contraindicated. By being aware of certain preparticipation issues and symptoms to watch for, school personnel can ensure a successful and safe experience for their athletes who have CF.

Specific Exercise and Conditioning Activities to Be Recommended

The best form of exercise for patients with CF is not yet known. What is known is that

- aerobic conditioning programs can improve aerobic fitness in patients with CF,
- high aerobic fitness is correlated with improved survival,
- upper body exercise may decrease lung overinflation,
- various forms of exercise may help clear excess mucus from the lungs, and
- patients with CF exercising in the heat will lose more (and replace less) fluid and salt than healthy youngsters.

Aerobic Activities

A graduated test to maximal tolerance with measurement of heart rate and oxygen saturation is helpful in setting up guidelines for an exercise program and for establishing a baseline against which progress or deterioration can be compared. The test is essential for patients with severe lung disease (i.e., those whose FEV_1 is less than 50% of FVC or less than 50% of predicted), since these are the patients who are at increased risk for developing desaturation during exercise (19). If a patient does desaturate, it will then be possible to identify the heart rate at which this occurs, and this can be taken into account. If desaturation occurs even at very low heart rates, it is advisable to prescribe supplemental oxygen to be used with the exercise program. Once the mode of exercise is selected (e.g., jogging, swimming, biking), guidelines should be given for frequency, intensity, and time (FIT). The frequency should probably be 3 to 5 times per week. Fewer sessions may not be effective, and more may not allow adequate musculoskeletal recovery, making injury more likely. Depending on the results of the exercise test regarding oxygen desaturation, the intensity should generally be great enough to elicit a heart rate that is 70-85% of maximal values. In healthy populations and cardiac rehabilitation programs these target heart rates are calculated from population norms based on age. Yet patients with cystic fibrosis (or other pulmonary disorders) may be limited by their ventilatory capacity and be at a truly maximal work rate with a heart rate that

has not yet reached 70% of their age-predicted maximal (40). Therefore, in prescribing exercise intensity based on a proportion of maximal heart rate, the maximal heart rate must be the patient's own maximal heart rate as actually measured, not predicted.

The duration of each session should ideally be 20 to 30 minutes. However, this may be a bit much for someone who is unfit to begin with, and it is better to start with whatever the patient can readily tolerate (e.g., 10 minutes), and gradually add time to the individual sessions as exercise tolerance improves. We have found the addition of 2 minutes each week to be tolerated by the majority of patients. Intermittent short sessions (i.e., of several minutes) may be easier for the very limited patient who has difficulty accomplishing prolonged continuous exercise. The overall program should probably be lifelong. Two months of the program are likely to be necessary before a change in maximal oxygen uptake will be seen, yet changing test results is not the goal. Rather, the goal is to increase and maintain exercise tolerance.

Relatively frequent contact between the patient and the physician or other medical personnel will let the physician stay informed about disease progression. Frequent contact will also help with patient compliance and will help demonstrate the physician's interest in the patient and the program. Periodic retesting will also serve to give the patient positive reinforcement for continuing the program. These guidelines for aerobic activities are virtually no different for youngsters with CF than for a healthy population. One must keep in mind only the greater fluid losses in the heat and the fact that some patients with CF will cough, become short of breath, or both, with exercise. Should there be prolonged exercise in the heat, the child with CF should be encouraged to drink more (either water or a sport electrolyte compound). Should youngsters have cough or shortness of breath, they should be allowed to decide if they need a brief rest, and to return to practice or competition as soon as they feel ready. The coach or teacher should not worry about harm being done by allowing youngsters back too soon, but should not force them before they feel ready.

Strength Training Activities

No special guidelines are needed for patients with CF to be able to participate in strength or flexibility training programs. Upper body strengthening programs may actually help lung function.

Activities to Be Avoided

Cystic fibrosis patients don't need to avoid any sport activities, with the possible exception of diving for the patient with very severe lung disease. Some experts feel that the underwater and inspired pressures could represent unwarranted risks for CF patients with severe disease. There is no agreement on this point, however, and individual consultation with the patient's physician should be made if this question arises.

Modification in Activities Due to Changes in the Clinical Stages of the Disease

As the lung disease of CF progresses exercise tolerance undoubtedly decreases, and youngsters will have difficulty tolerating activities they previously found easy. The specific symptoms are likely to be cough, including hard coughing spells, and shortness of breath. Patients should be allowed to slow down or take brief rest periods (literally, "breathers") until they are ready to resume. There are no situations specific to CF where the supervising adult will be able to tell better than the exercising patients that they need to stop. Importantly, there are also no situations where harm will be done if the youngster decides to continue playing or practicing through a coughing spell or an episode of shortness of breath. Furthermore, it is worth noting that the coughing patient poses no danger to other players.

Specific Sports to Be Recommended

As noted already, no sports are absolutely contraindicated for patients with CF. Individual aerobic sports (e.g., track, swimming, biking, and cross-country skiing) have many benefits, including excellent aerobic conditioning. Cystic fibrosis does not impose any limits on collision sports, except for the few patients with liver disease and an enlarged spleen (less than 3% of patients). No particular dominant motions are harmful for patients with CF, and no specific guidelines must be applied to CF patients based on static or dynamic activities.

Games such as tennis where skill plays a larger role than absolute strength or endurance provide a greater opportunity for the CF patient to achieve success, although CF patients have run marathons and competed successfully in Ironman-distance triathlons. The principal success to be sought should be the patient's own satisfaction. Team sports provide the CF patient opportunities to learn cooperation and teamwork, but individual sports do have some important advantages. If a youngster's disease worsens or is limiting to begin with, he or she will not be in the position of holding up or hurting the entire team (a hard coughing spell during the finals of an 8-person crew race might create problems for everyone). Nevertheless, no limitations should be placed on the CF patient who wants to compete at any level.

Once again, the main modification that needs to be made for sicker patients is that they should be allowed to take short breaks to catch their breath whenever they feel the need. A few patients might need to use supplemental oxygen, during rest breaks or even while they exercise. Some others will benefit from an inhalation or two of a bronchodilator medication from a small hand-held metered-dose inhaler.

Practical Summary of Recommendations for Sport Participation for Youngsters With Cystic Fibrosis

No sports (with the possible exception of scuba diving for the very severely affected patient) are contraindicated.

Preparticipation Issues

Preparticipation Testing. Exercise testing is essential for patients with severe lung disease (defined as $FEV_1 < 50\%$ of FVC or $< 50\%$ of predicted). This testing can identify those patients whose oxygen levels fall during exercise, and can also identify the heart rate at which this happens so that the patients may monitor their exercise heart rates and keep the intensity of exercise low enough that they do not exceed the maximum prescribed rate. Testing can also identify a patient's own maximum heart rate; the target heart rate should be 70–85% of this.

Preparatory Training Programs. No special preparations are needed for patients with CF before they enter a program. A possible exception is that if a CF patient is planning to join a hot-weather exercise program, being fairly fit will help him or her to tolerate the heat stress, and an aerobic training program might be recommended.

Dietary and Fluid Considerations. Patients with CF need more fluid during hot weather exercise than their healthy peers, but they will usually choose to drink less. Therefore, they should be encouraged to drink water, electrolyte solutions such as Gatorade, or both. They should never be denied the opportunity to drink before, during, or after exercise. Patients with CF often have difficulty maintaining their weight; thus, calories lost during exercise will need to be replaced with increased dietary intake. The only other diet consideration is that 90-95% of youngsters with CF need to take digestive enzyme capsules with their meals, and some may be shy about taking medicines in front of their peers. This is usually not an issue, but if there are separate training tables at a boarding school or college or if there is a road trip, arrangements must be made to allow the athlete to take his or her enzymes with meals.

Symptoms

The principal symptoms that youngsters with CF might experience during exercise are coughing and shortness of breath. They should be aware that should these occur during practice or competition, they will be able to stop to catch their breath with no penalty, overt or covert. Similarly, the CF patient should know that he or she will not be penalized for missing practices or competitions because of clinic visits or hospitalizations.

There are no exercise-related symptoms or signs specific to CF for which a call to the physician is needed. Certainly patients with CF can have medical emergencies related to their CF, and these would require prompt medical attention, but none of them are known to be brought on by exercise. Emergency symptoms include severe chest pain and shortness of breath that do not resolve with a short rest (from 1 to 5 minutes), and coughing or vomiting up very large amounts of blood. Any child, with or without CF, who exhibits these problems should receive prompt attention.

Expectations for School Personnel

Patients should be allowed to take their prescribed medications, including inhalers and digestive enzymes; to stop and rest if they have a hard coughing spell or shortness of breath; and to determine their own exercise intensity. School personnel should also encourage liberal fluid intake. This is generally all that is necessary to ensure a successful and safe program.

REFERENCES

1. Aitken, M.; Burke, W.; McDonald, G.; Shak, S.; Montgomery, A.; Smith, A. Recombinant human DNase inhalation in normal subjects and patients with cystic fibrosis: a phase 1 study. JAMA 267(14):1947-1951; 1992.
2. Andersen, D. Cystic fibrosis of the pancreas and its relation to celiac disease: a clinical and pathological study. Am. J. Dis. Child. 56:344-399; 1938.
3. Asher, M.I.; Pardy, R.L.; Coates, A.L.; Thomas, E.; Macklem, P.T. The effects of inspiratory muscle training in patients with cystic fibrosis. American Review of Respiratory Disease 126(5):855-859; 1982.
4. Auerbach, H.; William, M.; Kirkpatrick, J.; Colten, H. Alternate day prednisone reduces morbidity and improves pulmonary function in cystic fibrosis. Lancet 2:686-688; 1985.
4a. Bar-Or, O.; Blimkie, C.J.R.; Hay, J.A.; MacDougall, J.D.; Ward, D.S.; Wilson, W.M. Voluntary dehydration and heat intolerance in cystic fibrosis. Lancet 1992; 339:696-699.
5. Braggion, C.; Cornacchia, M.; Miano, A.; Schena, F.; Verlato, G.; Mastella, G. Exercise tolerance and effects of training in young patients with cystic fibrosis and mild airway obstruction. Pediatric Pulmonology 7(3): 145-152; 1989.
6. Burke, P.; Meyer, V.; Kocoshis, S.; Orenstein, D.; Chandra, R.; Nord, D. Depression and anxiety in pediatric inflammatory bowel disease and cystic fibrosis. J. Am. Acad. Child Adolesc. Psychiatry 28:948-951; 1989.
7. Cerny, F.J.; Cropp, G.J.; Bye, M.R. Hospital therapy improves exercise tolerance and

lung function in cystic fibrosis. American Journal of Diseases of Children 138(3):261-265; 1984.

8. Cerny, F.J.; Pullano, T.P.; Cropp, G.J. Cardiorespiratory adaptations to exercise in cystic fibrosis. American Review of Respiratory Disease 126(2):217-220; 1982.

9. Coates, A.L.; Boyce, P.; Muller, D.; Mearns, M.; Godfrey, S. The role of nutritional status, airway obstruction, hypoxia and abnormalities in serum lipid composition in limiting exercise tolerance in children with cystic fibrosis. Bulletin Europeen De Physiopathologie Respiratoire 15(2):341-342; 1979.

10. Corey, M.; Levison, H.; Crozier, D. Five- to seven-year course of pulmonary function in cystic fibrosis. Am. Rev. Respir. Dis. 114: 1085-1092; 1976.

11. Cropp, G.J.; Pullano, T.P.; Cerny, F.J.; Nathanson, I.T. Exercise tolerance and cardiorespiratory adjustments at peak work capacity in cystic fibrosis. American Review of Respiratory Disease 126(2):211-216; 1982.

12. di Sant' Agnese, P.; Darling, R.; Perera, G.; Shea, E. Abnormal electrolyte composition of sweat in cystic fibrosis of the pancreas. Pediatrics 12:549-563; 1953.

13. Drumm, M.; Pope, H.; Cliff, W.; et al. Correction of the cystic fibrosis defect in vitro by retrovirus-mediated gene transfer. Cell 62: 1227-1233; 1990.

14. Edlund, L.D.; French, R.W.; Herbst, J.J.; Ruttenburg, H.D.; Ruhling, R.O.; Adams, T.D. Effects of a swimming program on children with cystic fibrosis. American Journal of Diseases of Children 140(1):80-83; 1986.

15. Finkelstein, S.; Wielinski, C.; Elliott, G.; Warwick, W.; Barbosa, J.; Wu, S-C.; Klein, D. Diabetes mellitus associated with cystic fibrosis. J. Pediatr. 112:373-377; 1988.

16. FitzSimmons, S. Cystic fibrosis data registry report for 1992. Bethesda, MD: Cystic Fibrosis Foundation; 1993.

17. Godfrey, S.; Davies, C.; Wozniak, E.; Barnes, C. Cardiorespiratory response to exercise in normal children. Clin. Sci. 40:419-431; 1971.

18. Godfrey, S.; Mearns, M. Pulmonary function and response to exercise in cystic fibrosis. Archives of Disease in Childhood 46(246): 144-151; 1971.

19. Henke, K.; Orenstein, D. Oxygen saturation during exercise in cystic fibrosis. Am. Rev. Respir. Dis. 129:708-711; 1984.

20. Holzer, F.J.; Schnall, R.; Landau, L.I. The effect of a home exercise programme in children with cystic fibrosis and asthma. Australian Paediatric Journal 20(4):297-301; 1984.

21. Hortop, J.; Desmond, K.J.; Coates, A.L. The mechanical effects of expiratory airflow limitation on cardiac performance in cystic fibrosis. American Review of Respiratory Disease 137(1):132-137; 1988.

22. Hubbard, R.; McElvaney, N.; Birrer, P.; et al. A preliminary study of aerosolized recombinant human deosyribonuclease I in the treatment of cystic fibrosis. New England Journal of Medicine 326:812-815; 1992.

23. Keens, T.G.; Krastins, I.R.; Wannamaker, E.M.; Levison, H.; Crozier, D.N.; Bryan, A.C. Ventilatory muscle endurance training in normal subjects and patients with cystic fibrosis. American Review of Respiratory Disease 116(5):853-860; 1977.

24. Kerem, B-S.; Rommens, J.; Buchanan, J.; Markiewicz, D.; Cox, T.; Chakravarti, A.; Buchwald, M.; Tsui, L-C. Identification of the cystic fibrosis gene: genetic analysis. Science 345:1073-1080; 1989.

25. Kerem, E.; Corey, M.; Kerem, B-S.; Rommens, J.; Markiewicz, D.; Levison, H.; Tsui, L-C; Duric, P. The relationship between genotype and phenotype in cystic fibrosis—analysis of the most common mutation (delta F508). N. Engl. J. Med. 323:1517-1522; 1990.

26. Klinger, K. Genetics of cystic fibrosis. Semin. Respir. Med. 6:243-251; 1985.

27. Knowles, M.; Church, N.; Waltner, W.; Yanaskas, J.; Gilligan, P.; King, M. A pilot study of aerosolized amiloride for the treatment of lung disease in cystic fibrosis. N. Engl. J. Med. 322:1189-1194; 1990.

28. Knowles, M.; Stutts, M.; Yankaskas, J.; Gatzy, J.; Boucher, R. Abnormal respiratory epithelial ion transport in cystic fibrosis. Clin. Chest Med. 7:285-297; 1986.

29. Konstan, M.; Vargo, K.; Davis, P. Ibuprofen attenuates the inflammatory response to Pseudomonas aeruginosa in a rat model of chronic pulmonary infection. Implications for antiinflammatory therapy in cystic fibrosis. Am. Rev. Respir. Dis. 141:186-192; 1990.

30. Kraemer, R.; Rudeberg, A.; Hadorn, B.; Rossi, E. Relative underweight in cystic fibrosis and its prognostic value. Acta Paediatr. Scand. 67:33-37; 1978.

31. Landau, L.; Phelan, P. The variable effect of a bronchodilating agent on pulmonary function in cystic fibrosis. J. Pediatr. 82:863-868; 1973.

32. MacLusky, I.; McLaughlin, F.; Levison, H. Cystic fibrosis. Part I. Curr. Probl. Pediatr. 15(6):1-49; 1985.

33. MacLusky, I.; McLaughlin, F.; Levison, H. Cystic fibrosis. Part II. Curr. Probl. Pediatr. 15(7):1-39; 1985.

34. Marcotte, J.E.; Canny, G.J.; Grisdale, R.; Desmond, K.; Corey, M.; Zinman, R.; Levison, H.; Coates, A. L. Effects of nutritional status on exercise performance in advanced cystic fibrosis. Chest 90(3):375-379; 1986.

35. Marcotte, J.E.; Grisdale, R.K.; Levison, H.; Coates, A.L.; Canny, G.J. Multiple factors limit exercise capacity in cystic fibrosis. Pediatric Pulmonology 2(5):274-281; 1986.

36. McElvaney, N.; Hubbard, R.; Birrer, P.; Chernick, M.; Caplan, D.; Frank, M. Aerosol alpha-1 antitrypsin treatment for cystic fibrosis. Lancet 1:392-394; 1991.

37. Nielsen, O.; Thomsen, B.; Green, A.; Andersen, P.; Hauge, M.; Schiotz, P. Cystic fibrosis in Denmark 1945 to 1985. An analysis of incidence, mortality and influence of centralized treatment on survival. Acta Paediatr. Scand. 77:836-841; 1988.

38. Nixon, P.A.; Orenstein, D.M.; Curtis, S.E.; Ross, E. A. Oxygen supplementation during exercise in cystic fibrosis. American Review of Respiratory Disease 142(4):807-811; 1990.

38a. Nixon, P.A.; Orenstein, D.M.; Kelsey, S.F.; Doersluk, C.F. The prognostic value of exercise testing in patients with cystic fibrosis. New England Journal of Medicine 327:1785-1788; 1992.

39. O'Neill, P.; Dodds, M.; Phillips, B.; Poole, J.; Webb, A. Regular exercise and reduction of breathlessness in patients with cystic fibrosis. Brit. J. Dis. Chest 81:62-69; 1987.

40. Orenstein, D.; Henke, K.; Cerny, F. Exercise and cystic fibrosis. Physician Sports Med. 11:57-62; 1983.

41. Orenstein, D.; Henke, K.; Green, C. Heat acclimation in cystic fibrosis. J. Appl. Physiol. Respir. Environ. Exercise Physiol. 57:408-412; 1984.

42. Orenstein, D.; Nixon, P. Exercise performance and breathing patterns in cystic fibrosis: male-female differences and influence of resting pulmonary function. Pediatr. Pulmonol. 10:101-105; 1991.

43. Orenstein, D.; Nixon, P.; Ross, E.; Kaplan, R. Quality of well-being in cystic fibrosis. Chest 95:344-347; 1989.

44. Orenstein, D.M.; Franklin, B.A.; Doershuk, C.F.; Hellerstein, H.K.; Germann, K.J.; Horowitz, J.G.; Stern, R.C. Exercise conditioning and cardiopulmonary fitness in cystic fibrosis. The effects of a three-month supervised running program. Chest 80(4):392-398; 1981.

45. Orenstein, D.M.; Henke, K.G.; Costill, D.L.; Doershuk, C.F.; Lemon, P.J.; Stern, R.C. Exercise and heat stress in cystic fibrosis patients. Pediatric Research 17(4):267-269; 1983.

46. Park, R.; Grand, R. Gastrointestinal manifestations of cystic fibrosis: a review. Gastroenterol. 81:1143-1161; 1981.

47. Pattishall, E. Longitudinal response of pulmonary function to bronchodilators in cystic fibrosis. Pediatr. Pulmonol. 9:80-85; 1990.

48. Reisman, J.; Rivington-Law, B.; Corey, M.; Marcotte, J.; Wannamaker, E.; Harcourt, D. Role of conventional physiotherapy in cystic fibrosis. J. Pediatr. 113:632-636; 1988.

49. Riordan, J.; Rommens, J.; Kerem, B-S.; Alon, N.; Rozmahel, R.; Grzelczak, Z.; Zielenski, J.; Lok, S.; Plausik, N.; Chou, J-L.; Drumm, M.; Ianuzzi, M.; Collins, F.; Tsui, L-C. Identification of the cystic fibrosis gene: cloning and characterization of complementary DNA. Science 245:1066-1073; 1989.

50. Rosenstein, B.; Eigen, H. Risks of alternate-day prednisone in patients with cystic fibrosis. Pediatrics 87:245-246; 1991.

51. Roy, C.; Weber, A.; Morin, C.; LePage, G.; Brisson, G.; Yousef, I.; Lasalle, R. Hepatobiliary disease in cystic fibrosis: a survey of current issues and concepts. J. Pediatr. Gastroenterol. Nutr. 1:469-478; 1982.

52. Salh, W.; Bilton, D.; Dodd, M.; Webb, A.K. Effect of exercise and physiotherapy in aiding sputum expectoration in adults with cystic fibrosis. Thorax 44(12):1006-1008; 1989.

53. Scott, J.; Hutter, J.; Stewart, S.; Higenbottam, T.; Hodson, M.; Pemketh, A. Heart-lung transplantation for cystic fibrosis. Lancet 2:192-194; 1988.

54. Stanghelle, J.K. Physical exercise for patients with cystic fibrosis: a review. International Journal of Sports Medicine 1(6):6-18; 1988.

55. Stanghelle, J.K.; Hjeltnes, N.; Bangstad, H.J.; Michalsen, H. Effect of daily short bouts of trampoline exercise during 8 weeks on the pulmonary function and the maximal oxygen uptake of children with cystic fibrosis. International Journal of Sports Medicine 1(32):32-36; 1988.

56. Stanghelle, J.K.; Winnem, M.; Roaldsen, K.; Notgewitch, J.H.; Nilsen, B.R. Young patients with cystic fibrosis: attitude toward physical activity and influence on physical fitness and spirometric values of a 2-week training course. International Journal of Sports Medicine 1(25):25-31; 1988.

57. Stern, R.; Boat, T.; Doershuk, C.; Tucker, A.; Primiano, F.J.; Matthews, L. Course of cystic fibrosis in 95 patients. J. Pediatr. 89:406-411; 1976.

58. Stern, R.; Boat, T.; Wood, R.; Matthews, L.; Doershuk, C. Treatment and prognosis of nasal polyps in cystic fibrosis. Am. J. Dis. Child. 136:1067-1070; 1982.

59. Strauss, G.; Osher, A.; Wang, C-I; et al. Variable weight training in cystic fibrosis. Chest 92:273-276; 1987.

60. Thomassen, M.; Demko, C.; Doershuk, C. Cystic fibrosis: a review of pulmonary infections and interventions. Pediatr. Pulmonol. 3:334-351; 1987.

61. Upton, C.J.; Tyrrell, J.C.; Hiller, E.J. Two minute walking distance in cystic fibrosis. Archives of Disease in Childhood 63(12): 1444-1448; 1988.

62. Zach, M.; Oberwaldner, B.; Hausler, F. Cystic fibrosis: physical exercise versus chest physiotherapy. Archives of Disease in Childhood 57(8):587-589; 1982.

63. Zach, M.; Purrer, B.; Oberwaldner, B. Effect of swimming on forced expiration and sputum clearance in cystic fibrosis. Lancet 1:1201-1203; 1981.

CHAPTER 12

Chronic Blood-Borne Infections

Lawrence J. D'Angelo
Children's National Medical Center and George Washington University

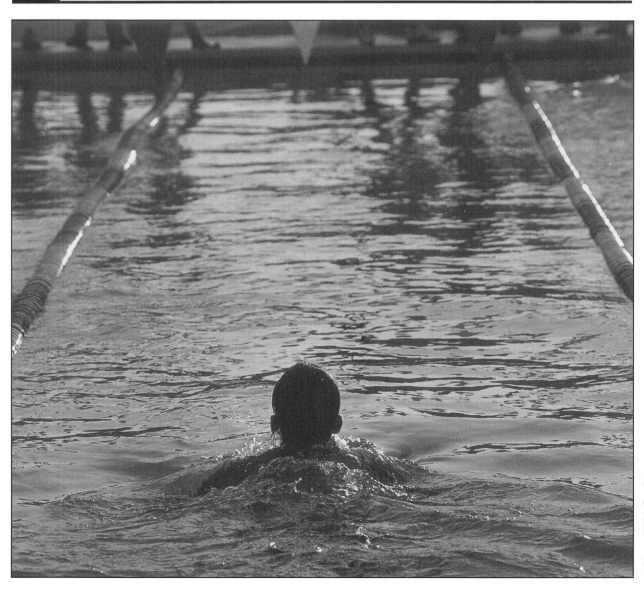

As prominent sport figures such as Earvin "Magic" Johnson and Arthur Ashe have made public their infection with the human immunodeficiency virus (HIV), the virus that causes Acquired Immunodeficiency Syndrome (AIDS), there has been much interest in the effect that this infection and other chronic blood-borne infections might have on young athletes. Of equal interest is the potential for infected athletes to transmit their infection to others as a result of the personal contact that is a part of some sporting events. This chapter will review the effect that blood-borne illnesses might have on an athlete, and the precautions appropriate for protecting the infected individual and others from either adverse consequences of illnesses or the possibility of transmission to others.

THE DISEASES: HIV INFECTION AND BLOOD-BORNE HEPATITIS

HIV Infection

Infection with the human immunodeficiency virus takes place via the exchange of bodily fluids, primarily blood or semen. Injection drug use and heterosexual or homosexual vaginal or anal intercourse are the most common modes of exposure to these infectious fluids. The virus can also be passed from an infected mother to her infant during pregnancy, at the time of delivery, or after delivery via breast milk. Blood or clotting factor transfusions were another prominent source of infection prior to 1985, but new production standards and screening techniques for HIV now make this mode of transmission highly unlikely. Nonetheless, there are a number of young athletes, particularly those with hemophilia, who might have been infected by transfusion therapy prior to this time who are still capable of passing the infection on to others through the more usual modes of transmission.

While transmission of HIV infection has occurred in a number of different settings, only a single case of possible transmission during a sporting event has ever been reported (16). This involved a violent collision between two soccer players where both individuals ostensibly bled profusely. One of the individuals was HIV-positive and the other individual seroconverted

to positive sometime after the accident. However, there was no way of determining whether the infection occurred as a result of the injury or as a result of some other exposure. The theoretical risk of infection during a sporting event exists, however, particularly during contact sports. For this reason, published guidelines for the participation of HIV-infected individuals in sport do recommend the voluntary avoidance of sports where blood exposure is likely (for example, boxing, wrestling, and football) (Table 12.1).

Transmission of HIV infection can occur through other activities that surround sport, including the use of injectable steroids to augment strength (15). The primary mode of HIV transmission in adolescents and young adults is unsafe sexual practices, including male-male and

Table 12.1   Summary of Recommendations for Participation in Sports by Individuals Infected With Blood-Borne Pathogens

1. Athletes infected with blood-borne pathogens should be allowed to participate in all competitive sports.[a]

2. Since a hypothetical risk for transmission of a blood-borne infection does exist when there is blood-to-blood or blood-to-mucous membrane exposure, athletes who are infected with a blood-borne pathogen should be advised of risk and urged to avoid participation in "Contact/Collision/Impact" sports.

3. Athletes with a blood-borne infection have a right to confidentiality. This includes not disclosing an individual's status to participants or staff.

4. All athletes should be informed that an athletic program is functioning under the rules cited above.

5. There is no medical or public health reason for routine or mandatory testing in sports activities.

6. Athletes and program staff should receive mandatory training on blood-borne pathogen transmission and its prevention.

7. During all athletic contests or practices, there should be strict adherence to universal precaution guidelines for preventing blood-borne infections.

8. All adolescent and young adult athletes at increased risk of Hepatitis B infection should receive Hepatitis B vaccine.[b]

[a]This recommendation is subject to review if new information concerning the transmission of blood-borne pathogens becomes available.
[b]See Table 12.3.
Adapted from the American Academy of Pediatrics Committee on Sports Medicine and Fitness (1991).

male-female sexual relations involving the exchange of bodily fluids without the use of barrier protection. These activities will more than likely remain the potential risk exposures posing the greatest challenge for athletes. Prevention of infection will require conscientious education of all young people and in particular those who are sexually active.

Initial infection with HIV can be totally without symptoms or can result in an acute febrile illness characterized by lymphadenopathy (swollen lymph nodes), sore throat, muscle aches, and headache. Fatigue and lethargy can be seen as well. These symptoms are common to many infections, particularly to those that occur frequently in adolescents and young adults such as infectious mononucleosis and various types of hepatitis. This illness usually occurs 2-4 weeks after infection by the virus. After this initial acute illness, the infection can enter a chronic phase where the infected individual has no symptoms whatsoever. This asymptomatic phase can last for as little as 1 to 2 years, or as much as 15 or 20 years, but the median time from infection to clinically significant illness is 8-12 years (2). Despite the lack of symptoms during this time, an infected individual may transmit infection to others via blood, semen, or theoretically, through other bodily fluids.

While the virus may infect a variety of cells in the body, its principle target is a certain population of blood lymphocytes (CD4 or "helper" lymphocytes). CD4 lymphocytes help regulate the immune system and are essential for activating both cellular and humoral immune responses. Dysfunction of these cells can result in development of infections with a wide variety of organisms, including a number of rare infections which usually have no effect on healthy individuals but which can cause serious, life-threatening illness ("opportunistic infections") in HIV-infected patients. The most common of these rare infections is a type of parasitic pneumonia, *Pneumocystis carinii* pneumonia. When one of these infections occurs, or when the count of helper lymphocytes drops below a certain level (<200 cells/mm3), an HIV-infected individual is then said to have AIDS. At this time many individuals are once again symptomatic with malaise and easy fatiguability, and these symptoms may reduce their exercise capacity.

While the infection is still in its asymptomatic phase or when an AIDS-defining illness or helper lymphocyte count has occurred, treatment with one of several antiviral medications may be prescribed. These medications in themselves may cause fatigue and muscle pain and result in decreased desire and ability to exercise (Table 12.2). Progression of illness in patients with definable AIDS may be as variable as the course of illness in patients with HIV infection. However, it is commonly accepted that once an individual develops AIDS, the invariable result

Table 12.2 Medications Commonly Taken by Individuals Infected With HIV

Medication category/ formal name	Also known as	Dose	Side effects
Antiretrovirals			
Zidovudine	Retroir, AZT, ZDV	200 mg TID	Headache, fatigue, nausea, anemia
Didanosine	Videx, DDI	150 mg BID	Headache, diarrhea, nausea, abdominal pain, pancreatitis, numbness, weakness (peripheral nerve damage)
Zalcitabine	DDC	0.75 mg TID	Numbness, weakness, rash
Pneumocystis prophylaxis			
Trimethoprim/ Sulfamethoxasole	TMP/SMX, Bactrim DS, Septra DS	1 tab 3 × per week	Rash, anemia
Pentamidine isethionate	Nebupent	300 mg Q4weeks (by nebulizer)	Cough, wheezing
Dapsone	Dapsone	50–100 mg QD	Anemia, nausea, vomiting, rash

is death from either progression of the chronic viral infection or from concomitant infection with one or more opportunistic pathogens. The time course of this progression is usually anywhere from 6 months to 5 years.

Blood-Borne Hepatitis

A variety of different viruses can cause hepatitis. However, the type of hepatitis that is usually transmitted by exposure to an infected individual's blood or other bodily fluids is *hepatitis B*, caused by the hepatitis B virus. Like HIV infection, this virus can be passed from one person to another via blood transfusions, sexual intercourse, injection drug use, and from infected mothers to their offspring at the time of delivery. Screening tests for blood products, testing of mothers prior to delivery, and the use of hepatitis B immune globulin and protective vaccination in exposed infants have significantly reduced the likelihood of transmission via these routes. Nonetheless, in 1989 8,794 cases of hepatitis B were reported to state health departments, with 80% of these reported cases occurring in individuals below the age of 40 years (5).

Transmission of hepatitis B has been documented to occur in athletic settings. Outbreaks have been documented, for example, in Swedish "orienteers" (14) and in Japanese Sumo wrestlers (10). As opposed to HIV infection, large amounts of infectious virus can be found in the blood and bodily secretions of a person infected with the Hepatitis B virus. For this reason, more casual forms of contact and potential secretion or blood exposure can result in the spread of the virus from an infected to a noninfected individual. Sports that involve close contact and potential blood or secretion exchange should be avoided by individuals who know that they are chronically infected with the virus.

Like HIV infection, hepatitis B infection can occur without any symptoms. This is particularly true when the infection is passed transplacentally or when it is contracted by young children. Beginning in adolescence, however, it is common for an acutely infected individual to develop clinical hepatitis. This usually occurs anywhere from 30 to 120 days after infection with the virus. Early symptoms include fever, headache, malaise, and loss of appetite. Between 10 and 20% of patients will additionally experience rash, arthralgia, and even painful joint swelling and inflammation. Within 5 to 10 days after the initial symptoms occur the patient may notice the onset of jaundice, light-colored stools and dark-colored urine. Abdominal discomfort or pain in the right upper quadrant associated with enlargement of the liver is very common. A small percentage of individuals will develop enlargement of the spleen, a definite contraindication to any sort of contact sport.

Laboratory tests will show elevation of the liver-associated enzymes alanine aminotransferase (ALT) and aspartate aminotransferase (AST), as well as elevation of serum bilirubin levels. These levels increase for the first 10 to 14 days and then begin a slow resolution. At the same time that the liver shows evidence of lessening inflammation, the patient's symptoms will begin to resolve; this may take 3 to 6 weeks overall. Other laboratory tests that are at times abnormal include the hemoglobin and hematocrit, which can be reduced, and the white blood cell count, which may be elevated and show the appearance of a moderate number of abnormal lymphocytes ("atypical" lymphocytes).

The role of exercise in acute hepatitis is controversial. While some observers claim that exercise and increased activity worsens the illness (11), others claim that is has no effect (6, 13). It is likely that patients with hepatitis will restrict their own activities while acutely ill. When patients notice an improvement in their symptoms and an improvement in their jaundice or other laboratory measures, they are most likely ready to resume exercising and training.

Ten percent of patients who develop acute hepatitis B infection will become carriers of the hepatitis B surface antigen (HbSAG), a marker of persistent infection with the virus. This group of individuals is at risk of long-term complications of chronic infection including persistent hepatitis, cirrhosis, and cancer of the liver. While these complications are rare, they warrant surveillance and concern. Regular medical follow-up is important.

No specific treatment is beneficial to patients with acute hepatitis. For patients with evidence of ongoing chronic infection, some studies have shown benefit from corticosteroids (7) and from human leukocyte interferon (HLI) (9). Chronic use of corticosteroids can result in muscle wasting and osteoporosis, making continued participation in athletics difficult, while treatment with

HLI causes fatigue, malaise, and hair loss. Luckily, few patients need either of these medical treatments.

Since 1980, a variety of vaccine products have been available to prevent hepatitis B. Hepatitis B Immune Globulin (HBIG) is prepared from plasma of individuals who have high levels of antibody to the virus circulating in their bloodstream. This product is administered to individuals who have had a known or probable exposure to the virus. This type of immunization is known as passive immunization because it does not depend on an active immunologic response on the part of the individual receiving it. It is meant to be used in combination with hepatitis B vaccine. This vaccine product relies on stimulating the recipient's immune response to the hepatitis B surface antigen produced by genetic engineering in bacteria. It is administered in 3 doses at 0, 1, and 6 months. The Centers for Disease Control currently recommend this vaccine for "all adolescents at high risk of infection because they are injecting drug users or have multiple sex partners (more than one partner/6 months)" (4). Vaccination of other selected high-risk groups is also urged (Table 12.3).

While the majority of cases of hepatitis B are either asymptomatic or self-limited, a small number of individuals will experience one of several more severe variants of this infection. One such variant is fulminant hepatitis accompanied by hepatic failure and encephalopathy. This manifestation of hepatitis B infection has a case fatality rate of over 50%; death usually occurs within 3 weeks. However, less than 1% of diagnosed cases of hepatitis B pursue this course. Other variants include prolonged acute hepatitis (where symptoms and laboratory findings may be abnormal for 4 to 6 months) and relapsing hepatitis, where initial recovery is interrupted by one or more episodes of symptoms suggesting the acute phase of infection. Again, these manifestations are seen in 2% and 1% of all reported cases, respectively.

EXERCISE AND CHRONIC BLOOD-BORNE INFECTIONS

Acute infection with HIV or hepatitis B will often cause symptomatic illness that will make it difficult for even elite athletes to either desire or be able to exercise. There is no research currently available to predict the consequences of exercise in individuals during the acute phase of either of these chronic blood-borne infections. However, extrapolating from studies on other viral illnesses that show that such acute illnesses reduce muscle strength and endurance (8) leads to the conclusion that it is probably best to advise that the acutely ill athlete with symptoms of fever, malaise, and myalgia due to either of these blood-borne infections not participate in strenuous exercise.

As acute symptoms resolve, the role of exercise in either of these infections becomes more controversial. Exercise stimulates the immune system and can increase the infected athlete's sense of well-being by stimulating endorphin production. Studies of patients with chronic asymptomatic HIV infection have shown increases in CD4 cell counts as well as in activity of natural killer (NK) cells when these patients are enrolled in an aerobic exercise program (12). The role of exercise in patients recuperating from hepatitis is controversial, with proponents of bed rest and controlled exercise both suffering from a lack of adequately controlled trials. Nonetheless, in the small population of hepatitis B patients that develop splenomegaly, contact sports should be strictly outlawed.

Table 12.3 Adult Candidates for Hepatitis B Vaccine

1. Persons with occupational risks (health care, public safety workers)
2. Clients and staff of institutions for the developmentally disabled
3. Hemodialysis patients
4. Recipients of certain blood products (hemophilia, etc.)
5. Household contacts and sex partners of HBV carriers
6. Adoptees from countries where HBV is endemic
7. International travelers to high-risk destinations for 6 or more months
8. Injecting drug users
9. Sexually active homosexual and bisexual men
10. Sexually active men and women who:
    a. have (an)other sexually transmitted disease(s)
    b. have had more than one sexual partner in the past 6 months
    c. are prostitutes
11. Inmates of long-term correctional facilities

Although the lack of data on the effects of exercise on chronic blood-borne infections precludes further speculation on how such activity might affect patients, consideration can also be given to the potential for nonmedical adverse effects associated with these chronic infections. Since neither infection is curable, the chronically infected individual must always be aware of the risk that he or she may pose for other participants. As mentioned earlier, this risk is probably more serious for the individual with chronic hepatitis B infection than for the individual with HIV infection. For both infections, however, the risk to others can be minimized by strict adherence to guidelines for limiting exposure to blood in athletic settings (Table 12.4). These guidelines are in keeping with those used in both hospital and emergency medical settings (3).

Of equal concern with the potential adverse physiological effects of exercise and competitive sports on patients with chronic blood-borne infections is the potential for adverse psychological effects. These will usually occur in two possible ways: 1) an athlete discovers that he or she is infected, not having previously known this,

or 2) an individual who knows of his or her infection status has the confidential nature of this information breached either knowingly or by accident by another person or institution. In the former case, the athlete may find out this information as part of a testing program run by the team. The potential catastrophic nature of the information, and its lack of relevance to anyone but the individual and the people with whom that individual is most intimately associated, is one of the reasons that virtually all organized sport groups as well as the World Health Organization advise against routine screening for HIV infection in athletic settings. The latter case is of even greater significance given the adverse publicity and unfounded concerns of personal risk that came to light when Magic Johnson first announced that he was HIV-infected. The unfounded concerns and negative feelings of others ultimately influenced his final decision to retire from organized sports.

In addition to the personal distress and lack of self-esteem that the chronically infected individual may feel, the potential for discrimination is of real concern. Given adequate precautions and adherance to the guidelines cited in Table 12.4, however, participation in any sport is possible and potentially beneficial to the infected athlete. For this reason, only those individuals involved with the immediate health and well-being of an individual should be privy to information concerning the presence of a chronic blood-borne infection.

While the potential physiological benefits of exercise on chronic blood-borne infections have already been mentioned, it is more difficult to gauge the psychological benefits of sport and exercise performance on children who are subjected to these infections. As with any chronic illness, children with chronic blood-borne infections by necessity often feel separated from their friends by the both real and imagined barriers that their illness creates. Participating in sports, particularly team sports, may mitigate this sense of estrangement. It will teach teamwork and life skills that will be important to the child, adolescent, or young adult facing the unknown challenge of a chronic illness whose course is difficult to determine. It will, moreover, improve the quality of life and relieve stress for both patient and family.

Table 12.4   Guidelines for Limiting Exposures to Blood-Borne Pathogens

1. When an injury occurs, if there is bleeding, the individual injured should be removed from participation until bleeding has been stopped, the wound cleansed with antiseptic, and covered securely or occluded.

2. If others are exposed to blood or other bodily fluids, this material should be removed with soap and running water.

3. Staff should use latex or vinyl gloves when handling material contaminated with blood or bodily fluids. If gloves are not available, the wound should be covered and the injured person transported to an area where the wound can be definitively and safely cared for. Emergency care, however, should not be delayed.

4. Objects covered with blood or bodily fluids should be cleaned with a solution of household bleach (1 part bleach, 100 parts water).

5. Equipment appropriate to allow for cardiopulmonary resuscitation without direct exposure to saliva (Ambu bags, oral airways) should be available.

6. All athletic staff should receive mandated training in HIV prevention as well as first aid and emergency care.

EXERCISE AND SPORT PROGRAMS FOR CHILDREN WITH CHRONIC BLOOD-BORNE INFECTIONS

The majority of children and adolescents with chronic blood-borne infections are asymptomatic. For this reason, participation in sports, particularly sports that involve aerobic activities, is not only allowed but encouraged.

As mentioned earlier, in one study a structured aerobic exercise program was associated with increased CD4 counts in patients with HIV infection. In this particular study the patients were asymptomatic; it is not clear whether similar benefits would accrue to patients who were symptomatic or at more advanced stages of disease as measured by CD4 level, but there is no reason to think that they would not.

The same is probably true of other blood-borne diseases. Little is known of the role of exercise on chronic hepatitis B infection, but once past the acute illness stage it is assumed that the benefits of exercise will outweigh any risks that convalescence will be prolonged.

Strength training activities need to only follow developmental guidelines and need not be adjusted because of the presence of a chronic blood-borne infection. The same is true for movement and flexibility training. Any activities to be avoided in these patients more likely involve those not related to the sporting or exercise activities as such but which have been associated with celebratory or social aspects of these activities. For this reason, this chapter also considers other issues such as the use of alcohol and drugs, as well as sexual behaviors.

Since alcohol can have an impact on the immune system and is obviously potentially toxic to the liver, patients with chronic blood-borne diseases should avoid the use of alcohol, as well as of illicit drugs. Even if the metabolic effects of alcohol and drugs do not make it more likely that a blood-borne infection will have a serious impact on the immune system, either of these agents can significantly alter the decision-making process and lead to risk-taking behaviors. These behaviors could ultimately place an athlete at increased risk either of transmitting or receiving a blood-borne infection. Therefore, individuals with chronic blood-borne diseases must either avoid sexual contact or activities that could possibly lead to the exchange of semen or blood, or use barrier protection (condoms and/or dental dams) to avoid and/or limit contact.

Since these barrier methods of protection are not 100% effective in preventing the exchange of potentially infected material, adolescents or young adults who are sexually active should be counseled about which types of sexual contact are less risky. Safe behaviors include body massage, hugging, petting, dry kissing, and mutual masturbation. Deeper, wet kissing is probably safe. Other behaviors that risk the exchange of blood, semen, or vaginal secretions are not safe, although the risk of any sexual encounter is reduced by the use of barrier protection methods such as condoms. Since such protective methods are irrelevant to the types of potential exposures that are experienced during athletic events, it is strongly suggested that individuals who are infected avoid collision sports such as

- boxing,
- wrestling,
- football, and
- rugby.

This will lessen their chances of sustaining an injury that could result in blood loss. In addition, since transmission will most often take place in the context of intimate contact, partners of patients with chronic blood-borne diseases should know of these infections so that they can make informed decisions concerning intimate contacts, as well as preventive therapies such as immunizations.

With the new recommendations for the widespread use of hepatitis B vaccine in children and adolescents, family and team members of an individual with chronic hepatitis B infection must be counseled concerning the indications for hepatitis B vaccine (see Table 12.3). Thought should be given to immunizing those at risk of regular blood or secretion exposure from the infected individual. While this will bring no immediate benefit to the person with the chronic infection, there may be profound psychological benefits for teammates and family members who will now feel that they can interact with the infected individual. Unfortunately, no vaccine is yet available to either prevent or ameliorate HIV infection.

Since universal precautions mandate that all blood exposures must be treated as if the blood is infectious, the following precautions have been put forward by the American Academy of Pediatrics as part of their comprehensive guidelines on the participation of individuals who are infected with HIV (1). These precautions should be taken by all teams and coaches:

- If a child's or adolescent's skin or mucous membrane is exposed to the blood or bodily fluid of another individual, the contaminated site should be promptly cleaned with soap and water, alcohol, moist towelettes, or the like.
- Water-impervious gloves should be available and utilized when handling blood, other bodily fluids, or objects contaminated with them. Hands should be washed after gloves are removed.
- Surfaces or objects contaminated with blood should be cleaned with a bleach solution (1 part bleach in 100 parts water).
- In sports where direct body contact may take place, any observed skin lesion should be cleaned and securely covered.
- If bleeding occurs, participation should be interrupted until the bleeding has stopped and the wound is cleaned and covered.
- Oral airways and breathing bags (Ambu bags) should be available for use in case of a cardiac or respiratory compromise.
- All coaches and trainers should receive training in emergency aid and prevention of transmission of HIV and other blood-borne illnesses.

If individuals with either hepatitis B infection or HIV infection begin to show signs of active progression of their illness, it is prudent to reconsider their activity and participation level. Blood-borne infections can result in fatigue that will limit performance. Rather than ceasing or radically altering exercise programs, cutting back on activities during times of symptoms is a good idea. In those rare patients that develop splenomegaly with either infection, all contact sports are to be curtailed for at least 3 weeks or until the spleen is normal in size. At this time there are no data to allow us to predict which, if any, patients with chronic blood-borne infections will be more symptomatic if they continue exercise or sport participation.

CONCLUSION

As already mentioned, with the exception of the aforementioned collision sports no exercise or sporting activity is contraindicated.

The precautions listed earlier for coping with any potential blood exposure during an athletic contest should be followed carefully. Adopting this as the standard of care for all athletes will relieve the potential pressure which would be felt by infected individuals knowing that special procedures would be implemented if they were involved in an incident that resulted in blood loss. This sort of approach would stigmatize them immediately and is to be avoided. If team members or officials do know about a patient's blood-borne infection they should not reveal this to anyone unless this has been approved by the patient.

With appropriate precautions, virtually all sporting activities and all forms of exercise should be safe and enjoyable for the individual with a blood-borne infection. Such activity will improve the sense of effectiveness and self-esteem that these children and adolescents so desperately need and deserve.

REFERENCES

1. American Academy of Pediatrics Committee on Sports Medicine and Fitness. Human immunodeficiency virus [acquired immunodeficiency syndrome (AIDS) virus] in the athletic setting. Pediatrics 88:640-641; 1991.
2. Bacchetti, P.; Moss, A.R. Incubation period of AIDS in San Francisco. Nature 338:251-253; 1989.
3. Centers for Disease Control. Guidelines for prevention of transmission of human immunodeficiency virus and hepatitis B virus to health-care and public-safety workers. MMWR 38(Suppl 6):5-15; 1989.
4. Centers for Disease Control. Hepatitis B virus: a comprehensive strategy for eliminating transmission in the United States through universal childhood vaccination: recommendations of the Immunization Practices Advisory Committee (ACIP). MMWR 40:1-24; 1991.
5. Centers for Disease Control. Hepatitis Surveillance Report No. 54. Atlanta: author; 1992.

6. Chalmers, T.C.; Eckhardt, R.D.; Reynolds, W.D.; et al. The treatment of infectious hepatitis: controlled studies of the effects of diet, rest and physical reconditioning on the acute course of disease and the incidence of relapses and residual abnormalities. J. Clin. Invest. 34:1163-1170; 1955.

7. Cook, C.G.; Mulligan, R.; Sherlock, S. Controlled prospective trial corticosteroid therapy in active hepatitis. Q. J. Med. 40:159-163; 1971.

8. Daniels, W.L.; Vogel, J.A.; Sharp, D.S.; et al. Effects of virus infection of physical performance in man. Mil. Med. 50:8-14; 1985.

9. Greenberg, H.B.; Pollard, R.B.; Lutwixk, L.I.; et al. Effect of human leukocyte interferon on hepatitis B virus infection in patients with chronic active hepatitis. N. Engl. J. Med. 295:517-521; 1976.

10. Kashiwagi, S.; Hayashi, J.; Ikematsu, H.; et al. An outbreak of Hepatitis B in members of a high school sumo wrestling club. JAMA 248:213-214; 1982.

11. Kirkler, D.M.; Zilberg, B. Activity and hepatitis. Lancet 2:1046-1048; 1966.

12. LaPerriere, A.; Fletcher, M.A.; Antoni, M.H.; et al. Aerobic exercise training in an AIDS risk group. Int. J. Sports Med. 12:853-857; 1991.

13. Repsher, L.H.; Freebern, R.K. Effects of early and vigorous exercise on recovery from infectious hepatitis. N. Engl. J. Med. 281:1393-1398; 1969.

14. Ringerz, M.B.; Zetterberg, B. Serum hepatitis among Swedish track finders. N. Engl. J. Med. 276:540-546; 1967.

15. Seltzer, D.G. Educating athletes on HIV disease and AIDS: the team physician's role. Phys. Sportsmed. 21:109-115; 1993.

16. Torre, D.; Sampietro, C.; Ferraro, G.; et al. Transmission of HIV-1 infection via sports injury. Lancet 335:1105; 1990.

CHAPTER 13

Hypertension

Bruce S. Alpert and Mary E. Fox
University of Tennessee, Memphis

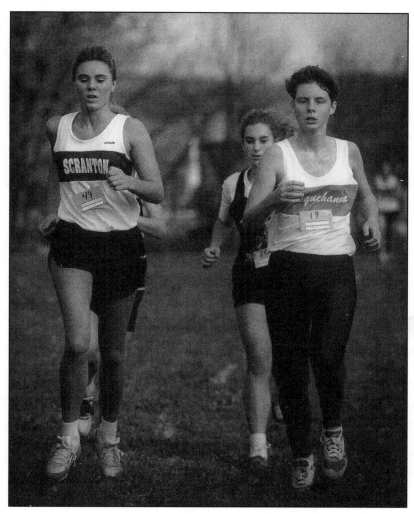

One of the major physiological responses to both dynamic and isometric exercise is the increase of systolic blood pressure (SBP). Children and adolescents who have hypertension, that is, elevated BP at rest, may be at risk for complications when they exercise and elevate BP even further. The purposes of this chapter are to review extant data which address: 1) the issue of safety of exercise in hypertensive children, and 2) the use of exercise as a nonpharmacological therapy for hypertension. To date there are not sufficient data to use exercise SBP in children as a predictor of later-onset hypertension, as has been done in adults.

The BP response to dynamic exercise (4) differs somewhat from that to isometric exercise. In dynamic exercise such as running, swimming, and soccer, large muscle groups undergo repetitive contraction (muscle shortening). Systolic BP rises linearly with increasing workload, as does cardiac output. Diastolic blood pressure (DBP), however, remains the same or decreases slightly. There is a significant fall in systemic vascular resistance in response to dynamic exercise.

In isometric (static) exercise such as wrestling, weightlifting, and football blocking, muscle length does not change (4). The increase in SBP is in proportion to the percent of maximal voluntary effort exerted by the specific muscle group, not the size of the contracting muscle mass. The rise in SBP is higher than that expected from the metabolic cost of the exercise performed, and generally continues to increase as the contraction is maintained. Diastolic BP also rises, and parallels the increase in SBP. Because of the perceived risk of stroke or myocardial ischemia, most clinicians are very wary of allowing hypertensive children and adolescents to participate in isometric exercise; thus, sports such as football, weightlifting, and wrestling are not recommended.

SAFETY OF EXERCISE

Five recent reports have been identified which address the hemodynamic responses to exercise of hypertensive children and adolescents. All of the reports include data from dynamic exercise; three also include data from isometric exercise. All describe laboratory rather than field evaluations.

Dynamic Exercise

Fixler and his coworkers (5) were the first to address the safety of exercise in a study of 109 juvenile hypertensives between the ages of 14 and 17 years. These authors compared the patient data to those of 74 control subjects within the same age range. The patients were heavier than the controls, but were similar with respect to height and habitual physical activity. The parents of the patients had a higher incidence of hypertension (40%) than the parents of the controls (14%).

At peak cycle ergometer exercise, 3% of the controls and 30% of the hypertensive patients had SBP values which exceeded 200 mmHg. The changes in SBP which occurred (exercise SBP – resting SBP) were essentially the same for both groups: 53 mmHg for the patients and 54 mmHg for the controls. None of the adolescents tested had any cardiac-related symptoms during exercise. There were 3 adolescents in whom ST-segment depression greater than 0.1 mV was recorded; 1 was a control and 2 were patients.

These findings were described as supporting the 1977 recommendation of the Task Force on Blood Pressure Control in Children (25), which states that dynamic exercise in hypertensive adolescents is safe. Fixler recommended that youth with hypertension be allowed to participate in sport activities in which the primary component is dynamic; he noted that no hypertensive patient developed "extreme hypertension," i.e., a value of exercise SBP > 230 mmHg or diastolic blood pressure DBP > 130 mmHg. The importance of these cutoffs is not clear; no adverse effects were recorded in either group.

Nudel and coworkers (20, 21) compared 10 adolescent essential hypertensives (fixed high values of blood pressure, group 1) with 8 youngsters with labile hypertension (variable values of blood pressure, group 2) and 10 age-matched normotensive controls (group 3). The hypertensive children had SBP ≥ 150 mmHg or DBP ≥ 95 mmHg, measured in the supine position. Group 1 patients had been hypertensive for 1 to 5 years and were not receiving antihypertensive medications. Cycle ergometer exercise was performed utilizing a 2-minute warm-up and 1-minute exercise stages.

As expected, peak SBP values were highest in the group 1 patients. The SBP values in the group 2 patients were similar to those in the controls (group 3), but since the pulse pressure (SBP – DBP) changes were less in group 2, the authors concluded that less vasodilation occurred in this group. As no patient developed any symptoms or complications, the maximal dynamic exercise stress was deemed safe. No ST changes occurred. The authors noted that only one group 1 patient developed "a dangerously high blood pressure during exercise" (p. 1077). This terminology refers to a value between 230 and 250 mmHg, which was published without clinical confirmation of reported complications in an American Academy of Pediatrics policy statement in 1977 (1). The authors added in a subsequent letter that, since no documented risk had been demonstrated, hypertensive adolescents should not be excluded from dynamic exercise (19). They suggested that the risk of a dangerously high exercise SBP could only be obtained through long-term follow-up studies on hypertensives who reach this level of SBP during dynamic exercise.

Schieken, Clarke, and Lauer (22) reported cycle ergometer dynamic exercise data from 264 Muscatine, Iowa children from the low, middle, and upper quintile of blood pressure distribution. The upper quintile children were heavier, had greater values for triceps skinfold thickness and body surface area, and included children with both normal and elevated BP. As in the studies described previously, the increase in SBP was essentially the same in each of the 3 groups, and the upper quintile children had the highest absolute values of dynamic exercise SBP.

The children in the highest quintile had the highest level of double product (SBP × heart rate), implying the highest level of myocardial oxygen consumption. As there were no complications noted in this group, the authors did not recommend any restriction of activity in children with elevated BP.

Klein, McCrory, Engle, Rosenthal, and Ehlers (16) studied not only exercise hemodynamics but also sympathetic nervous system activity as measured by epinephrine and norepinephrine values. Subjects included 8 hypertensives, 17 borderline hypertensives, and 21 controls. The peak SBP to treadmill exercise of the borderline hypertensive patients was higher (212 ± 7 mmHg) than that of the hypertensives (195 ± 11 mmHg). The authors noted that the patients with the highest SBP responses to exercise were also those who had the highest heart rate response. No patient experienced any ill effects from the exercise challenge. The hypertensive patients had the highest levels of exercise-induced epinephrine levels. The authors concluded that adolescents with borderline and significant hypertension have altered hemodynamic responses to dynamic exercise which is mediated by altered activity of the sympathetic nervous system.

Hansen, Hyldebrandt, Nielsen, and Froberg (10) studied 64 hypertensive children between 8 and 10 years of age and compared their results to those of a group of 68 age-matched controls. The exercise was performed on a cycle ergometer to exhaustion. The data demonstrated equivalent values for SBP and double product for the hypertensive group in comparison to the normotensive children. No complications occurred in either group.

It is interesting to note that no hypertensive patient reported in any study had any significant complication to dynamic exercise. While several authors have stated that dynamic exercise is safe in these patients, others have warned against exercise in children and adolescents with "excessively" or "dangerously high" levels of SBP. However, no data are extant which demonstrate any risk of dynamic exercise at any arbitrarily determined BP level in hypertensive children.

Isometric Exercise

The physiology of isometric exercise differs greatly from that of dynamic exercise. In dynamic exercise the large degree of vasodilation which occurs to deliver oxygen to exercising muscles is accompanied by large increases in cardiac output, heart rate, and oxygen consumption. In isometric exercise, the primary response is that of vasoconstriction (or lack of vasodilation), with only modest increases in oxygen consumption and heart rate. There is general agreement among clinicians that isometric exercise may represent an unacceptable risk for hypertensives because of the possibility of a central nervous system or cardiac complication.

The study by Fixler et al. (5) included data from a 4-minute 25% maximal isometric handgrip contraction in the supine position. There were no ST-T abnormalities recorded. The change in SBP from rest to exercise was essentially the same for the hypertensives (16 mmHg) as for the controls (18 mmHg). No hypertensive patient had a SBP > 190 mmHg, although about a fourth of the patients had DBP > 100 mmHg, and two patients had DBP values which exceeded 120 mmHg. Despite the lack of morbidity, the authors stated that they were: "reluctant to recommend that hypertensive adolescents be allowed to participate in weight lifting programs until additional studies have been done to determine whether this more strenuous exercise results in more pronounced changes in blood pressure" (p. 583).

Schieken et al. (22) also included data from handgrip isometric exercise in the supine position. Their subjects performed a 30% maximal handgrip for 3 minutes, avoiding the Valsalva maneuver. There was an increase in both SBP and DBP in all groups. The change from rest to exercise was the largest in the lowest quintile group for SBP. For DBP, however, the high-percentile group had the largest change.

Klein et al. (16) had their subjects perform a 30% maximal handgrip contraction for 90 seconds. Of the 46 subjects, 35 completed the isometric task. The increase in SBP and DBP which occurred was equivalent in all three groups. The patients with the highest resting BP (the significant hypertension group) had the highest peak values and highest increase from baseline for plasma epinephrine. These changes paralleled changes seen in heart rate in response to the handgrip exercise task. This difference in the sympathetic nervous system response was thought to be a valuable marker in the evolution of the pathophysiology of essential hypertension. No restriction from isometric exercise was recommended by these authors.

EXERCISE TRAINING AS THERAPY FOR HYPERTENSION

Six studies have been identified which have addressed the question of whether exercise training is effective in lowering BP for hypertensive children and adolescents.

Laird, Fixler, and Swanbom (17) reported data from a 2-month weightlifting program for 7 hypertensive boys. This short-term program produced no significant change in either SBP or DBP. There was also no increase in left ventricular mass or change in cardiac output. The authors concluded that neither deleterious nor therapeutic effects had occurred.

Hagberg et al. (8) designed an aerobic dynamic training program for hypertensive adolescents. The patients exercised 3 days per week, 30 to 40 minutes per day, for 6 (± 1) months. The exercises performed were either jogging, swimming, or cycling at 60-65% of maximal oxygen consumption. The patients ceased the training program and were assessed 9 ± 1 months later. Compliance with the program was > 90%. For the entire group of 25 patients, the exercise training led to a decrease in SBP from 137 ± 1 mmHg to 129 ± 1 mmHg (p < .01). After the program ceased BP returned to pre-training levels (139 ± 2 mmHg, p < .01 vs. values during training). There were parallel changes in DBP, from 80 ± 2 mmHg, to 75 ± 2 mmHg, to 78 ± 2 mmHg for untrained, trained, and detrained subjects, respectively. Those patients (n=16) who had normal DBP prior to training had no decrease in DBP as a result of the training period. The 9 patients with both S and D hypertension showed beneficial decreases in both SBP and DBP after the training period, but the values generally returned to pretraining levels after the 9-month period of detraining. Race did not correlate with BP response to training. The decrease in BP which occurred did not bring the SBP or DBP values into the normal range. The effects of exercise training were not long-lasting; they almost uniformly disappeared when the training ceased.

The same research group subsequently reported data from six hypertensive adolescents who underwent an initial endurance (dynamic) training program followed by a weight training protocol (7). The dynamic exercise training consisted of running at 60-75% of maximal oxygen consumption, 3 days per week, 30-50 minutes per day, for 5 months. Another 5 months were then spent doing weight training for 3 days each week. The weight training was performed either with free weights (n=3), or commercially available variable-resistance equipment (n=3). All subjects and controls (all hypertensive) were examined a year later, as well.

The dynamic exercise period led to an increase in maximal oxygen consumption. As expected, SBP decreased after training, but no change in

DBP was seen in this small group. The 2 patients with D hypertension, however, did experience a reduction in mean DBP from 93 to 79 mmHg.

The weight training led to a return to pre-dynamic training values for body weight, percent body fat, and maximal oxygen consumption. The SBP after weight training was 17 ± 4 mmHg (p < .01) lower than that prior to aerobic conditioning, and 4 ± 4 mmHg lower than following endurance training. The two patients with D hypertension maintained their reduced values of DBP. All BP values returned to the pre-intervention levels when either dynamic or weight training ceased.

Although the group of subjects was small (n= 6), the trend of hemodynamics was very favorable in response to the weight training. SBP and DBP, when elevated, were reduced. In addition, weight training led to a reduction of systemic vascular resistance in hypertensive adolescents. It should, however, be borne in mind that the exercise was weight training, not weightlifting. Weight training consists of repetitions of sub-maximal lifts, which is a primarily dynamic exercise. In weightlifting, the subject repeatedly attempts to lift maximal weights, giving an isometric stress in addition.

Hofman, Walter, Connelly, and Vaughan (12) studied the effects of physical fitness on BP in 2,061 fourth-grade children in the New York City area. The population included 58% whites, 27% blacks, 12% Hispanics, and 3% others. There were numerous significant correlations between assessments of fitness and SBP and DBP. As fitness increased, BP decreased. The authors did not specifically address the children in the highest levels of the BP distribution, but the large number of subjects and the consistency of the results make this study an important one for the present discussion.

Danforth et al. (2) used exercise as a treatment for hypertension in a selected population, black children with low socioeconomic status (SES). This population was targeted because it has higher BP values than most other populations. Low-SES individuals are less likely to be able to obtain medications than are high-SES patients, and nonpharmacological therapies are of greater importance in their overall treatment plans. Seven girls and 5 boys between the ages of 8 and 12 were studied; they performed walking/jogging or stationary cycling 3 days per week, increasing to 30 minutes per day. The program lasted 12 weeks. There were increases in measures of cardiovascular fitness and significant reductions of both SBP and DBP. The degree of success was not related to weight loss (average 1.1 kg) which occurred during endurance aerobic training. No complications of the program were reported. Thus, dynamic exercise was demonstrated to be an effective nonpharmacological therapy which can be of use in the low-SES black population without complications.

Most recently, Hansen, Froberg, Hyldebrandt, and Nielson (9) completed a prospective randomized controlled intervention trial of 69 hypertensives and 68 normotensives selected from a study population of 1369 children. The intervention consisted of an 8-month trial of 2 extra sessions per week of ordinary school physical education. Each session was 50 minutes long, with a 10-minute warm-up portion. The controls received the usual 2 periods per week of physical education. Assessments were performed after 3 months of the program, and again at the end of 8 months. The changes seen at 3 months were variable; by 8 months of training, however, there were significant reductions in SBP and DBP for both normotensive and hypertensive children. The fall in SBP which occurred in the normotensive group (6.5 mmHg) was similar to that which occurred in the hypertensive group (4.9 mmHg). BP response in boys was more consistent than that in girls. The fall in DBP was parallel to that of SBP. In the normotensive group, DBP decreased 4.1 mmHg, and in the hypertensive group, 3.8 mmHg.

This study points out that it may take a prolonged period of nonintense physical exercise to obtain a significant BP effect. The intervention described, a simple institution of daily school physical education, is a very low-cost and possibly highly effective health measure not only for the nonpharmacological treatment of elevated BP, but also as a possible primary prevention strategy. This activity could result in the adoption of life-long patterns of daily exercise, leading to lower risk for both essential hypertension and coronary disease. Until long-term studies on very large populations are completed, however, these prevention strategies remain hypothetical.

REVIEWS AND POLICY STATEMENTS REGARDING DYNAMIC OR ISOMETRIC EXERCISE

Several review articles have addressed the issue of safety of exercise (sport) and/or exercise testing in children with hypertension (3, 13, 26). Daniels and Loggie (3) noted that hypertensive adolescents who participated in competitive sports for several years showed "no short- or long-term ill effects" (p. 126). They summarized data from the 16th Bethesda Conference on Cardiovascular Abnormalities in the Athlete (6) by stating the following (p. 126):

- Patients who have severe uncontrolled hypertension (by adult standards) or target-organ involvement should not participate in competitive sports.
- Patients who have controlled hypertension and no target-organ disease may participate in competitive sports with moderate-to-high dynamic and low static demands.
- Patients who have controlled hypertension but evidence of left ventricular hypertrophy or renal functional impairment may participate in low-intensity activities such as bowling or golf.

The term *target organ damage* refers to deleterious changes in organs such as the heart (increased left ventricular mass), kidney (reduced creatinine clearance, microalbuminuria), eyes (severe vascular change), or central nervous system (transient ischemic attack, stroke). Daniels and Loggie (3) defined severe hypertension as SBP and/or DBP persistently > 99th percentile. Patients with BP levels in this range were thought by the participants at the Bethesda Conference to need initial treatment to reduce the BP prior to sport participation.

Tipton (26) has recommended that well supervised and monitored weightlifting or circuit-training programs should be performed to define the acute pressor effects of these events. When these exercises have been shown to be safe, programs may be recommended for hypertensive populations.

Most recently, the authors of the 1988 Report of the Joint National Committee on Detection, Evaluation, and Treatment of High Blood Pressure (13) stated that "uncomplicated elevated blood pressure, by itself, generally should not be a reason to restrict asymptomatic children from participating in sports and other physical activities" (p. 1034). We have been unable to find data from either dynamic or isometric exercise studies which document a measurable morbidity or risk of exercise of any specific level of resting or exercise SBP or DBP. It is generally accepted, although not supported by experimental data, that patients with preexisting target organ damage (e.g., renal dysfunction, or increased left ventricular mass by echocardiography) be excluded from strenuous dynamic or isometric exercise. We recommend, therefore, that before a hypertensive adolescent is cleared for sport activities the primary cause of the hypertension should be determined. We are unable to define at what BP value sport participation should be denied; more data from controlled studies are needed.

As early as 1976, Londe and Goldring (18) in St. Louis were concerned about isometric exercise in the child with high BP. They reviewed the evidence to date, of which there was a paucity, concerning the safety of isometric exercise. They stressed the need to recommend initial weight reduction for the obese child, and to withhold drug treatment for children with moderate hypertension. They advised the reduction of salt intake, if in excess. They did not wish to recommend a reduction of physical activity. There was a belief, however, that activities such as weight-lifting and nonmotorized lawn mowing might need to be prohibited.

An editorial by Strong (24) raised many critical questions. Many children diagnosed with hypertension will have their BP return to normal within 3 to 8 years, without treatment. Thus, what is the significance of this initial BP elevation? What is the role of the exercise test in the evaluation of the hypertensive child? Is there any contraindication to sport participation in the hypertensive child? Strong concluded that children with mild hypertension should be allowed to participate in athletics, and those with moderate hypertension should be allowed to participate in the absence of an underlying organic cause such as renal disease or coarctation of the aorta. If the physician chooses to treat a hypertensive child with pharmacological therapy, that child should undergo stress testing to confirm that exercise BP response is now in the acceptable range. Strong stated that the individual with severe hypertension should be thoroughly evaluated and treated appropriately. Competitive athletics are probably contraindicated because of the effect of severe blood pressure elevation on the kidney, brain, and heart (p. 694).

Strong also pointed out that many high school athletes have very large, muscular upper arms, and that care must be taken to ensure that the BP cuff is large enough.

The 1985 Task Force report which appeared in the *Journal of the American College of Cardiology* (6) reflected the existing differences of opinion with respect to the safety of athletic participation by hypertensive adolescents. The committee was aware that there was no evidence of any deleterious short- or long-term effects if several years of competitive sports are permitted during the adolescent years" (p. 1220). In the absence of target organ involvement or "severe" hypertension, participation was allowed.

In the most comprehensive article to date reviewing exercise and exercise training with respect to hypertension, Dlin (4) showed that normotensive trained youth tend to have higher BP responses to exercise than untrained normotensive or hypertensive youths. There were no data to suggest that this was an incremental risk factor for later-onset cardiovascular disease. He pointed out that stress testing in hypertensives may lead to abnormal ST-T changes, left ventricular strain, or an inappropriate BP rise. Dlin suggested that these be used as contraindications for exercise and chronic training.

Hofman and Grobbee (11) pointed out that in those individuals with high levels of circulating catecholamines, the combination of chronic athletic training and relaxation therapy is likely to be the most successful means of lowering BP. They also stressed the need for weight loss in obese hypertensives. It is not, of course, routine to measure catecholamines in hypertensive children.

The Task Force on Blood Pressure Control in Children (25) and the Second Task Force Report (23) have summarized data from over 70,000 children. These reports have defined and updated normal BP values by age and sex, but do not add any significant recommendations to those which have been discussed already. The members of the Task Force could define no risk of dynamic exercise or aerobic conditioning in any hypertensive youth who did not have renal involvement or increased left ventricular mass. Thus, testing renal and cardiac function is needed prior to clearing a hypertensive youth for athletics. Sport activities need be restricted only in those youth with severe hypertension in whom adequate response to therapy has not been achieved.

We should remember, as has most recently been pointed out by Kaplan (14) that there are other benefits to chronic exercise in addition to a direct effect on BP. These benefits include improvements in the lipid profile and in the glucose-insulin resistance relationship. Individuals who exercise tend not to smoke and are less obese. It is also generally thought that chronic exercisers have an improved sense of well-being. Exercise conditioning may be an effective antihypertensive nonpharmacological therapy, but its most important benefit may be the primary prevention of essential hypertension.

PRACTICAL RECOMMENDATIONS

A recent review (15) summarizes numerous committees' recommendations with respect to the evaluation of the hypertensive child. The physician must evaluate the child for

- target organ damage, such as retinal changes by ophthalmoscope exam,
- left ventricular mass by echocardiography, and
- renal damage by blood, urine, and imaging studies.

Those individuals with target organ damage are thought to be in need of restriction from isometric and high-contact dynamic sports (6). This presumably relates to transients (brief peaks) of SBP or DBP which may cause further target organ damage.

For patients in whom no target organ damage can be demonstrated, exercise evaluation prior to sport participation may be performed. The goal of this is to determine the level of BP during exercise, and whether there is either myocardial ischemia or dysrhythmia induced by exercise. The use of the level of SBP during dynamic exercise is controversial, but, as described earlier, many recommendations do include restriction from strenuous exercise for those hypertensive children with SBP maximal exercise values above 230 or 250 mmHg. However, there are no data of which we are aware that support the need for this restriction. In fact, since strenuous aerobic exercise may have a favorable effect on body weight, lipid levels, and psychological well-being, there may be direct benefits to allowing and even encouraging strenuous dynamic, aerobic exercise. However, unless the intensity of the exercise is sufficient, no training effect or benefit may be derived.

The sports which should be avoided in all children with severe untreated or unresponsive essential hypertension include those with high static demands in which there is a prolonged period of isometric stress. These sports are tabulated in Chapter 3. In addition, most recommendations have included a restriction from high-contact sports which might induce direct organ damage, as well as sports with high aerobic intensity such as basketball, boxing, football, ice hockey, karate, downhill skiing, soccer, weightlifting, and wrestling. There are, however, no data to suggest that children whose hypertension is under good control cannot participate in high-motion aerobic sports. The data presented earlier in this chapter suggest that they should be encouraged to do so.

If an individual child has a great deal of interest in a particular sport which involves a high isometric component but little in the way of contact, the physician may desire to do a prolonged handgrip stress and measure the child's SBP and DBP responses. The BP response is not determined by the volume of muscle mass involved in an anaerobic, isometric challenge, but by the percent of maximal effort which is sustained by the exercising muscles. Thus, a handgrip is as effective at inducing BP change as a weight lift using both legs. If the SBP and DBP responses are within the range acceptable to the physician (and there are no data to determine what that range might be), then the sport can be permitted.

SUMMARY

Because of the lack of any prospective data, specific recommendations cannot be made. We hope that investigators will collect the needed data in the next few years, but until then physicians must use their judgment in deciding whether to permit specific sports. In general, however, sports which contain little or no isometric (static) component and only limited collision (contact) should not only be permitted, but encouraged. The physiological and psychological benefits of these sports probably far outweigh the risks. Children with hypertension should be encouraged whenever possible to participate with their peers in daily life activities, of which sports are an important component.

REFERENCES

1. American Academy of Pediatrics. Cardiac evaluation for participation in sports (policy statement). Author; 1977.
2. Danforth, J.S.; Allen, K.D.; Fitterling, J.M.; Danforth, J.A.; Farrar, D.; Brown, M.; Drabman, R.S. Exercise as a treatment for hypertension in low-socioeconomic-status black children. J. Consult. Clin. Psychol. 58:237-239; 1990.
3. Daniels, S.R.; Loggie, J.M.H. Hypertension in children and adolescents. Physician. Sport Med. 20:121-134; 1992.
4. Dlin, R. Blood pressure response to dynamic exercise in healthy and hypertensive youths. Pediatrics 13:34-43; 1986.
5. Fixler, D.E.; Laird, W.P.; Browne, R.; Fitzgerald, V.; Wilson, S.; Vance, R. Response of hypertensive adolescents to dynamic and isometric exercise stress. Pediatrics 64:579-583; 1979.
6. Frohlich, E.D.; Lowenthal, D.T.; Miller, H.S.; Pickering, T.; Strong, W.B. Task Force IV: systemic arterial hypertension. J. Am. Coll. Cardiol. 6:1218-1221; 1985.
7. Hagberg, J.M.; Ehsani, A.A.; Goldring, D.; Hernandez, A.; Sincore, D.R.; Holloszy, J.O. Effect of weight training on blood pressure and hemodynamics in hypertensive adolescents. J. Pediatr. 104:147-151; 1984.
8. Hagberg, J.M.; Goldring, D.; Ehsani, A.A.; Heath, G.W.; Hernandez, A.; Schiechtman, K.; Holloszy, J.O. Effect of exercise training on the blood pressure and hemodynamic features of hypertensive adolescents. Am. J. Cardiol. 52:763-768; 1983.
9. Hansen, H.S.; Froberg, K.; Hyldebrandt, N.; Nielsen, J.R. A controlled study of eight months of physical training and reduction

of blood pressure in children: the Odense Schoolchild Study. BMJ 303:682-685; 1991.

10. Hansen, H.S.; Hyldebrandt, N.; Nielsen, J.R.; Froberg, K. Exercise testing in children as a diagnostic tool of future hypertension: the Odense Schoolchild Study. J. Hypertens. 7(suppl 1):S41-S42; 1989.

11. Hofman, A.; Grobbee, D.E. Non-pharmacological intervention in primary hypertension in childhood. Clin. Exp. Theory Prac. A8:813-822; 1986.

12. Hofman, A.; Walter, H.J.; Connelly, P.A.; Vaughan, R.D. Blood pressure and physical fitness in children. Hypertension 9:188-191; 1987.

13. Joint National Committee on Detection, Evaluation, and Treatment of High Blood Pressure. 1988 report. Arch. Intern. Med. 148:1023-1038; 1988.

14. Kaplan, N.M. Exercise for the treatment of hypertension: help or hype. Am. J. Hypertens. 5:574-576; 1992.

15. Kaplan, R.A.; Hellersteen, S.; Alon, U. Evaluation of the hypertensive child. Child. Nephrol. Urol. 12:106-112, 1992.

16. Klein, A.A.; McCrory, W.W.; Engle, M.A.; Rosenthal, R.; Ehlers, K.H. Sympathetic nervous system and exercise tolerance response in normotensive and hypertensive adolescents. J. Am. Coll. Cardiol. 3:381-386; 1984.

17. Laird, W.P.; Fixler, D.E.; Swanbom, C.D. Cardiovascular effects of weight training in hypertensive adolescents. Med. Sci. Sports Exerc. 11:78; 1979.

18. Londe, S.; Goldring, D. High blood pressure in children: problems and guidelines for evaluation and treatment. Am. J. Cardiol. 37:650-657; 1976.

19. Nudel, D.B. Is exercise testing worth it? Pediatrics 67:441; 1981.

20. Nudel, D.B.; Gootman, N.; Brunson, S.; Shenker, R.I.; Gauthier, B.G.; Stenzler, A. Exercise performance of adolescents with essential hypertension. Pediatr. Res. 12:366; 1978.

21. Nudel, D.B.; Gootman, N.; Brunson, S.C.; Stenzler, A.; Shenker, R.I.; Gauthier, B.G. Exercise performance of hypertensive adolescents. Pediatrics 65:1073-1078; 1980.

22. Schieken, R.M.; Clarke, W.R.; Lauer, R.M. The cardiovascular responses to exercise in children across the blood pressure distribution. Hypertension 5:71-78; 1983.

23. Second Task Force on Blood Pressure Control in Children Report. Pediatrics 79:1-25; 1987.

24. Strong, W.B. Hypertension and sports. Pediatrics 64:693-695; 1979.

25. Task Force on Blood Pressure Control in Children. Recommendations. Pediatrics 59(suppl):797-820; 1977.

26. Tipton, C.M. Exercise, training and hypertension: an update. Exerc. Sport Sci. Rev. 19:447-505; 1991.

27. Zahka, K.G. Adolescent hypertension update. Md. Med. J. 36:413-414; 1987.

CHAPTER 14

Congenital Heart Disease—Shunt Lesions and Cyanotic Heart Disease

John T. Fahey
Yale University School of Medicine

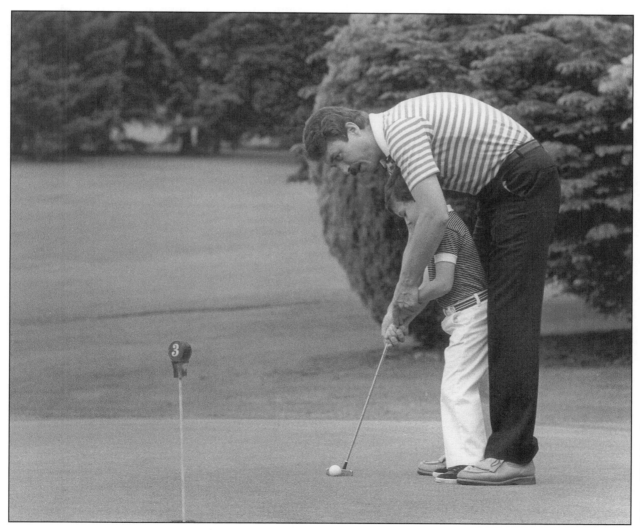

Blood exiting all body tissues but the lungs is relatively deoxygenated. It drains as systemic venous blood to the right heart, where it is pumped to the lungs and oxygenated. Fully oxygenated blood then drains as pulmonary venous blood to the left heart, which circulates the blood to the various body organs based on metabolic demands. The systemic and pulmonary circulations are normally separate, and blood moves serially through the right side of the heart to the lungs and then through the left heart to the systemic circulation. The blood flow through the right and left side of the heart is, therefore, the same and is referred to as the cardiac output. The lungs have a large vascular cross-sectional area, and the resistance to blood flow through the lungs is relatively low—normally, roughly one-tenth that of the systemic circulation. Since the blood flows are equal, the mean pulmonary artery pressure is correspondingly one-tenth that of the mean aortic pressure (based on the relationship pressure = flow × resistance).

Some forms of congenital heart disease allow communication between the left and right heart (or pulmonary and systemic circulations). If these communications are associated with obstruction to the flow of blood from the right ventricle to the pulmonary arteries or from the right atrium to the right ventricle, deoxygenated systemic venous blood will mix with the pulmonary venous blood. This is known as right-to-left shunting, and the result is systemic oxygen desaturation and cyanosis. If there is a communication between the left and right heart and no associated right heart obstruction (such as a ventricular septal defect or atrial septal defect), pulmonary venous blood entering the left ventricle will preferentially flow to the low-resistance pulmonary circulation (left-to-right shunting), leading to pulmonary overcirculation. Depending on the size of the communication and/or the severity of associated obstructions, children with shunt lesions may present very sick as newborns or may be completely asymptomatic.

Surgical techniques for even the most severe forms of congenital heart disease have improved greatly and can often restore heart function to normal or nearly normal. The goal of surgery is no longer merely to maintain survival: the expectation is that patients will become healthy and active children, adolescents, and adults with

little or no restrictions or limitations. More and more of these children will be participating in competitive and recreational activities and should be encouraged to do so, as long as it is safe. This chapter will present currently available information regarding risks and expectations of intensive exercise in children and adults with left-to-right shunt lesions (ventricular septal defects and atrial septal defects), as well as selected forms of cyanotic congenital heart disease with right-to-left shunts (tetralogy of Fallot, tricuspid valve atresia, and simple transposition of the great arteries).

VENTRICULAR SEPTAL DEFECTS

A ventricular septal defect (VSD) is a hole in the common wall (septum) between the left and right ventricles (Figure 14.1). This is the most common form of congenital heart disease.

Description of Ventricular Septal Defects

Pathophysiology

Normally, in the presence of VSD, the left ventricular systolic pressure is four to five times higher than the right ventricular systolic pressure. A VSD, therefore, exposes the high-pressure left ventricle to the low-pressure right ventricle, and blood will flow during systole from the left to right ventricle, a left-to-right ventricular-level shunt. The volume of blood shunted and the resulting symptoms are determined by the size of the VSD. Very small VSDs will transmit very little blood flow, allowing only a very small left-to-right shunt. These children will be asymptomatic. A very large VSD will allow equalization of the left and right ventricular systolic pressures, and blood will preferentially flow to the low-resistance pulmonary circulation, shunting blood away from the systemic circulation and resulting in a variable degree of congestive heart failure depending on the level of pulmonary vascular resistance.

With a VSD, the pulmonary blood flow is greater than the systemic blood flow, the difference being the left-to-right shunting of blood. Therefore, the pulmonary venous return (to the

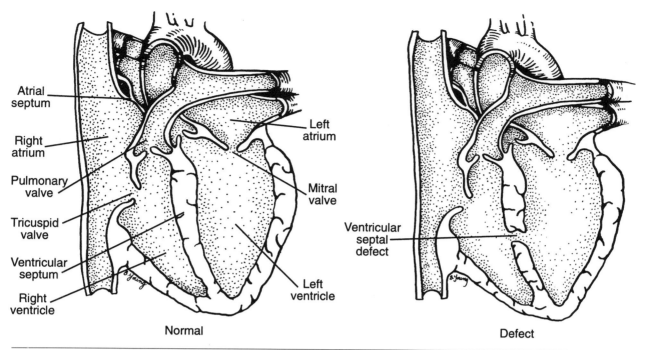

Figure 14.1 A structurally normal heart is shown schematically at left. There is no communication between the left and right heart. The figure at right shows a heart with a single large ventricular septal defect. The left-to-right shunt (left ventricle to right ventricle) is demonstrated by the shaded flow pattern.
Reproduced with permission. *If Your Child Has a Congenital Heart Defect*, 1991. Copyright © American Heart Association.

left atrium and ventricle) is greater than the systemic venous return (to the right atrium and ventricle), and the left ventricle pumps more blood than the right ventricle. The left ventricle must dilate to handle the extra volume load, which increases its volume work. Moderate and large VSDs will result in elevation of right ventricular pressure, increasing the pressure work of the right ventricle.

Physical Symptoms and Clinical Signs

Children with small and moderate VSDs are asymptomatic at rest. In general, large VSDs result in symptoms of congestive heart failure in infancy, which include poor feeding, reduced weight gain, and tachypnea. Physical exam shows normal to slightly increased precordial activity, depending on the volume of the left-to-right shunt. There is a holosystolic murmur, which is usually loudest at the lower left sternal border. The murmurs may be quite loud and may be associated with a left parasternal systolic thrill. If the shunt is significant, there may be a mid-diastolic low-pitched murmur at the cardiac apex, a so-called mitral rumble. This diastolic rumble is present when the pulmonary

blood flow is in the range of twice the systemic blood flow or greater. The rumble is caused by excessive flow (i.e., pulmonary venous return) across the normal mitral valve. The pulmonary component of the second heart sound is normal, as are perfusion and pulses.

Clinical and Laboratory Assessment

Children with small or moderate VSDs may present for preparticipation evaluation. These children may be seen by a pediatric cardiologist prior to competitive sport participation or evaluated by a knowledgeable primary care physician. An electrocardiogram and chest X ray should be obtained and would be expected to be normal. Any abnormality detected would warrant a referral to a pediatric cardiologist.

Any child with a characteristic holosystolic VSD murmur associated with a diastolic murmur should be evaluated by a pediatric cardiologist prior to any sport participation. The evaluation usually includes an electrocardiogram, chest X ray, and echocardiogram. The electrocardiogram will evaluate for the presence or absence of left or right ventricular hypertrophy or dilation and dysrhythmias. The presence of cardiomegaly on chest X ray would warrant further investigation. The echocardiogram will assess left ventricular chamber size and image the VSD, as well as predict the right ventricular pressure. Additionally, holosystolic murmurs may also be caused by tricuspid or mitral valve regurgitation and these can be ruled out by the echocardiogram. If the shunt is large and the right ventricular pressure is elevated, the child requires cardiac catheterization and, probably, surgical closure of the defect. An exercise stress test is usually not a part of the evaluation. However, any history of exercise limitation or related symptoms, regardless of the size of the VSD, requires further workup. The evaluation should include an exercise stress test as soon as the child is able to cooperate (usually at 5 years of age or older).

Following surgical closure of a ventricular septal defect, children require thorough evaluation before sport participation. Persistent holosystolic murmurs usually represent residual ventricular septal defects, but may also represent either tricuspid or mitral regurgitation. Evaluation before sport participation should include an electrocardiogram, chest X ray, echocardiogram, 24-hour ambulatory electrocardiography (Holter monitor), and exercise stress testing. Detectable abnormalities which may limit sport participation include

- significant residual left-to-right shunts,
- myocardial dysfunction, and
- resting or exercise-induced dysrhythmias.

Patients with preoperative pulmonary hypertension may require repeat cardiac catheterization.

Natural History

The ventricular septal defect either remains the same size or becomes smaller as the child grows. Most small defects present in infants close spontaneously either by muscular ingrowth or tricuspid valve tissue adherence. Moderate-sized defects are usually well tolerated in infancy and early childhood, and if there are no signs of congestive heart failure in infancy the children usually grow normally and are asymptomatic. Larger defects that cause congestive heart failure in infancy will require surgical closure. Even if congestive failure does not develop in infancy or

is controlled medically, the defects will require surgical closure if there is failure to thrive or if there is a significant volume load on the left ventricle still present at 12-18 months of age; however, practice varies from institution to institution. Large VSDs which are not closed surgically may lead to elevated pulmonary vascular resistance and pulmonary hypertension. If this state persists, the elevated pulmonary vascular resistance will become permanent and progressive, leading to pulmonary vascular obstructive disease. This elevated resistance will decrease the left-to-right shunt and, when severe, may actually reverse the shunting to right to left so that the children become cyanotic (so-called Eisenmenger's syndrome). Pulmonary vascular disease, once established, cannot be reversed by surgical VSD closure; the pulmonary vessels are permanently damaged, resulting in the eventual death of the child unless lung transplantation is undertaken.

Therapeutic Intervention

Infants who show signs of congestive heart failure from the left-to-right shunt are usually treated medically with a combination of digoxin, diuretics, and afterload reduction. If there are symptoms or poor growth in spite of medical management, surgical closure is undertaken. Most often the defects are closed via a right atrial incision, operating through the tricuspid valve and avoiding an incision in the muscular right ventricle. Surgery may be undertaken at a later date in response to poor weight gain or persistent cardiomegaly and left ventricular volume overload. For most VSDs which require closure, surgery will be performed before 2 years of age. However, there are many adolescents and adults who have had their VSDs closed at much older ages owing to prior unavailability of surgery. Many of these defects were closed via a right ventricular incision. Complications of surgery include

- residual ventricular septal defects,
- dysrhythmias, and
- depressed myocardial function.

Decreased myocardial function may result from a complication of the surgery or, in patients operated on at an older age, from the effects of chronic volume load on the left ventricle.

Morbidity and Mortality

Children with small VSDs should be asymptomatic, and, without associated cardiac problems, have a normal life span. The same expectancy was formerly felt to be true for persons with moderate ventricular septal defects. Recently, however, collaborative natural history study has shown a risk of sudden death in unoperated patients with small to moderate VSDs who do not meet the criteria for surgical closure (27). Whether these new data will change the indications for surgical closure is unknown. Similarly, it is not known whether surgical closure would have prevented these deaths. The surgical mortality from VSD closure is generally less than 2%. There is a small risk of sudden death in the postoperative group as well, usually related to associated dysrhythmias or poor ventricular function.

Children with Eisenmenger's syndrome (pulmonary vascular disease and right-to-left shunt) generally die as young adults.

Exercise and Ventricular Septal Defects

Since small VSDs transmit only a small left-to-right shunt volume at rest and the shunt remains small during exercise, these children should be asymptomatic with exercise (8). Data are available on the response to intense exercise in unoperated patients with moderate ventricular septal defects (21, 36). Patients were evaluated during cardiac catheterization and supine bicycle exercise; pulmonary blood flow increased more than systemic blood flow, the left-to-right shunt increased, and the patients were exercise-limited when compared to controls. Otterstad, Simmonsen, and Erikssen (36) found a subnormal increase in cardiac output with such exercise. Other reported abnormalities in this group of unoperated moderate VSDs include shorter endurance times (8), lower work levels at exhaustion (18), and lower maximal heart rates (22).

It is the hope of surgical VSD closure to return hemodynamics to normal or nearly normal. However, many studies have shown that even children with favorable resting hemodynamics after surgery may have detectable exercise limitations, including a blunted maximal heart rate

response (22, 39), decreased cardiac output response to exercise (32, 36, 39), subnormal work performance (36), and slightly lower than normal exercise duration (11). Interestingly, many or most postoperative patients have been able to achieve a normal maximal O_2 consumption. Age at operation seems to be an important variable for the inadequate increase in cardiac output seen after VSD closure, with surgical correction before the age of 10 years usually associated with a normal increase in cardiac output with exercise (32). Now that surgery for VSDs generally is being performed before the age of 2 years, it is the expectation that no exercise limitation will be detectable in this later group of postoperative patients (7, 19). However, careful evaluation as outlined earlier in all postoperative VSD patients is indicated before allowing participation in competitive athletics (34). Associated cardiac rhythm disturbances or decreased resting myocardial function will further complicate exercise responses.

An underlying question with all studies on either unoperated or postoperative children with VSD concerns the interpretation of the performance on fitness tests. Although clearly there are hemodynamic reasons for a subnormal response on exercise tests, a psychological component may also play a role. If children (or their parents) perceive themselves as abnormal or limited because they have a "hole in their heart" or a scar on their chest, they may be sedentary, poorly conditioned, or afraid to exercise. As long as there are no exercise-associated arrhythmias or resting myocardial dysfunction, however, there is no reason for these children not to exercise and participate normally; in fact, they should be encouraged to do so. Other than dysrhythmias, which will be dealt with in a separate chapter, there are no potential adverse effects from exercise for which these children are especially at risk or for which they need special observation. Benefits of exercise and fitness far outweigh any risks.

Recommendations for Sport Participation in Children With Ventricular Septal Defects

Recommendations for sport participation for children with VSD depend on the size and nature of the VSD. Symptoms that require either a rest period or termination of exercise are listed in Table 14.1.

Unoperated

Children with small VSDs and normal electrocardiogram and chest X ray can participate in all competitive sports without restriction. Children who have a history of a VSD which has undergone spontaneous closure (no murmur) should also be treated as normal children.

Most children with moderate VSDs will have surgical closure. If surgical closure is not undertaken, these children require a complete evaluation and special attention. The studies mentioned previously would predict that they will have a subnormal response to intense exercise. Because there seems to be a higher risk of sudden death in this group when observed over the long term (27), it probably is advisable to restrict these children from intense exercise, although this is controversial. Current recommendations (34) would allow only low-intensity sports with low static and low dynamic demands. However, each child should be closely followed by a pediatric cardiologist, and individual recommendations may be altered based on the clinical findings and laboratory assessment.

Children with Eisenmenger's syndrome are at particularly high risk for sudden death during sport activities, and should be restricted from all competitive sports. However, they should be encouraged to participate in nonsedentary activities for both physiological and psychological reasons.

Table 14.1 Symptoms in the Child With Cardiac Disease

---

1. Palpitations (irregular heartbeat)
2. Tachycardia (fast heart rate out of proportion to the level of exertion)
3. Lightheadedness
4. Syncope
5. Chest pain
6. Shortness of breath, "tightness" in chest with deep breath.

Note. Any of the above should lead to a rest period or termination of exercise, depending on the severity. Contact with or referral back to the cardiologist should be made.

Postoperative VSD Closure

These children should be restricted from competitive sport for 6 months following VSD closure (34). Prior to participation they must have a complete evaluation by a pediatric cardiologist. The evaluation should include physical exam, electrocardiogram, chest X ray, echocardiogram, 24-hour ambulatory electrocardiogram, and a maximal exercise stress test. In addition, patients with preoperative pulmonary hypertension who were operated at an older age (> 2 years) should probably have a postoperative cardiac catheterization to assess pulmonary artery pressure and pulmonary vascular resistance.

Children with no residual ventricular septal defect or a small residual septal defect and who have a normal evaluation (as just outlined) may participate in all competitive sports without restriction. Children with a moderate residual ventricular septal defect should be restricted from sports with a high aerobic intensity and encouraged to participate in low intensity sports with low static and dynamic demand.

Further evaluation is needed to determine the management of children who have postoperative dysrhythmias, either at rest or with exercise. Restrictions are made based on the type of dysrhythmia and are detailed in chapter 16. Children who have postoperative ventricular dysfunction and dilated left ventricles also require further evaluation. Restrictions are based on the degree of myocardial dysfunction and are detailed in chapter 17.

ATRIAL SEPTAL DEFECTS

An atrial septal defect (ASD) is an abnormal communication between the left and right atrium. Although most defects are centrally located in the middle portion of the interatrial septum (so-called secundum atrial septal defects), defects may be located anywhere along the interatrial septum.

Description of Atrial Septal Defects

Pathophysiology

Normally left atrial pressure is slightly higher (by 1-3 mmHg) than right atrial pressure. This occurs because the left ventricle generates higher pressures than the right ventricle and is therefore thicker and stiffer (less compliant). Thus the left ventricle requires higher filling pressures compared to the right ventricle.

An ASD, therefore, allows blood to flow from the left atrium to the right atrium and represents a left-to-right shunt. As seen with VSD, the volume of the left-to-right shunt depends on the size of the defects and the ratio between pulmonary and systemic resistance. Large ASDs allow equalization of pressure between the left and right atrium, and blood will preferentially flow during diastole (ventricular filling) to the more compliant right ventricle. However, as left and right atrial pressures are low, blood is not forced under high pressure towards the right ventricle (as opposed to VSD shunting), and the left-to-right shunt is more a passive event.

In the presence of an ASD, the pulmonary blood flow is greater than the systemic blood flow, the difference being the left-to-right shunt. However, since the left-to-right shunt is at the atrial level, flow across the tricuspid valve to the right ventricle is greater than flow across the mitral valve to the left ventricle, and the right ventricle pumps more blood than the left ventricle. The right ventricle must dilate to handle the extra volume load. Unlike with VSD, the burden of extra work is on the right ventricle. As the left-to-right atrial shunt is not forced at high pressure to the right ventricle, right ventricular pressure, even with large ASDs, is usually normal or only slightly elevated.

Physical Symptoms and Clinical Signs

Infants and children with small, moderate, and large ASDs are most often asymptomatic at rest. It is unusual for an infant to manifest signs of congestive heart failure or failure to thrive even with large left-to-right atrial shunts. If the right ventricle is dilated, the physical exam will show increased precordial activity. These children classically have a pulmonary flow murmur represented by a systolic ejection murmur at the upper left sternal border. This results from excessive flow and increased right ventricular ejection across a normal pulmonary valve. As flow from the left atrium to the right atrium is with a minimal or no pressure difference, there is no turbulence and, therefore, no murmur due to

flow across the ASD. With a large-volume left-to-right atrial shunt, there may be a mid-diastolic low-pitched murmur at the lower left sternal border (tricuspid rumble). The rumble is due to excessive flow across the normal tricuspid valve. The classic finding on physical exam for children with large ASDs involves the second heart sound. It has wide splitting due to delayed pulmonic closure. In addition, the second heart sound has fixed splitting, i.e., no respiratory variation in the degree of splitting. The systemic perfusion and pulses are normal.

Clinical and Laboratory Assessment

Children with a pulmonary ejection murmur and a hyperdynamic precordium should be evaluated. There must be a high clinical suspicion of an ASD with such an examination and a referral to a pediatric cardiologist is indicated. The electrocardiogram may show right ventricular hypertrophy or a right bundle branch block, but may also be normal. A chest X ray may show cardiomegaly, or may be relatively normal even with a large ASD. An echocardiogram is diagnostic and will be obtained if the clinical suspicion is high.

Any child with a pulmonary flow murmur, dynamic precordium, and the addition of a diastolic murmur should be referred to a pediatric cardiologist prior to any sport participation. The workup includes an electrocardiogram, chest X ray, and echocardiogram. The electrocardiogram will evaluate the presence or absence of right ventricular hypertrophy as well as assess the cardiac rhythm, which may be abnormal in children with ASD. The chest X ray will assess heart size, right ventricular dilation, and pulmonary flow markings. The echocardiogram is the best means to identify the ASD and its size and location. The left-to-right shunt can be documented by Doppler and color flow analysis. The degree of right heart dilation can be measured. Mitral valve prolapse, which is present in approximately 10% of young people with ASD (29), can also be diagnosed. If the ASD is large and there is a significant left-to-right shunt and right ventricular volume overload, the child will require surgical or transcatheter closure. Small ASDs with low-volume shunts and no right heart dilation usually do not require intervention. An exercise stress test is usually not a part of the workup.

Children who have had surgical closure of an ASD should be evaluated prior to competitive sport participation. Workup, in addition to a physical exam, should include an electrocardiogram, chest X ray, and a 24-hour ambulatory electrocardiogram monitor. Any persistent cardiomegaly should be further evaluated by echocardiogram to assess ventricular function and size, as well as to detect residual defects and left-to-right shunts. In the event of any tachyarrhythmias or evidence of sinus node dysfunction, further evaluation should be conducted, which may include exercise stress testing.

Natural History

Most children with ASDs are asymptomatic and the diagnosis is suspected on routine evaluation, most commonly between 2 and 5 years of age. Small defects which do not impart a significant right ventricular volume load do not require surgical closure. Moderate to large defects which have an associated significant right ventricular volume load will be referred for elective closure between 2 and 4 years of age, or upon diagnosis if detected at an older age. Children and adolescents with unoperated large ASDs may have mild exercise intolerance but may be completely asymptomatic. The long-term complications of a large atrial septal defect include atrial arrhythmias, right ventricular dysfunction, and elevated pulmonary vascular resistance and pulmonary vascular obstructive disease with pulmonary hypertension.

Therapeutic Intervention

Surgical closure obviously involves open heart surgery on a heart-lung bypass machine. The surgery is performed via a right atrial incision. Most defects are primarily sewn closed, although very large defects may require patch closure. There are currently clinical trials ongoing in which selected secundum ASDs may be closed during cardiac catheterization using an implantable closure device and avoiding surgery. The results are promising and this may be the treatment of choice in the near future (31).

Morbidity and Mortality

Children with small and moderate ASDs should be asymptomatic and have a normal life span.

The same is true for unoperated large ASDs unless there are associated dysrhythmias, or reduced right ventricular function or pulmonary vascular disease with pulmonary hypertension. There is probably a slightly higher than normal risk of paradoxical emboli and stroke, although an accurate assessment of this risk is not available. The mortality of surgical closure of an ASD is small, generally less than 1%.

Exercise and Atrial Septal Defects

Children with ASDs usually have normal or nearly normal exercise capacity. These children can usually attain normal values of maximal O_2 consumption (40). The behavior of the left-to-right shunt in response to exercise is variable, and may increase (21), decrease (3, 40), or stay the same (3, 40). There may be a smaller than normal increase in systemic blood flow with ASDs, but this does not seem to be limiting (3).

A variety of abnormalities with exercise have been reported following surgical ASD closure. Postoperative patients may have a smaller than normal increase in cardiac output in response to intense upright exercise, even in the absence of residual shunts, arrhythmias, or pulmonary artery hypertension (12). Perrault et al. found that during maximal exercise testing using bicycle ergometry, postoperative ASD closure patients had lower than normal maximal heart rates as compared to controls (39). There was no difference, however, in the attained maximal O_2 consumption between the two groups. Interestingly, all children in this study were operated on before the age of 5 years. In a subsequent study, Reybrouck, Weymans, Stijns, and van der Haywaert found that children who had surgical closure of an ASD after the age of 5 years had lower than normal ventilatory thresholds, while those operated upon before the age of 5 had normal ventilatory thresholds (41). Associated cardiac rhythm disturbances may further complicate exercise responses (5, 43).

Overall, abnormalities detected in children with either unoperated or surgically closed ASDs are usually minor and do not result in limitations in exercise ability. Unless arrhythmias are a complication, children with these defects should be encouraged to exercise and participate in all sports, at all levels. A formal exercise stress test prior to sport participation is not necessary unless indicated by symptoms or associated problems such as dysrhythmias.

Recommendations for Sport Participation in Children With Atrial Septal Defects

Unoperated

Children with atrial septal defects of any size should be allowed to participate in all competitive sports unless there is documented or suspected pulmonary hypertension. Young adults with pulmonary hypertension will be restricted to low-intensity sports (low static and low dynamic demands) or restricted from all competitive sports based on the degree of pulmonary hypertension.

Operated

Children or adults who have undergone surgical ASD closure should be restricted from all competitive sports for 6 months postoperatively. After this period no restrictions are necessary (34). Anyone who has had preoperative pulmonary hypertension requires a cardiac catheterization to ensure that the pressures have returned to normal prior to exercise recommendations.

Children who have postoperative dysrhythmias require further evaluation. Restrictions will be based on the type of dysrhythmia as outlined in chapter 16.

TETRALOGY OF FALLOT

Two major structural abnormalities in tetralogy of Fallot account for physiological disturbances: 1) a large ventricular septal defect and 2) obstruction to pulmonary blood flow.

Description of Tetralogy of Fallot

Pathophysiology

In tetralogy of Fallot, the ventricular septal defects are large and unrestrictive, allowing equalization of left and right ventricular pressures (see the previous discussion of ventricular septal defects). The obstruction to pulmonary blood flow (i.e., flow from the right ventricle to the pulmonary arteries) is variable and may be mild, moderate, severe, or complete (pulmonary atresia). The severity of obstruction to pulmonary blood flow determines the magnitude of the lung blood flow. If the obstruction is mild there may be left-to-right shunting of blood, and the pulmonary blood flow may be greater than the systemic blood flow. Most often, however, the obstruction to pulmonary blood flow is moderate or severe. In these cases lung blood flow will be decreased, and some or most of the desaturated systemic venous return which enters the right ventricle will course through the VSD to the aorta, i.e., a right-to-left shunt. Desaturated blood entering the aorta (systemic circulation) leads to desaturation of the systemic arterial blood and results in peripheral cyanosis. The greater the obstruction to lung blood flow, the larger the right-to-left shunt and the more severe the resulting cyanosis and systemic desaturation (Figure 14.2).

The obstruction to pulmonary blood flow may occur at two levels. The obstruction may be only within the outflow from the right ventricle (the right ventricular infundibulum) to the pulmonary valve, with a long segment of muscular narrowing. In this case the pulmonary valve and main pulmonary artery may be normal in size. Alternatively, the right ventricular outflow may be nearly normal with only mild obstruction, and the major obstruction to pulmonary blood flow may be caused by a small or malformed pulmonary valve. Most commonly both forms of obstruction are present, with a narrowed right ventricular outflow and a small pulmonary valve annulus and main pulmonary artery.

Standard treatment of tetralogy of Fallot is surgical repair in infancy or early childhood. It would be highly unlikely that a child with unoperated tetralogy of Fallot would be evaluated for sport participation, and only brief mention of the unoperated child will be made where appropriate.

Surgical repair of tetralogy of Fallot is straightforward and serves to correct the two major defects: the VSD must be closed and the obstruction to pulmonary blood flow must be relieved or bypassed. The VSD is closed with a patch which eliminates the communication between the left and right ventricles. Repair of the

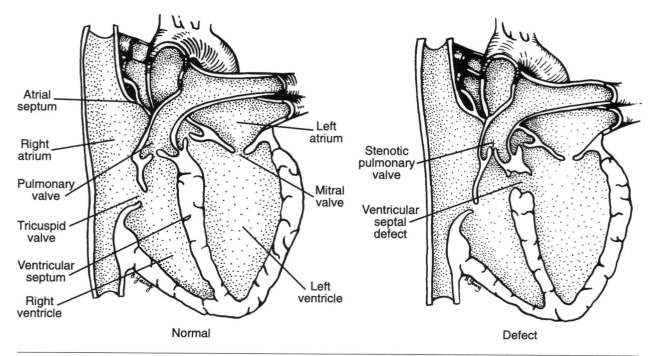

Figure 14.2 Tetralogy of Fallot is shown schematically at right, demonstrating a ventricular septal defect and pulmonary stenosis. The right-to-left shunt (right ventricle to left ventricle) is shown by the shaded flow pattern. As in Figure 14.1, a normal heart is shown for comparison in the figure at left.
Reproduced with permission. *If Your Child Has a Congenital Heart Defect*, 1991. Copyright © American Heart Association.

obstruction to pulmonary blood flow is dictated by the level of obstruction. If there is only obstruction in the right ventricular outflow and the pulmonary valve is normal, the obstruction is relieved by making an incision in the right ventricular outflow; obstructing muscle is then excised and the outflow is patch enlarged. This should not distort the pulmonary valve, and the valve should be competent postoperatively. If the obstruction is only at the valve itself, the surgery may only require a reparative valve procedure to relieve the obstruction.

If the obstruction to pulmonary blood flow involves both the right ventricular outflow and the pulmonary valve, an incision must be made along the right ventricular outflow and extended across the pulmonary valve annulus into the main pulmonary artery. Obstructing muscle is excised and the right ventricular outflow is patch enlarged, with the patch extending to the main pulmonary artery. Although this relieves the obstruction, the pulmonary valve is no longer competent and there are varying degrees of pulmonary valve insufficiency as a sequellae of the repair. If the obstruction to pulmonary blood flow is complete and the pulmonary valve is atretic, the surgical repair will require placement of a valved conduit from the right ventricle

to the main pulmonary artery, bypassing the obstruction.

Physical Symptoms and Clinical Signs

Infants with milder forms of tetralogy of Fallot may have no symptoms other than cyanosis. The physical exam will reveal varying degrees of cyanosis, both central and peripheral. The cardiac exam will have a single second heart sound, as the pulmonic closure sound is absent or reduced. There is a harsh systolic ejection murmur along the left sternal border produced by the pulmonic stenosis. There may be an associated parasternal thrill. There is usually no diastolic murmur. The perfusion and pulses should be normal.

The examination of the postoperative patient will be quite different. There is no longer any cyanosis, as the right-to-left shunt is eliminated with closure of the VSD. The surgery is performed through a midline sternotomy. The cardiac exam usually shows increased precordial activity, especially if there is significant pulmonary insufficiency. The second heart sound will be single. There is usually a systolic ejection murmur of residual pulmonic stenosis. In addition, there is usually a diastolic decrescendo murmur of variable intensity representing pulmonary insufficiency.

Clinical and Laboratory Assessment

Following surgery for tetralogy of Fallot, children will be followed by a cardiologist for their lifetime. The name and phone number of the attending cardiologist should always be readily available to caretakers, coaches, and supervisors during school and athletic activity.

Survival without symptoms is common in this group of patients, and questions regarding athletic participation have become frequent. Persisting abnormalities which may limit sport participation include

- residual pulmonic stenosis,
- pulmonary insufficiency,
- residual ventricular septal defects
- myocardial dysfunction, and
- ventricular dysrhythmias.

There is a small risk of sudden death. Therefore, a complete evaluation in the postoperative patient must be undertaken before making a decision regarding sport participation. This workup should include a chest radiograph, electrocardiogram, echocardiogram, 24-hour ambulatory electrocardiography, and exercise stress testing. The echocardiogram is most important in detecting the severity of residual pulmonic stenosis, the magnitude of pulmonary insufficiency, ventricular function, and residual ventricular septal defects. Children with significant residual pulmonic stenosis (predicted right ventricular pressure greater than 40 mmHg or greater than 1/2 systemic pressure) or significant residual ventricular septal defects should undergo cardiac catheterization before a decision can be made regarding sport participation.

Natural History, Morbidity, and Mortality

As mentioned earlier, the vast majority of children with tetralogy of Fallot undergo surgical repair before 2 years of age. Surgical mortality is fairly low, ranging from 2 to 8% (28). There is usually some degree of residual right ventricular outflow obstruction following operation, and pulmonary insufficiency is present in the majority of cases. Reoperation is required in a minority

of patients, usually for significant residual outflow obstruction or ventricular septal defects. Most children are in sinus rhythm, and surgical complete heart block is rare. Postoperative right bundle branch block is the rule because of the right ventricular incision. Ventricular ectopy is common, and frequent ventricular ectopy is usually treated aggressively (13).

There is a risk of sudden unexpected death in the postoperative patient (15, 23). The precipitating event is probably a dysrhythmia, but residual hemodynamic abnormalities probably also enhance the risk of death. Ventricular ectopy appears to correlate with sudden death as well, and it is presumed that sustained ventricular tachycardia is the cause in these cases. Sudden death is more likely if ventricular ectopy is accompanied by high right ventricular pressures (caused by significant residual pulmonic stenosis) or myocardial dysfunction. Treatment of ventricular ectopy may result in a reduction in the frequency of sudden death (14).

However, long-term survival is the rule, and most patients are active and asymptomatic. Survival without late events (symptomatic dysrhythmias, reoperation, congestive heart failure, or sudden death) occurs in 91-96% of patients (26).

Exercise and Tetralogy of Fallot

Children with unoperated tetralogy of Fallot will very rarely need to be evaluated for sport participation, as the vast majority will have had corrective surgery in infancy. However, previous studies have found that children with unoperated tetralogy exhibit severe exercise limitations. This is due to the fact that exercise induces an increase in the pressure gradient across the stenotic area, leading to increase in the right-to-left shunt and severe systemic desaturation. In fact, exercise can lead to a four-fold increase in the right-to-left shunt, with marked acute cyanosis rapidly limiting exercise (16).

Postoperative children who are felt to have "good" surgical results (no significant residual ventricular septal defect, a pressure drop between the RV and pulmonary artery of less than 20 mmHg, and an RV pressure less than 40 mmHg) generally are asymptomatic at rest. A variety of hemodynamic abnormalities, however, may be brought out by intensive exercise. These include

- high right ventricular pressure, with values as high as 100 mmHg during maximal exercise, caused by progressively increasing pressure gradients between the right ventricle and the pulmonary artery (12),
- blunted increases in stroke volume (12) and heart rate (39, 45), and
- appearance of ventricular dysrhythmias (13).

In spite of these abnormalities after tetralogy of Fallot repair children and adolescents usually do fairly well on exercise testing with only mild impairment in exercise capacity. Maximal O$_2$ consumption ranges from 84% (35, 42) to 100% (39) of control values. Exercise duration ranges on average between 82% (45) to 92% (42) of controls, with many attaining normal values. In addition, Goldberg et al. (17) have shown that with training, postoperative tetralogy patients may attain a 25% improvement in maximal work capacity.

Approximately 5-10% (13) of postoperative tetralogy patients will have ventricular ectopy on routine resting electrocardiography. In addition, 20-58% of patients will have exercise induced ventricular arrhythmias (13, 24, 42, 44, 45). Resting ventricular ectopy may or may not be suppressed with exercise, and ventricular ectopy may occur only during exercise or only during recovery from exercise (13). The ventricular ectopy seems to correlate with a poor hemodynamic surgical result, specifically with right ventricular pressures greater than 60 mmHg at rest. In addition, ventricular ectopy may occur late following surgery, and ventricular ectopy has been shown to increase in frequency as the time from surgery increases. Exercise-induced complex ventricular arrhythmias (multiform premature ventricular complexes, ventricular couplets, or nonsustained ventricular tachycardia) may occur in as high as 16% of patients undergoing stress testing (42).

Sudden death in these patients has been reported both at rest and during exercise (23). Exercised-induced complex ventricular arrhythmias have been highly associated with sudden death. Resting or exercise-induced ventricular arrhythmias (including unifocal premature ventricular contractions) in combination with high resting right ventricular pressures are also felt to be a risk factor for sudden death (14, 15).

Recommendations for Sport Participation in Children With Tetralogy of Fallot

McNamara et al. (34) make the following recommendations for children with unoperated tetralogy of Fallot and those who have undergone tetralogy repair.

Unoperated

Children with unoperated tetralogy of Fallot may participate only in low-intensity sports.

Operated

As mentioned, most children after tetralogy repair have good hemodynamic results and are asymptomatic. They may participate even in strenuous and competitive athletics, and many have done so (24, 45). However, participation may be allowed only after extensive evaluation. In addition, as arrhythmias may present late after surgical repair, this group will also need repeated evaluations.

After repair of tetralogy of Fallot patients should be permitted participation in all competitive sports provided that the following criteria are met:

- Low right ventricular pressure (<40 mmHg), as documented by cardiac catheterization or predicted by cardiac echo-Doppler.
- No residual right-to-left shunts and normal systemic saturations.
- Only a small (or no) residual ventricular septal defect, documented by catheterization or echo-Doppler, with small left-to-right shunt (ratio of pulmonary to systemic blood flow less than 1.5).
- No ventricular arrhythmia with maximal exercise stress test. No or infrequent ventricular ectopy (less than 30 per hour) of single morphology on routine ambulatory 24-hour monitor.
- Normal ventricular function by echocardiogram, nuclear scan, or angiography.

Children meeting all five of the above criteria are considered to have "good" surgical results and probably represent 50 to 70% of postoperative patients (13). However, children should be reevaluated yearly prior to sport participation. Since ventricular arrhythmias may appear late (many years) after surgery, these children should have maximal exercise stress tests every 2-3 years.

Patients should be restricted from all sport participation if:

- The right ventricular pressure at rest is elevated to greater than 60 mmHg.
- There is poor left or right ventricular function.
- There is a large left-to-right shunt via a residual ventricular septal defect (pulmonary to systemic flow ratio greater than 1.5 to 1).
- There are resting or exercise-induced complex ventricular arrhythmias (multiform premature ventricular complexes, ventricular couplets, or ventricular tachycardia).

Obviously, there will be a large group of patients who do not meet the criteria either for "good" surgical results or for exclusion from all sports. Children who have mild residual defects (pulmonary stenosis, pulmonary insufficiency, or small ventricular septal defects) require individual consideration and careful testing by their cardiologists. A special group includes those patients with a good hemodynamic result but unifocal ventricular ectopy. There is no evidence that patients with ventricular ectopy (either at rest or with exercise) and normal right ventricular pressures, normal ventricular function, and no significant ventricular septal defects are at risk for sudden death. While strict adherence to the consensus from the Bethesda Conference (34) would require restriction from all but low-intensity sports for this group, this is probably too restrictive and recommendations for such patients should be made after extensive evaluation and thorough discussions between the cardiologist, patient, and parents.

OTHER CYANOTIC LESIONS

Two other forms of cyanotic congenital heart disease, transposition of the great arteries and tricuspid valve atresia, will be discussed in much less detail as they are relatively uncommon. However, improved surgical techniques may palliate or repair these conditions so that children may participate in sport.

Transposition of the Great Arteries

Pathophysiology and Surgical Approach

In simple transposition of the great arteries (TGA), the aorta arises from the right ventricle and the pulmonary artery arises from the left ventricle. This results in severe cyanosis as the desaturated systemic venous blood is pumped via the right atrium and ventricle back to the aorta and systemic organs, bypassing the lungs. Similarly, the pulmonary venous return is pumped via the left atrium and left ventricle back to the lungs. The blood is already fully saturated and the lungs can add no more oxygen to the blood. Early intervention is usually required for survival. Early palliative procedures allowing mixing between the systemic and pulmonary circulations include maintaining patency of the ductus arteriosus by prostaglandin infusion, and creation of an atrial septal defect using a balloon septostomy technique.

Early surgical attempts at anatomic correction of these defects were unsuccessful. This included transsection of the aorta and pulmonary artery and switching these connections so that the aorta arose from the left ventricle and the pulmonary artery arose from the right ventricle. However, the coronary arteries arise from the aorta and these had to be excised and translocated with the aorta so that they could receive arterial blood. In the early years of surgery, manipulation and reanastomosis of such small arteries was universally unsuccessful and this approach was abandoned.

The surgical approach to TGA from the late 1960s to the early 1980s involved baffling or rerouting of the systemic venous return (from the superior vena cava and inferior vena cava) to the mitral valve and left ventricle. The desaturated blood would then be pumped to the pulmonary artery (arising from the LV) to the lungs. The interatrial septum was removed and the pulmonary venous return drained to the tricuspid valve and right ventricle, where it was pumped to the aorta. Such atrial switching procedures, either the Mustard operation or Senning operation, left the right ventricle as the systemic ventricle and the left ventricle as the pulmonary ventricle. The major problems with this surgery resulted from (1) extensive atrial incisions, and (2) leaving the right ventricle as the systemic ventricle. Long-term problems included sinus node dysfunction, slow junctional rhythms, supraventricular tachycardia, depressed right ventricular function, right ventricular failure, tricuspid valve insufficiency, and sudden death (37).

With the advent of microsurgical techniques and improved heart-lung bypass methods to allow open heart surgery in the immediate newborn period, anatomic correction for TGA, the arterial switch operation, was again attempted in the 1980s with excellent success (25). While reimplantation of the coronary arteries remains the most technically difficult part of the operation, this makes the circulation nearly normal as the left ventricle becomes the systemic ventricle and the right ventricle the pulmonary ventricle. As this is a relatively new surgical approach no long-term follow-up has yet been carried out. Problems encountered thus far center upon the coronary anastomoses, either of which may become stenotic (2). Occlusion of a coronary artery and myocardial infarction have been reported. Myocardial dysfunction and arrhythmias appear not to be a common problem, at least to date.

Response to Exercise and Exercise Recommendations

Exercise testing following atrial switching procedures (Mustard or Senning operations) has detected a variety of abnormalities even in those asymptomatic at rest. Decreased endurance times and lower peak heart rates and O_2 consumption have been reported (20, 33, 38). When the response of the right ventricle to exercise was assessed by nuclear angiography, more than half of the patients had either no change or a decrease in the RV ejection fraction. This brings the suitability of the RV as the systemic ventricle into question. A variety of arrhythmias may also be provoked by exercise, including junctional rhythm, premature atrial contractions, and premature ventricular contractions (both unifocal and multifocal). In fact, exercise testing has been advocated as a sensitive method to detect sinoatrial node dysfunction in postoperative children (20). In addition to these abnormalities, potentially detrimental effects of training in these patients have been reported (34). Whether the right ventricle can dilate and hypertrophy in response to training, as does the left ventricle

in highly trained young athletes, is unknown. Similarly, whether the increased vagal tone and bradycardia associated with training increase the risk of sinus node dysfunction in a patient following Mustard or Senning operation is unknown. This is especially important since the risk of sudden death in these patients is related to sinus node dysfunction and to supraventricular dysrhythmias.

For these reasons, high physically intense isometric or aerobic sports are not recommended for children and adults who have undergone an atrial switching procedure. Thorough evaluation before participation in moderate- and low-intensity sports is mandatory and should include chest X ray, electrocardiogram, echocardiogram, 24-hour ambulatory electrocardiographic monitoring, and maximal exercise stress testing. As for tetralogy patients, the name and phone number of the attending cardiologist should be readily available.

Specific Recommendations

Patients with a Mustard or Senning operation may be permitted to participate in sports of low intensity (34). Selected patients may participate in selected sports of high to moderate dynamic and low static demands only if

- There is no cardiac enlargement on chest X ray.
- Resting electrocardiogram shows sinus rhythm. Conduction disturbances, junctional rhythms, or atrial arrhythmias would be causes for limitation of athletic activity.
- Normal or nearly normal RV function and size by angiography, nuclear studies, or echocardiogram.
- No supraventricular tachycardia or severe sinus bradycardia is found on 24-hour electrocardiographic monitoring.
- No ventricular or supraventricular dysrhythmias occur during exercise and no bradycardia occurs after exercise.

Periodic reevaluations at yearly intervals are recommended as arrhythmias may develop late.

As mentioned, follow-up for the arterial switch operation for TGA is limited at this time. However, it appears that rhythm disturbances are not a problem. The main focus is on the coronary artery anastomoses and whether these anastomotic sites, made in the immediate newborn period, will be compromised with growth. Obviously, repetitive exercise testing to detect coronary insufficiency will be exceedingly important in this group prior to sport participation.

Tricuspid Valve Atresia

Pathophysiology and Surgical Approach

With tricuspid valve atresia, not only is the tricuspid valve absent but also the inflow portion of the right ventricle. Most children with this defect have a hypoplastic right ventricle which receives blood only from a VSD. The pulmonary valve and main pulmonary artery may also be hypoplastic. The only outlet from the right atrium is via the foramen ovale to the left atrium. These children present cyanotic as newborns and do not survive without intervention.

The right ventricle cannot be used to sustain pulmonary blood flow, and the surgical approach is to bypass the right ventricle by connecting the right atrium directly to the pulmonary artery and closing the foramen ovale (Fontan operation). Systemic venous blood drains via the superior vena cava and inferior vena cava to the right atrium, which then drains directly to the pulmonary arteries. There is no muscular pumping chamber and blood flows to the pulmonary arteries mainly by gravity and the pumping action of peripheral skeletal muscles. The left ventricle is usually normal or slightly dilated, and the pulmonary venous return to the left atrium is pumped normally to the body. Since all of the systemic venous blood returns to the pulmonary arteries after the Fontan operation, the children are no longer cyanotic and should have normal resting oxygen saturations.

Long-term complications in postoperative Fontan patients include supraventricular tachyarrhythmias, junctional rhythm, heart block, exercise limitation, elevated central venous (right atrial) pressures with resultant hepatic congestion or protein-losing enteropathy, and sudden death. However, long-term survival is expected, and 5-year survival was greater than 70% in early studies (6) and more optimistic in more recent reports (30).

Response to Exercise and Exercise Recommendations

As would be predicted in children with an inadequate systemic venous pumping chamber, the majority of postoperative Fontan patients have significant exercise limitations (1). These include decreased duration of exercise (in the range of 60% of normal) and decreased maximal O_2 consumption (in the range of 50% of normal) (10). They have been found to have blunted maximal heart rates (8) and diminished increases in stroke volume (4, 9). Driscoll et al. (10) showed these patients to have low resting cardiac outputs and inadequate increases in cardiac output with exercise. In addition, this study also demonstrated a 38% incidence of dysrhythmias during or immediately following exercise. This included both atrial and ventricular dysrhythmias.

For these reasons, sport participation is necessarily limited but not completely discouraged. A complete evaluation is mandatory before recommendations regarding sport participation and activity can be made. This should include electrocardiogram, chest X ray, 24-hour ambulatory electrocardiographic monitoring, echocardiogram with assessment of left ventricular function, and maximal exercise stress testing.

Specific Recommendations

Patients who have undergone the Fontan operation and who have normal left ventricular function and no dysrhythmias should be permitted to participate in low-intensity sports. Selected children may be permitted to participate in sports with moderate static and dynamic demands provided that there is (34)

- Nearly normal duration of exercise using a standard protocol.
- No dysrhythmias at rest or during exercise.
- No supraventricular tachycardia, significant sinus bradycardia, or significant ventricular dysrhythmias on 24-hour electrographic monitoring.
- No signs of peripheral venous congestion.
- No severe O_2 desaturation (<80%) with maximal exercise.
- Normal left ventricular function.

Obviously, at least yearly evaluations by the attending cardiologist are indicated, and any changes in exercise recommendations must be made in consultation with parents, patients, cardiologist, and the people responsible during the activity.

REFERENCES

1. Alpert, B.S. Exercise testing in tricuspid atresia. In: Rao, P. S., ed. Tricuspid atresia. 2d ed. Mount Kisco, NY: Futura Publishing, Inc.; 1992.
2. Arensman, F.W.; Sievers, H.H.; Lange, P.; Radley-Smith, R.; Bernhard, A.; Heintzen, P.; Yacoub, M.H. Assessment of coronary and aortic anastomoses after anatomic correction of transposition of the great arteries. J. Thorac. Cardiovasc. Surg. 90:597-604; 1985.
3. Bay, G.; Abrahamsen, A. M.; Müller, C. Left-to-right shunt in atrial septal defect at rest and during exercise. Acta Med. Scand. 190:205-209; 1971.
4. Ben Shachar, G.B.; Fuhrman, B.P.; Wang, Y.; Lucas, R.V.; Lock, J.E. Rest and exercise hemodynamics after the Fontan procedure. Circulation 65:1043-1048; 1982.
5. Bink-Boelkens, M.T.; Velvis, H.; van der Heide, J.J.; Eygelaar, A.; Hardjowijono, R.A. Dysrhythmias after surgery in children. Am. Heart J. 106:125-129; 1983.
6. Cleveland, D.C.; Kirklin, J.K.; Naftel, D.C.; Kirklin, J.W.; Blackstone, E.H.; Pacifico, A.D.; Bargeron, L.M. Surgical treatment of tricuspid atresia. Ann. Thorac. Surg. 38:447-457; 1984.
7. Cordell, D.; Graham, T.P.; Atwood, G.F.; Boerth, R.C.; Boucek, R.; Bender, H.W. Left heart volume characteristics following ventricular septal defect closure in infancy. Circulation 54:294-298; 1976.
8. Cumming, G.R. Maximal exercise capacity of children with heart defects. Am. J. Cardiol. 41:613-619; 1978.
9. DelTorso, S.; Kelly, M.J.; Kalff, V.; Venables, A.W. Radionuclide assessment of ventricular contraction at rest and during exercise following the Fontan procedure for either tricuspid atresia or single ventricle. Am. J. Cardiol. 55:1127-1132; 1985.
10. Driscoll, D.J.; Danielson, G.K.; Puga, F.J.; Schaff, H.V.; Heise, C.T.; Staats, B.A. Exercise tolerance and cardiorespiratory response to exercise after the Fontan operation for tricuspid atresia or functional single ventricle. J. Am. Coll. Cardiol. 7:1087-1094; 1986.
11. Driscoll, D.J.; Wolfe, R.R.; Gersony, W.M.; Hayes, C.J.; Keane, J.F.; Kidd, L.; O'Fallon, W.M.; Pieroni, D.R.; Weidman, W.H. Cardiorespiratory responses to exercise of patients with aortic stenosis, pulmonary stenosis, and ventricular septal defect. Circulation (Suppl I) 87:102-113; 1993.
12. Epstein, S.E.; Beiser, G.D.; Goldstein, R.E.; Rosing, D.R.; Redwood, D.R.; Morrow, A.G. Hemodynamic abnormalities in response to mild and intense upright exercise following operative correction of an atrial septal defect or tetralogy of Fallot. Circulation 47:1065-1075; 1973.
13. Garson, A.; Gillette, P.C.; Gutgesell, H.P.; McNamara, D.G. Stress-induced ventricular arrhythmia after repair of tetralogy of Fallot. Am. J. Cardiol. 46:1006-1012; 1980.
14. Garson, A.; Randall, D.C.; Gillette, P.C.; Smith, R.T.; Moak, J.P.; McVey, P.; McNamara, D.G. Prevention of sudden death after repair of tetralogy of Fallot: treatment of ventricular arrhythmias. J. Am. Coll. Cardiol. 6:221-227; 1985.
15. Gillette, P.C.; Yeoman, M.A.; Mullins, C.E.; McNamara, D.G. Sudden death after repair of tetralogy of Fallot. Circulation 56:566-571; 1977.
16. Godfrey, S. Exercise testing in children. Philadelphia, PA: W. B. Saunders Co.; 1974.
17. Goldberg, B.; Fripp, R.R.; Lister, G.; Loke, J.; Nicholas, J.A.; Talner, N.S. Effect of physical training on exercise performance of children following surgical repair of congenital heart disease. Pediatrics 68:691-699; 1981.
18. Goldberg, S.J.; Mendes, F.; Hurwitz, R. Maximal exercise capability of children as a function of specific cardiac defects. Am. J. Cardiol. 23:349-353; 1969.
19. Graham, T.P. Ventricular performance in adults after operation for congenital heart disease. Am. J. Cardiol. 50:612-620; 1982.
20. Hesslein, P.S.; Gutgesell, H.P.; Gillette, P.C.; McNamara, D.G. Exercise assessment of sinoatrial node function following Mustard operation. Am. Heart J. 103:351-357; 1982.
21. Hugenholtz, P.G.; Nadas, A.S. Exercise studies in patients with congenital heart disease. Pediatrics 32:769-775; 1963.
22. Hurwitz, F.A.; Goldberg, S.J. Maximal cardiac rate before and following repair of cardiac lesions. J. Sports. Med. 10:165-168; 1970.

23. James, F.W.; Kaplan, S.; Chou, T. Unexpected cardiac arrest in patients after surgical correction of tetralogy of Fallot. Circulation 52:691-695; 1975.

24. James, F.W.; Kaplan, S.; Schwartz, D.C.; Chou, T.C.; Sandker, E.T.; Naylor, V. Response to exercise in patients after total surgical correction of tetralogy of Fallot. Circulation 54:671-679; 1976.

25. Jatene, A.D.; Fontes, B.F.I.; Souza, L.C.B.; Paulista, P.P.; Abdulmassih Neto, C.; Sousa, J.E.M.R. Anatomic correction of transposition of the great arteries. J. Thorac. Cardiovasc. Surg. 83:20-26; 1982.

26. Katz, N.M.; Blackstone, E.H.; Kirklin, J.W.; Pacifico, A.D.; Bargeron, L.M. Late survival and symptoms after repair of tetralogy of Fallot. Circulation 65:403-410; 1982.

27. Kidd, L.; Driscoll, D.J.; Gersony, W.M.; Hayes, G.J.; Keane, J.F.; O'Fallon, W.M.; Pieroni, D.R.; Wolfe, R.R.; Weidman, W.H. Second natural history study of congenital heart defects. Results of treatment of patients with ventricular septal defects. Circulation 87(Suppl I): 38-51; 1993.

28. Kirklin, J.W.; Blackstone, E.H.; Kirklin, J.K.; Pacifico, A.D.; Aramendi, J.; Bargeron, L.M. Surgical results and protocols in the spectrum of tetralogy of Fallot. Ann. Surg. 198:251-265; 1983.

29. Leachman, R.D.; Cokkinos, D.W.; Cooley, D.A. Association of ostium secundum atrial septal defects in mitral valve prolapse. Am. J. Cardiol. 38:167-199; 1976.

30. Lee, C.N.; Schaff, H.V.; Danielson, G.K.; Puga, F.J.; Driscoll, D.J. Comparison of atriopulmonary versus atrioventricular connections for modified Fontan/Kreutzer repair of tricuspid valve atresia. J. Thorac. Cardiovasc. Surg. 92:1038-1043; 1986.

31. Lock, J.E.; Rome, J.J.; Davis, R.; VanPraagh, S.; Perry, S.B.; VanPraagh, R.; Keane, J.F. Transcatheter closure of atrial septal defects: experimental studies. Circulation 79:1091-1099; 1980.

32. Maron, B.J.; Redwood, D.R.; Hirshfeld, J.W.; Goldstein, R.E.; Morrow, A.G.; Epstein, S.E. Postoperative assessment of patients with ventricular septal defect and pulmonary hypertension. Response to intense upright exercise. Circulation 48:864-874; 1973.

33. Mathews, R.A.; Fricker, F.J.; Beerman, L.B.; Stephenson, R.J.; Fischer, D.R.; Neches, W.H.; Park, S.C.; Lenox, C.C.; Zuberbuhler, J.R. Exercise studies after the Mustard operation in transposition of the great arteries. Am. J. Cardiol. 51:1526-1529; 1983.

34. McNamara, D.G.; Bricker, J.T.; Galioto, F.M.; Graham, T.P.; James, F.W.; Rosenthal, A. Task Force I: Congenital heart disease. JACC 6:1200-1208; 1985.

35. Mocellin, R.; Bastanier, C.; Hofacker, W.; Bühlmeyer, K. Exercise performance in children and adolescents after surgical repair of tetralogy of Fallot. Eur. J. Cardiol. 4:367-374; 1976.

36. Otterstad, J.E.; Simmonsen, S.; Erikssen, J. Hemodynamic findings at rest and during mild supine exercise in adults with isolated, uncomplicated ventricular septal defects. Circ. 71:650-662; 1985.

37. Paul, M.H. Complete transposition of the great arteries. In: Adams, F.H.; Emmanouilides, G.C.; Riemenschneider, T.A., eds. Moss Heart disease in infants, children, and adolescents. 4th ed. Baltimore, MD: Williams and Wilkins; 1989.

38. Paul, M.H.; Wessel, H.O.; Muster, A.J.; Idriss, F.S. Exercise and ventricular function studies in transposition of the great artery patients 10 years after atrial (Mustard) repair. Am. J. Cardiol. 60:637 (Abstr); 1987.

39. Perrault, H.; Drblik, S.P.; Montigny, M.; Darignon, A.; Lamarre, A.; Chartrand, C.; Stanley, P. Comparison of cardiovascular adjustments to exercise in adolescents 8 to 15 years of age after correction of tetralogy of Fallot, ventricular septal defect, or atrial septal defect. Am. J. Cardiol. 64:213-217; 1980.

40. Petersson, P.O. Atrial septal defect of secundum type. A clinical study before and after operation with special reference to hemodynamic function. Acta Paediatrica Scandinavica 174 (Suppl): 71-85; 1967.

41. Reybrouck, T.; Weymans, M.; Stijns, H.; van der Haywaert, L.G. Ventilatory anaerobic threshold for evaluating exercise performance in children with congenital left-to-right intracardiac shunt. Pediatr. Cardiol. 7:19-24; 1986.

42. Rowe, S.A.; Zahka, K.G.; Manolio, T.A.; Horneffer, P.J.; Kidd, L. Lung function and pulmonary regurgitation limit exercise capacity in postoperative tetralogy of Fallot. J. Am. Coll. Cardiol. 17:461-466; 1991.

43. Vetter, V.L.; Horowitz, L.N. Electrophysiologic residua and sequelae of surgery for congenital heart defects. Am. J. Cardiol. 50:588-604; 1982.

44. Webb Kavey, R.E.; Blackman, M.S.; Sondheimer, H.M. Incidence and severity of chronic ventricular dysrhythmias after repair of tetralogy of Fallot. Am. Heart J. 103:342-350; 1982.

45. Wessel, H.V.; Cunningham, W.J.; Paul, M.H.; Bastanier, C.K.; Muster, A.J.; Idriss, F.S. Exercise performance in tetralogy of Fallot after intracardiac repair. J. Thorac. Cardiovasc. Surg. 80:582-693; 1980.

CHAPTER 15

Congenital Obstructive and Valvular Heart Disease

Thomas W. Rowland
Baystate Medical Center, Springfield, MA

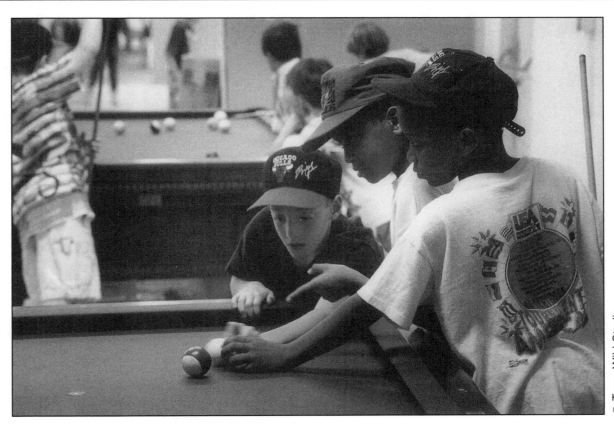

Misadventures in normal cardiac embryogenesis which result in obstruction to blood flow and valvular dysfunction are commonly encountered by the pediatric cardiologist. Aortic valve stenosis, pulmonary valve stenosis, and coarctation of the aorta consistently rank among the top 10 most common forms of congenital heart disease, and are typically identified early in life by primary health care providers from their characteristic physical findings. Mitral valve prolapse, a lesion not uncommonly observed in young adult females, becomes increasingly apparent in the teenage population. These abnormalities are highlighted in this chapter because of particular concern over risks that may be assumed by these patients from participation in sport activities.

Many forms of athletic competition draw on maximal cardiac reserve; indeed, the desire of the athlete, coach, parents, and fans is often for that "supramaximal" effort that is the hallmark of the superb sport competitor. Whether this type of physiological intensity is safe in the child or adolescent with a cardiac anomaly which restricts blood flow or predisposes to dysrhythmias is an important question which deserves careful consideration. Concern that such abnormalities may 1) create a risk for sudden death during sports play, or 2) be adversely affected by high cardiac demands from athletic competition and training need to be balanced by the positive physical and emotional benefits that these youngsters can gain from sport participation.

As usual, a paucity of scientific data exists upon which well-informed exercise guidelines can be created for these conditions. This chapter will present that information which is available regarding risks of intensive exercise in athletes with congenital valvular and obstructive cardiac anomalies, and endeavor to present acceptable safe guidelines for sport participation.

AORTIC VALVE STENOSIS

Congenital stenosis of the aortic valve results from varying amounts of fusion of the valve commissures, which limits leaflet mobility and diminishes the size of the valve orifice. The effect is a narrowing which restricts left ventricular outflow, placing demands on the left ventricle in direct proportion to the degree of stenosis.

Since adequate cardiac output is obligatory, the left ventricular myocardium must generate a higher pressure to eject blood past the stenotic valve. This "pressure work" is accomplished through the adaptive response of ventricular hypertrophy.

The difference between the systolic pressure within the left ventricle and that in the ascending aorta (the left ventricular outflow tract gradient) in patients with aortic valve stenosis serves as a numerical indicator of the severity of the valve obstruction. In the child with a normal heart, little or no gradient exists; in patients with a normal cardiac output and a gradient of over 70 mmHg, valvular aortic stenosis is considered severe, and surgical or balloon valvuloplasty is generally indicated. Such intervention is also often instituted in those with at least a 50 mmHg gradient who have either symptoms (angina, syncope) or electrocardiographic ischemic changes (ST depression). Patients with gradients of less than 50 mmHg typically have normal electrocardiograms, experience no symptoms, and require no intervention.

The long-term natural course of valvular aortic stenosis characteristically consists of slowly progressive valve thickening and narrowing, with increasing left ventricular outflow tract gradient, left ventricular hypertrophy, and, often, valvular insufficiency. Except in small infants with critical levels of obstruction, however, the left ventricle is capable of adapting to even severe degrees of aortic stenosis during the childhood and adolescent years without evidence of significant myocardial dysfunction. Such compensation has its limits, however, and untreated severe aortic stenosis may result in congestive left ventricular failure in the adult years.

While the child with aortic stenosis is spared the risk of congestive heart failure, severe valve narrowing is associated with a small chance of sudden death (probably no greater than 1-3% of all patients with this anomaly) (21). The risk of endocarditis is also small, but this complication is particularly devastating for patients with aortic valve disease, since infection may lead to serious acute worsening in valve function.

Clinical Evaluation

Valvular aortic stenosis is usually readily identified by its typical physical findings. The patient is well-nourished and shows no signs of tachypnea or cyanosis. A left ventricular lift may be present, but in the absence of aortic valve incompetence, the apical impulse is not displaced to the left. A systolic thrill is noted over the carotid arteries and in the suprasternal notch in all patients with more than very mild degrees of obstruction, and those with significant stenosis demonstrate a thrill at the right upper sternal border as well. A constant early systolic ejection click is evident, usually heard best at the apex. A harsh systolic ejection murmur is most audible at the right upper sternal border with radiation into the neck, and an associated diastolic decrescendo blowing murmur of aortic valve insufficiency is often heard along the middle left sternal border. Unless the obstruction is severe, the peripheral pulses are usually normal.

While the identification of patients with aortic valve stenosis is not usually difficult, the quantification of the severity of the obstruction by clinical examination can be more problematic. While patients who have no or little thrill with a grade 2/6 murmur can be presumed to have small left ventricular outflow gradients, estimates of severity in those with more dramatic findings can be fraught with error. Electrocardiographic changes of left ventricular hypertrophy and/or ischemic ST depression over the left precordial leads are generally confined to those patients who have severe valve stenosis, but the absence of such changes provides no comfort that a serious degree of obstruction does not exist.

Since the only definitive means of determining the left ventricular outflow gradient in a patient with aortic stenosis is by cardiac catheterization, the search for a noninvasive means of accurately identifying those with significant obstruction has long occupied pediatric cardiologists. The list of once-promising but ultimately discarded tools has included vectorcardiography, systolic time intervals, phonocardiography, pulse wave analysis, and M-mode electrocardiography. Currently, Doppler echocardiographic estimates of left ventricular outflow gradients by measurement of velocity of blood across the stenotic aortic valve have shown good correlation with those determined at the time of cardiac catheterization. This technique has proved a reliable means of identifying patients with significant valve obstruction. A normal exercise test (showing no ischemic changes with a normal blood pressure response) is also helpful in identifying those with serious outflow obstruction (1, 4).

Treatment

Surgical valvotomy for relief of aortic valvar obstruction has been effective in significantly reducing left ventricular outflow gradients with low mortality rates. Surgery for aortic valve stenosis must be considered palliative, however, since recurrence of obstruction, often with valvular insufficiency, is common and often leads ultimately to prosthetic valve replacement.

In recent years, percutaneous balloon aortic valvuloplasty has become the initial approach to relieving valvular aortic stenosis in many centers. Early results indicate that balloon dilation of the stenotic valve is at least as effective in decreasing obstruction as surgery, with a similar degree of resulting aortic valve incompetence (19). This technique, likewise, is palliative, and close long-term follow-up of these patients is important after either balloon catheter or surgical approach.

Exercise and Aortic Stenosis

The basic anatomic problem confronting the patient with aortic valve stenosis is a fixed obstruction to left ventricular outflow. As a consequence, adequate cardiac output is contingent on an elevation of left ventricular systolic pressure, which is generated by the development of left ventricular hypertrophy. The physiological stresses placed on the left ventricular myocardium from these events are magnified during exercise.

Normal Responses to Exercise

When an individual with a normal heart undergoes dynamic exercise, as during a progressive treadmill stress test, left ventricular and aortic systolic pressure rise (without a significant valve gradient), while diastolic pressure remains the same or falls slightly. Maximal systolic pressure at exhaustion is approximately 35-60% greater than that at rest.

The increased oxygen demands of exercising muscle are met through an augmentation in cardiac output, which rises at maximal dynamic exercise to levels 3-5 times that at rest. Most of that increase is met by a nearly threefold rise in heart rate, while stroke volume increases about 40%. During the tachycardia of exercise, the duration of ventricular systole and diastole are not only shortened, but the relationship between the two also changes. At rest, diastole is 1.5 to 2 times longer than systole. Studies in exercising adults indicate that when heart rate rises from 66 to 158 bpm, the duration of diastole is shortened from 550 to 161 milliseconds (70% fall), while systole decreases from 356 to 219 milliseconds (a 38% decline). At moderate levels of exercise, then, the duration of ventricular diastole becomes considerably shorter than that of systole (11).

The energy demand of the left ventricular myocardium (determined as the myocardial oxygen uptake) is dictated by the left ventricular pressure, heart rate, and contractile state, all of which rise with progressive dynamic exercise. The increase in myocardial oxygen uptake during exercise is achieved through dilation and increased perfusion of the coronary arteries. Because ventricular contraction mechanically interferes with coronary perfusion, the volume of coronary flow is about 2.5 times greater in diastole than in systole (2). The subendocardial region of the ventricle is most susceptible to limitations of coronary flow, since the intramyocardial compressive forces are greatest in this area.

Resistance exercise such as weightlifting triggers a different cardiovascular response from dynamic exercise such as running or cycling. Resistance exercise is characterized by significant increases in both systolic and diastolic pressures with only small increases in heart rate and cardiac output. While blood pressure levels as high as 480/350 mmHg with maximal lifts have been described in adult weightlifters, values of 180/140 are more typical in children (16). These forms of activity pose a transient but significant afterload stress on myocardial function.

Responses to Exercise With Aortic Stenosis

Physiological responses to dynamic exercise in patients with aortic valve stenosis usually differ little from normal until outflow tract gradients of at least 40 mmHg are reached. Those with more severe obstruction may demonstrate a blunted stroke volume response to exercise, as

well as diminished rise in blood pressure. The increase in left ventricular pressure are exaggerated, and the left ventricle-aorta pressure gradient is increased (6). Cueto and Moller (5) demonstrated that moderate exercise in children with aortic stenosis elevated the left ventricular outflow tract gradient in approximate relationship to the increase in cardiac output. These observations presumably reflect the impact of a fixed outlet obstruction upon demands for increasing cardiac output during exercise.

Exercise in children with significant aortic stenosis may seriously strain the relationship between the demand for myocardial perfusion and the supply of coronary blood flow. The exaggerated rise in left ventricular pressure and increased ventricular muscle mass combine to escalate myocardial oxygen uptake, which is further increased by the fast heart rate and augmented contractility during exercise. At the same time, shrinking of diastolic coronary flow time to one-fourth of resting values may seriously impair ventricular perfusion, particularly to the subendocardial layers (13). The resulting perfusion supply/demand mismatch may predispose to ischemia and ventricular dysrhythmias.

Clinical Expressions of Aortic Valve Obstruction

Symptoms and laboratory findings in patients with significant aortic valve stenosis are clinical expressions of the physiological difficulties posed by the fixed left ventricular outflow already outlined. In many cases, as would be expected, these difficulties are initiated or exacerbated during exercise.

Decreased exercise tolerance is typically observed in patients with high outflow tract gradients, presumably reflecting limitations in the cardiac output that can be generated through an obstructed valve orifice (5, 6). Exercise studies in children with aortic stenosis have usually involved only moderate-intensity exercise, but these have failed to reveal any evidence of myocardial dysfunction to account for impaired limits to cardiac output. Diminished peripheral skeletal muscle aerobic function from limitation of physical activity in these subjects may contribute to exercise intolerance.

Syncope in patients with severe aortic valve stenosis may result from several mechanisms.

Carotid sinus reflex hyperreactivity, dysrhythmias, acute left ventricular failure, and left ventricular baroreceptor activation have all been suggested as contributory. Monitoring of exercising adult subjects with aortic stenosis during near-syncopal episodes has revealed marked drops in systemic and pulmonary artery pressure without abnormal heart rhythms, suggesting stimulation of left ventricular baroreceptors from the sudden rise in intracavitary pressure during exercise as the most likely etiology (18).

Life-threatening dysrhythmias have also been observed in adult patients with aortic valve stenosis during syncopal episodes (20). It is therefore not clear whether the mechanisms for syncope with aortic stenosis are identical to those which cause myocardial ischemia and sudden death.

Angina pectoris is also observed only in patients with serious valve obstruction. Chest pain with exercise reflects myocardial ischemia from imbalance of myocardial perfusion supply and demand, and typically indicates an outflow gradient of over 50 mmHg. Symptoms are often accompanied by ischemic changes on the electrocardiogram (ST depression over the left precordial leads) during exercise testing.

It should be noted that while symptoms of angina, ease of fatigue with exercise, dizziness, and overt syncope are confined to patients with significant aortic valve gradients, the converse is not true. Many children with serious degrees of left ventricular outflow obstruction remain symptom-free, yet may be at increased risk for sudden death during sport participation.

Sudden Death With Aortic Stenosis

It has long been recognized that aortic valve stenosis poses a risk for sudden unexpected death in children as well as adults. While initially risks of this catastrophe were felt to be as high as 7% of all children with aortic valve obstruction, more recent studies indicate an incidence of about 1% during the childhood years.

The etiology for sudden death with aortic valve stenosis is unclear. As many of the features of severe valve stenosis mimic those of adults with coronary artery disease (including angina and ischemic EKG changes), a model of relative coronary insufficiency with ischemia and terminal dysrhythmia has been most frequently assumed (Figure 15.1). The causes of coronary perfusion supply/demand imbalance with aortic stenosis have been outlined above. The role of left ventricular baroreceptors causing hypotension and syncope in these patients as an alternative mechanism for sudden death is uncertain.

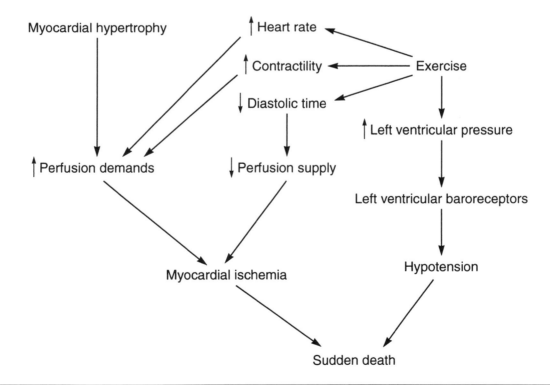

Figure 15.1   Possible mechanisms for sudden death with intensive physical activity with aortic valve stenosis.

In most cases sudden death in young patients with aortic stenosis has not been associated with sport participation. In their review of such cases, Doyle, Arumugham, Lara, Rutkowski, and Kiely (7) noted that among 19 patients, 8 died during vigorous physical activity (football, swimming), 6 during mild exertion (walking home from school), and 5 at rest (sleeping, watching television). It seems apparent, though, that a disproportionate number of these deaths do occur during intense physical activity.

Doyle et al. (7) and Glew, Varghese, Krovetz, Dorst, and Rowe (8) have analyzed reported cases of sudden death in children with aortic stenosis in an attempt to identify premonitory features. Many of these cases lack full clinical information, but based on the available data, certain patterns emerge. Of the 64 cases reviewed by Doyle et al., resting electrocardiograms were available on 35. Ischemic left ventricular changes were observed in 24 (70%); 8 (21%) had left ventricular hypertrophy or conduction delay; and 3 (9%) were normal. Twenty-eight of 31 reported symptoms of angina, syncope, or dyspnea. Outflow gradients at cardiac catheterization were seldom available in these reports, but values over 60 were measured in all known cases.

Wagner, Ellison, Keane, Humphries, and Nadas (22) described the course of 294 children and adolescents followed with aortic valve stenosis over an 8-year period. Three sudden unexpected deaths were observed: a 9-year-old with a 55-mm gradient and left ventricular ischemic changes on the electrocardiogram; a 15-year-old with a 46-mm gradient and ischemic EKG changes; and a 16-year-old with a 68-mm gradient and normal EKG. Reid, Coleman, and Stevenson (17) described 8- and 15-year old boys with aortic stenosis who died suddenly during sport (football, swimming) without prior symptoms. Their electrocardiograms showed left ventricular hypertrophy but no ischemic changes. Outflow gradients were unknown.

Based on these data, it can be concluded that sudden unexpected death is extremely unlikely in children and adolescents with aortic valve stenosis who have all three of the following conditions:

- a left ventricular outflow gradient less than 40-50 mmHg,
- normal resting electrocardiogram, and
- absence of symptoms (angina, dizziness, syncope, exercise fatigue).

Exercise Recommendations for Patients With Aortic Valve Stenosis

As noted previously, myocardial dysfunction is not a typical feature of children and adolescents with aortic valve stenosis. Similarly, there is no information to suggest that early intensive athletic training and competition in these patients impairs heart muscle function or hastens the progression to a congestive picture in adult years.

Significant valve obstruction does, however, impose a small but distinct risk of sudden unexpected death, and these tragedies appear to be more commonly associated with vigorous physical activity. For this reason, restrictions from sport participation have traditionally been placed on children and adolescents with particular degrees of valve stenosis and clinical characteristics. The rarity of episodes of sudden death and the paucity of predictive clinical markers has led to a good deal of subjectivity in creating such recommendations. Moreover, most cases of sudden death from aortic stenosis do not occur with sport participation, and there is no evidence that restriction from athletics is truly effective in avoiding these events.

Any possible preventive value of exercise restriction in these patients needs to be weighed against potential benefits that might be gained from sport participation, both at competitive and recreational levels. No specific cardiovascular benefit from physical activity has been recognized in youngsters with aortic stenosis; still, unnecessary limitation of exercise in these patients may rob them of the emotional, social, and physical gains that can be expected from involvement in sport activities. How these benefits may be particularly helpful to those with chronic illness has been outlined elsewhere in this book.

Every patient with aortic valve stenosis requires careful assessment by a pediatric cardiologist before sport participation. The decision regarding clearance for athletics needs to be individualized for each youngster and is contingent upon a knowledge of the patient's degree and progression of obstruction, symptoms, and findings on laboratory evaluation. The latter generally includes echocardiography (or cardiac catheterization), electrocardiogram, and exercise stress testing.

Guidelines have been proposed to assist physicians in the decision regarding athletic participation in children and adolescents with aortic stenosis. A consensus conference sponsored by the American College of Cardiology in 1984 (14) recommended that for patients with unoperated aortic stenosis, participation in all forms of competitive athletics was allowed if

- the resting valvar outflow gradient was <20 mmHg,
- the resting electrocardiogram was normal,
- an exercise stress test was unremarkable (no dysrhythmia or ischemic EKG changes; normal blood pressure response),
- there was no cardiomegaly,
- an echocardiogram, angiogram, or nuclear study revealed no left ventricular dysfunction, and
- the patient had no evidence of dysrhythmia.

These recommendations included the prohibition of all competitive sports for patients with a resting gradient >40 mmHg. For those with a gradient between 20 and 40 mmHg (and fulfilling the other criteria above), low-intensity sports (such as bowling and golf) were permitted, and in selected cases patients could also participate in sports defined as those with high to moderate static and low dynamic demands (gymnastics, judo). According to these recommendations, then, competitive activities such as cycling, football, hockey, wrestling, soccer, baseball, basketball, distance running, tennis, and swimming would not be allowed for patients with a gradient between 20 and 40 mmHg (and no other indicators of complications).

Such guidelines are highly conservative; it is difficult to conclude that strict adherence to these recommendations would place any patient with aortic stenosis at risk from sport participation. On the other hand, they also disallow patients with a mild to moderate gradient (20-40 mmHg) and no complicating factors (even at maximal exercise) the benefits from participating in the major forms of interscholastic sport. As the data reviewed above suggest that risk of sudden death for this group is extremely low, physicians may wish to allow patients in this category full athletic participation as well.

The consensus guidelines were created in reference to participation in organized competitive sport teams, considering the high intensity associated with such training and competition. Similar guidelines for participation in recreational sports (sandlot games and intramural sports) and physical education classes have not been formulated. A conservative approach might be employed using the consensus guidelines for these types of activities. Alternatively, it might be assumed that since these forms of activity rarely demand the physical intensity of interscholastic competition, limitations on certain patients with aortic stenosis might be liberalized. This author usually permits recreational sport in those with a moderate gradient (40-50 mmHg) if the patient has no symptoms, has a normal exercise stress test, and is free of ischemic ST changes on the resting electrocardiogram. However, exhaustive exercise (e.g., mile-run testing in physical education classes) is prohibited.

Summary

Vigorous physical activity poses a small but definite risk for sudden death in patients with moderate to severe aortic stenosis because of myocardial perfusion supply/demand mismatch. Symptoms of significant left ventricular outflow obstruction such as angina, dizziness, and shortness of breath with exercise therefore deserve particular attention. Identification of such patients through clinical evaluation should lead to their exclusion from participation in competitive sport.

Patients with aortic stenosis who have at least a moderate degree of obstruction (over 40-50 mmHg gradient) should be prohibited from all forms of organized competitive athletics and should be cautioned regarding participation in vigorous recreational sports that lead to physical exhaustion. Those with lesser gradients who are asymptomatic and have a normal electrocardiogram, exercise stress test, and ventricular function on echocardiogram, without cardiomegaly or dysrhythmia, can be considered for all forms of competitive athletics. Patients with aortic stenosis require regular follow-up assessment, since obstruction tends to progress slowly with time and may lead to changes in recommendations for sport participation.

PULMONARY VALVE STENOSIS

Pulmonary valve stenosis shares many of the anatomic, physiological, and clinical features of its aortic counterpart. However, differences in hemodynamic effect and natural history alter the risks associated with obstruction of outflow to the pulmonary circulation. These aspects may influence recommendations for athletic participation.

Like aortic stenosis, pulmonary valve stenosis is always congenital in children and usually results from fusion of the valve commissures. The resulting pressure overload on the right ventricle is dealt with by myocardial hypertrophy and generation of augmented right ventricular systolic pressure. This adaptation is sufficient to maintain normal cardiac output—at least at rest—throughout the growing years, even in the face of marked degrees of outflow obstruction, but congestive heart failure from myocardial dysfunction may eventually appear in the adult years in untreated cases.

Contrary to aortic stenosis, however, the severity of pulmonary valve stenosis is rarely progressive, and restenosis is highly unlikely after surgical or balloon valvuloplasty relief of obstruction. The effectiveness and safety of pulmonary balloon valvuloplasty has led to routine intervention in patients with even moderate gradients (40-60 mmHg).

Sudden unexpected death has not been recognized as a feature of patients with pulmonary valve stenosis. Typical symptoms of dyspnea and fatigue with exertion are limited to those with severe obstruction, and presumably reflect an impaired rise in stroke volume across the fixed right ventricular outflow obstruction during vigorous activity (9).

Clinical Evaluation

Findings of pulmonary valve stenosis, even when severe, generally occur in a well-appearing patient who has no evidence of undernutrition, tachypnea, or cyanosis. A right ventricular lift and systolic thrill are palpable at the upper left sternal border. In that area a variable early systolic click precedes a harsh systolic ejection murmur. No diastolic murmur is usually heard. The second sound splits widely but moves appropriately with respirations, and

the pulmonary valve closure (P2) is soft. The electrocardiogram displays right axis deviation and right ventricular hypertrophy. On the chest X ray the heart is of normal size, and the only finding may be prominence (post-stenotic dilation) of the main pulmonary artery.

As opposed to aortic stenosis, the clinical findings in patients with pulmonary obstruction typically provide a good guide to the severity of stenosis. The degree of lift and thrill, softness of P2, length and loudness of the systolic murmur, and electrocardiographic changes all vary directly with the right ventricular outflow gradient. Doppler echocardiography also provides an accurate means of estimating the degree of obstruction.

Exercise Recommendations for Patients With Pulmonary Valve Stenosis

Strenuous exercise will increase right ventricular pressure and diminish cardiac output reserve in patients with serious pulmonary valve stenosis, but these effects are not known to 1) pose a risk for sudden death, or 2) promote progressive right ventricular myocardial dysfunction. Limitations to sports participation in these patients are therefore related not to identifiable risks but rather to impairment of performance.

The consensus conference (15) recommended that patients with pulmonary stenosis be permitted to participate in all sports if the outflow gradient was less than 50 mmHg and right ventricular function was normal. This author suggests that a normal exercise stress test be included in these criteria as a means of assuring that 1) the patient has appropriate fitness for the desired sport, and 2) no dysrhythmias occur with intense exercise.

Patients with a gradient of over 50 mmHg are usually candidates for relief of their obstruction by balloon valvuloplasty or surgery. Athletic participation may be allowed if appropriate reduction of gradient and normal right ventricular function can be demonstrated 6 months later.

Summary

Vigorous exercise in patients with moderate to severe pulmonary stenosis may markedly increase right ventricular pressure and limit exercise capacity. Surgical or balloon valvuloplasty relief of valvar obstruction is recommended before approval for participation in any organized competitive sport team if the gradient exceeds 50 mmHg at rest. Asymptomatic patients with lesser gradients may be permitted participation in all sports if right ventricular function is normal and no dysrhythmias are observed on exercise stress testing.

MITRAL VALVE PROLAPSE

Mitral valve prolapse is a generally benign condition, not uncommonly detected among young adult females. However, the recognized association of mitral valve prolapse with both atrial and ventricular dysrhythmias, as well as with rare cases of sudden death, has led to a consideration of risks that might be imposed by sport participation in these patients. Among young athletes with prolapse, factors which might identify a patient as being at risk are very unusual, and full participation in sport is almost always permissible.

Clinical Features

Mitral valve prolapse is a bowing of one or both mitral leaflets backward toward the left atrium during ventricular systole. This movement typically creates a mid-systolic click heard best at the cardiac apex, and if prolapse is sufficiently pronounced, the leaflets become unopposed and a late systolic murmur of mitral insufficiency is audible in the same area.

Mitral prolapse is unusual in small children but the frequency in the young adult female population may be as high as 6%. Among any large group of high school athletes, then, the finding of an apical midsystolic click of mitral valve prolapse is not unexpected, particularly in girls. Prolapse has been reported to be more common with idiopathic scoliosis and is a typical feature of patients with Marfan's syndrome.

The great majority of children and adolescents with mitral valve prolapse are asymptomatic and remain free of complications. Arrhythmias, recurrent chest pain, endocarditis, progressive mitral regurgitation, and sudden death have all been reported in large groups of adults with prolapse, but the incidence of these problems is very low during the pediatric years (3).

The potential for an increased incidence of ventricular and atrial arrhythmias is the most common consideration in these patients. Kavey, Blackman, Sondheimer, and Brum (12) reported premature ventricular contractions in 43 of 103 pediatric patients with prolapse who were evaluated by treadmill testing and 24-hour electrocardiogram recordings. In no case, however, did these dysrhythmias appear to be clinically significant.

The incidence of sudden death appears to be increased in patients with mitral prolapse and is presumably related to ventricular tachyarrhythmias and ventricular fibrillation. These catastrophes, however, are largely limited to older adults with serious mitral regurgitation. Jeresaty (10) noted in 1986 that only 60 such cases had been reported, including only 4 under the age of 20 years. Of the total group, death occurred during vigorous physical activity in only 3: mowing the lawn (aged 39 years), after a game of tennis (aged 40), and during a football scrimmage (aged 17). From these data it appears that any small risk of sudden death with prolapse is not increased by sport participation.

Exercise Recommendations for Patients With Mitral Valve Prolapse

Very few young patients with mitral valve prolapse require restriction from sport activities. A resting electrocardiogram is indicated in the initial assessment, but exercise testing and 24-hour electrocardiogram are not necessary in the asymptomatic patient. These tests are important, however, in evaluating those with a history of unexplained tachycardia, palpitations, dizzy spells, syncope, or chest pain.

Jeresaty (10) offered the following criteria for disqualifying patients with mitral valve prolapse from competitive athletics, and these were adopted by the consensus conference (14) as well:

- history of syncope
- family history of sudden death with mitral valve prolapse
- chest pain exacerbated by exercise
- repetitive forms of ventricular ectopic activity or sustained supraventricular tachycardia, particularly if worsened by exercise
- significant mitral valve insufficiency
- associated Marfan's syndrome

Summary

Identification of mitral valve prolapse should rarely affect unrestricted recommendations for athletic participation. History, physical examination, and resting electrocardiogram constitute an appropriate assessment before approving involvement in sports. The unusual findings outlined above preclude participation in sports high in dynamic and static demand (see chapter 3), but certain low-demand activities may be permissible in these patients.

COARCTATION OF THE AORTA

Congenital narrowing or coarctation of the aorta typically occurs as a lateral infolding of the intimal and medial layers just distal to the origin of the left subclavian artery. Since collateral vessels form to bypass the obstruction, flow to the lower half of the body, although often nonpulsatile, remains adequate. Instead, the pathophysiology principally involves proximal hypertension with left ventricular afterload. In times prior to recognition and surgical repair of aortic coarctation, the ultimate prognosis during adulthood was poor, with death often occurring from stroke, left ventricular failure, aortic rupture, or infectious endarteritis.

Clinical Features

Coarctation of the aorta may present clinically as congestive heart failure (often associated with intracardiac anomalies) during infancy, but the diagnosis is not uncommonly initially made in the asymptomatic older child found to have systemic hypertension on a routine examination. These patients will have diminished or absent femoral pulses, increased brachial pulses, and a systolic murmur heard loudest over the left back. Upper-extremity systolic blood pressure typically will exceed femoral pressure by at least 20-30 mmHg, but because of the potential influence of collateral blood flow, the height of the brachial artery systolic pressure may not accurately reflect the severity of obstruction.

Treatment

Surgery for coarctation of the aorta typically involves resection of the stenotic aortic segment with end-to-end anastomosis. Longer segment narrowing may, however, require interposition of prosthetic material to enlarge the aortic diameter. Balloon dilation for aortic coarctation has largely been utilized for patients who experience a reobstruction of the coarctation site after surgery, but techniques to safely allow balloon relief of "native" coarctations have been developed in some centers as well.

With elimination of the coarctation, systemic blood pressure typically falls to the normal range. However, in some patients, often those who are operated on beyond early childhood, elevation in blood pressure persists to some degree despite the absence of a significant residual aortic gradient.

Exercise With Coarctation

Exercise is normally a hypertensive event. Isolated rises in systolic blood pressure are typically observed during dynamic activities (running, swimming) while dramatic increases in both systolic and diastolic pressure often accompany resistance exercises (such as weightlifting). Patients with a coarctation of the aorta before surgery, a postoperative residual gradient, or hypertension following surgical relief of their stenosis all may have exaggerated blood pressure responses to physical activity. The specific risk of this response has not been clearly defined, but it is considered prudent to limit activities or provide pharmacological management for patients with an exaggerated elevation in blood pressure with exercise (see chapter 13).

Exercise Recommendations for Patients With Coarctation of the Aorta

The principal consideration regarding sport participation in patients with coarctation of the aorta are risks related to systemic hypertension (see chapter 13). The would-be athlete who is discovered to have a significant coarctation of the aorta should be referred for surgical repair or balloon angioplasty before clearance for sport participation. Decision making for the physician therefore usually involves the question of athletic competition in patients following either of these procedures.

The consensus conference (15) agreed that patients should be allowed full sport participation

6-12 months after repair of coarctation of the aorta if there is no resting arm-to-leg blood pressure gradient, normal blood pressure responses are observed on exercise testing, and no residual ventricular hypertrophy or enlargement is evident. This conservative recommendation would prevent patients with mild residual gradients from participating in athletic competition. As adverse effects from sport participation have not been demonstrated in patients with mild degrees of systemic hypertension, clearance for athletic participation may be considered in postoperative coarctation patients whose gradient is not sufficiently severe to warrant reoperation or balloon intervention.

Summary

The potential risks of sport participation for the patient with coarctation of the aorta are related to those of systemic hypertension. Surgical or balloon relief of aortic obstruction is therefore recommended before approval for athletics. Those with mild hypertension postoperatively may be considered for all forms of sport participation but deserve evaluation for exaggerated blood pressure responses with exercise and left ventricular dysfunction prior to clearance.

REFERENCES

1. Alpert, B.S.; Kartodihardjo, W.; Harp, R.; Izukawa, T.; Strong, W.B. Exercise blood pressure response—a predictor of severity of aortic stenosis in children. J. Pediatr. 98:763-765; 1981.
2. Astrand, P-O; Rodahl, K. Textbook of work physiology. 2d ed. New York: McGraw-Hill Book Company; 1977.
3. Bisset, G.S.; Schwartz, D.C.; Meyer, R.A.; James, F.W.; Kaplan, S. Clinical spectrum and long-term followup of isolated mitral valve prolapse in 119 children. Circulation 62:423-429; 1980.
4. Chandramouli, B.; Ehmke, D.A.; Lauer, R.M. Exercise-induced electrocardiographic changes in children with congenital aortic stenosis. J. Pediatr. 87:725-730; 1975.
5. Cueto, L.; Moller, J.H. Haemodynamics of exercise in children with isolated aortic valvular disease. Br. Heart J. 35:93-98; 1973.
6. Cyran, S.E.; James, F.W.; Daniels, S.; Mays, W.; Shukla, R.; Kaplan, S. Comparison of the cardiac output and stroke volume response to upright exercise in children with valvular and subvalvular aortic stenosis. JACC 11:651-658; 1988.
7. Doyle, E.F.; Arumugham, P.; Lara, E.; Rutkowski, M.R.; Kiely, B. Sudden death in young patients with congenital aortic stenosis. Pediatrics 53:481-489; 1974.
8. Glew, R.H.; Varghese, P.J.; Krovetz, L.J.; Dorst, J.P.; Rowe, R.D. Sudden death in congenital aortic stenosis. A review of 8 cases with an evaluation of premonitory clinical features. Am. Heart J. 78:615-625; 1969.
9. Howitt, G. Haemodynamic effects of exercise in pulmonary stenosis. Brit. Heart J. 28:152-160; 1966.
10. Jeresaty, R.M. Mitral valve prolapse: definition and implications in athletes. JACC 7:231-6; 1986.
11. Karpman, V.L. Cardiovascular system and physical exercise. Boca Raton, Florida: CRC Press; 1987.
12. Kavey, R.W.; Blackman, M.S.; Sondheimer, H.M.; Brum, C.J. Ventricular arrhythmias and mitral valve prolapse in childhood. J. Pediatr. 105:885-890; 1984.
13. Lewis, A.B.; Heymann, M.A.; Stanger, P.; Hoffman, J.I.E.; Rudolph, A.M. Evaluation of subendocardial ischemia in valvar aortic stenosis in children. Circulation 49:978-984; 1974.
14. Maron, B.J.; Gaffney, F.A.; Jeresaty, R.M.; McKenna, W.J.; Miller, W.W. Task force III: Hypertrophic cardiomyopathy, other myopericardial diseases and mitral valve prolapse. JACC 6:1215-1217; 1985.
15. McNamara, D.G.; Bricker, J.T.; Galioto, F.M.; Graham, T.P.; James, F.W.; Rosenthal, A. Task force I: Congenital heart disease. JACC 6:1200-1208; 1985.
16. Nau, K.L.; Katch, V.L.; Beekman, R.H.; Dick, M. Acute intraarterial blood pressure response to bench press weight lifting in children. Pediatr. Exerc. Science 2:37-45; 1990.
17. Reid, M.J.; Coleman, N.E.; Stevenson, J.G. Management of congenital aortic stenosis. Arch. Dis. Child. 45:201-205; 1970.
18. Richards, A.M.; Ikram, H.; Nicholls, M.G.; Hamilton, E.J.; Richards, R.D. Syncope in

aortic valvular stenosis. Lancet 327:1113-1116; 1984.

19. Roth, S.J.; Keane, J.F. Balloon aortic valvuloplasty. Prog. Pediatr. Cardiol. 1:3-16; 1992.

20. Schwartz, L.S.; Goldfischer, J.; Sprague, G.J.; Schwartz, S.P. Syncope and sudden death in aortic stenosis. Am. J. Cardiol. 23:647-658; 1969.

21. Selzer, A. Changing aspects of the natural history of valvular aortic stenosis. N. Engl. J. Med. 317:91-98; 1987.

22. Wagner, H.R.; Ellison, R.C.; Keane, J.F.; Humphries, J.O.; Nadas, A.S. Clinical course in aortic stenosis. Circulation 56 (Suppl I):47-56; 1977.

CHAPTER 16

Dysrhythmic Heart Disease

Reginald Louis Washington
Rocky Mountain Pediatric Cardiology, Denver, CO

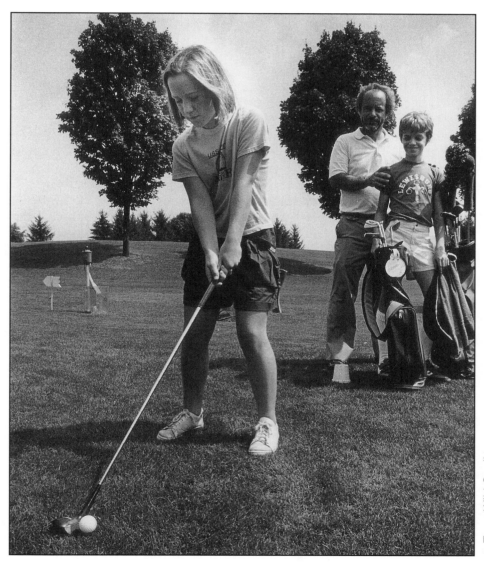

A dysrhythmia is an irregularity in the normal rhythm of the heart. This irregularity has also been termed an arrhythmia. In the strictest sense, however, an arrhythmia is the absence of a heart rate; hence, the term dysrhythmia will be used throughout this chapter. Irregularities in heart rate are very common in children, and most dysrhythmias are benign. This chapter will discuss the physical activity that is allowed in individuals who have been diagnosed with a dysrhythmia.

THE ELECTRICAL CONDUCTION SYSTEM OF THE HEART

Normal Anatomy and the Regulation of the Heart Rate

Cardiac muscle is unique in the body because it has the capability of creating and maintaining its own rhythm. When left to its own inherent rhythm, the heart will beat steadily between 70 and 80 times per minute (this is the case in a transplanted heart where all of the external nerves have been severed). Ordinarily, external controls of cardiac function (nerves and chemical regulation) cause the heart to speed up or slow down during daily activities.

The normal heart consists of four chambers. Situated in the back wall of the right upper chamber is a mass of specialized tissue known as the sinoatrial node or S-A node (Figure 16.1). This specialized tissue generates a small amount of electricity that exits the sinus node and spreads very rapidly into the muscle cells of the right and left atria, causing them to contract. For this reason, the S-A node is often referred to as the pacemaker of the heart. The electrical activity then moves into the junction between the atria and the ventricles and passes through another specialized structure known as the atrioventricular node or A-V node. The A-V node serves as a relay station taking the signal that comes from the upper chambers, delaying it slightly, and then passing the signal on to the lower chambers. Once the electrical impulse passes through the A-V node, special pathways rapidly carry the signal to both ventricles, resulting in a contraction of the lower chambers.

The Regulation of the Heart Rate During Exercise

Several reviews are available that discuss in detail the regulation of the heart rate during exercise (6, 7). The highlights of these regulatory mechanisms will be presented here.

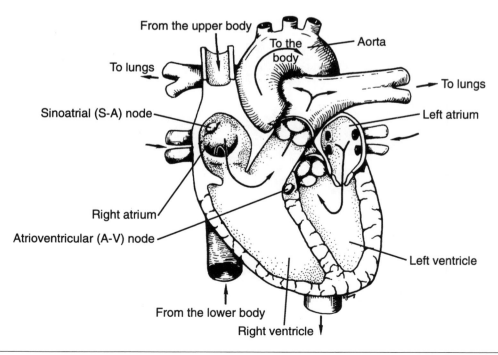

Figure 16.1 The normal heart.

During exercise, the quantity of blood pumped by the heart must change in accordance with the increased oxygen demand. Changes in heart rate involve factors that influence the S-A and A-V nodes. The two most prominent factors are the parasympathetic and sympathetic nervous systems. The parasympathetic fibers originate in the brain and are transmitted by the vagus nerve to the heart. These fibers make contact with both the S-A and the A-V nodes. When stimulated, these nerve endings release a substance known as acetylcholine, which causes a decrease in the activity of both the S-A and the A-V nodes. This results in a reduction in heart rate. In other words, the parasympathetic nervous system acts as a braking system to slow down the heart rate.

Studies have shown that the initial increase in heart rate that occurs during exercise (up to approximately 100 beats per minute) is due to a withdrawal of parasympathetic impulses, as just described (6). Stimulation of the S-A and A-V nodes by the sympathetic nervous system is also responsible for increases in heart rate. These special sympathetic fibers release norepinephrine, which causes an increase in both heart rate and the force of muscle contraction of the heart.

At rest, there is a normal balance between the parasympathetic and sympathetic activity to the heart that is regulated by the brain. The brain receives information from various parts of the circulatory system and monitors important parameters including, but not limited to, blood pressure, pH, and blood oxygen content. Another regulatory reflex involves special pressure receptors that are located in the right atrium. In this case, an increase in right atrial pressure signals the brain that an increase in venous return of blood to the heart has occurred. In order to prevent a backup of blood in the venous system, an increase in cardiac output must occur. The brain responds by sending sympathetic nerve impulses to the heart, which results in an increase in heart rate and an increase in cardiac output. This in turn lowers right atrial pressure back to normal.

Heart rate may also be influenced by changes in body temperature. An increase in body temperature results in an increase in heart rate, while a lowering of body temperature causes a reduction in heart rate (8).

DYSRHYTHMIAS

Physical Signs and Symptoms of Dysrhythmias

Many subjects who have dysrhythmias are asymptomatic; however, when symptoms are present, they are variable. The most common complaint is palpitations, which are often described as "the heart beating hard" or, in some instances, "fast." The common feature is that the child will notice his or her heart beating, which is an unusual sensation to be noticed. Dizziness is not commonly associated with palpitations, but, if it is present, a cardiac dysrhythmia should be considered.

Presyncope is a vasovagal collection of symptoms in which the patient does not feel well and may experience dizziness or light-headedness. The patient is cold and sweaty with a thready pulse and may experience low blood pressure. In presyncope there is no loss of consciousness, but in syncope these symptoms are followed by loss of muscle tone as well as of consciousness. If presyncope or syncope occur during physical activity, the individual may be injured.

There are several causes for presyncope and syncope, including the vasodepressor faint. The mechanism for this reaction begins when there is reduced left ventricular filling that is secondary to the pooling of blood in the lower parts of the body. This usually occurs with sudden changes in body position (e.g., from supine to standing), or upon prolonged standing. The reduction in left ventricular volume results in the stimulation of left ventricular mechanoreceptors. The stimulation of these receptors causes a reflux slowing of the heart rate and vasodilation. This paradoxical bradycardia and vasodilation may result in an exaggerated vasodepressor response and is then termed neurocardiogenic syncope. Another cause of syncope is a sudden blockage in the A-V node that results in an elimination of the contraction of the ventricles.

Chest pain is not commonly associated with dysrhythmias, but younger children may describe palpitations as chest pain.

Clinical and Laboratory Assessment of Individuals Suspected of Having Dysrhythmias

A detailed review of the evaluation of a child suspected of having dysrhythmias is beyond the scope of this book and will only be highlighted here. When a child is suspected of having a dysrhythmia, a careful history should be obtained. Questions that should be explored include

- the number, frequency, and duration of episodes,
- the time of day when episodes occur,
- the relationship to meals or exercise,
- the severity of symptoms,
- recent medications,
- caffeine intake,
- possible drug use or abuse, and
- associated symptoms (including but not limited to headache, nausea, vomiting, incontinence, tingling of extremities, and loss of vision).

A detailed family history should also be obtained to determine whether any other family members or close relatives have had similar complaints. A family history should include

- sudden death,
- syncope,
- presyncope,
- seizures,
- accidental death,
- Wolff-Parkinson-White syndrome,
- prolonged QT syndrome,
- hypertrophic cardiomyopathy,
- congestive cardiomyopathy, and
- arrythmogenic right ventricular dysplasia.

Diagnostic Tools Commonly Used to Diagnose Dysrhythmias

A variety of modalities are available and are used to diagnose dysrhythmias. The most important modality is a careful history and physical examination. Once the physician has obtained these and the presence of a dysrhythmia is suspected, an electrocardiogram (ECG) is obtained. The electrocardiogram can be used to monitor the activity of both the atria and the ventricles. The electrocardiogram also will provide information regarding the function of the S-A and A-V nodes. If the dysrhythmia involves electrical activity originating from other places within the heart, the electrocardiogram is helpful in pinpointing the origin of these abnormal

ectopic foci. The ECG also informs the physician about the frequency of the electrical activity through the heart (i.e., whether it is normal, slow, fast, or irregular).

Another modality that is often used is an exercise test which involves walking or running on a treadmill or pedaling a cycle. This test evaluates how well the heart is working and also determines how the heart rate increases with physiological stimulation (exercise). It should be done while an electrocardiogram is in place so that the electrical activity of the heart may be recorded. If a patient has started on medication to treat a dysrhythmia, this test is often repeated to evaluate the effectiveness of the medication. A negative result does not exclude the possibility of an exercise-induced dysrhythmia. For example, the test may be negative if the exercise test does not mimic the physical activity that induced the dysrhythmia. Other factors such as the time of day and relationship to meals must also be considered when interpreting the results of an exercise test.

The Holter monitor is a device that records heart rate and heartbeats continuously during a 24-hour period. An event monitor or transient arrhythmia monitor (TAM) is used to record a heart rate or rhythm for brief periods of time. The TAM is activated by the patient and the heart rate is recorded for 15-30 seconds. This information can then be transmitted via telephone to the physician for evaluation. The TAM is particularly useful if the symptoms are experienced in a very irregular fashion, and allows the physician to compare the symptom simultaneously with the heart rate and rhythm. If a patient does not experience dysrhythmias in a regular and predictable manner, the 24-hour Holter monitor often gives negative results and must be repeated several times before useful information is obtained. If the patient experiences a symptom while the Holter is in place and the heart rate and rhythm are normal, that information can be extremely valuable in evaluating the cause of the symptoms (i.e., by eliminating dysrhythmias as a possibility). When using either the Holter monitor or the TAM, the subject should engage in routine physical activities which are known to cause symptoms.

An electrophysiological cardiac catheterization may also be performed. During this procedure electrodes are introduced into the heart, various portions of the heart are electrically stimulated, and the response to this electrical stimulation is recorded. Often dysrhythmias may be induced using these techniques, and this information is valuable to electrophysiologists not only for the diagnosis of dysrhythmias but also for formulating a treatment plan.

Therapeutic Interventions Used to Treat Dysrhythmias

The treatment of dysrhythmias is beyond the scope of this book. Children who have been evaluated by a physician and diagnosed as having a dysrhythmia may be treated with a variety of medications that are designed to suppress abnormal electrical foci. Certain dysrhythmias will require special pacemakers that are designed to suppress the irregular rhythm and readjust the heart rate back to a normal rhythm. When these medications or other treatment modalities are being utilized, everyone involved with the care of the child should be familiar with the specific treatment.

Congenital Heart Disease and Dysrhythmias

Dysrhythmias may occur at any age. Some children are unaware that they are having dysrhythmias until they are informed by their physician. Others come to the attention of the physician because of symptoms such as those outlined previously. It must be emphasized that not all patients with congenital heart disease have dysrhythmias, and patients with similar disorders should not be compared to one another. The occurrence of dysrhythmias in individuals is variable. Table 16.1 includes the most common congenital heart defects that may be associated with dysrhythmias (4). This is not intended to be an exhaustive list, and all individuals with the listed disorders do not experience dysrhythmias. The incidence of dysrhythmias in these individual conditions is variable, and the patients should be evaluated by a cardiologist if the presence of a dysrhythmia is suspected.

EXERCISE AND DYSRHYTHMIAS

The most common dysrhythmias are listed in Table 16.2. An abnormal rhythm usually starts

Table 16.1 Common Congenital Defects Associated With Dysrhythmias

Acyanotic heart disease	
Aortic stenosis—postop	Ventricular septal defect—postop
Pulmonary stenosis—postop	Atrial septal defect—postop
Ebstein's anomaly	Mitral insufficiency pre- and postop

Cyanotic lesions	
Tetralogy of Fallot	Tricuspid atresia
Transposition of the great vessels	Single ventricle
Corrected transposition of the great vessels	

Note. Postop = patients who have undergone corrective surgery.

Table 16.2 Common Dysrhythmia

Premature ventricular contractions
Premature supraventricular contractions
Atrial flutter and fibrillation
Premature A-V node complexes
Supraventricular tachycardia
Congenital complete heart block

at a site other than the sinus node. All tissue of the heart is capable of initiating a heartbeat under certain conditions; thus, when an abnormal rhythm occurs it is important to determine the origination of the impulse. Some dysrhythmias originate from the ventricles, others originate from the atria, and still others originate in special pathways between the atria and the ventricles which can either be external to the A-V node or reside in the A-V node itself. The most common dysrhythmias are discussed in the following section.

Premature Ventricular Contractions (PVCs)

These are extra beats that originate in the ventricles, and are fairly common. Patients with no structural heart disease in whom PVCs disappear during exercise may participate in all competitive sports (10). Patients in whom PVCs increase in frequency or occur in pairs during exercise should be further evaluated by a physician before being allowed to participate in competitive sport. The extent of this evaluation is left to the discretion of the physician, but will usually include at least a resting ECG, as well as a stress ECG, echocardiogram, and perhaps a Holter monitor. After evaluation these individuals may be cleared to participate in sports with low dynamic or static demands (10). Patients with structural heart disease who are in high-risk groups (including patients with a right ventriculotomy, significant aortic stenosis, aortic insufficiency, coronary artery disease, or cardiomyopathies) should be excluded from high- to moderate-intensity competitive sport with or without treatment (10).

Occasionally, patients who have been diagnosed with premature ventricular contractions are found to have prolongation of the QT interval. This is often variable, however, and may in fact be normal at times. It should be determined whether there is a family history of this syndrome or history of syncope or near syncope. Minor degrees of QT prolongation should not be overinterpreted. Evaluation of this cardiovascular abnormality is required and includes but is not limited to an electrocardiogram, exercise test, and Holter monitor. Some patients with prolonged QT interval syndrome are at risk for sudden death with physical activity; such patients should be restricted from all competitive sports (10).

Premature Supraventricular Contraction

Extra beats may originate in the upper chambers. This type of dysrhythmia is termed premature supraventricular contraction (also known as premature atrial contraction or PAC). This is the most common dysrhythmia that is described as "skipping a beat." In reality the heart does not skip a beat; rather, some area of the heart other than the S-A node generates an electrical signal that causes the heart to beat early, before the next regularly scheduled beat occurs. This is followed by a short pause, which causes the next beat to be more forceful. It is this forceful beat that the patient recognizes.

Premature beats of this variety are very common in normal children and teenagers (all of whom have probably had them at some time), and this dysrhythmia is easily recognized by the electrocardiogram. Unless a careful history and physical examination suggests the presence of structural heart disease and there are symptoms other than the occasional palpitation, no evaluation is necessary other than a 12-lead ECG. These patients may participate in all competitive sports (10).

Atrial Flutter and Atrial Fibrillation

These dysrhythmias involve the chaotic and very fast heart rate initiated in the atria. Sustained atrial flutter and fibrillation is uncommon in patients without structural heart disease. Therefore, an evaluation by a cardiologist is mandatory before these individuals may be cleared to participate in physical activities. Their level of participation must be individually determined (10).

Premature A-V Node Complexes

This dysrhythmia originates in the A-V node. It is easily diagnosed by the 12-lead ECG. Often, however, a Holter monitor is necessary to determine the heart's behavior over a 24-hour period. Occasionally, further tests will be ordered by a physician.

Patients who have a structurally normal heart, without evidence of a sustained tachycardia (rapid beats for more than several seconds), may participate in all sports. Patients with a structurally abnormal heart may possibly be permitted to participate in activities with low static and low dynamic demands, but the approval of their personal physician is needed (10).

Supraventricular Tachycardia

Supraventricular tachycardia (SVT) is also known as paroxysmal atrial tachycardia (PAT). This dysrhythmia occurs when the normal gatekeeper function of the A-V node is circumvented. The result is a very rapid heart rate that has a sudden onset and termination. This rapid heart rate often occurs in bursts, hence the term paroxysmal. The diagnosis is readily apparent on 12-lead ECG. However, as the episodes often occur in paroxysms they may not be visualized at the time the ECG is performed. These individuals often require a Holter monitor, an event monitor, or an exercise test to make the diagnosis.

Individuals with reproducible exercise-induced supraventricular tachycardia may participate in all competitive sports if prevention of recurrences has been achieved via medication (10).

Individuals who do not have an exercise-induced supraventricular tachycardia but who suffer from sporadic reoccurrences should have an attempt made at prevention. These individuals may participate in low-intensity competitive sports if they have no structural heart disease and if their ventricular rate remains less than 200-250 beats per minute (depending on age). However, because of the unpredictable nature of the tachycardia they should not participate in more vigorous activities (10).

Patients who have suffered from syncope or who have significant structural heart disease should not participate in any sports with high static or dynamic demands until they have been adequately controlled and until no recurrence has been demonstrated (e.g., by history, ECG, or Holter) for a minimum of 6 months. These patients should remain under the care of a cardiologist.

Congenital Complete Heart Block

In these individuals there is no transmission of the electrical impulse from the upper chambers to the lower chambers. In other words, the lower chambers are contracting independently of the upper chambers. These patients should be evaluated by a cardiologist before being cleared to participate in physical activities. In many cases cardiac activity should be evaluated by a stress test before participation is allowed. Patients with symptoms of fatigue or syncope often require a pacemaker before being allowed to participate in any competitive activities. The degree of participation should be determined by the cardiologist.

Dysrhythmias and Sudden Death

The deleterious effects of dysrhythmias during exercise have been reviewed by Bricker and Ross, and the results of their review will be summarized here (2). Most young athletes who die suddenly are not known to have a cardiac abnormality, and most young individuals with cardiac disease who die suddenly and unexpectedly do not do so during exercise. In fact, sudden unexpected death in children with heart disease has been related to exercise or physical activity in only 10% of cases (5). Garson found a 0.004% incidence of sudden death in a large cardiac clinic over a 25-year period; 22% of these were related to activity or exercise (3). If a dysrhythmia is properly diagnosed and treated, the risk of sudden unexpected death declines.

Many of those who experience sudden cardiac death have cardiac abnormalities that are inapparent prior to death, even despite thorough preparticipation physical examinations. Disorders such as hypertrophic cardiomyopathy or anomalies of the coronary arteries are two of the more common cardiac causes of sudden unexpected death. These patients are thought to ultimately die from a dysrhythmia. The abuse of drugs, particularly cocaine and amphetamines, may also result in a fatal dysrhythmia.

In summary, patients with structural heart disease and/or symptoms compatible with a dysrhythmia should be further evaluated by a physician before being granted clearance to participate in athletics, as sudden death can occur during exercise. This evaluation should include, but not necessarily be limited to,

- a thorough medical history,
- a family history,
- a physical examination, and
- appropriate laboratory studies.

Fortunately, sudden unexpected death is not a common event.

Dysrhythmias and the Risk of Injury

Dysrhythmias can occur in which the individual is only mildly symptomatic during the dysrhythmia and is, therefore, thought to be at low risk for sudden death. However, the possibility exists that symptoms occurring during play may cause injury to the patient or others. A partial list of these potentially dangerous activities includes snow skiing, rock climbing, race car driving, sky diving, scuba diving, and swimming.

Individuals who complain of symptoms compatible with dysrhythmias may not be at risk for sudden unexpected death but may nevertheless be of some risk to themselves and others. They, too, should be further evaluated before participation is allowed.

Summary

Any individual with symptoms or physical complaints compatible with a dysrhythmia should be further evaluated by a physician. The clearance to participate in individual sports must be individualized. Patients who are known to have a structural cardiac defect deserve special attention, and may require an evaluation by a pediatric cardiologist before being allowed to participate in sports. Not all individuals with a particular cardiac defect should be categorized in a similar fashion, however. Some individuals with a particular defect may have no dysrhythmia at all and can, therefore, be cleared to participate in all physical activities. However, other individuals with the same structural problems may exhibit signs or symptoms compatible with a serious dysrhythmia, and may require further evaluation and/or treatment before being allowed to participate in physical activities. It should also be remembered that some individuals with significant dysrhythmias are asymptomatic. Schools, athletic teams, and recreational centers should require appropriate documentation and clearance from a qualified physician before allowing these children to participate.

EXERCISE AND SPORT PROGRAMS FOR CHILDREN WITH DYSRHYTHMIAS

Benefit of Exercise on the Disease

A sedentary lifestyle is a known risk factor for future cardiovascular disease. The risk in an individual who participates in physical activity with a known dysrhythmia cannot be precisely known. Likewise, the benefit of participating in physical activity in this individual also is difficult to accurately predict. Therefore, the responsibility for the decision about sport participation for the potential athlete with a dysrhythmia should be shared by the athlete, the athlete's family, and the physician involved. A risk-free environment cannot be assured even for the athlete without known disease. It should be noted, however, that the vast majority of athletes with dysrhythmias do not die suddenly.

The psychological benefits of sport participation are obvious, and participation in athletics can improve the young individual's self-confidence and self-image (1). This is particularly true in the adolescent whose self-image has been negatively affected by the presence of a cardiac defect. Thus, patients most likely to benefit from sport participation are often individuals who have been diagnosed with heart disease. In select individuals, cardiac rehabilitation programs have proven beneficial in not only increasing physical fitness but also in improving an individual's confidence and sense of self-worth (9).

Individual Evaluation

Any potential athlete suspected of having a dysrhythmia must be further evaluated. The responsibility for requesting this evaluation rests on the individual who suspects the dysrhythmia. The assumption should never be made that the dysrhythmia is of no consequence.

The results of this individual evaluation should be shared with the patient, his or her family, his or her coach, and any other individuals responsible for the child's well-being during athletics participation (e.g., physical education teacher, classroom teacher, youth league sports coach, camp director). It is helpful for the personal physician to communicate with all of the above individuals in writing, and this communication should include specific recommendations. If medications are being used they should also be included in this documentation.

Standard cardiopulmonary resuscitation (CPR) should be available in any setting where athletes are participating in an organized fashion (in other words, for example, all coaches should have CPR training). Suffice it to say that a dysrhythmia may occur in any individual at any given time. While it is true that individuals with previous symptoms or cardiovascular disease are at increased risk for dysrhythmias, any child may have them. For this reason, all coaches, teachers, athletic personnel, athletic trainers, and physicians and other allied health personnel should be experienced in CPR.

Occasionally, an athlete with a serious dysrhythmia will continue to participate in physical activities against the advice of one or more physicians. These athletes are usually either professional or highly regarded amateurs, and they seek the advice of multiple physicians in order to find one who will allow them to participate. In some circumstances, these athletes are provided with sophisticated anti-arrhythmic equipment to be used in the field. Unfortunately, this practice has resulted in several instances of sudden death while participating in physical activities. When there are conflicting opinions among physicians regarding the safety of participation, both the athlete and the individuals responsible for his or her well-being must carefully weigh all the evidence before making a decision regarding participation.

SUMMARY

The majority of dysrhythmias diagnosed in children are benign, and these children will be allowed to participate in most if not all activities. If an individual is diagnosed with a dysrhythmia that is not benign, certain guidelines should be followed when deciding how much or what activity is safe (10). It is the responsibility of all individuals involved with the young athlete to make sure that he or she has been properly evaluated and treated, if necessary, before being allowed to participate. Physical activity is vital to the well-being of all individuals, and the ultimate goal should be to control the dysrhythmia to whatever extent possible so that the activity, although limited in some, is safe.

REFERENCES

1. Bailey, D.A. The growing child and the need for physical activity. In: Albinson, J.G.; An-
drew, G.M., ed. Sport and physical activity international series on sports sciences. Baltimore: University Park Press; 1976:81-93.
2. Bricker, J.T.; Ross, B. Arrhythmias in sports. In: Gillette, P.C.; Garson, A., ed. Pediatric arrhythmias: electrophysiology and pacing. Philadelphia: W.B. Saunders; 1990:617-629.
3. Garson, A. Sudden death in a pediatric cardiology population, 1958-1983: relation to prior arrhythmias. Journal of the American College of Cardiology 5:138B-141B; 1985.
4. Garson, A. Chronic postoperative arrhythmia. In: Gillette, P.C.; Garson, A., ed. Pediatric arrhythmias: electrophysiology and pacing. Philadelphia: W.B. Saunders; 1990: 667-678.
5. Lambert, E.C.; Menon, B.A.; Wagner, H.R. Sudden unexpected death from cardiovascular disease in children. American Journal of Cardiology 34:89-96; 1974.
6. McArdle, W.D.; Catch, F.I.; Catch, B.L. Exercise physiology—energy, nutrition and human performance. Philadelphia: Lea and Febiger; 1991:314-319.
7. Powers, S.K.; Howley, E.T. Exercise physiology, theory and application to fitness and performance. Dubuque, Iowa: William C. Brown; 1990:186-188.
8. Rubin, S. Core temperature regulation of heart rate during exercise in humans. Journal of Applied Physiology 62:1997-2002; 1987.
9. Washington, R.L. Cardiac rehabilitation programs in children. Sports Medicine 14:164-170; 1992.
10. Zipes, D.P.; Garson, A. 26th Bethesda Conference: recommendation for determining eligibility for competition in athletes with cardiovascular abnormalities. Task Force VI: Arrhythmias. Journal of the American College of Cardiology 24:892-899; 1994.

CHAPTER 17

Carditis, Cardiomyopathy, and Marfan's Syndrome

David S. Braden
University of Mississippi Medical Center

William B. Strong
Medical College of Georgia Hospital and Clinics

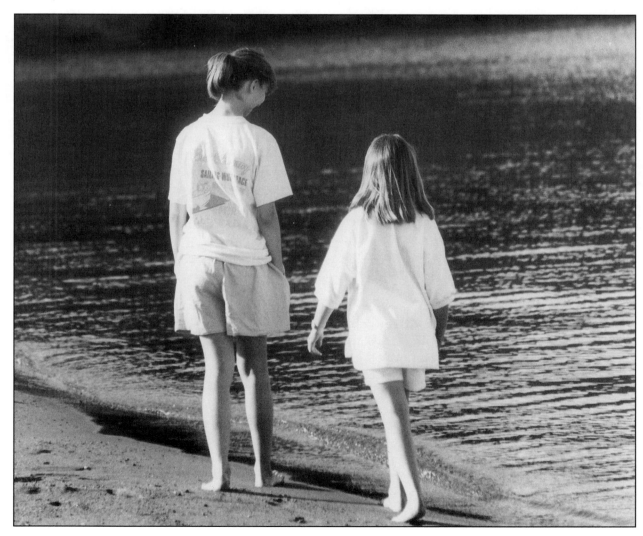

This chapter will focus on three cardiovascular disease entities which have consistently been associated with sudden unexpected death, especially among competitive athletes. Although sudden death in young athletes is rare, with 1 to 2 cases reported per 200,000 athletes (3, 9, 34), the tragic and unexpected nature of these events lends to great concern and often great publicity. Two main disease entities, hypertrophic cardiomyopathy and aortic dissection in association with Marfan's syndrome, comprise the bulk of athletes at risk for sudden death. Hypertrophic cardiomyopathy is far and away the leading cause, with estimates varying from 10 to 48% (22, 30, 45). In a recent review of the literature, McCaffrey, Braden, and Strong (34) noted that 6 of 87 reported cases of sudden death in young athletes were secondary to complications of Marfan's syndrome (19, 22, 27). And, although rare, sudden death has also been reported to occur secondary to chronic myocarditis or dilated cardiomyopathy (22, 45). Therefore, it behooves the clinician to be familiar with the diagnosis and management of young athletes with these conditions.

MARFAN'S SYNDROME

In 1896 a French pediatrician named Antoine Bernard-Jean Marfan described a young girl with a constellation of unusual clinical features, including scoliosis and contractures of the knees, elbows, fingers, and toes, and loose wrist and ankle joints (40). She had long, tapered extremities and "spiderlike" digits, a condition he termed *dolichostenomelia* (40). She had normal intelligence and lacked cardiovascular and ocular abnormalities. Although this was the original description of "Marfan's syndrome," Beals and Hecht later suggested that this original patient may actually have had congenital contractural arachnodactyly (2, 19). Nevertheless, reports in the early 1900s clarified Marfan's syndrome as a hereditary disorder involving bones, joints, eyes, heart, and blood vessels. The involvement of the cardiovascular system was documented in 1943, and the extent of the cardiovascular involvement is now accepted to be the primary index of the severity of the disorder.

Description of Marfan's Syndrome

Pathophysiology

Although the cause of Marfan's syndrome is unknown, it has long been assumed to occur secondary to an inborn error of protein metabolism, particularly of collagen or elastin (49). The prevalence of classic Marfan's syndrome is 4-6:100,000 people, without gender, racial, ethnic, or geographic predilection (49). Marfan's syndrome is inherited in an autosomal dominant manner in 65-75% of cases; thus, each affected person has a 50% chance of passing the mutant gene to his or her offspring (47). The mutant gene exerts a pleiotrophic effect, i.e., multiple and seemingly unrelated phenotypic features stem from a single genetic alteration (47). Although the syndrome is not felt to skip generations, there is both interfamilial and intrafamilial variability (47). Between 25 and 35% of all cases of Marfan's syndrome occur sporadically, often in cases of advanced paternal age. Infants with the sporadic form of the disease may be more severely affected than many infants with familial transmission (40).

Pathologically, arterial wall defects are found in the aorta as well as the pulmonary, carotid, and other systemic arteries (59). Grossly, there may be saccular and "flask"-shaped aneurysms with chronic dissections, transverse arterial tears, and degeneration and thinning of the arterial walls (20). These changes are reflected microscopically as fragmentation of elastic fibers, disorganization and increased deposition of collagen fibers, and disorganized smooth muscle in the media and cystic medial necrosis (51). In the aorta, this process begins at the level of the sinuses of Valsalva, propagating distally and enlarging secondary to shearing forces generated by cardiac contraction and progressively increasing wall tension. The mitral valve is also typically involved with ballooning; redundancy and fenestrations of the leaflets; annular dilatation and incompetence; and thinning and elongation of the chordae. The conducting system may also be affected secondary to degenerative changes of the walls of the nutrient arteries of the sinoatrial and atrioventricular nodes.

Physical Symptoms and Clinical Signs

Classical Marfan's syndrome may involve the eyes, the joints, the heart and large arteries, the

Table 17.1 Diagnostic Features of Aortic Dissection (Marfan's)

Family history (autosomal dominant)
Ophthalmologic, skeletal, and cardiac examination (wrist sign; thumb sign)
Lower body segment → upper body segment
2D echocardiography

skin, and the lungs; see Table 17.1 for the syndrome's diagnostic features. Ocular abnormalities are found in at least 70% of affected individuals, and perhaps more if a careful slit-lamp examination is performed. Ocular findings are more common in males (83%) than in females (53%). Ectopic lentis, caused by dysfunction of the normal suspensory apparatus, occurs in 60% of patients, and is usually present at the first detailed opthalmalogic examination. The dislocation is typically upward and outward with preservation of normal accommodation, in contrast to that found in homocystinuria, in which the lenses dislocate downward with inadequate accommodation (49). Affected individuals may also have increased axial lengths of the globes, causing a tendency to myopia and an increased risk of retinal detachment (49). The corneas of affected individuals may also be relatively flat, with keratometer readings several standard deviations below the population mean.

As many as 60% of individuals with Marfan's syndrome have ausculatory evidence of cardiovascular involvement, including diastolic murmurs suggestive of aortic insufficiency and systolic clicks and/or murmurs of mitral valve origin. However, most are asymptomatic until the third or fourth decade of life. Symptoms that are described are those caused by acute and/or chronic aortic dissection, congestive heart failure secondary to valvular insufficiency, and occasionally arrhythmias. Syncope, nonanginal chest pain, orthostatic phenomena, and fatigue are not uncommon.

Affected individuals are usually tall, with arm span typically greater than height. They exhibit dolichostenomelia or increased limb length as compared with trunk length (49). This is best estimated by dividing the lower segment length (top of pubic ramus to floor) into the upper segment length (height minus lower). This ratio varies with age during normal growth development, but in individuals with Marfan's syndrome, it is usually at least two standard deviations greater than the mean for age, race, and sex. Normal values for this ratio are as follows:

- 0.92 (SD=.04) in whites
- 0.85 (SD=.03) in blacks

This ratio may be further decreased by scoliosis.

Although in large part a subjective finding, arachnodactyly is also common. Simple maneuvers such as the Steinberg thumb sign (37) (positive if the thumb, when completely opposed with a clenched hard fist, projects beyond the ulnar border [Figure 17.1]) and the Walker-Murdoch wrist sign (37) (positive if the distal phalanges of the first and fifth digits of one hand overlap when unwrapped around the opposite wrist [Figure 17.2]) are helpful but also somewhat subject to observer interpretation (49). Common thoracic and vertebral column deformities include

- pectus excavatum,
- pectus carinatum,
- kyphoscoliosis,
- spina bifida,

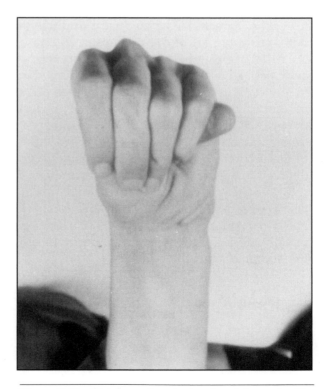

Figure 17.1 Steinberg thumb sign in adolescent with Marfan's syndrome.

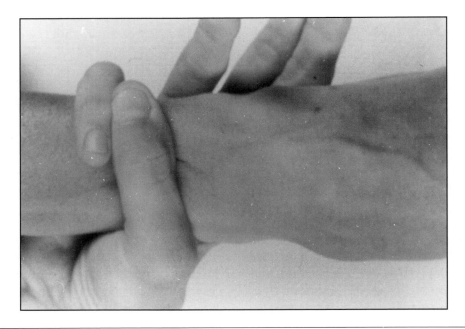

Figure 17.2   Walker-Murdoch wrist sign in adolescent with Marfan's syndrome.

- spondylolithesis, and
- the loss of the normal thoracic curvature (49).

Inguinal hernias are not uncommon. Less common findings include characteristic facial features, malocclusion of the teeth, and deformities of the ankle or knee.

Poorly characterized pulmonary findings do not constitute part of the diagnostic criteria or the usual clinical presentation. Their prevalence and pathogenesis are unknown. Pulmonary manifestations may include spontaneous pneumothorax, bullous emphysema, aneurysms, or dissections of the pulmonary artery. Lung volumes and capacities may be decreased either in accordance with or out of proportion to the degree of chest wall and spinal deformities.

Stria distensae caused by involvement of the connective tissue of the dermis are found in about one quarter of cases (20, 37). These are usually most conspicuous on the upper thorax, the abdomen, and the buttocks.

Diagnostic Evaluation

Once Marfan's syndrome is suspected a complete diagnostic evaluation should be performed, including:

- a thorough physical examination, including the measurement of body proportions,

- a detailed ophthalmologic evaluation utilizing a slit-lamp with pupillary dilation,
- a chest X ray, and
- an echocardiogram (49).

Utilizing this as a minimal workup, the diagnosis can be made or rejected in greater than 90% of cases (49). In order to make the diagnosis, positive features are required in two systems if the family history is positive (as defined by involvement in a first-degree relative); or in the skeletal system and at least two other systems if the family history is negative (47). More reliance is placed on hard features, i.e., those features common in Marfan's syndrome but uncommon in the general population (ectopia lentis, aortic dilation, severe kyphoscoliosis, and anterior thorax deformities) than on so-called soft features (myopia, mitral valve prolapse, tall stature, joint laxity, and arachnodactyly).

No specific changes are seen on the electrocardiogram in Marfan's syndrome (49), although a left ventricular strain pattern may be found with significant aortic insufficiency, or left atrial enlargement with significant mitral insufficiency. These findings may also be reflected on chest X ray, as may scoliosis and pectus deformities. Aortic root enlargement is often not evident on chest X ray until already pronounced and often not until dissection or insufficiency has occurred, because the part of the aorta to dilate first is usually within the cardiovascular silhouette (49).

The echocardiogram is far more sensitive than a chest X ray in the early detection of aortic root dilation. It has also enhanced the early detection of cardiovascular abnormalities and has improved both the diagnosis and management of individuals with Marfan's syndrome. Additionally, two-dimensional echocardiography may confirm the presence of mitral value prolapse. Doppler evaluation is useful in the evaluation of aortic and mitral insufficiency.

Cardiac catheterization and angiography has traditionally been utilized for defining the extent and severity of aortic dilation and aortic insufficiency, as well as aiding in deciding the timing of surgical intervention and documenting aortic root dissection (38). However, the reliability of aortography in documenting the presence of aortic insufficiency is often less than optimal. Transthoracic echocardiography may be equal to catheterization and angiography for defining the extent of aortic root dilation and the degree of aortic insufficiency. Recently, transesophageal echocardiology has proven to be very helpful, especially when biplane imaging is available. Aortic root involvement can also be satisfactorily documented by computed tomography and magnetic resonance imaging (7, 16, 56).

Natural History

Several studies have suggested that aortic root dilation may appear early in life, possibly even in utero. Aortic root complications, however, are rare in early stages. Aortic insufficiency usually begins when annular dilation reaches 6.0 cm, and progressively worsens with increasing strain on the left ventricle and an increasing evidence of heart failure. Hemodynamically significant aortic insufficiency is rare if the aortic root is less than 5.0 cm, but invariably occurs when aortic root diameter exceeds 6.5 cm. Aortic dissection also occurs with an increasing frequency in later life as the aortic root exceeds 5.0 cm.

Mitral valve prolapse (MVP) is usually benign in the early stages of the disorder. While 25% of affected individuals may develop serious valve dysfunction with an unpredictable rate of progression (48), serious mitral insufficiency may be observed at all ages and is the most common indication for cardiac surgery in children with Marfan's sydrome (7).

Management

Once the diagnosis of Marfan's syndrome has been made, management is aimed at preventing life-threatening complications. Affected children should have regular evaluations at 6- to 12-month intervals. Each evaluation should include

- a general medical examination with cardiovascular emphasis,
- an ophthalmologic examination,
- scoliosis screening,
- orthopaedic evaluation (if indicated), and
- echocardiography (47).

Bracing should be considered early for scoliosis, with instrumentation considered for curves more severe than 40 degrees (16). Repair of chest wall deformities, however, should not be performed until late adolescence unless necessitated by cardiopulmonary compromise (47, 49).

If severe mitral insufficiency occurs secondary to MVP, surgical intervention may be required. Repair is preferable to mitral valve replacement because of the long- and short-term concerns about anticoagulation (54). All children with Marfan's syndrome and valvular insufficiency should also be considered to be at risk for endocarditis and should receive prophylaxis for all potential bacteremic procedures.

There is some evidence suggesting that beta blockers may retard aortic root dilation by negative inotropic effects in decreasing the intensity of left ventricular ejection (63). Aortic root dilation is defined as an aortic annulus diameter exceeding the 95th percentile for body surface area. Beta blockade is recommended if there are no contraindications (e.g., bronchospasm) in children with evidence of aortic root dilation (49). Although both propranolol and atenolol are acceptable, atenolol (12.5 mg/10 kg body weight, given in two divided doses daily) is probably the better choice because of its cardioselectivity and lower incidence of adverse effects (1). In adolescents with Marfan's syndrome, aortic root complications become more frequent as the aortic root diameter exceeds 5.0 cm. More frequent echocardiographic evaluation may be necessary at that point. Prophylactic composite graft repair is recommended when the aortic root attains a diameter of 6.0 cm (47). Postoperative patients are maintained on both warfarin sodium and beta blocker. In those patients repaired utilizing an aortic homograft, salicylates alone may be adequate for anticoagulation. Continued annual follow-up may also involve computed tomography or magnetic resonance imaging.

Mortality and Morbidity

Death is estimated to occur in one third of patients with Marfan's syndrome during the first 32 years of life, and in two thirds by the age of 50 years (41). Mortality is usually cardiovascular in nature, usually secondary to aortic dissection or aortic insufficiency in children. These vascular lesions may also contribute to significant morbidity by causing congestive heart failure and dysrythmias. Chest wall deformities and kyphoscoliosis may also contribute to morbidity by causing pulmonary compromise. As noted earlier, ocular causes of morbidity center around decreased visual acuity and an increased risk of retinal detachment.

Exercise and Marfan's Syndrome

Children and adolescents with minimal evidence of Marfan's syndrome may have normal responses to both aerobic and isometric exercise. In fact, the reader is probably quite familiar with excellent competitive athletes with Marfan's syndrome—for example, Olympic volleyball star Flo Hyman, an elite athlete who died suddenly and tragically of an aortic dissection (5). However, those affected individuals with significant aortic or mitral valvular insufficiency may have varying degrees of exercise impairment (1, 8, 21). Abnormalities observed in these individuals include decreased exercise capacity, as evidenced by historical complaints of easy fatigability and dyspnea on exertion. Correlating exercise parameters might include decreases in physical working capacity (PWC), endurance time, and maximal oxygen consumption ($\dot{V}O_2$max) (1, 8, 21). The maximal heart rate (HR max) may be decreased, and the peak systolic blood pressure (SBP max) may be blunted or decreased (1, 8, 21). The child may have chest pain and/or ischemia (1, 8, 21) on ECG if there is significant aortic insufficiency. Physical performance may also be limited in some children because of poor muscular development, joint laxity, and thoracic and spinal abnormalities

(47). Pectus deformities may limit the ventilatory capacity and adversely affect exercise performance (Figure 17.3).

The most serious adverse effect of exercise in the individual with Marfan's syndrome is sudden death secondary to aortic dissection (37, 41, 42). This risk, as has been stated, is most marked in those adolescents and young adults with aortic diameters greater than or equal to 6.0 cm. Obviously, the echocardiogram serves as the primary screening tool for aortic root dilation. In those individuals with aortic diameters greater than the 95th percentile for body surface area, we generally recommend the avoidance of competitive strenuous athletics, isometric activities, resistance training, and exercise to the point of exhaustion. Children in this category should be encouraged to be as active as possible in alternative types of activities. The school should be encouraged to establish appropriate exercise programs in lieu of standard physical education. Although no data support the benefits of limited exercise on physical fitness in children with Marfan's syndrome, there is little question that totally precluding their participation in physical activity may cause them to be ostracized by their peers and thus hinder their psychosocial development. In other words, it is good to balance the risks of activity with the benefits of participation, thereby increasing the quantity of life without unnecessarily hampering the quality of life.

Exercise and Sport Programs for Children With Marfan's Syndrome

The Bethesda Conference in 1984 specifically recommended the avoidance of the following activities in children with Marfan's syndrome (see chapter 3):

- sports with the danger of body collision,
- sports with high to moderate aerobic and static demands, and
- sports with high-to-moderate static and low dynamic demands (39).

It is the authors' opinions that in the absence of cardiovascular disease (as evidenced by a complete echocardiogram, including an aortic diameter less than the 95th percentile), or of significantly compromising ophthalmologic or musculoskeletal abnormalities, the child, adolescent, or young adult with Marfan's syndrome

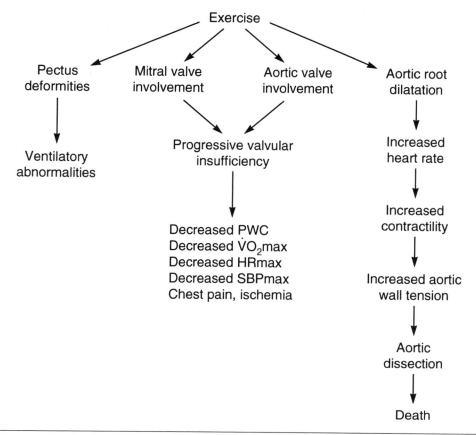

Figure 17.3 Presumed pathophysiology in exercise in patient with Marfan's syndrome.

should not be restricted from sport participation, except those sports where high-impact collisions are likely. As children with Marfan's syndrome develop strength, coordination, and an interest in sports, they should probably be directed toward noncompetitive sports such as recreational swimming and bicycling (47). Guiding them toward noncompetitive endeavors early in life may preclude the unpleasant necessity of restricting a previously competitive athlete at a later date. Moreover, children previously allowed unlimited participation should be redirected toward those activities if cardiovascular involvement progressess. Otherwise, recommended allowable sports are based primarily on dynamic and static demands (39). Those individuals with significant aortic root dilation or mitral insufficiency may be allowed to participate in competitive sports with low dynamic and low static demands, such as bowling, cricket, golf, archery, and riflery (39). In selected cases individuals may be allowed to participate in some sports with high dynamic and low static demands, such as badminton, baseball, basketball, field hockey, lacrosse, ping-pong, race walking,

racquetball, distance running, soccer, squash, swimming, tennis, and volleyball (39). These are only recommendations, of course, and clinicians may vary in their adherence to them. Table 17.2 suggests possible guidelines for sport participation based on the degree of cardiovascular involvement. However, if exceptions are made, the athlete should not have significant cardiac involvement and must undergo regular medical assessment (5).

DILATED CARDIOMYOPATHY

Dilated cardiomyopathy is defined as a disease process in which myocardial pathology is the dominant feature without a gross structural basis for cardiac disability (6).

Description of Dilated Cardiomyopathy

The revised World Health Organization classification divides the cardiomyopathies into three main categories:

Table 17.2   Sports Participation in Marfan's Syndrome (See Chapter 3)

Cardiovascular (CV) involvement	Activities contraindicated	Activities permitted	Other considerations
1. No evidence of CV disease by echocardiogram	Danger of body collision	All other sports	Participation only if no significant arrhythmias or symptoms (chest pain, syncope)
2. Mild AI/MI with aortic diameter <95% for BSA or <5.0 cm.	Body collision High-moderate dynamic/static High-moderate static/low dynamic	Low intensity High-moderate dynamic/low static	Low intensity only if arrhythmias present
3. Moderate-severe AI/MI with aortic diameter >95% or >5.0 cm.	All competitive sports	Low intensity	Low intensity permitted if no arrhythmias or symptoms (chest pain, syncope)

Note. AI = aortic insufficiency; MI = mitral insufficiency; BSA = body surface area; CM = centimeters.

- dilated,
- hypertrophic, and
- restrictive (62).

However, any given individual may show characteristics of more than one category.

Pathophysiology

This section will address dilated cardiomyopathy, which is characterized by congestive heart failure caused by impaired biventricular systolic function—usually predominant left ventricular dysfunction. The following section will discuss hypertrophic cardiomyopathy, in which marked left ventricular hypertrophy, in the absence of hypertension or aortic valve stenosis, is associated with impaired left ventricular filling and, in some cases, left ventricular outflow tract obstruction. Restrictive cardiomyopathy, in which ventricular filling is restricted secondary to endocardial or myocardial disease, is rarely seen in pediatric patients and will not be discussed.

The prevalence of dilated cardiomyopathy in the United States is approximately 0.02% per year, with an annual incidence of 6 new cases per 100,000 individuals. Males are more frequently affected, and the age of onset is variable. While there are no recent reliable data regarding the prevalence of dilated cardiomyopathy in children, between 1973 and 1987, 367 patients presented to the Children's Hosptial in Boston with

primary myocardial disease (dilated cardiomyopathy, myocarditis, or endocardial fibroelastosis), comprising 2.5% of cardiac admissions (6). A report from the Mayo Clinic in 1985 reported 24 children with myocarditis over a 10-year period (14). The reported etiologies of dilated cardiomyopathy are numerous and diverse, but unfortunately are rarely substantiated. Recent evidence has pointed toward chronic viral myocarditis and autoimmune mechanisms. The evidence for these mechanisms remains inconclusive, however, and most cases continue to be classified as idiopathic in nature (6).

Pathologically, there is significant enlargement of one or both ventricles, and not infrequently all four cardiac chambers are enlarged (48). The left ventricular wall thickness may be normal or decreased, but may thicken with time. There may be areas of softening of the endocardium, and endocardial fibroelastosis (EFE) may be present in the infant (18). On postmortem examination thrombi are found in one third of cases, most often in the left ventricular apex and the left atrial appendage. Microscopically, there is considerable variation among the various disease processes (6); however, degeneration of the sarcolemma or myocytosis is a fairly consistent feature. There may also be variability in the sizes of the remaining muscle cells (6). Other common features on histological examination include myocyte hypertrophy, interstitial fibrosis, and EFE (18).

Physical Symptoms and Clinical Signs

Patients often present with signs and symptoms of varying right and/or left ventricular failure—often in association with a recent viral upper respiratory infection (6). These symptoms seen in children and adolescents include varying degrees of dyspnea on exertion, orthopnea, fatigue, and paroxysmal nocturnal dyspnea. Other less frequent complaints include syncope, seizures, vomiting, abdominal pain, and chest pain. A positive family history of dilated cardiopathy may be present.

Physical findings vary with the severity and chronicity of the disease process. Signs of congestive heart failure are common, including tachypnea, tachycardia, diaphoresis, pallor, and hepatomegaly. The skin may be cool and clammy with diminished peripheral pulses. Jugular venous distention may be visible. Edema and ascites are less common and may reflect protein malnutrition secondary to chronic cardiac failure. Auscultation of the lungs may reveal rales at lung bases. Heart sounds may be muffled, and typically a third and/or fourth heart sound may be auscultated. Murmurs of mitral and tricuspid insufficiency are common, and pulmonic closure will be accentuated if there is pulmonary hypertension. A readily palpable precordial impulse may be present secondary to a diffuse and/or displaced left ventricular impulse.

Clinical and Laboratory Assessment

The electrocardiogram (ECG) shows a variety of abnormalities in dilated cardiomyopathy. The majority have ST-T changes, especially in the lateral and left precordial leads, with flattened or inverted T waves and ST segment depression, left atrial enlargement, and generalized low-voltage QRS complexes may be present (6). The ECG may occasionally mimic myocardial infarction with localized Q wave abnormalities and elevated ST segments. Arrhythmias are not uncommon (17), including:

- atrioventricular block, bundle branch block, fascicular block.
- atrial or ventricular ectopy,
- ventricular or supraventricular tachycardia.

The chest X ray typically demonstrates cardiomegaly when hemodynamic deterioration occurs. There is also pulmonary vascular plethora or redistribution, interstitial and alveolar edema, pleural effusions, and atelectasis.

Two-dimensional echocardiography is virtually diagnostic and reveals a dilated, thin-walled, and globally hypokinetic left ventricle (6, 46). Less frequently there is predominant right ventricular dilation or segmental dyskinesis. There may also be left and right atrial enlargement with a dilated vena cava and pulmonary veins. M-mode echocardiography confirms the chamber dilation and diminished ventricular function, as well as providing an estimate of wall stress. Color flow mapping is useful in quantifying the degree of mitral and tricuspid insufficiency, and conventional Doppler can be used to provide an estimate of pulmonary hypertension, using the velocity of the tricuspid insufficiency jet. Echocardiography is useful in excluding obstructive lesions or an anomalous left coronary artery arising from the pulmonary artery.

Radionuclide ventriculography demonstrates dilated ventricular chambers and a diminished ejection fraction. Cardiac catheterization reveals elevated left atrial and left ventricular end-diastolic pressures. Pulmonary arterial pressure may be modestly elevated. There is typically a reduced cardiac index with angiographic evidence of hypokinesis, mitral regurgitation, and occasionally filling defects secondary to a thrombus. Aortography and occasionally selective coronary arteriography are useful in excluding coronary pathology. Although there is controversy regarding its usefulness, catheterization is often accompanied by endomyocardial biopsy of the right or left ventricle in an effort to identify active inflammation.

Natural History

The prognosis for children with dilated cardiomyopathy varies (13, 15, 17, 57). Classically, if patients are not separated by age of presentation or presumptive diagnosis, approximately one third improve, one third remain unchanged, and one third die (17). Factors associated with the poorer outcome include:

- a positive family history,
- arrhythmias, and
- persistent cardiomegaly (18).

Management

Therapy for dilated cardiomyopathy begins with the treatment of the underlying disease, if known. Moderate salt restriction is indicated in conjunction with diuretic therapy (58). Anticoagulant drugs are important in preventing systemic and pulmonary embolism. Aspirin, Persantine, and warfarin have all been used. Lanoxin has traditionally been used in the treatment of dilated cardiomyopathy but its effectiveness may be limited. Whether lanoxin is more toxic and arrhythmogenic in dilated cardiomyopathy is controversial.

Angiotension converting enzyme inhibitors (ACE inhibitors) are the mainstay of treatments in adults and are becoming increasingly important in the treatment of dilated cardiomyopathy in infants and children. ACE inhibitors have been shown to improve cardiac performance, relieve signs and symptoms of congestive heart failure, and improve survival (50).

Although arrhythmias should be treated, caution needs to be exercised, since many antiarrhythmics have negative inotropic and/or proarrhythmic effects. If the endomyocardial biopsy reveals active inflammation, treatment with steroids or other immunosuppressive therapy is probably indicated. The studies supporting this are controversial, however.

Cardiac transplantation is indicated in acceptable candidates. Among studies in children, there has been a progressive decrease in short-term mortality (43). However, there remain some long-term concerns regarding the issue of premature and accelerated coronary artery disease in children who have undergone cardiac transplantation.

Exercise and Dilated Cardiomyopathy

The degree of exercise impairment in the child with dilated cardiomyopathy is dependent upon the degree of cardiac compromise imposed by the disease process. Those well compensated may not have any apparent impairment of their exercise capacity. However, most individuals have at least moderate impairment, evidenced historically by dyspnea on exertion, easy fatigability, chest pain, and occasionally syncope (50). On exercise testing, impairment is evidenced by decreased endurance time, a decreased $\dot{V}O_2max$,

and a blunted blood pressure response (60, 35). The chronotropic response at maximal exercise may be blunted, or there may be heart rates in excess of what would be expected at each stage of exercise.

There is usually subjective improvement in exercise performance after cardiac transplantation in patients with dilated cardiomyopathy. The transplanted heart is a denervated heart, and this is reflected in an increased resting heart rate (RHR) in adults who have been assessed following transplantation (44). Post-transplant patients also demonstrate increases in respiratory exchange ratio, minute ventilation, peak ventilatory equivalent, and lactate levels upon maximal exercise testing (53).

Those patients with dilated cardiomyopathy may also be at risk of sudden death during exertion, presumably from exercise-induced ventricular arrhythmias (39). Prior to being allowed to participate in exercise, they should undergo a thorough assessment of systolic and diastolic cardiac function by echocardiography and stress testing and, if necessary, radionuclide angiography or cardiac catheterization. However, studies in adults have shown no consistent correlation between measures of ventricular function and measures of exercise capacity (55). Prior to exercise each patient should also have an assessment of ventricular and supraventricular irritability by 24-hour ambulatory electrocardiography and a baseline clinical exercise test. Consideration should be given to close monitoring of each exercise session (55).

In spite of these risks, data suggest that careful exercise and training may have a beneficial effect on adult patients with dilated cardiomyopathy and congestive heart failure. Rehabilitation can augment the patient's exercise capacity and improve the comfort with which submaximal exercise can be carried out. One study at Duke University documented a 26% increase in $\dot{V}O_2max$ and an 18% increase in exercise duration after a 16-24-week training program (55). It remains to be determined whether there is an adverse effect on prognosis.

Exercise and Sport Participation for Children With Dilated Cardiomyopathy

Recommendations are limited regarding sport participation in children with dilated cardiomyopathy. While those children significantly affected will to a large extent limit their own participation, they may also need to be restricted. Because of the risk of sudden death secondary to arrhythmia, these children are generally advised against participation in strenuous sports (39). However, those children with less significant cardiac dysfunction may participate in sports with lower dynamic and static demands, and may also safely tolerate other activities.

After transplantation, restrictions on the avoidance of competitive athletics may be relaxed to varying degrees. In fact, there is one example of a soccer player competing at the highest international level after transplantation. Table 17.3 summarizes recommendations for sport participation in children with dilated cardiomyopathy.

HYPERTROPHIC CARDIOMYOPATHY

Hypertrophic cardiomyopathy (HCM) is a primary myocardial disease that is genetically transmitted in a pattern consistent with an autosomal dominant trait (25).

Description of Hypertrophic Cardiomyopathy

Pathophysiology

Although up to 55% of HCM cases have been found to have evidence of familial transmission, the exact percentages of autosomal dominant transmission are unknown. Certainly, a reasonable percentage of cases appear to be sporadic in nature—probably representing either new mutations or an autosomal recessive inheritance with reduced gene penetrance. Genetic heterogeneity exists within families, with a gene penetrance having a risk of transmission of future offspring that may approach 50% but in other families probably below 25%. Cardiomyopathies characterized by left ventricular hypertrophy may also be found in a number of noncardiac conditions such as pheochromocytoma, tuberous sclerosis, neurofibromatosis, lentiginosis, Friedreich ataxia, Pompe's disease, Turner and Noonan Syndromes, and hyperthyroidism.

Pathologically, hypertrophic cardiomyopathy is characterized grossly as a hypertrophied and nondilated left ventricle. This occurs in the absence of a coexisting cardiac or systemic disease capable of producing left ventricular hypertrophy, e.g., aortic stenosis or systemic hypertension (25). The left ventricular cavity is usually small or normal in size, and the increased left ventricular mass is caused almost totally by an increase in left ventricular wall thickness. The distribution of the left ventricular hypertrophy is variable—mild and localized in some patients but more diffuse in others (25). Histologically, the disease is characterized by cardiac muscle-cell disorganization, myocardial scarring, and abnormalities of the small intramural arteries

Table 17.3   Sports Participation in Dilated Cardiomyopathy (See Chapter 3)

Cardiovascular (CV) involvement	Activities contraindicated	Activities permitted	Other considerations
1. Mildly diminished LV function with mild-moderate valvular insufficiency	High-moderate dynamic/static	Low intensity Other activities of higher intensity as determined by LV function, symptoms & ± arrhythmias	Participation largely determined by symptoms (chest pain, syncope, palpitations & LV function)
2. Moderate-severe LV dysfunction and/or severe valvular insufficiency	All competitive sports	Recreational walking and cardiac rehabilitation	
3. Posttransplantation	None unless prohibited by arrhythmias, deconditioning or noncardiac reasons	All activities as tolerated	

(25, 58). Ninety-five percent of patients have some degree of cellular disorganization contributing to impaired diastolic or systolic function and possibly serving as a nidus for ventricular dysrhythmia (25). Myocardial scarring varies from patchy interstitial fibrosis to extensive and grossly visible transmural scars. Small intramural coronary arteries are abnormal in about 80% of cases with thickened vessel walls and narrowed lumens. There may be a causal relationship between the abnormal coronary vessels and the myocardial scarring, suggesting a form of "small vessel" disease contributing to the myocardial ischemia and necrosis seen in some patients.

Obstruction to left ventricular outflow may occur secondary to subaortic septal hypertrophy and/or to systolic anterior motion of the mitral valve (25). Left ventricular inflow is often impaired secondary to altered left ventricular relaxation and distensibility. The altered coronary circulation and the thickened myocardium may cause myocardial ischemia via an imbalance between myocardial oxygen supply and demand.

Physical Symptoms and Clinical Signs

The primary symptoms in HCM are exertional chest pain, dyspnea, fatigue, lightheadedness, near-syncope, and syncope (26). Other symptoms found in adults include orthopnea, paroxysmal nocturnal dyspnea, and palpitations. Commonly, there are no symptoms, or the initial symptom is sudden unexpected death (34). In children and infants, HCM is often diagnosed when the child is referred for the evaluation of a murmur. Unfortunately there is no consistent relationship between symptomatology and obstructive phenomena. Physical findings are variable and related in large measure to the hemodynamic state. The classic findings found in the obstructive form of HCM include an increased apical impulse that may be double or triple in nature. The carotid pulse may be bifid in nature. Patients with obstruction have a medium-pitched systolic murmur heard best at the lower left sternal border in two-thirds of cases, and at the upper left sternal border in one third. The intensity of the murmur varies with the severity of left ventricular outflow obstruction, as well as with different physical maneuvers. Some individuals may also have an apical diastolic

Table 17.4   Physiological and Pharmacological Maneuvers That Affect the Murmur of HCM

Maneuver	Murmur intensity	Effect on LVOT/volume
Squatting	↓	↓/↑
Upright posture	↑	↑/↓
Exercise	↑	↑/−
Amyl nitrite	↑	↑/↓

rumbling murmur, probably related to impaired left ventricular compliance (Table 17.4).

Clinical and Laboratory Assessment

The electrocardiogram (ECG) may show a wide variety of abnormalities, varying from subtle to more overt. Patients with normal ECGs usually have the nonobstructive form of HCM. No particular pattern is characteristic but the most common abnormalities include

- left ventricular hypertrophy,
- S-T segment alterations,
- inverted T waves,
- left atrial enlargement,
- abnormal Q waves, and
- absent R waves in the lateral precordial leads.

The chest X ray has limited diagnostic usefulness in HCM. An increased cardiac silhouette is sometimes present, usually secondary to increased left ventricular mass and left atrial enlargement. However, if one has an index of suspicion, echocardiography is diagnostic. Two-dimensional echocardiography reveals the characteristic left ventricular hypertrophy. This is usually asymmetrical in nature; that is, the septum is thicker than the free wall of the left ventricle. However, even with echocardiography there may be some degree of overlap between the physiological and usually concentric hypertrophy seen in certain athletes, and the abnormal hypertrophy of HCM. M-mode echocardiography confirms the typical systolic anterior motion of the mitral valve (Figure 17.4). Finally, Doppler interrogation may confirm left ventricular outflow obstruction or an abnormal left ventricular filling pattern.

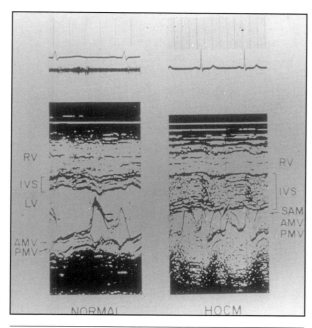

Figure 17.4 M-mode echocardiogram of patient with hypertrophic cardiomyopathy.

Natural History

The clinical course of affected individuals with HCM is variable, with some progressively deteriorating and others remaining stable for decades. Progression of the disease process may develop along several pathways, including left ventricular outflow obstruction, impaired left ventricular filling, and possibly myocardial ischemia (26). The onset of important symptoms in early childhood usually indicates early disease progression.

Therapeutic Intervention

Treatment of HCM may be medical or surgical. Beta blockers have been the primary agents used in HCM since the mid-1960s (12). They can relieve all of the principal cardiac symptoms, including angina, dyspnea, lightheadedness, and syncope. Some also recommend the use of beta blockers in asymptomatic patients to try to retard progression or prevent sudden death, especially in those patients with a positive family history of premature sudden death, marked left ventricular hypertrophy on echocardiography, and abnormal ECG (24). However, it is not universally accepted that anything is effective in preventing sudden death. Verapamil also improves cardiac symptoms and exercise capacity in most patients with HCM, probably by reducing heart rate and blood pressure (26), or by improving left ventricular filling.

Surgery (septal myotomy or myectomy) has been recommended for severely affected individuals whose symptoms resist medical treatment and whose resting or provacated left ventricular outflow gradients are greater than or equal to 50 mmHg. Although surgery may decrease symptoms and improve the quality of life, there is no evidence that it prolongs life (25, 61). More recently, the use of dual-chamber pacing has been found to be an effective alternative to surgery in most patients with obstructive HCM and drug refractory symptoms (10).

Other measures employed include the judicious use of diuretic agents for pulmonary edema, medical treatment of arrhythmias, and endocarditis prophylaxis.

Morbidity and Mortality

Premature cardiac death is common in HCM, with an annual mortality rate of 2-4% (25), increasing to 8% in affected individuals with documented ventricular tachycardia. Death is sudden and unexpected in 85% of cases, and is particularly common in children and young adults between 12 and 35 years of age (28, 30). HCM is the leading cause of sudden death (Table 17.5) among young athletes (27, 30, 32), and one third of sudden death cases occur during strenuous physical activities (29). Risk factors for sudden death in HCM include

- young age,
- ventricular tachycardia on 24-48-hour ambulatory ECG (36),
- family history of sudden death in more than one first-degree relative with HCM (28), and
- marked and diffuse left ventricular hypertrophy conferring a predisposition for

Table 17.5 Most Common Causes of Sudden Death in the Young Athlete

1. HCM
2. Aberrant coronary artery
3. Aortic dissection (Marfan's)
4. Premature atherosclerotic disease

potentially life-threatening dysrhythmias and possibly sudden death (61).

Syncope and severe dyspnea are the only symptoms predictive of sudden death (34).

The mechanism of sudden death has not been definitely identified. However, the common final pathway is most likely ventricular dysrhythmia (25, 34).

Exercise and Hypertrophic Cardiomyopathy

Because many individuals with hypertrophic cardiomyopathy (HCM) are asymptomatic, there is often no history of exercise intolerance, dyspnea on exertion, or chest pain (24). Exertional syncope or palpitations may be present and should be considered significant (31, 63, 24). Individuals with significant left ventricular outflow tract obstruction may have objective evidence of exercise intolerance by exercise testing, including chest pain or syncope, ischemic changes on ECG, excessive heart rate response for workload, and exercise-induced ventricular dysrhythmias (4) (Figure 17.5).

A history of palpitations is also worrisome and warrants 24-hour ambulatory ECG and possibly an electrophysiological study (EPS). EPS may help identify arrhythmic causes for cardiac arrest and syncope. In the absence of syncope,

induction of sustained ventricular dysrhythmia may aid in identifying patients at risk for sudden death and possibly predict the need for the use of an implantable cardioverter defibrillator device (11). The Bethesda Conference recommends that young people with HCM be excluded from participation in strenuous athletics if any of the following exist (28):

- marked left ventricular hypertrophy on echocardiogram (absolute ventricular thickness greater than or equal to 20 mm), either of the interventricular septum or the left ventricular free wall;
- evidence of significant left ventricular outflow obstruction under basal conditions, estimated by echocardiogram or catheterization (peak systolic gradient greater than 50 mmHg);
- important ventricular or atrial arrhythmias on ambulatory ECG (e.g., ventricular tachycardia, couplets, frequent premature ventricular or atrial contractions, atrial fibrillation, or atrial tachycardia);
- history of sudden death in relatives with HCM, particularly if less than 40 years of age;
- history of syncope.

There are few or no data on the beneficial effects of exercise in children and adolescents

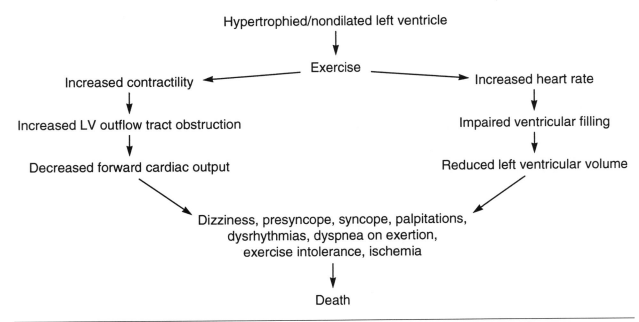

Figure 17.5 Presumed pathophysiology in exercise in patient with hypertrophic cardiomyopathy.
Data from American Academy of Pediatrics (1971).

with HCM. As mentioned with Marfan's syndrome, it is important not to limit participation unnecessarily so as not to hinder the child's general level of physical fitness or self-image.

Exercise and Sport Programs for Children With Hypertrophic Cardiomyopathy

The guidelines for sport restriction were outlined in the preceding section. Those athletes with none of the risk factors previously mentioned may be considered for participation in some low-intensity competitive sports, as may some with one or more risk factors if there are no symptoms (chest pain, syncope, or palpitations), or no minimal left ventricular outflow obstruction and no documented arrhythmias. After medical and surgical treatment, the child is usually subject to the same restrictions.

REFERENCES

1. Alpert, B.S.; Moes, D.M.; DuRast, R.H.; et al. Hemodynamic responses to ergometer exercises in children and young adults with left ventricular perssure or volume overload. Am. J. Cardiol. 52:563-567; 1983.
2. Beals, R.K.; Hecht, F. Congenital contractural arachnodactyly. J. Bone Joint Surg. 53-1:987-993; 1971.
3. Braden, D.S.; Strong, W.B. Preparation screening for sudden cardiac death in high school and college athletes. Phys. Sports Med. 16:128-140; 1988.
4. Canedo, M.I.; Frank, M.J.; Abdulla, A.M. Rhythm disturbances in hypertrophic cardiomyopathy: prevalence, relation to symptoms and management. Am. J. Cardiol. 45:848-855; 1980.
5. Cantwell, J.D. Marfan's syndrome: detection and management. Phys. Sports Med. 14:51-55; 1986.
6. Colan, S.D.; Spevak, P.S.; Parness, I.A.; Wadar, A.S. Cardiomyopathies. In: Fuler, D.C. ed. Pediatric cardiology. Philadelphia: Hanleu and Belfus; 1992:329-361.
7. Crawford, E.S.; Caselli, J.S. Marfan's syndrome: combined compositive valve graft replacement of the aortic and transaortic

mitral valve replacement. An. Thorac Surg. 45:296-302; 1988.
8. Cumming, G.R. Maximal exercise capacity of children with heart defects. Am. J. Cardiol. 42:613-619; 1978.
9. Epstein, S.E.; Maron, B.J. Sudden death and the competitive athlete: perspectives on preparticipation screening studies. J. Am. Coll. Cardiol. 7(1):220-230; 1986.
10. Fananapazir, L.; Cannon, R.O.; Tripodi, D.; Panza, J.A. Impact of dual-chamber permanent pacing patients with obstructive hypertrophic cardiomyopathy with symptoms refractory to verapamil and β-adrenergic blocker therapy. Circulation 85:2149-2161; 1992.
11. Fananapazir, L.; Chang, A.C.; Epstein, S.E.; McAreavey, D. Prognostic determinants in hypertrophic cardiomyopathy. Prospective evaluation of a therapeutic strategy based on clinical, holter, hemodynamic, and electrophysiological findings. Circulation 86:730-740; 1992.
12. Flamm, M.D.; Harrison, D.C.; Hancoch, E.W. Muscular subaortic stenosis: prevention of outflow obstruction with propanolol. Circulation 38:846-858; 1986.
13. Fuler, D.C.; Buckley, L.P.; Hellerbrand, W.E.; et al. Report of the New England Regional Infant Cardiac Program. Pediatrics 65:375-461; 1980.
14. Fuster, V.; Geush, B.J.; Gulliani, E.R.; et al. The natural history of idiopathic dilated cardiomyopathy. Am. J. Cardiol. 47:525-531; 1981.
15. Gillium, R.F. Idiopathic cardiomyopathy in the United States, 1970-1982. Am. Heart J. 111:752-755; 1986.
16. Godwin, J.D. Examination of the thoracic aorta by computed tomography. Chest 858:564-567; 1984.
17. Greenwood, R.D.; Wadas, A.S.; Fuler, D.C. The clinical course of primary myocardial disease in infants and children. Am. Heart J. 42:549-560; 1976.
18. Griffin, M.I.; Hernandez, A.; Martin, T.C.; et al. Dilated cardiomyopathy in infants and children. JACC 111:139-144; 1988.
19. Hecht, F.; Beals, R.K. "New" syndrome of congenital contractural arachnodactyly originally described by Marfan in 1896. Pediatrics 40:574-579; 1971.

20. Hirst, A.E.; Gore, T. Marfan's syndrome: a review. Prog. Cardiovasc. Dis. 16:187-198; 1973.

21. James, F.W.; Donner, R.; Kaplan, S. Exercise responses in children with progressive aortic regurgitation. Am. J. Cardiol. 41:389; 1978.

22. Kramer, M.R.; Drori, Y.; Lev, B. Sudden death in young soldiers, high incidence of syncope prior to death. Chest 93:345-347; 1988.

23. Lambert, E.C.; Vijeyan, A.M.; Wagner, H.R.; Vlad, P. Sudden unexpected death from cardiovascular disease in children, a cooperative international study. Am. J. Cardiol. 34:89-96; 1974.

24. Maron, B.J. Cardiomyopathies in Heart Disease in Infants, Children, and Adolescents. In: Adams, F.H.; Emmesouilides, G.G.; Reimerschneider, T.A., ed. Williams and Williams, 1989; 940-964.

25. Maron, B.J.; Bonow, R.O.; Cannon, R.O.; et al. Hypertrophic cardiomyopathy interventions of clinical manifestations, pathophysiology, and therapy. Part I. N. Engl. J. Med. 316:780-789; 1987.

26. Maron, B.J.; Bonow, R.O.; Cannon, R.O.; et al. Hypertrophic cardiomyopathy interventions of clinical manifestations, pathophysiology, and therapy. Part 2. N. Engl. J. Med. 316: 844-852; 1987.

27. Maron, B.J.; Epstein, S.E.; Roberts, E.C. Causes of sudden death in competitive athletes. J. Am. Coll. Cardiol. 7:204-214; 1986.

28. Maron, B.J.; Lipson, L.C.; Roberts, W.C.; et al. "Malignant" hypertrophic cardiomyopathy: identification of a subgroup of families with unusually frequent premature death. Am. J. Cardiol. 41:1133-1140; 1978.

29. Maron, B.J.; Roberts, W.C.; Epstein, S.E. Sudden death in hypertrophic cardiomyopathy: profile of 78 patients. Circulation 65:1394; 1982.

30. Maron, B.J.; Roberts, W.C.; McAllister, H.A.; et al. Sudden death in young athletes. Circulation 62:218-229; 1980.

31. Maron, B.J.; Savage, D.D.; Wolfson, J.K.; et al. Prognostic significance of 24-hour ambulatory electrocardiographic monitoring in patients with hypertrophic cardiomyopathy: a prospective study. Am. J. Cardiol. 48: 252-257; 1981.

32. Maron, B.J.; Tajik, A.S.; Ruttenberg, H.D.; et al. Hypertrophic cardiomyopathy in infants: clinical features and natural history. Circulation 65:7-17; 1982.

33. Maron, B.J.; Wolfson, J.K.; Epstein, S.E.; Roberts, W.C. Intramural ("small vessel") coronary artery disease in hypertrophic cardiomyopathy. JACC 8:545-557; 1986.

34. McCaffrey, F.M.; Braden, D.S.; Strong, W.B. Sudden cardiac death in young athletes: a review. Am. J. Dis. Child. 145:177-183; 1991.

35. McElroy, P.A.; Janicki, J.S.; Weber, K.T. Cardiopulmonary exercise testing in congestive heart failure. Am. J. Cardiol. 62:35A; 1988.

36. McKenna, W.J.; England, D.; Doi, Y.L.; et al. Arrhythmia in hypertrophic cardiomyopathy. I. Influence as prognosis. Br. Heart J. 46:168-172; 1981.

37. McKusik, V.A. Heritable disorder of connective tissue. 4th ed. St. Louis: C.V. Mosby; 1972:61-201.

38. Missri, J.C.; Swett, D.D. Marfan syndrome: a review. Cardiol. Rev. Rep. 3:1645-1653; 1982.

39. Mitchell, S.H.; Maron, B.J.; Epstein, S.E. Sixteenth Bethesda Conference: cardiovascular abnormalities in the athlete: recommendations regarding eligibility for competition. JACC 6:1186-1224; 1984.

40. Moose, R.P.; Rockenmacher, S.; Pyevitz, R.E.; Sanders, S.P.; Bieber, F.R.; Lin, A.; MacLead, P.; Hall, B.; Graham, J.M., Jr. Diagnosis and management of infantile Marfan syndrome. Pediatrics 86:888-895; 1990.

41. Murdoch, J.L.; Walker, B.A.; Halpen, B.L.; et al. Life expectancy and causes of death in the Marfan Syndrome. N. Engl. J. Med. 286-304; 1972.

42. Oakley, C.M. Clinical decisions in the cardiomyopathies. Hosp. Prac. (Oct): 41-60; 1985.

43. Pennington, D.G.; Sarafian, J.; Swartz, M. Heart transplantation in children. Heart Transplant 4:441-445; 1985.

44. Pflugfelder, P.W.; Purves, P.D.; McKenzie, F.N.; et al. Cardiac dynamics during supine exercise in cyclosporin treated orthopid heart transplant recipients: assessment by radionuclide angiography. JACC 10:336-341; 1987.

45. Phillips, M.; Robinowitz, M.; Higgins, J.R.; et al. Sudden cardiac death in Air Force recruits, a 20 year review. JAMA 256:2696-2699; 1986.

46. Pinamant, B.; Alberti, E.; Cigalotti, A.; et al. Echocardiogram findings in myocarditis. Am. J. Cardiol. 62:285-291; 1988.

47. Pyeritz, R.E. The Marfan syndrome. Am. Fam. Phys. 34:83-94; 1986.

48. Pyeritz, R.E. Heritable disorders of connective tissue. In: Fortin, N.J., ed. Current therapy in cardiovascular disease. Philadelphia: Decker; 1987:274-276.

49. Pyeritz, R.E.; McKusick, V.A. The Marfan syndrome: diagnosis and management. N. Engl. J. Med. 300:722-777; 1979.

50. Rezkalla, S.; Kloner, R.A. Myocarditis and cardiomyopathy. Cardiovasc. Rev. Rep. 48-66; 1991.

51. Roberts, W.C. Congenital heart disease in adults. Philadelphia: F.A. Davis, 1979:443-449.

52. Roberts, W.C.; Ferrons. Pathologic anatomy of the cardiomyopathies: idiopathic dilated and hypertrophic types, infiltrate types, and endomyocardial disease with and without eosinophilia. Hum. Pathol. 6:287-342; 1975.

53. Savin, W.M.; Haskell, W.I.; Schroeder, T.S.; Stinson, E.B. Cardiorespiratory response of cardiac transplant patients to graded, symptom-limited exercise. Circulation 62: 55-60; 1980.

54. Sisk, H.E.; Zahka, K.G.; Pyeritz, R.E. The Marfan syndrome in early childhood: analysis of 15 patients diagnosed at less than 4 years of age. Am. J. Cardiol. 52:353-358; 1983.

55. Smith, L.K. Exercise in patients with heart failure. In: Shephard, R.J.; Miller, H.S., ed. Exercise and the heart in health and cardiac disease. New York: Marcel Dekker; 1992: 397-412.

56. Soulen, R.L.; Fishman, E.K.; Pyeritz, R.E.; et al. Marfan syndrome: evaluation with MR imaging versus CT. Radiology 165:697-701; 1987.

57. Talerico, C.P.; Seward, J.B.; Driscoll, D.J.; et al. Idiopathic dilated cardiomyopathy in the young: clinical profile and natural history. JACC 6:1126-1131; 1985.

58. Treave, D. Asymmetrical hypertrophy of the heart in young adults. Br. Heart J. 20:1-8; 1958.

59. Wagenroort, C.A.; Neufeld, H.W.; Edwards, J.E. Cardiovascular system in Marfan's syndrome and in idiopathic dilation of the ascending aorta. Am. J. Cardiol. 9:496-507; 1962.

60. Weinder, D.A. Clinical significance of abnormal blood pressure response during exercise stress testing. Practical. Cardiol. 10:37-45; 1984.

61. Wigle, E.D.; Sassan, Z.; Henderson, M.A.; et al. Hypertrophic cardiomyopathy. The importance of the site and the extent of hypertrophy. A review. Prog. Cardiovasc. Dis. 28:1-83; 1985.

62. World Health Organization. Report of the WHO/IFSC task force on the definition and classification of cardiac myopathies. Br. Heart J. 44:672-673; 1980.

63. Zahka, K.G.; Hansley, C.; Glesby, M.; Pyeritz, R.E. The impact of medical and surgical therapy on the cardiovascular prognosis of the Marfan syndrome in early childhood (abstract). JACC 13:119A; 1989.

CHAPTER 18

Chronic Renal Disease

Thomas L. Kennedy III
Bridgeport Hospital, Bridgeport, CT

Norman J. Siegel
Yale University School of Medicine

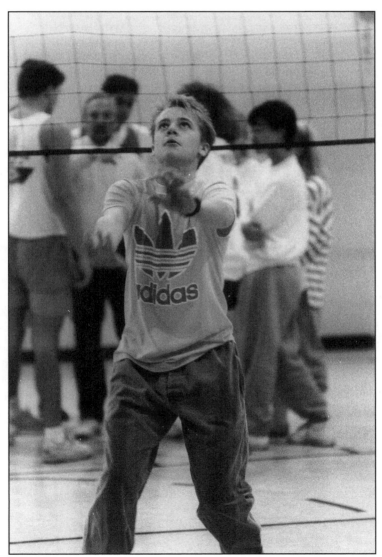

The outlook for the child or adolescent with renal failure is very good and continues to improve. Prompt and accurate diagnosis should lead to measures that recognize, treat, and prevent some complications of renal disease. When renal failure is severe and irreversible, replacement therapy by kidney transplant may permit the recipient to lead a long and active life. Nevertheless, the potential for problems is great and includes such major concerns as undernutrition, growth failure, anemia, hypertension, risk of infection, skeletal demineralization, acidosis, and electrolyte abnormalities. Any of these may lead to limitation of physical activity and a decrease in fitness, unless the importance of exercise is recognized and made part of the patient's treatment plan and lifestyle.

DESCRIPTION OF CHRONIC RENAL DISEASE

Chronic renal insufficiency is an irreversible reduction in kidney function. Although there is no firmly established level of function which defines chronic renal failure, a decrease of 60% or more is used. The course and rate of progression may vary, but renal insufficiency predictably leads to a level of dysfunction which is inadequate to maintain fluid, electrolyte, and excretory balance. This generally occurs when renal function declines to less than 5% of normal, and is called end-stage renal disease (ESRD). At this point some form of renal replacement therapy must be instituted, either dialysis or transplantation. In children, transplantation is virtually always the treatment of choice because it permits a more independent and active lifestyle. If dialysis is begun, there are two alternatives, peritoneal dialysis or hemodialysis. Among adolescents 3 years after the onset of ESRD, 60% have received transplants, 10% are on peritoneal dialysis, and 30% are on hemodialysis (28). Most children on peritoneal dialysis carry out either continuous ambulatory peritoneal dialysis (CAPD) or continuous cycling peritoneal dialysis (CCPD). In both forms the patient has a reservoir of dialysate in the peritoneal cavity throughout the day. Thus, children and adolescents considered in this chapter who are broadly characterized as having chronic renal failure include three groups:

- those with significantly reduced renal function,
- those with ESRD who are on dialysis, and
- those with ESRD who have received a kidney transplant.

Renal disease and dysfunction are generally considered synonymous with the diminished ability of the kidneys to filter and remove nitrogenous waste products from the blood—that is, a decrease in the glomerular filtration rate (GFR). Although glomerular filtration is an essential function of the kidney and is easily measured clinically, it is only one of many tasks which are disturbed in renal failure and which may have significant clinical implications.

In health the kidneys act to maintain fluid, electrolyte, and acid-base balance, help to regulate blood pressure, and serve as endocrine organs through their role in the metabolism of Vitamin D, the production of erythropoietin, and the secretion of renin, prostaglandins, and kinins. With renal failure the disruption of these multiple functions can profoundly affect the health and activity of the child by causing volume and electrolyte abnormalities, acidosis, hypertension, bone disease, growth failure, anemia, and malnutrition. Any attempt at optimizing the child's lifestyle, including physical activity and exercise, must address the impact as well as the treatment and prevention of these abnormalities.

Incidence

The incidence of ESRD in the pediatric population (ages 19 years or less) in the United States is 11 per million annually (28), or approximately 830 cases per year. About 85% of these are 5 years or older and 55% are adolescents, defining the population for which an exercise and sport program is most realistic. Males outnumber females 1.5:1 and there is no strong racial predominance, except that African-Americans between 15 and 19 years of age have an annual incidence of 42 per million.

Causes

The causes of pediatric ESRD vary somewhat by location and also change with age. Nationally, acquired glomerulonephritis accounts for about

33% of cases, congenital or heritable conditions for about 25%, systemic disease (e.g., systemic lupus erythematosus, hemolytic uremic syndrome) for about 10%, and obstructive nephropathy for about 10% (19). The causes are significant for the following reasons:

- renal disease which is present at birth and throughout childhood is much more likely to interfere with growth;
- renal disease caused by or associated with urologic abnormalities (e.g., posterior urethral valves) may be complicated by the persistence of urologic problems even after transplantation;
- renal disease associated with systemic disease (e.g., systemic lupus erythematosus) may be complicated by extrarenal involvement (e.g., neurological, cardiac), which may affect exercise capacity; and
- some causes of acquired pediatric ESRD may lead to recurrent disease in an allograft.

Pathophysiology

The pathological appearance of the end stage kidney and the clinical syndrome of ESRD are remarkably similar, independently of the underlying cause(s). The mechanism of injury, however, varies considerably. For example, in renal dysplasia the kidney tissue is intrinsically disorganized and dysfunctional. In a severe ischemic, hypoxemic insult, there is widespread cell death and loss of functional renal tissue. In glomerulonephritis, renal injury is immune-mediated through the inflammatory release of mediators which damage kidney tissue. These examples and others share in common the reduction in functioning nephrons in the face of a continuing excretory load, thus placing increased requirements on remaining nephrons. Much of what is known of the pathophysiology of chronic renal failure is derived from the long-standing clinical observation that major reduction in renal function may occur without serious disturbances in body fluid composition or clinical consequences, until the GFR falls to levels of less than 10% of normal. That is, the remaining nephrons make a series of compensatory adaptations, functioning at an increased level and bearing the relatively increased excretory load, which contributes significantly to their eventual demise.

The compensatory changes exact their own price, however, long before ESRD is reached. One example frequently cited is the renal handling of phosphorus. As the GFR declines the decrease in the filtered load of phosphorus will lead to hyperphosphatemia unless the reabsorption of phosphate is also reduced. In order to achieve this, the parathyroid responds with increased secretion of parathormone (PTH), which increases phosphaturia. Increased PTH, however, contributes to the bone disease of renal disease—renal osteodystrophy—thus creating a "trade-off" for the compensation it provides.

Presentation

Pediatric patients with chronic renal insufficiency may present in many different ways. Some clinical patterns are predictable and are directly associated with symptoms referable to the kidneys or urinary tract, while others are quite nonspecific. For example, the child presenting with abnormalities in urine output may have oliguria (because of a severely reduced GFR), or polyuria (because of the inability of the kidneys to concentrate the urine). Renal insufficiency may be discovered as an incidental finding during a routine physical examination in connection with elevated blood pressure, an abnormal urinalysis (e.g., hematuria, proteinuria), or an abdominal mass (e.g., hydronephrosis or distended bladder). Alternatively, the presentation may be dramatic, with the sudden onset of seizures related to electrolyte disturbances or severe hypertension. The presentation of CRF may also be subtle with the complaint or discovery of fatigue, poor appetite, slowed growth, weight loss, or anemia.

Assessment

Important in the clinical assessment of the child with CRF is the determination of blood pressure. This should be obtained on several occasions when the child is relaxed with a stable, resting heart rate; an appropriately sized cuff should also be used. Because ESRD may be associated with autonomic dysfunction and abnormal intravascular volume, it is important to obtain blood pressures in both the recumbent and the standing positions. Other important clinical signs of renal disease include edema, pallor, abdominal distention or tenderness, decreased muscle strength, and poor nutritional status. Edema may reflect salt and water retention caused by a greatly diminished GFR, or a very low serum albumin caused by heavy proteinuria. Abdominal tenderness is especially significant in the child on peritoneal dialysis since peritonitis is the most important complication of this therapy, and in the child with a transplant since tenderness around the allograft is an important sign of rejection. Motor strength may be decreased because of poor nutrition, deconditioning stemming from inactivity, myopathy secondary to steroid therapy, peripheral neuropathy associated with the uremic state, and bone pain related to renal osteodystrophy.

Laboratory assessment should be directed at identifying the many and common abnormalities accompanying CRF (see Table 18.1). These include anemia, hyperkalemia, hyponatremia, metabolic acidosis, hyperphosphatemia, hypocalcemia, hypoalbuminemia, and hyperuricemia. Serial assessment of renal function through the determination of the creatinine clearance tends to overestimate the extent of residual GFR as renal disease progresses, although it remains the best test that is easily available. An alternative method of quickly and accurately assessing GFR without a time urine collection is the formula:

$$GFR = 0.55\ Ht\ (cm)\ /\ P_{cr}$$

where GFR is the estimated glomerular filtration rate corrected for body surface area to $1.73M^2$, Ht is the body height in centimeters, and P_{cr} is the serum creatinine in mg/dl (26).

The status of parathyroid function should be assessed periodically by an assay of PTH that is not affected by GFR (e.g., intact or N-terminal PTH). In children with some residual renal function, it is important to exclude any problem that could hasten the progression to ESRD. For example, the physician should obtain a urine culture to exclude infection, and an initial renal ultrasound to exclude urinary tract obstruction. In the child who is not oliguric it is important to know whether the kidneys have the ability to concentrate the urine. If not, under conditions of excessive fluid losses (e.g., heat, exercise) continued obligate renal water loss could lead to dehydration. Therefore, adequate fluids must be continuously available.

Table 18.1 Clinical Findings Associated With Renal Insufficiency in Childhood

Presentation	Abnormality	Laboratory study	Therapy
Pallor, fatigue	Anemia	Hematocrit, Retic Ct. Serum Fe, Ferritin	Erythropoietin
Tachypnea, hyperpnea	Metabolic acidosis	Serum bicarbonate	Alkali
Muscle weakness	Hyperkalemia	Serum potassium	Restrict intake; K'-resin binder
Lethargy, malaise	Hyponatremia	Serum sodium	Fluid restriction
Bone pain/fractures	Osteodystrophy	Serum Ca', Phos, PTH, Alkaline Phosphatase	Ca' supplements; PO binders; vitamin D
Poor growth/weight gain	Poor appetite	Serum Albumin, Pre-albumin, calorie count	Caloric supplements Nutrition consultation
Rapid weight gain	Edema, fluid excess	Serum albumin, sodium	Restrict NaCl, water intake; diuretics
Headaches, irritability	Hypertension	Monitor blood pressure	Diet, exercise, restrict NaCl; medication
Seizures	Hypertension, hyponatremia	Monitor blood pressure Serum sodium	Medication, Na' supplements; dialysis

Natural History

The typical course in a child who is discovered to have chronic renal insufficiency is a relentless progression to ESRD. Although the rate of progression may vary for different conditions and may span many months or years, the need for renal replacement is usually required. Early in the course the child may be totally asymptomatic, even with substantial loss of renal function (e.g., 60-70%). Attention must be directed at subclinical abnormalities such as the earliest signs of renal osteodystrophy. This disorder, which was formerly a major cause or morbidity in pediatric ESRD but is now totally preventable, results from a combination of factors including inadequate levels of 1,25-dihydroxyvitamin D, chronic acidosis, and hyperparathyroidism. Although abnormalities should also be identified and addressed in order to avoid later morbidity, overt symptoms including the vague complex of constitutional complaints known as the uremic syndrome (e.g., malaise, fatigue, anorexia, somnolence, and pruritus) are usually not evident until the GFR is reduced to less than 10% of normal. If careful attention is given to the progression of the CRF, overt symptoms can be prevented and avoided through treatment and the timely institution of some form of replacement therapy.

Intervention

The ultimate intervention in ESRD is the institution of replacement therapy, either dialysis or transplantation. Before these therapies are required, however, the physician can attempt to prevent or correct the problems which frequently accompany chronic renal insufficiency.

First, an aggressive program to provide adequate nutrition should be started. Calorie counts should be determined routinely because the anorexia caused by CRF frequently causes deficient intake. Carbohydrate and lipid calories should be maximized because they do not increase renal solute load and stress the kidney. The composition of fat-derived calories must be monitored, however, since the child with renal disease and the nephrotic syndrome generally has hyperlipidemia with an unfavorable lipid profile (high LDL, low HDL). Protein calories, which are metabolized to nitrogenous wastes, must be excreted by the kidneys; thus, their consumption must be regulated. Clinical studies have suggested that dietary protein restriction can slow the decline in renal function, while unrestricted protein consumption hastens the progression of CRF. Although a firm recommendation for protein restriction is not available, a reasonable goal is an intake of 1-2 gm/kg/day. Increased allowances must be made for children with unremitting nephrotic-range proteinuria.

One of the most recent and important interventions in CRF is the treatment of anemia. Anemia is almost always present in chronic renal disease and is a major contributor to the fatigue and decreased physical activity in children with ESRD. The causes of the anemia are multiple. Nutritional deficiencies of iron and folate, uremic bleeding diathesis, and a slight decline in erythrocyte survival all contribute to the anemia, but the most important cause is a deficiency of erythropoietin (Epo), the renal hormone which stimulates marrow red blood cell production. The clinical availability of recombinant Epo has dramatically altered the therapy of the anemia of CRF, which was previously treated with blood transfusions and their attendant risks. Regular injections of Epo are very successful in correcting the anemia, and have been free of side effects except for hypertension resulting from increased intravascular volume.

Hypertension commonly accompanies CRF and may occur on a volume and/or renin-dependent basis. Treatment frequently requires one or more antihypertensive agents, although careful control of salt intake and diuretic therapy may also be helpful. Hypocalcemia, hyperphosphatemia, and renal osteodystrophy may be prevented by administration of Vitamin D, usually in the form of 1,25-dihydroxyvitamin D, and by administration of oral calcium carbonate, which serves as a calcium supplement and as a phosphate binder in the gut when given with meals. Acidosis, when severe, may be corrected by the administration of alkali, either as bicarbonate or citrate.

Morbidity and Mortality

The typical child with CRF has pallor, fatigue, lassitude, weakness, anorexia, weight loss, growth failure, and pruritus. Other problems have included bone pain, edema, headaches, and seizures. With early recognition of CRF, therapy with the interventions discussed previously, and appropriate institution of dialysis or transplantation, most of the typical problems can be avoided or attenuated. The morbidity of ESRD is related to inadequate nutrition, anemia, hypertension, osteodystrophy, and fluid and electrolyte disturbances. Also important, however, are problems related to therapeutic agents, especially glucocorticoids and immunosuppressive agents. The most frequent and significant side effects include increased risk of infections, growth failure, and avascular necrosis of bone. Prednisone, the most commonly used steroid for several types of renal disease, may contribute significantly to limitations in physical activity since it may cause muscle weakness, induce osteopenia and fractures, and increase adipose tissue (Cushingoid changes) and bruising. Long-term problems with peritoneal dialysis include infections in the peritoneal cavity or of the peritoneal catheter. Also important is family and patient fatigue, since the procedure of peritoneal dialysis requires great time and attention. Long-term problems with hemodialysis include difficulty with vascular access, and infectious and thrombotic complications with shunts and fistulae. Although it requires less time than CAPD, hemodialysis must be done for approximately 4 hours, 3 times a week, and significantly interferes with independence and a normal lifestyle.

Survival with ESRD is very good and continues to get better. Cyclosporine has had a significant and beneficial effect on graft survival and morbidity. Despite concerns about the side effect of nephrotoxicity, cyclosporine has permitted substantial reductions in the doses of other immunosuppressive agents, including prednisone. Considerations of mortality must differentiate children on peritoneal dialysis, children on hemodialysis, and children with allografts. Survival statistics with transplantation must include both patient and graft survival. Important variables are the donor source, either from living relatives or cadavers, and the ages of the donor and recipient. In general, allografts from relatives (usually from a parent) account for about 40% of pediatric transplants and have a better survival rate than cadaveric grafts. Children transplanted with cadaver kidneys after age 4 do better than younger children, and kidneys harvested from cadavers beyond infancy function longer. Other important variables include

differences among transplant centers, HLA histocompatibility matching, and the underlying disorder which caused the ESRD. Emotional and psychological issues remain important after transplantation, and noncompliance is a significant cause of allograft loss. Although the leading cause of mortality in children with transplants is infection resulting from immunosuppression, the leading cause of death in ESRD is cardiovascular disease, thus presenting a rationale for promoting exercise and some degree of fitness.

EXERCISE AND END-STAGE RENAL DISEASE

It is predictable that the uremic child who is chronically fatigued, weak, and anorexic, with little interest in physical activity of any kind, will have impaired exercise tolerance and sport performance. What is surprising, however, is that this impairment also occurs in asymptomatic individuals with significant renal disease. Understanding the factors which limit exercise capacity in chronic renal failure helps to make reasonable recommendations and set realistic goals for these children.

There are several clinical studies which address the issue of fitness and exercise performance in patients with CRF. Most of the studies consider small groups of adults on hemodialysis. Unfortunately, direct application of data from adults to children and adolescents is not warranted, for several reasons:

- Less than one quarter of children with ESRD receive maintenance hemodialysis.
- Many adults with ESRD have complicating conditions, including atherosclerotic cardiovascular disease.
- The common causes of CRF in adults, specifically diabetic nephropathy, are very different than those in childhood.

Nevertheless, the causes of exercise limitation may be shared by children and adults and may be important and relevant when considering a pediatric population. There are some studies which have looked at exercise in children with ESRD, but they are few and consider small numbers of children (2, 3, 21, 27).

The causes of decreased exercise tolerance in children with renal failure are multiple. The exact contribution of each cause may differ in relative importance from child to child. The compromise in exercise capacity also may vary for a given child, becoming progressively worse as ESRD develops, improving with the onset of dialysis, becoming more pronounced with prolonged dialysis, and ultimately improving significantly with successful transplantation (23).

The causes of impaired exercise capacity and decreased physical activity in children with renal failure include inadequate nutrition, anemia, hypertension, electrolyte and acid-base disturbances, metabolic deficiencies causing impairment of both skeletal muscle and myocardial performance, impaired carbohydrate metabolism, obesity in post-transplantation patients, and mental depression. Side effects of medications may also limit exercise.

Inadequate Nutrition

Inadequate caloric intake leads to a catabolic state with muscle loss and negative nitrogen balance. For those patients with heavy proteinuria and those on peritoneal dialysis, there is additional protein loss. Decreased strength results, which impairs the child's ability and desire to be active and participate in sport. The inadequate nutrition is largely the result of anorexia which accompanies the uremic state. Occasionally, dietary restrictions and limits on salt intake also play a role. Because of anorexia and nausea, attempts at increasing caloric intake are difficult and should aim to maximize the foods the child finds palatable and supply at least 70% of the recommended dietary allowance of calories and 1.0-2.0 gm/kg of protein per day. The consultation and regular input of a pediatric nutritionist is very helpful in achieving an optimal diet.

Anemia

Anemia is a major contributing factor in decreased exercise tolerance because it limits oxygen transport to muscles. As a general rule, the hematocrit is proportional to the GFR and anemia becomes very common when the glomerular filtration rate (GFR) declines to one quarter of normal (approximately 30 ml/min/1.73M^2). Furthermore, exercise capacity is inversely proportional to the degree of anemia (21, 27). Correction of the anemia through the use of human recombinant erythropoietin leads to significant improvement in peak exercise capacity (2, 18, 24, 27).

Hypertension

Hypertension is another common problem in patients with ESRD. When blood pressure is poorly controlled and of long duration, hypertension can lead to cardiac septal hypertrophy and impair cardiac output. Abnormalities of vascular resistance can also affect maximal exercise capacity. Exercise, however, has a beneficial effect on lowering blood pressure in children and adolescents with hypertension (16, 20). Physical activity, therefore, in conjunction with appropriate antihypertensive medication, should be encouraged in children with ESRD and elevated blood pressure (14).

Electrolyte and Acid-Base Disturbances

Electrolyte disturbances and metablic acidosis frequently occur in chronic renal failure and include abnormalities of sodium, potassium, calcium, and phosphorus. These abnormalities can adversely influence exercise performance through their negative effects on cardiac contractility and rhythm. These and other abnormalities of cardiac function in pediatric patients with ESRD are well summarized in a review by O'Regan (22).

Metabolic Deficiencies

There has been speculation that metabolic deficiencies and toxicities play important roles in the uremic syndrome, including the weakness and fatigue that frequently occur. It has been shown that altered skeletal muscle function contributes to impaired exercise tolerance in adults with uremia (9). Recent work has focused on carnitine, which is important in normal muscle metabolism during exercise and appears to be deficient in patients with ESRD on hemodialysis (1, 15). Carnitine infusion and replacement improves exercise tolerance in these patients (2). Other unidentified deficiencies or accumulation of toxic metabolites may also prove to have similar negative effects on exercise tolerance.

Impaired Carbohydrate Metabolism

Abnormal carbohydrate metabolism may also impair physical performance in uremia. Castellino, Bia, and DeFronzo (6) showed that the rate of hepatic gluconeogenesis and peripheral uptake of glucose during exercise are decreased in adults with ESRD on hemodialysis.

Medication Side Effects

Medication side effects may occasionally interfere with physical activity. With the use of beta blockers as antihypertensives, it is important to measure the pulse during physical activity to be certain that the heart rate can increase in response to the need for greater cardiac output. Prednisone, which is used chronically in the treatment of several diseases which cause ESRD in children (for example, nephritis associated with systemic lupus erythematosus) and for the prevention of rejection in recipients of renal allografts, may also cause proximal muscle weakness which can interfere with exercise capacity. Studies in animals have shown that regular exercise involving specific muscle groups can effectively prevent myopathy during chronic steroid use (8). Recent studies suggest that steroid-related muscle atrophy is mediated through antagonism of a subset of hormone responsive genes. In experimental animals, the atrophy which results from the molecular effects of gene regulation can be overcome by regular exercise (10). Prednisone may also lead to obesity, a predictable effect when long-term, high-dose daily therapy is necessary. The obesity may limit exercise, but an exercise program may be the most important factor in preventing or resolving it.

Deconditioning

Another factor which limits exercise capacity in children with chronic renal failure is the adverse effect of inactivity on physical performance, so-called deconditioning (7). The child with a life-long history of renal and/or urologic disease is much more likely to experience the limitation of deconditioning than one who has lost renal function over a short period of time.

In general, children and adolescents with CRF have difficulty with activities which require quick, maximal bursts of energy, and also with those which involve prolonged, intense exercise and stamina. Because many children with CRF are retarded in growth and have decreased muscle mass, they have difficulty participating in sports which require strength to excel. They become fatigued more easily, and because of electrolyte abnormalities are more prone to muscle cramps.

There are exceptions to these generalizations, however, and the physical status of the pediatric patient with ESRD can be extremely variable depending on the etiology and duration of the renal disease. For example, two 13-year-old children may present with ESRD. One may have been previously healthy and developed renal failure as a result of an acute insult such as hemolytic uremic syndrome. This child may have been in the 95th percentile for height and weight and very active in sports prior to becoming ill. The other patient may have been born with dysplastic kidneys and had a long, slow progression of renal insufficiency. This patient is likely to have retarded growth, little muscle mass, a long history of hypertension, and delayed puberty. Clearly, the exercise capacity and potential of these two patients will be very different.

Potential Adverse Effects of Sports and Exercise

The potential adverse effects from sports and exercise on children with chronic renal disease vary with the status of the child. Regular and clear communication among the physician, parents, and those directing the exercise and sport programs is essential. Potential adverse effects that can result from sport and exercise in children with renal disease include dehydration, electrolyte disturbances, seizures, syncope, reactive airway disease, and injury to a catheter, vascular access site, or allograft. In a child with significant osteodystrophy (renal rickets or bone disease), the risk of traumatic fractures are greater than in other children.

In the child with progressive renal insufficiency, fluid and electrolyte abnormalities are a potential concern before the need arises for dialysis or transplantation. Because the kidneys frequently are unable to concentrate the urine, under conditions of excessive fluid loss dehydration is more likely to occur, especially if access to water is limited. Also, because the kidneys are unable to regulate electrolyte concentrations in the blood as precisely as normal, significant loss of sodium and potassium in perspiration may result in abnormalities. Because very strenuous exercise can lead to transcellular movement of potassium and elevate serum levels in healthy subjects, the child with chronic renal insufficiency and risk of hyperkalemia who exercises should be followed carefully and treated to maintain a normal serum potassium. In the few pediatric ESRD patients who have little or no residual urine output and who are observing strict fluid limits, strict regulation of fluid intake must be carefully monitored to avoid fluid overload or dehydration. In the child with a normally functioning allograft, fluid and electrolyte balance is usually no different than in healthy children.

Children with ESRD are more likely to experience seizures for several reasons, including

- electrolyte disturbances, especially hypocalcemia or hyponatremia;
- uncontrolled hypertension; and
- the uremic state itself (11).

Syncope may result from a cardiac dysrhythmia associated with electrolyte disturbances (e.g., hypokalemia). Syncope may also be secondary to hypotension, hypovolemia, or severe anemia. Reactive airway disease with wheezing may be induced by exercise in some patients, and is associated with the use of β-adrenergic blocking agents.

Perhaps the most common adverse effect is injury to the peritoneal catheter, the vascular access catheter, or to an arteriovenous fistula or renal allograft. Peritoneal catheters are located on the lower abdominal wall below the umbilicus and are tunneled beneath the skin. Arteriovenous fistulae are created on an extremity, usually the forearm. A vascular access catheter may be located on the upper chest below the clavicle. Renal transplants are positioned on either side of the lower abdomen just beneath the abdominal wall, and are therefore more susceptible to injury than a native kidney. In any sport or activity where the potential for trauma is even remote, precautions may be taken to try to avoid renal injury.

Another important potential adverse effect of sport participation is the feeling of failure. The emotional status of children with ESRD is often very fragile (4, 12, 25), and although participation in a sport or exercise program can have very positive psychosocial effects it is important to avoid a situation where the achievement of some success is remote.

Precautions to avoid adverse effects involve close observation of the child during exercise, and continuous communication with the physician to learn of changes in the child's general condition, renal function, or medication. Other specific precautions include permitting the child free access to fluids based on thirst. Fluids which supply a carbohydrate source as well as appropriate electrolyte replacement are usually adequate when exercise involves vigorous activity or perspiration; commonly available solutions are listed in Table 18.2. These fluids are also indicated for a child who develops muscle cramps and are effective in helping to prevent the fluid and electrolyte disturbances which could lead to seizures or syncope. Injury prevention to the graft, catheter, or fistula is achieved by adequate padding and protection, and by avoiding activities in which there is high likelihood of trauma.

The response to adverse effects involves the use of common sense once an understanding of ESRD is achieved. The response to trauma to an arteriovenous fistula is to inspect the site for bleeding, apply ice, and send the child to the nephrologist. In the case of a peritoneal catheter injury the site should be inspected and wrapped, and the child referred to the nephrologist. With trauma to an allograft the transplant surgeon should be consulted immediately.

The appropriate response to a seizure or syncope is no different from that for other children.

Table 18.2 Approximate Composition of Commonly Used Sports Drinks (Amounts Expressed per Quart)

Drink	Sodium	Potassium	Calories[a]
Gatorade	18.9 mEq	2.6 mEq	200
10-K	9.5 mEq	3.1 mEq	240
Snapple Snapup	10 mEq	5.1 mEq	320
Sqwincher	20.8 mEq	3.7 mEq	260
Power Burst	6.1 mEq	5.6 mEq	230

[a]All of the calories are from carbohydrate.

With a seizure the child should be placed on one side on a surface where no injury can occur. If there is emesis, it is important to ensure that the airway is clear, although nothing should be placed in the mouth. With syncope, the child should be placed flat and the legs elevated. The pulse rate should be determined, and if the child does not respond and awaken promptly or if the pulse remains irregular an ambulance should be called, since intravenous fluids and glucose may be needed.

Benefits of Sport and Exercise

Physical activity has clear and significant benefits for pediatric patients with ESRD. One of these is to avoid or reduce the threat of cardiovascular disease, which is the leading cause of mortality in adults with ESRD. Exercise can also help to reduce hypertension, which is an important risk factor in hastening the decline of residual renal function and causing later cardiovascular disease. Exercise may also help to normalize the lipid profile, which is frequently unfavorable in ESRD. Although there are data to suggest that exercise favorably affects lipid levels in adults on hemodialysis (11), little is known about a similar effect in children.

Children with chronic renal failure, especially those on dialysis, may suffer from depression and anxiety, and tend to have increased psychosocial problems in the areas of self-esteem, dependence, and peer interaction and acceptance (4, 12, 25). It is reasonable to expect that sport participation and physical fitness will improve self-esteem, encourage feelings of independence, and increase peer contact (5).

EXERCISE AND SPORTS RECOMMENDATIONS

Recommendations for specific exercises and activities depend not only on the patient, but also on the physician. Factors of significance for the patient include duration of disease and physical inactivity, body stature and muscle mass, extrarenal organ system involvement, and presence and type of renal replacement therapy. Recommendations by the physician depend largely on personal experience and attitudes toward physical activity and sport.

In order to determine what pediatric nephrologists recommend for their patients with chronic renal disease, the authors sent a questionnaire to pediatric nephrologists from 110 different pediatric renal centers in the United States. Information was received from 54 (49%), and reflects experience with approximately 4100 children and adolescents. About one half of the reported patients had received transplants, and 15% were on dialysis. Most nephrologists strongly encourage an exercise program and ask about physical activity at visits, but only 2% prescribe a specific exercise program. An additional 20% do not routinely discuss exercise with their patients.

To initiate a fitness program, the patient's current capabilities, level of activity, and sport interests should be determined. Formal exercise testing should be obtained for those whose status is uncertain and who wish to participate in strenuous activities or sports (17). Testing measures current exercise capacity, serves as a baseline to assess the effectiveness of a fitness program, determines the presence of cardiovascular disease, and permits recommendations for initial activity. Approximately one half of pediatric nephrologists obtain exercise testing for some of their patients.

Recommendations should set realistic goals that will allow some measure of success and satisfaction and encourage the child to continue. The physician must work closely with the parents and physical education instructors to formulate advice, structure programs, set goals, and elicit support and cooperation. In this regard, only one third of nephrologists view parents as allies in encouraging their children to become active or participate in sport, while 45% believe that parents are anxious to restrict activity. School officials fare even less well: only 6% of physicians feel that schools are supportive of sport and exercise for children with ESRD, and 75% view them as generally anxious to restrict activity. The perception of the schools' reluctance to permit exercise and sport may relate to inadequate communication, since only 20% of nephrologists report that they either "always" or "frequently" interact with coaches or instructors, while 33% "occasionally," 40% "seldom," and 7% "never" communicate.

Recommendations by nephrologists for children with CRF mainly emphasize aerobic activity, since this promotes cardiovascular fitness and may help to reduce elevated blood pressure and serum lipid levels. Aerobic activities also allow the child to gradually increase the intensity and duration of exercise and generally are not associated with risk of injury. Commonly encourged aerobic activities include exercise and dance classes, walking, jogging, biking, and swimming. Aerobic exercise and dance classes provide the benefits of movement and flexibility training, which are also considered important by nephrologists. Strength training, on the other hand, is encouraged by less than 10% of nephrologists, even for children with functioning transplants. Strength training is frequently equated with weightlifting, which is traditionally discouraged in hypertensive patients because it may further elevate blood pressure. It should be noted, however, that at least one well-designed study questions this belief (13). If weight training is undertaken, multiple repetition exercises with lighter weights should be used and the blood pressure should be followed closely. Caution is important when considering weight-lifting for children on peritoneal dialysis, since straining may increase intra-abdominal pressure and lead to hernias.

Physicians' recommendations concerning activities to be avoided are based primarily on the risk of injury to the child or to a renal transplant. Important considerations for sports include the child's body size, as well as the presence and location of bone disease. Seventy percent of pediatric nephrologists base their choice of activity on concerns regarding injury or excessive demands, while 30% recommend participation in any sport in which the child has an interest and demonstrated prowess.

Modifications in activities may be required as a result of progression of the renal disease or of changes in therapy including institution of dialysis, change in type of dialysis, renal transplantation, or change in the level of function of an allograft. The most significant changes are brought about by a successful transplant: while exercise capacity and energy increase, so do concerns regarding potential trauma to the transplanted kidney. Nephrologists report that established fitness and exercise programs are most commonly modified because of inadequately controlled hypertension, osteodystrophy (renal bone disease), or poor nutrition. Less common reasons for limiting activity include anemia, side effects of medication, and systemic disease.

Specific sports participation recommendations depend largely on the physician's personal experience with other children, since there are no published reports of children with ESRD and sport. Table 18.3 shows the relative importance of several factors which influence nephrologists' recommendations for involvement in specific sports. Collision potential and risk of injury remains the leading concern, and is greatest for the child with a kidney transplant.

Table 18.4 shows specific sports and activities that are usually permitted by pediatric nephrologists for their patients with chronic renal disease. It is notable that fewer restrictions are placed on children prior to the need for dialysis and in turn before transplantation, especially with respect to contact and collision sports. The fact that 75% permit football in children with CRF and 19% continue to permit it following transplantation is surprising; in general, the diminutive size and stature of the ESRD population will limit the opportunity for success in sports such as football and will result in the selection of sports that do not require great strength. In the limited contact and noncontact categories, only weightlifting is restricted by a large number of physicians, mainly because of concerns regarding hypertension.

Swimming is a sport approved by all nephrologists, since it promotes cardiovascular fitness, presents no danger from contact or collision, and is relatively free of injury. There is some concern, however, regarding the risk of infection in children with peritoneal catheters or external vascular access. The risk appears to be much smaller if the swimming is done in chlorinated pools rather than lakes and rivers.

Table 18.3   Percent of Pediatric Nephrologists Who Base Recommendations for Specific Sports on the Following Factors

Collision/injury potential	65%
Aerobic demands	54%
Isometric activity	41%
Dynamic activity	38%
Expected ability to participate for extended period	29%
Opportunity to achieve success	23%
Level of competition	19%

Table 18.4 Percent of Pediatric Nephrologists Who Usually Permit Participation in a Sport

	CRF children with no dialysis	Children on dialysis	Children with transplant
Contact/Collision/Impact			
Basketball	98	95	92
Cycling	100	100	100
Field hockey	96	91	75
Football	75	43	19
Gymnastics	95	96	87
Ice hockey	87	68	57
Karate/Judo	89	64	45
Lacrosse	95	85	70
Skiing	96	96	96
Soccer	93	93	85
Waterskiing	95	88	88
Wrestling	77	57	38
Limited contact			
Baseball	98	98	96
Cheerleading	100	100	100
Ice skating	95	98	98
Softball	96	98	98
Volleyball	98	98	98
Weightlifting	77	57	38
Non-contact			
Aerobics	100	100	100
Dance	100	100	100
Golf	100	100	100
Running	98	100	100
Swimming	98	100	100
Tennis	98	98	98
Walking	100	100	100

Table 18.5 Competitive Sports of the 1992 United States Transplant Games

Badminton	
Bowling	1-kilometer time trial
Bicycling	20-kilometer road race
Golf	
Road race	
Table tennis	
Tennis	Doubles
	Singles
Track and field	Long jump
	Shotput
	Softball throw
	High jump
	50-meter dash
	400-meter race
	1500-meter race
	1500-meter racewalk
Swimming	50-meter breaststroke
	50-meter freestyle
	50-meter backstroke
	50-meter butterfly
	100-meter breaststroke
	100-meter freestyle
	100-meter backstroke
	100-meter butterfly
	500-meter freestyle
	4 × 25–meter relay
	4 × 50–meter relay

Children who show no desire to compete will do best if they begin with a noncompetitive activity and are permitted to attain a measure of self-satisfaction before progressing to competition. Even children who wish to compete are best placed in a recreational situation initially and later allowed to join an organized team if their exercise capacity and stamina are shown to be adequate. In order to make these judgments, the physician must maintain close communication with the child's parents and physical education instructor or coach.

That people who have received a transplant can successfully participate in sport is illustrated by the competitions which are held on the regional, state, national, and international levels.

The United States Transplant Games are administered by the National Kidney Foundation and are held biennially for transplant recipients of all ages, including children and adolescents. The games, first held in 1982, most recently involved 875 athletes and included 529 kidney transplant recipients and 82 athletes under the age of 18. The athletes compete in 10 sports for men and women, which are listed in Table 18.5. The stated purposes of the event include the desire to demonstrate that people with transplants are able to lead active lives, and to provide an organized event which promotes the successful rehabilitation of transplant recipients.

CONCLUSION

Everyone who participates in the life of a child with chronic renal disease hopes not only for normal renal function following successful transplantation, but also for a normal and active life. An active lifestyle presumes some level of fitness, which is best obtained by participation in a fitness program or a sport which the child enjoys. It is essential that the physician, parents, and school or sport officials work closely to assure that the exercise and activity occur without unnecessary restrictions and within an environment where success and satisfaction may be achieved. The vast majority of nephrologists report that in their experience, exercise programs and sport participation play a significant role in their patients' overall feelings of well-being and self-esteem, as well as contributing significantly to their health.

REFERENCES

1. Ahmad, S.; Robertson, H.T.; Golper, T.A.; Wolfson, M.; Kurtin, P.; Katz, L.A.; Hirschberg, R.; Nicora, R.; Ashbrook, D.W.; Kopple, J.D. Multicenter trial of L-carnitine in maintenance hemodialysis patients. II. Clinical and biochemical effects. Kidney Int. 38:912-918; 1990.

2. Baraldi, E.; Montini, G.; Zanconato, S.; Zacchello, G.; Zacchello, F. Exercise tolerance after anaemia correction with recombinant human erythropoietin in end-stage renal disease. Pediatr. Nephrol. 4:623-626: 1990.

3. Bonzel, K.E.; Wildi, B.; Weiss, M.; Scharer, K. Spiroergometric performance of children and adolescents with chronic renal failure. Pediatr. Nephrol. 5:22-28; 1991.

4. Brownbridge, G.; Fielding, D.M. Psychosocial adjustment to end-stage renal failure: comparing haemodialysis, continuous ambulatory peritoneal dialysis and transplantation. Pediatr. Nephrol. 5:612-616; 1991.

5. Carney, R.M.; McKevitt, P.M.; Goldberg, A.P.; Hagberg, J.; Delmez, J.A.; Harter, H.R. Psychological effects of exercise training in hemodialysis patients. Nephron. 33:179; 1983.

6. Castellino, P.; Bia, M.; DeFronzo, R.A. Metabolic response to exercise in dialysis patients. Kidney Int. 32:877-883; 1987.

7. Coyle, E.R.; Martin, W.H.; Bloomfield, S.A.; et al. Effects of detraining on responses to submaximal exercise. J. Appl. Physiol. 59: 853; 1985.

8. Czerwinski, S.M.; Kurowski, T.G.; O'Neill, T.M.; Hickson, R.C. Initiating regular exercise protects against muscle atrophy from glucocorticoids. J. Appl. Physiol. 63:1504-1510; 1987.

9. Diesel, W.; Noakes, T.D.; Swanepoel, C.; Lambert, M. Isokinetic muscle strength predicts maximum exercise tolerance in renal patients on chronic hemodialysis. Am. J. Kid. Dis. 16:109-114; 1990.

10. Falduto, M.T.; Young, A.P.; Hickson, R.C. Exercise interrupts ongoing glucocorticoid-induced muscle atrophy and glutamine synthetase induction. Am. J. Physio. 263 (Endocrinol. Metab. 26): E1157-1163; 1992.

11. Goldberg, A.P.; Geltman, E.M.; Hagberg, J.M.; Gavin, J.R.; Delmez, J.A.; Carney, R.M.; Naumowicz, A.; Oldfield, M.H.; Harter, H.R. Therapeutic benefits of exercise training for hemodialysis patients. Kidney Int. 24 (Suppl. 16):S303-S309; 1983.

12. Grupe, W.E.; Greifer, I.; Greenspan, S.I.; Leavitt, L.A.; Wolf, G. Psychosocial development in children with chronic renal insufficiency. Am. J. Kid. Dis. 7:324-328; 1986.

13. Hagberg, J.M.; Ehsani, A.A.; Goldring, D.; Hernandez, A.; Sinacore, D.R.; Holloszy, J.O. Effect of weight training on blood pressure and hemodynamics in hypertensive adolescents. J. Peds. 104:147-151; 1984.

14. Hagberg, J.M.; Goldberg, A.P.; Ehsani, A.A.; Heath, G.W.; Delmez, J.A.; Harter, H.R. Exercise training improves hypertension in hemodialysis patients. Am. J. Nephrol. 3:209-212; 1983.

15. Hiatt, W.R.; Koziol, B.J.; Shapiro, J.I.; Brass, E.P. Carnitine metabolism during exercise in patients on chronic hemodialysis. Kidney Int. 41:1613-1619; 1992.

16. Hofman, A.; Walter, H.J.; Connelly, P.A.; Vaughan, R.D. Blood pressure and physical fitness in children. Hypertension 9:188-191; 1987.

17. Klein, A.A. Pediatric exercise testing. Pediatr. Ann. 16:546-558; 1987.

18. Lundin, P.A.; Akerman, M.J.H.; Chesler, R.M.; Delano, B.G.; Goldberg, N.; Stein, R.A.; Friedman, E.A. Exercise in hemodialysis patients after treatment with recombinant human erythropoietin. Nephron. 58:315-319; 1991.

19. McEnery, P.T.; Stablein, D.M.; Arbus, G.; Tejani, A. Renal transplantation in children.

A report of the North American Pediatric Renal Transplant Cooperative Study. N. Engl. J. Med. 236:1727-1732; 1992.

20. Nudel, D.B.; Gootman, N.; Brunson, S.C.; Stenzler, A.; Sheuker, I.R.; Gauthier, B.G. Exercise performance of hypertensive adolescents. Peds. 65:1073; 1980.

21. Ono, M. Exercise capacity of children with chronic renal failure. Japan. J. Nephrol. 21:1089; 1979.

22. O'Regan, S. Cardiovascular abnormalities in pediatric patients with ESRD. In: Fine, R.N.; Gruskin, A.B., ed. End stage renal disease in children. Philadelphia: W.B. Saunders Co.; 1984:359-374.

23. Painter, P.; Hanson, P.; Messer-Rehak, D.; Zimmerman, S.W.; Glass, N.R. Exercise tolerance changes following renal transplantation. Am. J. Kid. Dis. 10:452-456; 1987.

24. Robertson, H.T.; Haley, N.R.; Guthrie, M.; Cardenas, D.; Eschbach, J.W.; Adamson, J.W. Recombinant erythropoietin improves exercise capacity in anemic hemodialysis patients. Am. J. Kid. Dis. 15:325-332; 1990.

25. Rosenkranz, J.; Bonzel, K.E.; Bulla, M.; Michal, K.; Offner, G.; Reichwald-Klugger, E.; Schärer, K. Psychosocial adaptation of children and adolescents with chronic renal failure. Pediatr. Nephrol. 6:459-463; 1992.

26. Schwartz, G.J.; Haycock, G.B.; Edelmann, C.M.; Spitzer, A. A simple estimate of glomerular filtration rate in children derived from body length and plasma creatinine. Peds. 58:259; 1976.

27. Ulmer, H.E.; Greiner, H.; Schuler, H.W.; Scharer, K. Cardiovascular impairment and physical working capacity in children with chronic renal failure. Acta. Paediatr. Scand. 67:43-48; 1978.

28. U.S. Renal Data System. USRDS 1991 annual data report. Bethesda, MD: The National Institutes of Health, National Institute of Diabetes and Digestive and Kidney Diseases. August 1991. (Reprinted as ESRD in children. Am. J. Kid. Dis. 18(Suppl. 2):79-88; 1991.)

CHAPTER 19

Anemia

Arnold T. Sigler and William H. Zinkham
Johns Hopkins University School of Medicine

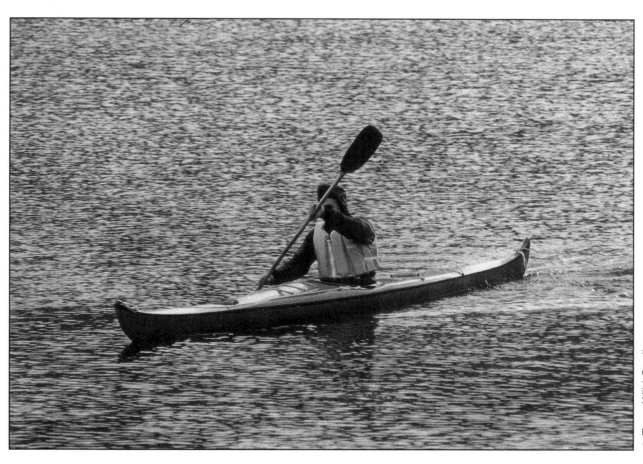

One of the most common abnormalities of the blood is anemia, a condition in which there is a reduction in the mass of circulating red cells. Since one of the primary functions of the red cells is delivery of oxygen to tissues, any disease associated with anemia, especially those that are chronic in nature, could affect the physical activity of affected individuals.

As illustrated in Figure 19.1, anemia may be secondary to a variety of mechanisms. In this illustration the needle of the pan balance points to a hematocrit value of 40, a number that represents the percentage of red cells in whole blood. Of all the biological values in man, those for the hematocrit are the most constant. For this to be so, production of red cells must equal red cell destruction, such that for each young red cell (reticulocyte) entering the circulation, a red cell exits at the end of its life span of 120 days. Disruption of this equilibrium may be secondary to any of three major events: a failure of red cell production as in iron deficiency anemia; an increased rate of destruction, as in sickle cell anemia; or a catastrophic combination of both events—cessation of red cell production in a patient with a red cell destructive disorder. Thus, anemia is not a disease per se but a condition for which an etiology, and the disease with which it is associated, must be determined.

PHYSIOLOGICAL MECHANISMS

The primary physiological functions of the red cell are twofold. One is the transport of oxygen to tissues, a function that is mediated by hemoglobin, the major protein constituent of the red cell; the other is the transport of carbon dioxide from tissues to the lungs. Both of these functions involve a complex series of events, the nature of which has been elucidated by many different investigators (14).

A quantitative expression of oxygen delivery to tissues is the Fick equation,

$$VO_2 = 0.139 \cdot Q \cdot Hb \cdot S_A O_2 - S_V O_2$$

In this equation VO_2 is the volume of oxygen released to tissues per unit of time (l/min), 0.139 represents the amount of oxygen bound to one gram of hemoglobin (Hb), Q is a measure of blood flow (l/min), Hb is the amount of hemoglobin in the blood, and $S_A O_2$ and $S_V O_2$ are arterial and mixed venous oxygen saturations, respectively. As indicated by the equation, a decrease in hemoglobin would impair delivery of oxygen to tissues and in turn affect physical activities. Evidence for this relationship has been provided by measuring the effects of acute and chronic anemia on maximal oxygen consumption and exercise performance (115). When

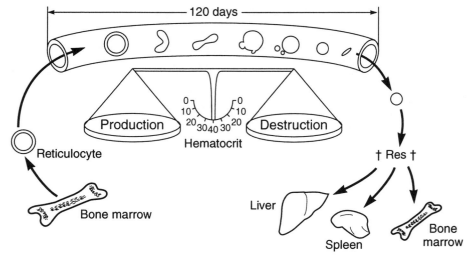

Figure 19.1 The mechanistic approach to anemia.

hemoglobin concentration decreases by only 1 to 2 g/dl, these parameters decrease proportionately. Conversely, increases in hemoglobin concentrations in healthy subjects may improve performance.

Factors other than those expressed in the Fick equation are also important determinants of tissue oxygen delivery. One of these is the affinity of hemoglobin for oxygen, a relationship that is expressed as P_{50}, the partial pressure of oxygen at which hemoglobin is half oxygenated. Although this measurement provides information regarding the halfway point, it does not express the overall shape of the oxygen-dissociation curve. As illustrated in Figure 19.2, a variety of factors may affect the shape and position of the curve. The normal oxygen dissociation curve is the middle of the three curves. Shifting the curve to the right may accompany any one or more of three major environmental changes: an acid environment ($\downarrow$pH), an increase in 2,3-diphosphoglycerate ($\uparrow$DPG), or an elevation of temperature ($\uparrow$Temp). Changes opposite to these result in a leftward shifting of the curve. At any given oxygen tension or pressure, designated O_2 tension (mmHg) in the figure, a greater amount of oxygen will be released from hemoglobin to tissues for a rightward shifted curve as compared to the normal or the left-shifted curve. For example, at a normal O_2 tension of 26 mmHg, the amount of hemoglobin containing oxygen (oxyhemoglobin) for a leftward shifted curve is approximately 58% and for a rightward shifted curve, 42%, demonstrating that 16% more oxygen would be released from hemoglobin to tissues under these conditions.

An important metabolic product of glucose metabolism by the red cell is 2,3-disphosphoglycerate (2,3-DPG). Binding of 2,3 DPG to hemoglobin reduces its affinity for oxygen, thereby improving tissue oxygen delivery. In most types of anemia, levels of 2,3-DPG are increased. Evidence for the physiological importance of this phenomenon is a report in which patients with similar degrees of anemia exhibited markedly different degrees of exercise tolerance (78). In one patient an inherited abnormality of glucose metabolism by the red cell, a deficiency of the enzyme hexokinase, resulted in decreased levels of 2,3-DPG, a left-shifted oxygen dissociated curve, and markedly decreased exercise tolerance. A different type of enzyme defect in the red cells of the other patient, a deficiency of pyruvate kinase, caused a marked elevation of 2,3-DPG, a rightward shifting of the oxygen dissociation curve, and a normal response to graded exercise.

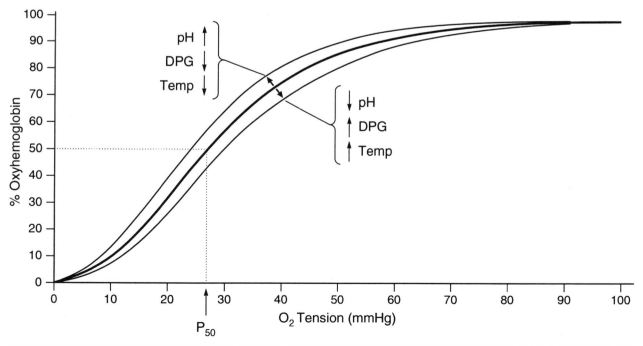

Figure 19.2 Factors affecting the oxygen-dissociation curve.
Reprinted with permission from M. Delivoria-Papadopoulos, F.A. Oski, and A.J. Gottlieb, "Oxygen-Hemoglobin Dissociation Curves: Effect of Inherited Enzyme Defects of the Red Cell," *Science*, **165**, pp. 601-2, 1969. Copyright 1969 American Association for the Advancement of Science.

Another factor affecting the position of the oxygen-dissociation curve is the presence of an abnormal hemoglobin with either an increased or decreased affinity for oxygen. Those hemoglobinopathies with an increased oxygen affinity result in a leftward shift of the curve, while those with decreased oxygen affinity cause a rightward shift with the consequent favorable impact on tissue oxygen delivery.

In summary, a variety of physiological mechanisms determine the rate of delivery of oxygen to tissues, chief among these being rate of blood flow, hemoglobin values, and the unloading of oxygen from the red cells. By definition, anemia is characterized by a reduction in hemoglobin values. Therefore, in most anemic states, oxygen delivery to tissues may be impaired. Even so, compensatory physiological mechanisms vary according to the type and degree of the anemia. Consequently, individual assessment of each anemic patient is required in order to gauge the impact of anemia on the patient's exercise performance.

EXERCISE AND ANEMIA

There is ample evidence to support the thesis that anemia adversely affects exercise tolerance and therefore performance. Although limitations in performance are clearly related to the degree of hemoglobin reduction, any disability—either as perceived by the athlete or as measured by scientific means—varies greatly with each individual (Table 19.1). In general, the anemic state will affect the individual's maximal aerobic capacity. Maximal aerobic capacity is equal to the highest oxygen uptake that the exercising subject can process during a progressively difficult exercise test, a value that is expressed as $\dot{V}O_2$max. In anemic individuals, exercise at or near the point of maximal oxygen

Table 19.1   Severity of Anemia Based on Hemoglobin Concentration g/dl (Lower Limits of Normal) 8 Years and Older

Mild anemia (Normal males > 12.5) (Normal females > 12.0)	10-12.5
Moderate anemia	7-10
Severe anemia	< 7

consumption can be sustained for only a relatively short period of time (32).

Most of the information concerning the effect of anemia on exercise capacity is derived from studies on naturally occurring iron-deficient humans or from experiments in which animals and human subjects are made anemic by artificial blood withdrawal. In humans there is a positive correlation between reduction in hemoglobin value, maximal oxygen consumption, and exercise capacity (26, 115). Changes as small as 1 to 2 g/dl are associated with a concomitant fall in maximum oxygen consumption but only minor changes in cardiopulmonary parameters (37). Similarly, there is a 20% decrease in exercise capacity on the treadmill in patients with hemoglobin levels of 11.0 to 11.9 g/dl as compared to control subjects with hemoglobin levels above 13 g/dl (44). In subjects with more severe acute or established anemia there is a linear relationship between arterial O_2 content and maximal exercise capacity (115). Thus, it is not surprising that many reports have noted a deleterious effect of anemia on physical work capacity, both clinically and experimentally (5, 22, 33, 75, 110).

Conversely, when a normal athlete's total hemoglobin is increased by 10% to 20%, the result is an improvement in maximal oxygen consumption and performance. Consequently, elite endurance athletes—especially marathon runners, skiers and cyclists—have pursued methods to increase their red cell mass, and thus their oxygen-carrying capacity. The physiological method of training at high altitudes stimulates red cell production in response to the hypoxic stimulus. Similarly, artificially induced erythrocythemia, generally known as blood doping, is produced by increasing hemoglobin mass by intravenous transfusions of red blood cells, and more recently by the use of genetically engineered erythropoietin (r Hu Epo) which is now available as a licensed drug (8).

It has been known since 1972 that reinfusion of autologous red cells, withdrawn three months earlier and stored, can significantly improve an athlete's $\dot{V}O_2$max and endurance (37). Other recent studies demonstrate that the effects of r hu epo and transfusions are similar and both improve maximal aerobic power ($\dot{V}O_2$max) in healthy males (1, 36, 102). Blood doping and the use of r Hu epo are illegal in NCAA and Olympic sports, and their ergogenic use may be extremely hazardous. Use of r epo raises the hematocrit and with it the viscosity of the blood—an effect that continues for several days after discontinuance of the drug. With unsupervised use, hematocrits that rise above the 50-55% level result in exponential increases in viscosity, which can result in coronary or cerebral vascular occlusions, deep venous thrombosis, and pulmonary embolism (51, 111).

Normal subjects compensate for anemia during exercise with increases in stroke volume, heart rate, and ventilation, or with decreases in peripheral resistance (10, 109). These events occur even when accompanied by a compensatory rise in erythrocyte 2, 3-diphosphoglycerate concentration in red blood cells and a shift to the right in the O_2 dissociation curve (7, 56, 80). However, some anemic individuals may be unable to adequately compensate during exercise, and the oxygenation of tissues and production of CO_2 is markedly curtailed (104).

The effect of anemia on exercise capacity has also been studied in animals. In the rat, acute isovolemic anemia decreased exercise capacity by 25% for each 20% drop in hemoglobin (33).

Iron Deficiency and Exercise

Iron deficiency anemia, as well as the iron-deficient state without anemia, may be associated with an abnormal capacity for work and exercise. Many patients, and especially children with mild iron-deficiency anemia, seldom have complaints severe enough to bring them to a physician, a phenomenon that is attributable to cardiovascular adjustments that result in increased blood flow to tissues (22). During exercise, tissue hypoxia develops as the rate of blood flow fails to meet oxygen demands in spite of greater cardiac output. Accordingly, the clinical symptomatology of iron-deficiency anemia ranges from fatigue and decreased exercise capacity to cardiac failure (44).

Important manifestations of mild iron-deficiency anemia include impaired work capacity and reduced exercise performance. Female workers in Sri Lanka with hemoglobin levels between 11.0 and 11.9 g/dl exhibited a 20% diminution in work performance as compared to women with a hemoglobin above 13.0 g/dl (45). In a similar study of Guatemalan agricultural laborers, minimal degrees of anemia resulted in

impaired performance on the Harvard Step Test. The hemoglobin level as well as the exercise performance rapidly improved when anemic workers were treated with iron (110).

Additional studies to substantiate these findings have been reported in the literature (25, 26, 75). In one of these (75), hemoglobin and maximal work time in 20 iron-deficient men and women (ages 21 to 72) increased significantly within 4 days after iron treatment and continued to increase up to 16 days as compared to the placebo group. Heart rates at a given exercise level were lower with iron treatment groups than in control subjects who had the same hemoglobin levels but had not been treated with iron.

Although iron deficiency with anemia unequivocally impairs exercise capacity, the impact of the nonanemic iron deficiency state on exercise is widely debated. By definition, iron deficiency without anemia is a condition characterized by normal hemoglobin values and decreased iron stores as measured by serum ferritin values. Depletion of the body's iron stores reduces myoglobin and cytochrome levels as well as iron-containing enzymes in many different tissues, especially muscle including the heart (23). Even though the total iron content of these and other tissue components is small (only 5% of total body iron), their metabolic functions are essential for normal physical activity.

Data derived from animal studies have shown that nonanemic iron depletion also impairs exercise performance. Nonanemic iron-deficient rats had diminished endurance on the treadmill, with performance improving after iron therapy (43). In two other studies, the iron-deficient state in rats resulted in abnormal exercise performance as well as a decrease in the concentration of cytochromes, myoglobin, and other enzymes essential for normal muscle metabolism (27, 28).

The effects of nonanemic iron deficiency on the exercise performance of human subjects is less clear. Forty adult women with hemoglobin levels over 12 g/dl and ferritin levels below 20 ng/ml were evaluated before and after 8 weeks of treatment with ferrous sulfate or placebo (72). Tests performed included the Wingate Cycle ergometer test for short-burst, high-intensity exercise; an anaerobic speed test; ventilatory theshhold; maximum oxygen uptake; and maximal velocity during the treadmill test. Since no significant differences in test performance were observed, the investigators concluded that a serum ferritin level of less than 20 ng/ml in someone with normal hemoglobin values does not impair exercise performance.

Similarly, other investigators have been unable to show any deleterious effect of nonanemic iron deficiency on treadmill endurance or maximal oxygen uptake in male adults after phlebotomy-induced iron deficiency (15). In another study, there was no improvement in exercise performance following iron therapy to 11 adult female marathon runners who had normal hemoglobin concentrations and ferritin levels less than 40 ng/ml. A deficiency in this study, however, was the fact that the group's mean ferritin value of 30 ng/ml prior to therapy was above the range that is usually considered diagnostic of depleted iron stores (66).

In contrast, a double-blind study of a group of female high school cross-country runners with nonanemic iron deficiency characterized by ferritin levels of less than 20 ng/ml and normal hemoglobin values demonstrated favorable effects with iron repletion (92). Pertinent to this experience is the fact that almost 50% of female high school long-distance runners have low serum ferritin levels without anemia, suggesting that nonanemic iron deficiency may be very common in these athletes (92).

Several additional studies in humans also support the notion that the nonanemic iron deficient state may impair exercise performance. Maximal exercise lactate concentrations decreased in nonanemic female college athletes with low ferritin levels following treatment with iron (96). In addition, the treatment of another group of iron-deficient, anemic individuals resulted in improved work capacity and lower heart rates that could not be accounted for by the increase in hemoglobin (75).

A variety of causes may underlie the iron-deficient state, the recognition of which is important for the development of preventive and therapeutic approaches. One of these is "sports anemia," a phenomenon that has been described in both distance runners and individuals who suddenly increase the intensity of their usual exercise routines. Acute forms of sports anemia are usually secondary to increased plasma volume resulting in an artificial lowering of hemoglobin and hematocrit levels. A less common cause is destruction of red cells; both of these

events are independent of iron status. In the longer term, sports anemia may be associated with iron deficiency as demonstrated by low serum ferritin values. In these subjects, diminished iron stores may be secondary to inadequate dietary intake in female athletes and gastrointestinal blood loss in distance runners (6, 50, 63).

Definitive answers to questions regarding the management of iron-deficient states in athletes are unavailable. For example, does the small but significant improvement in treadmill exercise after iron therapy correlate with improved performance in endurance athletes? Furthermore, can data which have been collected in adolescents and adults be applied to younger children? Another question relates to the improved exercise performance observed in nonanemic endurance athletes (runners, swimmers, cross-country skiers) after iron therapy—especially since these same athletes may have a worsening iron-deficient state as the competitive season progresses (91).

Even though answers to some of these questions are unavailable, the spectrum of severity of iron depletion in some athletes favors a vigorous preventive as well as therapeutic approach. In accordance with this suggestion is the observation that athletes with low ferritin values and normal or borderline hemoglobin levels may develop frank anemia while training. Even athletes with persistent nonanemic iron deficiency have compromised exercise performance because of the other effects of iron deficiency, including abnormal intellectual performance, behavior, motivation, and attention span (77, 79).

Those athletes at risk for developing iron deficiency anemia include menstruating females, adolescents during their growth spurt, and athletes who regularly restrict calories such as dancers, gymnasts, figure skaters, and wrestlers (32). Other risk groups include high school runners and possibly female high school swimmers who may become iron-deficient as the season of competition progresses (93). Amenorrheic females need about 10 mg of iron each day. In growing adolescent males and menstruating females, the recommended dietary allowance is 18 mg of iron per day.

Athletes should be encouraged to eat an iron-rich diet, including enough calories to maintain weight. Breakfast is important and should include cereals and/or breads that are enriched with iron. A vitamin C food such as a glass of orange juice at each meal improves iron absorption. Pastas fortified with iron are ideal foods for iron enhancement of the diet, as are lean red meat and the dark meat of chicken and turkey. Athletes should be aware that iron in animal protein (heme-meat) is more readily absorbed than nonheme iron (96).

Other foods rich in iron such as green vegetables, liver, and shellfish may not be popular with teenagers. Also, the recent emphasis on high-energy starches rather than red meats for the athlete may add to iron depletion (74). Since the dietary habits of many adolescents are unusual and unpredictable, the short-term increase in calories and/or iron from diet alone may be difficult to achieve.

Adolescent athletes with low hemoglobin values or with serum ferritin values less than 12 ng/ml should be treated with oral iron, 3 mg/kg/day of elemental iron divided into two doses. During therapy hemoglobin values should be obtained every 4 to 6 weeks until testing indicates iron sufficiency.

Since data supporting the deleterious role of nonanemic iron deficiency on athletic prowess is not yet proven, each athlete should be individually assessed for iron deficiency even if anemia is not present. A more convincing and lasting service to every athlete is a pretraining examination that includes measurements of hemoglobin and serum ferritin where indicated, as well as education regarding appropriate nutrition. If preventive supplementation or iron therapy is indicated, then the dose of iron should be about 105 mg elemental iron per day—the amount that prevented iron deficiency in female high school cross country runners (73).

Controversy exists regarding the necessity of hemoglobin/hematocrit determinations as components of the presport examination. Even very recent authoritative guidelines are ambiguous regarding screening for anemia and the iron-deficient state (32). Every child should have a hemoglobin determination some time prior to participation in actual sports. In high-risk adolescent athletes such as menstruating females and endurance athletes, more frequent surveillance for iron deficiency is recommended.

Since peripheral blood values may be normal in mild iron deficiency, other laboratory tests are necessary to diagnose the iron-deficient state. Of these, the serum ferritin is the most sensitive indicator of iron stores. In general, a serum ferritin value of less than 10 ng/dl in children or 12 ng/dl in adults indicates that iron stores are depleted. Measurement of serum ferritin is recommended in the nonanemic athlete whose exercise performance does not meet expectations initially or appears to be deteriorating over time (90). If the ferritin value is low, a course of iron therapy should be administered. Because of concerns about the potential harm from increased bodily iron stores in carriers of the hemochromatosis gene (10% of the Caucasian population) (34), as well as the possible risk of other serious diseases in genetically normal individuals (18, 94, 105), the prolonged use of prophylactic iron supplements without documentation of the iron-deficient state should be discouraged.

Sickle-Cell Disease and Exercise

The term sickle-cell disease encompasses several different clinically important syndromes, each of which is defined most often by hemoglobin electrophoresis: sickle-cell anemia (Hb SS); sickle-cell–hemoglobin C disease (Hb SC); and S or C hemoglobin variants combined with thalassemic disorders. The steady-state hemoglobin levels in these disorders are variable; their ranges in the two most common forms are 6-10 gm/dl (for Hb SS disease), and 9-14 gm/dl (for Hb SC disease).

In general, the clinical severity of sickle-cell disease is related to the percentage of sickle hemoglobin in the red cells. Patients with Hb SS disease have 80-90% sickle hemoglobin and 2-20% fetal hemoglobin which is unevenly distributed between the red cells. Patients with sickle-cell trait are usually asymptomatic with only 40% sickle hemoglobin. In some variants, a less severe clinical course may be secondary to the presence of Hb A or elevated levels of Hb F, which is evenly distributed among the red cells. The even distribution of fetal hemoglobin prevents irreversible sickling and confers a benign clinical course. Hence the precise nature of the type, amount, and distribution of the abnormal hemoglobin should be determined in any patient with a hemoglobin variant or a thalassemic disorder prior to strenuous exercise.

The effects of sickle-cell disease on exercise tolerance and sport performance are complex and difficult to study. The chronic hemolytic state is often complicated by infections, painful crises, and, in some patients, multi-organ disease. Crises may occur weekly or monthly, or as infrequently as once a year. Otherwise patients may be entirely free of symptoms. Occasionally, the hemoglobin and hematocrit level in these disorders may quickly fall as a result of an aplastic, hyperhemolytic, or sequestration crisis. Hence, the course of sickle-cell anemia is unpredictable.

The impact of Hb SS disease on physical activity is quite variable. Some patients are capable of a variety of sports (Tables 19.2 and 19.3) whereas others are so incapacitated that even minimal exercise is impossible. However, patients with sickle-cell disease variants usually exhibit milder courses and may not be detected until adulthood.

Multi-organ disease may also interfere with exercise tolerance. In sickle-cell disease and some sickle-cell variants, pneumonia and pulmonary infarction may lead to chronic lung disease with a resting arterial PO_2 of 65 to 85 mmHG in asymptomatic children. There may be large alveolar-arterial PO_2 differences in room air, findings consistent with increased pulmonary shunting (12, 41, 69, 112). In addition, the increase in the arterial-alveolar gradient in patients with sickle-cell anemia is greater than what would be expected on the basis of anemia alone (103, 104).

Another factor contributing to defective exercise performance in sickle-cell anemia consists of abnormalities of the heart. With mild exercise, heart rate increases are similar to those in normal controls, but Hb SS subjects exhibit much greater increases in stroke volume and cardiac index (61). With maximal exercise, however, the heart rates of children and adolescents with sickle-cell anemia are lower than in healthy black controls (3, 21).

Furthermore, with maximal exercise, the cardiac output of a sickle-cell patient increases

Table 19.2   Sports Selection for Children and Teenagers With Anemia

	Contact		Noncontact				
	Full	Limited	Aerobic high and moderate	Aerobic low	Dynamic high	Dynamic low	High static
Iron deficiency							
No anemia	yes	yes	yes	yes	yes	yes	yes
Mild to moderate	yes	yes	yes	yes	yes	yes	yes
Severe anemia	no	yes	no	yes	no	yes	no
Sickle-cell trait	yes	yes	yes	yes	yes	yes	yes
Sickle-cell anemia	no	no	no[b]	yes	no	yes	no
Thalassemia minor	yes	yes	yes	yes	yes	yes	yes
Thalassemia major	no	no	no	yes	no	yes	no
Hemolytic disorders							
With splenomegaly	no	no	no	yes	no	yes	no
Without splenomegaly	yes[a]	yes[a]	yes[a]	yes	yes[a]	yes	yes[a]
Chronic productive disorders							
Pure red cell and							
aplastic anemia	no	yes[a]	yes[a]	yes	yes[a]	yes	yes[a]
Anemia of chronic disease							
Rheum. arthritis	no	yes	yes[a]	yes	yes[a]	yes	no
Other collagen vasc. dis.	no	yes	yes[a]	yes	yes[a]	yes	no
Renal disease	no	yes	yes[a]	yes	yes[a]	yes	no
Chronic infection	no	yes	yes[a]	yes	yes[a]	yes	no

[a]May be contraindicated for severe anemia.

[b]May be exceptions.

Table 19.3 Sports Classification for Children and Teenagers With Anemia

Full contact/collision

Basketball	Field hockey	Karate/Judo	Rugby
Boxing	Football	Lacrosse	Skiing—downhill
Cycling	Gymnastics	Mountain climbing	Skiing—jump
Diving	Handball—team	Polo	Water polo
Equestrian	Hockey—ice	Rodeo	Waterskiing
			Wrestling

Full contact, high and moderate aerobic, high dynamic

Basketball	Football	Mountain climbing	Skiing—jump
Boxing	Gymnastics	Polo	Soccer
Cycling	Handball—team	Rope climbing	Water polo
Diving	Hockey—ice	Rugby	Wrestling
Field hockey	Lacrosse	Skiing—downhill	

Limited contact

Baseball	Paddleball	Skating—speed	Surfing
Cheerleading	Racquetball	Skiing—cross-country	Volleyball
Field hockey	Skating—figure	Softball	Weightlifting
Jai alai	Skating—roller	Squash	

Limited contact, high and moderate aerobic, high dynamic

Baseball	Jai alai	Skating—figure	Skiing—cross-country
Cheerleading	Paddleball	Skating—roller	Softball
Field hockey	Racquetball	Skating—speed	Volleyball

Noncontact, high and moderate aerobic, high dynamic

Aerobic dance	Crew rowing	Race walking	Scuba diving
Badminton	Dance	Rope jumping	Swimming
Ballet	Fencing	Running—distance	Table tennis
Canoeing	Handball	Running—sprint	Tennis

Noncontact, low aerobic, low dynamic

Archery	Camping	Darts	Horseshoes
Billiards	Cricket	Fishing	Riflery
Boccie	Croquet	Golf	Sailing
Bowling	Curling	Hiking	Shuffleboard
Bridge/Chess			

Limited contact, high and moderate aerobic, high static

Field events	Field hockey	Skiing—cross-country	Weightlifting

twofold as compared to a threefold increase in normal adults (21, 64). The left ventricular ejection fraction normally increases with exercise, but in Hb SS patients the volume is less than in normal controls. Therefore, the cardiac output response to exercise in sickle-cell patients is abnormal, thereby diminishing their ability to maintain a normal level of physical activity (21).

Although typical myocardial infarction and coronary disease are uncommon in sickle-cell disease, a more subtle myocardiopathy may be present (40, 65, 89, 108). Also, there is evidence that one third of Hb SS children have decreased left ventricular contractility (86), and 15% have an ischemic type of electrocardiographic response to exercise (3, 21). In another study, however, sickle-cell patients with hemoglobin levels equal to or greater than 8.5 g/dl performed mild to moderate levels of exercise without evidence of myocardial ischemia. In contrast, 36 percent of sickle-cell patients with hemoglobin levels less than 8.5 g/dl developed asymptomatic ST-segment depression (EKG evidence of decreased oxygen supply) at similar workloads (67). These studies confirm that the working capacity and therefore exercise tolerance of patients with Hb

SS disease are decreased, and that patients with the lowest hemoglobin levels have the highest occurrence of cardiac ischemia with acute exercise.

As in other forms of anemia, blood transfusions increase the exercise capacity of patients with sickle-cell anemia. In one study, following isovolemic partial exchange transfusion with normal blood, the percent of Hb A rose from 9% to 55%, but the total Hb value increased by only 1.4 g/dl and in 2 patients decreased. Results of this study suggested that improved exercise capacity was unrelated to the rise in hemoglobin (68). Most studies, however, indicate that the improvement in exercise capacity is secondary to the subsequent increase in hemoglobin concentration and improvement in oxygen transport, rather than to changes in the percent of sickle cells in the patient's blood (17). There is little evidence to indicate that blood flow to muscles is decreased in patients with sickle-cell anemia, although very low O_2 tensions have been recorded in the femoral vein during exercise (31).

An additional hazard to patients with Hb SS disease is exercise-induced shear hemolysis of dehydrated, irreversibly sickled red cells. As a result, intravascular hemolysis and hemoglobinuria may occur (82).

Patients with sickle-cell disease and some of the sickle variants may experience difficulty during high and moderate aerobic exercise because of hypoxia, dehydration, and acidosis, events that may potentiate sickling. In addition, both aerobic and anaerobic exercise in cold air or water (87) or at high altitudes (above 7200 feet) pose additional risks. In spite of the potential lethal consequences of intense exercise, death in sickle-cell disease is usually not exercise related, but is caused by infection, splenic sequestration, stroke, acute chest syndrome, or chronic organ failure; it may also occur suddenly without obvious cause (53a, 98, 107).

Some patients with Hb SC disease and some other variants may exercise and even play competitive sports without incident for many years prior to diagnosis. One 18-year-old boarding school student with Hb SC disease first presented to us with gross hematuria and mild anemia, having played field hockey and lacrosse without apparent incident. Nevertheless, measures to prevent dehydration, exhaustion, and

hypoxia should be emphasized. Oxygen and fluids should always be available and used liberally. Avoidance of strenuous exercise under conditions of increased heat and humidity as well as cold is advisable (53). Those patients with sickle-cell disease who elect to play high-intensity sports should have hemoglobin, hematocrit, and reticulocyte determinations as well as hemoglobin electrophoresis to identify the sickling disorder. This information together with the past medical history allows the physician to counsel the sickle-cell disease patient regarding the occurrence of sports-related morbidity.

With proper education and supervision, patients with sickle-cell disease should be encouraged to participate in all sport activities (Tables 19.2 and 19.3). Each athlete must learn his or her limits, and this personal assessment (Table 19.4) will in turn determine which sports are appropriate.

Sickle-Cell Trait and Exercise

Because sickle-cell trait (Hb AS) has most often been regarded as clinically harmless, these individuals have been encouraged to pursue normal lives including full participation in all sports without restrictions (Table 19.2 and 19.3). However, occasional reports of sudden death in previously healthy individuals with sickle-cell trait during exercise indicates that a reevaluation of the risk of participation in sport is merited (16, 30, 52, 58, 96, 100). Despite these sporadic reports of a deleterious association between strenuous exercise and sickle cell trait (some at high altitudes), larger surveys demonstrate that aerobic capacity and the cardiovascular response to strenuous exercise are normal in sickle-cell trait (2, 88).

The frequency of Hb AS is approximately 7%, suggesting that millions of students, many unidentified, have participated in strenuous sports without incident. Most reports of disaster associated with sickle-cell trait have been uncontrolled case reports and clinical anecdotes. Furthermore, the diagnosis of sickle-cell trait has not always been confirmed by electrophoresis (97).

Nevertheless, in previously healthy military recruits with sickle-cell trait, sudden death has occurred during physical training. In one report there was a 28% increase in sudden unexplained

Table 19.4 Effect of Type of Anemia on Sports-Related Characteristics

	Muscular strength	Flexibility	Coordinated skill	Aerobic capacity	Movement	Skeletal abnormalities	Splenomegaly
Iron deficiency with							
1. Mild to mod. anemia	±	0	0	±	0	0	0
2. Severe anemia	++	0	0	+++	0	0	0
Sickle-cell trait	0	0	0	0	0	0	0
Sickle-cell anemia	±	0	0	++ to +++	0	±	±
Thalassemia minor	0	0	0	0	0	0	0
Thalassemia major	±	0	0	+++	0	+	+++
Hemolytic disorders							
1. With splenomegaly	±	0	0	±	0	0	+++
2. Without splenomegaly	±	0	0	±	0	0	0
Chronic productive disorders							
Pure red cell and aplastic anemia	±	±	±	+ to +++	0	++	0
Anemia of chronic disease	±	±	±	+ to +++	±	±	±

Note. 0 = none; + = mild; ++ = moderate; +++ = marked; ± = variable.

deaths among black military recruits with sickle-cell trait as compared to black recruits without the trait. Most of the deaths occurred during very strenuous basic training (53), and may have resulted from exertional heat stroke (53a).

The relevance of these observations to the typical student athlete is unclear, but it is generally assumed that the risk of sudden death is extremely small. Therefore, the same advice and precautions given to all athletes should be especially stressed in athletes with sickle-cell trait, including

- gradual conditioning,
- gradual acclimatization, especially at high altitudes,
- maintenance of hydration, and
- moderation of exertion in hot, humid environments (53).

In addition, some sports such as scuba diving or snorkeling may be hazardous for persons with sickle-cell trait (as in normals); thus, proper conditioning and training are also essential (54).

Recently it has been suggested that a central registry for athletic deaths, including autopsy results, be developed in the United States (80).

As part of this registry, screening for hemoglobinopathies would ascertain the true incidence of hemoglobin-related complications. At this time, the rare and unlikely chance of death due to sickle-cell trait does not justify restricting these individuals from athletic competition.

Thalassemia Major and Exercise

Thalassemia major is one of a group of hereditary disorders caused by a defect in hemoglobin synthesis and associated with persistent severe anemia. Thalassemia minor is the corresponding heterozygous, asymptomatic, state in which only mild anemia occurs. Thalassemia intermedia patients may have moderately severe anemia, splenomegaly, and iron overload, but are usually able to maintain their hemoglobin levels above 7 g/dl without chronic transfusions. As childhood progresses, patients with untreated thalassemia major develop bony changes, iron overload due to periodic blood transfusions, and marked hepatosplenomegaly as a result of chronic hemolysis and extra medullary hematopoiesis. Prior to initiation of a chronic transfusion program, hemoglobin values range between 5 and 6 g/dl.

With the advent of blood transfusions designed to maintain hemoglobin concentrations above 10 g/dl, the symptoms and physical abnormalities of thalassemia major have abated and early mortality has been prevented. However, multiple transfusions cause excess iron deposition, which is associated with functional abnormalities of the cardiovascular, hepatic, and endocrine organs (38).

Progressive iron deposition in heart muscle is associated with fibrosis and necrosis, a phenomenon that can be measured by echocardiogram (60). If cardiac hemochromatosis is uncontrolled, cardiac output fails to meet the demands of exercise, and cardiac failure ensues (39).

The cardiorespiratory response to exercise is abnormal in patients with thalassemia major (48). As noted in other forms of anemia, the adequacy of oxygen for the demands of exercise depends on gas exchange in the lungs, the amount and distribution of blood flow, the hemoglobin concentration, and the affinity of hemoglobin for oxygen (42, 116). Even in stable transfused patients with thalassemia major, peak oxygen consumption is low and heart rate and cardiac output are high for the amount of oxygen consumed (48, 59, 70, 104). Pulmonary function abnormalities in thalassemia patients receiving transfusions have also been described (55). Many of these patients hypoventilate during exercise with concomitant slight increases in alveolar PCO_2 and reduction of PO_2. None of these respiratory abnormalities have improved after transfusion (48, 89).

In other forms of chronic anemia, hyperventilation is typical of the ventilatory response to exercise (104, 116). In thalassemic patients mild hypoxemia is present at rest (39), and more significant hypoxemia occurs during exercise (19, 49, 55).

Another complication of thalassemic subjects on a chronic transfusion program is the failure of the post-transfusion red cells to elevate 2,3-DPG levels (78). In contrast, in patients receiving monthly transfusions for congenital hypoplastic anemia, 2,3-DPG levels have increased as the degree of anemia worsens (29).

In recent years, programs of iron chelation therapy with desferrioxamine delay complications of a chronic transfusion program and provide a longer, symptom-free life. With this improved prognosis, patients have a greater opportunity to be involved in sport. Unfortunately, chelation treatment does not appear to reverse or prevent cardiac disease in patients with thalassemia major when treatment is started after 5 years of age (38, 76). Studies are still in progress to determine whether chelation therapy initiated early in life will prevent the onset of heart disease and congestive heart failure, and in turn improve survival.

In contrast to thalassemia major, there is no significant abnormality of cardiopulmonary function or exercise performance in subjects with thalassemia minor (Table 19.4). The variants of thalassemia, including thalassemia intermedia with moderate anemia and iron overload, might be expected to be associated with mild exercise abnormalities in proportion to their hemoglobin concentrations, but this observation has not been formally studied.

Congenital Hemolytic Anemia and Exercise

Hemolytic anemias such as hereditary spherocytosis and hereditary elliptocytosis may sometimes pose problems regarding the appropriate selection of exercise programs. The characteristic features of hereditary spherocytosis with an incidence of 1:5000 are anemia, splenomegaly, and sometimes jaundice. However, occasionally patients are not anemic and the condition may be so mild as to be undetected. In fact, over 75-85% of patients have hemoglobin levels greater than or equal to 10 g/dl, although younger children may be more severely anemic, and occasional patients (<5%) may be transfusion-dependent (57, 62). The primary treatment of hereditary spherocytosis is splenectomy, a procedure that is followed by disappearance of the anemia in most patients.

In general, exercise capacity is related to the degree of anemia, since most mildly affected patients have little or no disability (114). However, precipitous falls in hemoglobin may occur as a result of decreased production (aplastic crisis) or increased destruction of red cells (hyperhemolytic crisis). These crises frequently are secondary to intercurrent infections such as Ebstein Barr virus–induced infectious mononucleosis and disease due to human parvovirus 19 (46, 47).

In many hemolytic states the increased mechanical fragility of the red cells is associated with worsening of the anemia during strenuous exercise (11, 47). This phenomenon may occur in patients with low-grade, insignificant hemolysis, especially during physical activities such as running, swimming, recurrent trauma to local areas of the body (104), karate (106), rowing (35), weightlifting (13), marathon running, and prolonged marching—sometimes called "march hemoglobinuria" or "foot strike hemolysis" (24). Other factors which may potentiate exercise-related hemolysis include abnormalities of the aortic and mitral valves, synthetic prosthesis in the heart (84, 101), and primary aortic disease (85). Anemic athletes need to be aware of these additional hazards which may worsen their anemia.

Another reason for limiting the selection of a specific sport in individuals with hemolytic anemia may be the presence of splenomegaly. Enlarged spleens in congenital hemolytic anemia as well as in thalassemia and sickle-cell disease may be subject to rupture during contact sports and some noncontact high-aerobic sports, as indicated in Tables 19.2 and 19.4.

A much less common condition known as hereditary xerocytosis is also associated with mechanically fragile cells. A 21-year-old world-class competitive freestyle swimmer with xerocytosis and a hematocrit of 50 developed recurrent intravascular hemolysis during atraumatic swimming (83). This case illustrates again that nonanemic athletes with well-compensated hemolytic disorders may occasionally experience severe hemolysis and anemia during certain types of exercise.

Chronic Productive Disorders: Hypoplastic and Aplastic Anemias and Exercise

This group of disorders is complex because white cells as well as red cells may be affected. In contrast, pure red cell aplasia (Diamond-Blackfan anemia) and the chronic anemia seen with end-stage renal disease have impaired exercise capacity which is mainly attributable to the reduction in hemoglobin concentration.

In these disorders, untreated patients may have hemoglobin levels less than 6 gm/dl. Based on experience with other types of anemia of this severity, aerobic exercise and activities with moderate or high dynamic demands could be

hazardous. However, successful therapy and normalization of hemoglobin levels should enable these individuals to participate in all levels of sports. Even so, other physical problems exhibited by some of these patients may result in reduced exercise tolerance (4).

EXERCISE AND SPORT PROGRAMS FOR CHILDREN AND ADOLESCENTS WITH ANEMIA

As is now evident, exercise and aerobic athletic capacity may be compromised in any athlete with anemia. Nevertheless, the child or adolescent with reasonably stable chronic anemia can develop a state of physical fitness that is compatible with his or her degree of anemia. In many chronic anemic states without associated cardiopulmonary involvement, fitness should especially emphasize cardiovascular and muscular development to an appropriate level for each individual. This recommendation implies that the anemic individual's maximal O_2 consumption should increase to a level that is comfortably and reasonably attained. Just as the normal subject compensates during submaximal exercise with relative increases in cardiac output, heart rate and ventilatory response, the anemic patient responds in similar fashion up to an individual maximum, a state that is extremely variable.

In most anemic patients, improved exercise capacity and increased $\dot{V}O_2$max correlate with an improved state of physical fitness (17). In addition to cardiopulmonary conditioning, the concept of fitness for the anemic child and adolescent should ideally include optimal muscle strength, flexibility, and body composition (32). As in normal individuals, there are many personal factors, both genetic and environmental, that determine athletic success for anemic individuals. Therefore, there is no specific hemoglobin level that absolutely excludes participation in either casual informal athletics or in competitive sport. Although there are no supporting data, most children with chronic anemia experience less exercise than their physical status merits, a phenomenon that occurs even in normal, nonanemic children.

Since severe clinical symptoms of anemia begin to appear in children when hemoglobin levels decrease to 6 g/dl, exercise tolerance can diminish rapidly at this level (115) (Table 19.1). Nevertheless, according to the histories given by parents, hematologists have observed some young children with slowly developing, severe iron deficiency who appear to have relatively normal physical activity. Similarly, the authors presently care for a slightly jaundiced 18-year-old Nigerian youth with Hb SS disease and a hematocrit in the 23-27% range who is now entering college in the U.S.A. as a competitive soccer player. He now runs about 2 miles each day in preparation for the soccer season, a sport that he has avidly played throughout childhood. Although he suffers painful crises, this highly motivated student and athlete is able to overcome some of the complications of his disease and to successfully compete. Unfortunately, most patients with sickle-cell anemia will never achieve athletically at such a high level.

In contrast, physical fitness in subjects with uncomplicated chronic anemia can be improved by aerobic cardiovascular conditioning with exercise of submaximal intensity. Aerobic exercise features large muscle groups which are used continuously and rhythmically in sports such as swimming, jogging, bike riding, brisk walking, cross-country skiing, and rowing. The emphasis in these aerobic sports is on continuous rather than on stop-and-go activity; thus, the intensity and duration of the exercise must be initially limited and gradually increased within individual tolerance levels.

Individual rather than competitive team sports are usually preferable for individuals with severe anemia. Under these conditions the athlete will be able to modify or terminate the activity in response to his or her own early signals of trouble (Table 19.2 and 19.3). Another of the author's patients, a 17-year-old with severe chronic hemolytic anemia caused by pyruvate kinase deficiency and a hemoglobin level in the 6 g/dl range, plays noncompetitive tennis and also maintains a walking and hiking program. She reports that the emotional benefit is significant and provides her with a sense of accomplishment and well-being, but only if she is able to self-direct and limit the pace and duration of each exercise. Fatigue and light-headedness are symptoms that signal to her that it is time to rest. This patient has a very high 2,3-DPG level, which probably explains her surprisingly good exercise tolerance.

Older children and teenagers with severe varieties of anemia can improve their bodily flexibility with stretching activities. In these individuals, muscle strength and power can be safely increased with appropriate weight training—either free weights or Nautilus-type apparatus. However, during weight lifting heart rate and blood pressure increase with little increase in O_2 consumption. As a result, myocardial oxygen demand may increase in the face of inadequate myocardial oxygen supply. Although this is not a threat to the normal individual, the severely anemic child with decreased oxygen delivering capacity might be at risk. Nevertheless, in the severely affected adolescent, tailored and monitored weightlifting programs might hold great appeal, not only because of the strength enhancement but also for the ego boost provided by having big muscles.

It is impressive that youngsters with long-standing anemias may learn to adjust to very low hemoglobin levels in the 6-8 g/dl range. Some of these children report that they are able to play such aerobically demanding sports as basketball, usually at a pace which they learn to tolerate and limit as necessary. As expected, behavioral as well as physiological compensation occurs. The main physiological compensatory mechanisms include an increased circulation of blood to energy-demanding tissues and a larger removal of oxygen from hemoglobin (110). When physiological compensation reaches a maximum and becomes insufficient, the individual is forced to modify the exercise or complete the activity. In chronic anemia, the remarkable physiological adaptation and behavioral patterns that often occur during sport and exercise may be very efficient but are not easily measured by standard tests under laboratory conditions.

On the other hand, the paucity of scientific data reporting life-threatening effects of exercise in chronic anemia suggests that young patients gradually acquire insight into their own physical limitations. Our responsibility as physicians, nurses, trainers, coaches, physical therapists, and parents is to

- encourage participation in an appropriate sport or exercise program so as to establish reasonable fitness,
- educate the individual and family as to the potential adverse conditions to avoid, and

- monitor and record the positive as well as negative effects of the exercise program.

RECOMMENDATIONS FOR SPECIFIC SPORTS AND EXERCISE PARTICIPATION BY INDIVIDUALS WITH ANEMIA

Predictably, on the basis of the data already presented, recommendations for specific exercise and conditioning activities as well as specific sports vary with both the type and severity of chronic anemia (Tables 19.2 and 19.3). Pertinent to all types of chronic anemia, however, are several general observations. Prior to elementary school, if given the opportunity and encouragement, anemic children will usually be active enough without an organized or professionally supervised exercise program. Emphasis should be on normal social interaction, which in turn will encourage flexibility, movement, and strength development.

In elementary and middle school, the chronically anemic child needs encouragement and support to be physically active, rather than to be made fearful and inactive because of his or her disorder. Most children of all ages seem capable of modifying or limiting their exercise if they experience significant symptoms due to anemia.

Adolescents with anemia may need the most guidance regarding a reasonable exercise and sports program. Their aspirations to be heroic in stature and speed may produce frustration and hostility and may result in unhealthy athletic overachievement. As in all age groups, the challenge is to help the individual select a sport or physical activity that is realistic, not only in terms of potential proficiency and achievement but also to avoid unnecessary discomfort or potential hazard. The goal should be to prevent frustration and the ultimate "turning off" of the youngster to all kinds of physical activity.

Precise recommendations for appropriate sport and exercise routines for each individual with anemia are impossible. Genetically determined athletic "talent", motivation, conditioning, and acclimatization will influence functioning at each hemoglobin level as well as within

each type of anemia. Thus, there can be no minimally acceptable hemoglobin level for participation in a given sport. Rather, some guidelines and general recommendations can be made on the basis of the likelihood of serious complications (Table 19.2 and 19.3). At one end of the severity spectrum is the iron-deficient state without anemia. In spite of the physiological abnormalities already described, it is very unlikely that any serious complications will occur in this condition, and affected athletes can continue to exercise and participate in all sports. Hopefully, they will be diagnosed and informed of their iron deficiency and made to realize that they may lose their competitive edge or that mild unrecognized symptoms may occur. Some competitive athletes with chronic or recurrent iron deficiency should be followed medically, particularly if the athlete falls into a high-risk group. Risk factors may include menstrual blood loss, inappropriate nutritional intake in either sex, and engaging in sports associated with iron loss, such as distance running.

Today, children with severe, chronic anemia caused by iron deficiency are seen much less frequently in the United States than in other areas of the world, and when diagnosed and treated, usually promptly improve. Until severe iron deficiency anemia (Table 19.1) is corrected, however, sports moderate or high in aerobic intensity should be curtailed (e.g., competitive distance running) (Table 19.2 and 19.3). Most sports with high dynamic demand, as well as some sports with high static demand, also involve high aerobic demand and may also be inadvisable (Table 19.2 and 19.3). However, some team sports with high aerobic and dynamic demands (e.g., baseball) can be modified in some instances to allow for limited but enjoyable participation (swinging the bat, catching, and throwing). Improvement in the hemoglobin level should then allow for expanded involvement.

Children with severe anemia stemming from other causes may be unable to engage effectively in sports with high and moderate aerobic demand. Even some sports with low dynamic demands (weight lifting) and low static demands (swimming) are inadvisable since the related aerobic demands may be excessive. In contrast, neuromuscular (skill) functions, motion, and dynamics are usually normal in uncomplicated anemia (Table 19.4). Flexibility and agility are also normal. Therefore, individual sports with low aerobic demands such as golf, horseback riding, bowling, archery, and some hiking should be ideal for patients with severe anemia. However, local muscular strength may be adversely affected as the hemoglobin level falls (5, 22, 33, 75, 110). Individual trials will determine the extent of sport and exercise possible for the individuals with moderate anemia, since some athletes will do well as the hemoglobin concentration rises toward 10 g/dl. Those individuals with moderate or severe anemia who are interested in pursuing competitive individual or team sports should have formal fitness testing. Even though the direct measurement of O_2 uptake ($\dot{V}O_2$max) is expensive, this procedure may be indicated in some instances. An inexpensive cycle ergometer or portable step apparatus together with a heart rate monitor may, using progressively increased workloads, be helpful in the formulation of a more formal sport program. Even with this testing, in patients with mild or moderate anemia the results may be difficult to apply to performance in individual sports. Communication with a knowledgeable sport supervisor or physician will often provide the most useful information.

In general, individuals with mild or moderate anemia may participate in all sports, although some will be unable to successfully compete in moderately or highly aerobic team sports such as football, basketball, soccer, and water polo. On the other hand, athletes in these categories can safely play tennis, softball or baseball, table tennis, dance, badminton, or downhill skiing after acclimatization. That is not to say that a moderately anemic but otherwise talented place kicker could not succeed in competitive football; the limiting factor would likely be the athlete's natural ability and the availability of an appropriate conditioning program, which may require less rigorous cardiopulmonary training.

The selection of exercise and sports for sickle-cell anemia patients is hindered by a lack of scientific data as to how these patients fare during basketball or baseball games, or even during sports with high static demands such as weightlifting. Patients with Hb SS and cardiopulmonary abnormalities should be advised not to participate in competitive highly and moderately aerobic sports such as basketball, football, or competitive swimming. In addition, the risk of

bone marrow embolism, pulmonary infarction, or ruptured spleen precludes participation in contact sports, either competitive or noncompetitive. Whether sports-related trauma initiates painful crises in sickle-cell disease is unknown, but this risk also makes participation in contact/collision sports hazardous.

Thalassemia major patients prior to splenectomy should not play contact sports since splenic rupture is a major risk factor. In addition, the potential for cardiac failure, even during a transfusional program, should alert the patient to the risks of highly aerobic and contact/collision sports. However, it is possible that some patients with thalassemia major who receive early treatment will tolerate highly or moderately aerobic team sports.

Recommendations given for sport and exercise programs to children with other forms of hemolytic disease, such as hereditary spherocytosis, should depend entirely on the severity of anemia and the stability of the disorder. Children with the very common variety of mild hereditary spherocytosis (no clinical symptoms and little or no anemia because of compensated hemolysis) may participate in all sports. However, some patients with mild to moderate splenomegaly may be susceptible to splenic rupture following trauma (Table 19.2).

CONCLUSION

Participation in sport and exercise by youngsters with chronic productive disorders will depend on the degree of anemia and the type of therapy that they are receiving. Children with anemia secondary to chronic disease may be more limited by the overall effects of the disease than by the degree of anemia. Recommendations for sport and exercise in this group should stress maintenance of flexibility and reasonable aerobic conditioning.

REFERENCES

1. Adamson, J.; Vapnek, D. Recombinant erythropoietin to improve athletic performance. N. Engl. J. Med. 324:698-699; 1991.
2. Alpert, B.S.; Flood, N.L.; Strong, W.B.; Blair, J.R.; Levy, A.L. Responses to exercise

in children with sickle cell trait. Am. J. Dis. Child. 136(11):1002-1004; 1982.

3. Alpert, B.S.; Gilman, P.A.; Strong, W.B.; Ellison, M.F.; Miller, M.D.; McFarlane, J.; Hayashidera, T. Hemodynamic and ECG responses to exercise in children with sickle cell anemia. Am. J. Dis. Child. 135(4):362-366; 1981.

4. Alter, B.P. Childhood red cell aplasia. Am. J. Pediatr. Hematol. Oncol. 2:121-139; 1980.

5. Anderson, H.T.; Borkve, H. Iron deficiency and muscular work performance. Scand. J. Clin. Lab. Invest. 25(suppl. 114): 3-62; 1970.

6. Anonymous. "Anemia" in athletics (editorial). Lancet i:1490-1491; 1985.

7. Austin, P.L.; Stegink, L.D.; Gisolfi, C.V.; Lauer, R.M. The effect of exercise on red blood cell 2, 3 diphosphoglycerate in children. J. Pediatr. 83:41-45; 1973.

8. Baraldi, E.; Montini, G.; Zanconato, S.; Zacchello, G.; Zacchello, F. Exercise tolerance after anaemia correction with recombinant human erythropoietin in end-stage renal disease. Pediatr. Nephrol. 4:623-626; 1990.

9. Barrett, O.; Saunders, D.E.; McFarland, D.E.; Humphries, J.O. Myocardial infarction in sickle cell anemia. Am. J. Hematol. 16:139-147; 1984.

10. Bishop, J.M.; Donald, R.W.; Wade, O.L. Circulatory dynamics at rest and on exercise in the hyperkinetic states. Clin. Sc. 14:329-360; 1955.

11. Blum, S.F.; Sullivan, J.M.; Gardner, F.H. The exacerbation of hemolysis in PNH by strenuous exercise. Blood 30:513-517; 1967.

12. Bromberg, P.A. Pulmonary aspects of sickle cell disease. Arch. Intern. Med. 133:652-657; 1974.

13. Bula, B.; Ziobro, E.; Sutylo, Z. Myogenic causes of hemolysis (in Polish). Physical Education and Sport. 2:33-38; 1966.

14. Bunn, H.F.; Forget, B.G. Hemoglobin: molecular, genetic, and clinical aspects. 2d ed. Philadelphia: W.B. Saunders Co.; 1986.

15. Celsing, F.; Blomstrand, E.; Werner, B.; Pihlstedt, P.; Ekblom, B. Effects of iron deficiency on endurance and muscle enzyme activity in man. Med. Sci. Sports Exerc. 18:156-161; 1986.

16. Charache, S., editor. Sudden death in sickle trait. Am. J. Med. 84:459-460; 1988.

17. Charache, S.; Blecker, E.R.; Bross, D.S. Effects of blood transfusion on exercise capacity in patients with sickle cell anemia. Am. J. Med. 74:757-764; 1983.

18. Cook, J.D. The effect of endurance training on iron metabolism. In: Spivak, J.L., ed. Sports hematology; seminars in hematology 31:146-154; 1994.

19. Cooper, D.M.; Mansell, A.L.; Weiner, M.A.; Berdon, W.E.; Chetty-Baktaviziam, A.; Reid, L.; Mellins, R.B. Low lung capacity and hypoxemia in children with thalassemia major. Am. Rev. Respir. Dis. 121(4):639-646; 1980.

20. Correra, A.; Graziano, J.H.; Seaman, C.; Piomelli, S. Inappropriately low red cells 2,3-diphosphoglycerate and P50 in transfused B-thalassemia. Blood 63:803-806; 1984.

21. Covitz, W.; Eubig, C.; Balfour, I.C.; Jerath, R.; Alpert, B.S.; Strong, W.B.; DuRant, R.H. Exercise-induced cardiac dysfunction in sickle cell anemia. Am. J. Cardiol. 51(3):570-575; 1983.

22. Dallman, P.R. Manifestations of iron deficiency. Seminars in Haematology 19:19-30; 1982.

23. Dallman, P.R.; Beutler, E.; Finch, C.A. Effects of iron deficiency exclusive of anaemia. Brit. J. Hematology. 40:179-184; 1978.

24. Davidson, R.J.L.; Robertson, J.D.; Maughan, R.J. Hematological changes associated with marathon running. International J. of Sports Med. 8:19-25; 1987.

25. Davies, C.T.M.; Chukweumeka, A.C.; Von Haarin, J.P.M. Iron deficiency anaemia: its effect on maximum aerobic power and responses to exercise in African males ages 17-40 years. Clin. Science. 44:555-562; 1973.

26. Davies, C.T.M.; Von Haarin, J.P.M. Anemia: effect of therapy on responses to exercise. Proc. of the Physiologic Society 36-37; Sept. 1972.

27. Davies, K.J.A.; Donovan, C.M.; Refino, C.J.; Brooks, G.A.; Packer, L.; Dallman, P.R. Distinguishing effects of anemia and muscle iron deficiency on exercise bioenergetics in the rat. Am. J. Physiol. 246:E535-E543; 1984.

28. Davies, K.J.A.; Maguire, J.J.; Brooks, G.A.; Dallman, P.R.; Packer, L. Muscle mitochondrial bioenergetics, oxygen supply, and work capacity during dietary iron deficiency and repletion. Am. J. Physiol. 242: E418-E427; 1982.

29. Dickerman, J.D.; Ostrea, E.M.; Zinkham, W.H. In vivo aging of transfused erythrocytes and 2,3-diphosphoglycerate levels. Blood 42:9-15; 1973.

30. Diggs, L.W. The sickle cell trait in relation to the training and assignment of duties in the armed forces: III Hyposthuria, hematuria, sudden death, rhabdomyolysis and acute tubular necrosis. Aviat. Space Environ. Med. 55:358-364; 1984.

31. Doll, E.; Keul, J. pO, pH, and pCO_2 in the coronarvenous and femoral-venous blood during exercise and hypoxia. In: Biochemistry Exercise Medicine Sport, (Volume 3). Basel: S. Karger; 1969:35-40.

32. Dyment, P.G., editor. Sports medicine: health care for young athletes. 2d. ed. Elk Grove, IL: Amer. Acad. Pediatr.; 1991.

33. Edgerton, V.R.; Bryant, S.L.; Gillespie, C.; Gardner, G.W. Iron deficiency anemia and physical performance and activity of rats. J. Nutr. 102:381-399; 1972.

34. Edwards, C.Q.; Griffen, L.M.; Goldgar, D.; Drummond, C.; Skolnick, M.H.; Kushner, J.P. Prevalence of hemochromatosis among 11,065 presumably healthy blood donors. N. Engl. J. Med. 318:1355-1362; 1988.

35. Eichner, E.R.; Strauss, R.H.; Sherman, W.M.; Dernbach, A.; Lamb, D.R. Intravascular hemolysis in elite college rowers. Abstract No. 466. Medicine and Science in Sports and Exercise. 21 (2 suppl):S78; 1989.

36. Ekblom, B.; Berglung, B. Effect of erythropoietin administration on maximal aerobic power. Scand. J. Med. Sci. Sports 1:88-93; 1991.

37. Ekblom, B.; Goldbarg, A.N.; Gullbring, B. Response to exercise after blood loss and reinfusion. J. of Applied Physiology. 33:175-180; 1972.

38. Engle, M.A. Cardiac involvement in Cooley's anemia. Ann. N.Y. Acad. Sci. 119:694-702; 1964.

39. Engle, M.A.; Erlandson, M.; Smith, C.H. Late cardiac complications of chronic severe, refractory anemia with hemochromatosis. Circulation 30:698-705; 1964.

40. Falk, R.H.; Hood, W.B., Jr. The heart in sickle cell anemia. Arch. Intern. Med. 142: 1680-1684; 1982.

41. Femi-Pearse, D.; Gazioglu, K.M.; Yu, P.N. Pulmonary function studies in sickle cell disease. J. Appl. Physiol. 28:574-577; 1970.

42. Finch, C.A.; Lenfant, C. Oxygen transport in man. N. Engl. J. Med. 286:407-415; 1972.

43. Finch, C.A.; Miller, C.R.; Inamdar, A.R.; Person, R.; Seilder, K.; Mackler, B. Iron deficiency in the rat: physiological and biochemical studies of muscle dysfunction. J. Clin. Invest. 58:447-453; 1976.

44. Gardner, G.W.; Edgerton, V.R.; Bernard, R.J.; Bernauer, E.M. Cardiorespiratory, hematological and physical performance responses of anemic subjects to iron treatment. Am. J. Clin. Nutr. 28:982-988; 1975.

45. Gardner, G.W.; Edgerton, V.R.; Senewiratne, B.; Ohira, Y. Physical work capacity and metabolic stress in subjects with iron deficiency anemia. Am. J. of Clin. Nutr. 30:910-917; 1977.

46. Gehlbach, S.H.; Cooper, B.A. Haemolytic anemia in infectious mononucleosis due to inapparent congenital spherocytosis. Scand. J. Haematol. 7:141-144; 1970.

47. Godal, H.C.; Refsum, H.E. Haemolysis in athletes due to hereditary spherocytosis. Scand. J. Haematol. 22:83-86; 1979.

48. Grant, G.P.; Graziano, J.H.; Seaman, C.; Mansell, A.L. Cardiorespiratory response to exercise in patients with thalassemia major. Am. Rev. Resp. Dis. 136(1):92-97; 1987.

49. Grant, G.P.; Mansell, G.L.; Graziano, A.L.; Mellins, R.D. The effect of transfusions on lung capacity, diffusing capacity and arterial oxygen saturation in patients with thalassemia major. Pediat. Res. 20:20-23; 1986.

50. Halvorsen, F.A.; Lyng, J.; Ritland, S. Gastrointestinal bleeding in marathon runners. Scan. J. Gastroenterology 21:493-497; 1986.

51. Jones, M.; Pedoe, D.S.T. Blood doping: a literature review. Br. J. Sports Med. 23:84-88; 1989.

52. Jones, S.R.; Binder, R.A.; Donowho, E.M. Sudden death in sickle cell trait. N. Engl. J. Med. 282:323-325; 1970.

53. Kark, J.A.; Posey, D.M.; Schumacher, H.R.; Ruehle, C.J. Sickle cell trait as a risk factor for sudden death in physical training. N. Engl. J. Med. 317:781-787; 1987.

53a. Kark, J.A.; Ward, F.T. Exercise and hemoglobin S. In: Spivak, J.L., ed. Sports hematology; seminars in hematology. 31:181-225; July, 1994.

54. Kats, B.A. Decompression disease and the sickle cell trait. Can. Med. Assoc. J. 116:475-476; 1977.

55. Keens, T.G.; O'Neal, M.H.; Ortega, J.A.; Hyman, C.B.; Platzker, A.C. Pulmonary function abnormalities in thalassemia patients on a hypertransfusion program. Pediatrics 65:1013-1017; 1980.

56. Klocke, R.A. Oxygen transport and 2,3 diphosphoglycerate. Chest 62(5):79S-85S; 1972.

57. Krueger, H.C.; Burgert, E.O. Hereditary spherocytosis in 100 children. Mayo Clin. Proc. 41:821-830; 1966.

58. Lane, P.A.; Githens, J.H. Splenic syndrome at mountain altitudes in sickle cell trait. Its occurrence in non-black persons. JAMA 253:2251-2254; 1985.

59. Leight, L.; Snider, T.H.; Clifford, G.O.; Hellems, H.K. Hemodynamic studies in sickle cell anemia. Circulation 10:653-662; 1954.

60. Leon, M.B.; Borer, J.S.; Bacharach, S.L.; Green, M.V.; Benz, E.J., Jr.; Griffith, P.; Nienhuis, A.W. Detection of early cardiac dysfunction in patients with severe beta-thalassemia and chronic iron overload. N. Engl. J. Med. 301(21):1143-1148; 1979.

61. Lonsdorfer, J.; Bogui, P.; Otayeck, A.; Bursaux, E.; Poyart, C.; Cabannes, R. Cardio-respiratory adjustments in chronic sickle cell anemia. Bull. Eur. Physiopathol. Respir. 19(4):339-344; 1983.

62. MacKinney, A.A., Jr.; Morton, N.E.; Kogower, N.S.; Schilling, H.F. Ascertaining genetic causes of hereditary spherocytosis by statistical analysis of multiple laboratory tests. J. Clin. Invest. 41:554-567; 1962.

63. Magnusson, B.; Hallberg, L.; Rossonder, L.; Swolin, B. Iron metabolism and sports anemia: II. A hematological comparison of elite runners and control subjects. Acta Med. Scand. 216(2):157-164; 1984.

64. Manno, B.V.; Burka, E.R.; Hakki, A.H.; Manno, C.S.; Iskandrian, A.S.; Noone, A.M. Biventricular function in sickle cell anemia: radionuclide angiographic and thallium-201 scintigraphic evaluation. Am. J. Cardiol. 52(5):584-587; 1983.

65. Martin, C.R.; Cobb, C.; Tatter, D.; Johnson, C.; Haywood, L.J. Acute myocardial infarction in sickle cell anemia. Arch Int. Med. 143(4):830-831; 1983.

66. Matter, M.; Stittfall, T.; Graves, J.; Myburgh, K.; Adams, B.; Jacobs, P.; Noakes, T.D. The effect of iron and folate therapy on maximal exercise performance in female marathon runners with iron and folate deficiency. Clin. Sci. 72(4):415-422; 1987.

67. McConnell, M.E.; Daniels, S.R.; Lobel, J.; James, F.W.; Kaplan, S. Hemodynamic response to exercise in patients with sickle cell anemia. Pediatr. Cardiol. 10:141-144; 1989.

68. Miller, D.M.; Winslow, R.M.; Klein, H.G.; Wilson, K.C.; Brown, F.L.; Statham, N.J. Improved exercise performance after exchange transfusion in subjects with sickle cell anemia. Blood 56(6):1127-1131; 1980.

69. Miller, G.J.; Serjeant, G.R. An assessment of lung volumes and gas transfer in sickle anaemia. Thorax 26:309-315; 1971.

70. Miller, G.J.; Serjeant, G.R.; Sivapragasam, S.; Petch, M.C. Cardio-pulmonary responses and gas exchange during exercise in adults with homozygous sickle cell disease (sickle cell anemia). Clin. Sci. 44(2):113-128; 1973.

71. Modell, B.; Letsky, E.; Flynn, D.M.; Peto, R.; Weatherall, D.J. Survival and desferrioxamine in thalassemia major. Br. Med. J. 284(6322):1081-1084; 1982.

72. Newhouse, I.J.; Clement, D.B.; Taunton, J.E.; McKenzie, D.C. The effects of prelatent/latent iron deficiency on physical work capacity. Med. Sci. Sports Exerc. 21(3):263-268; 1989.

73. Nickerson, H.J.; Holubets, M.C.; Tripp, A.D.; Pierce, W.E. Decreased iron stores in high school female runners. Am. J. Dis. Child. 139(11):1115-1119; 1985.

74. Nickerson, H.J.; Holubets, M.C.; Weiler, B.R.; Haas, R.G.; Schwartz, S.; Ellefson, M.E. Causes of iron deficiency in adolescent athletes. J. Pediatr. 114(4, Pt 1):657-663; 1989.

75. Ohira, Y.; Edgerton, V.R.; Gardner, G.W.; Senewiratne, B.; Barnard, R.J.; Simpson, D.R. Work capacity, heart rate and blood lactate responses to iron treatment. Br. J. Haematol. 41(3):365-372; 1979.

76. Olivieri, N.; Freedman, M.H.; Saunders, F.; Greenberg, G.M.; Rose, V. Uncertain efficacy of conventional desferoxamine chelation in thalassemic heart disease. Ped. Res. 17:240A; 1983.

77. Oski, F.A. The nonhematologic manifestations of iron deficiency. Am. J. Dis. Child. 133:315-322; 1979.

78. Oski, F.A.; Gottlieb, A.J.; Miller, W.W.; Delivoria-Papdopoulos, M. The effect of deoxygenation of adult and fetal hemoglobin on the synthesis of red cell 2,3 diphosphoglycerate and its in vivo consequences. J. Clin. Invest. 49:400-407; 1970.

79. Oski, F.A.; Honig, A.S. The effects of therapy on the developmental scores of iron-deficient infants. J. Pediatr. 92:21-25; 1978.

80. Oski, F.A.; Marshall, B.E.; Cohen, P.J.; Sugerman, H.J.; Miller, L.D. The role of the left-shifted or right-shifted oxygen-hemoglobin equilibrium curve. Ann. Intern. Med. 74(1):44-46; 1971.

81. Pearson, H.A., editor. Sickle cell trait and competitive athletics: is there a risk? Pediatrics 83:613-614; 1989.

82. Platt, O.S. Exercise-induced hemolysis in sickle cell anemia: shear sensitivity and erythrocyte dehydration. Blood 59:1055-1060; 1982.

83. Platt, O.S.; Lux, S.E.; Nathan, D.G. Exercise-induced hemolysis in xerocytosis: red cell dehydration and shear sensitivity. J. Clin. Invest. 68:631-638; 1981.

84. Rasmussen, K.; Anders, A.; Myhre, E.; Hillestad, L. Hemolysis during acute exercise in patients with aortic ball valve prostheses. Acta Med. Scand. 188(4):281-286; 1970.

85. Ravenel, S.D.; Johnson, J.D.; Sigler, A.T. Intravascular hemolysis associated with coarctation of the aorta. J. Pediatr. 76:67-73; 1969.

86. Rees, A.H.; Stefadouros, M.A.; Strong, W.B.; Miller, M.D.; Gilman, P.; Rigby, J.A.; McFarlane, J. Left ventricular performance in children with homozygous sickle cell anaemia. Br. Heart J. 40(6):690-696; 1978.

87. Resar, C.M.; Oski, F.A. Cold water exposure and vaso-occlusive crises in sickle cell anemia. J. of Pediatrics 118:407-409; 1991.

88. Robinson, J.R.; Stone, W.T.; Asendorf, A.C. Exercise capacity of black sickle cell trait males. Med. Sci. Sports 8(4):244-245; 1976.

89. Ross, R.D.; Wessel, H.V.; Paul, M.H. Reduced ventilatory response to graded exercise in patients with thalassemia major. Fed. Proc. 43:634; 1984.

90. Rowland, T.W. Iron deficiency in the young athlete. Ped. Clin. of N.A. 37:1153-1163; 1990.

91. Rowland, T.W.; Black, S.A.; Kelleher, J.F. Iron deficiency in adolescent endurance athletes. J. of Adoles. Health Care. 8:322-326; 1987.

92. Rowland, T.W.; Deisroth, M.A.; Green, G.M.; Kelleher, J.F. The effect of iron therapy on the exercise capacity of nonanemic iron-deficient adolescent runners. Am. J. Dis. Child. 142(2):165-169; 1988.

93. Rowland, T.W.; Kelleher, J.F. Iron deficiency in athletics—insights from high school swimmers. Am. J. Dis. Child. 143:197-200; 1989.

94. Salonen, J.T.; Nyyssonen, K.; Korpela, H.; Tuomliehto, J.; Seppanen, R.; Salonen, R. High stored iron levels are associated with excess risk of myocardial infarction in Eastern Finnish men. Circulation 86:803-811; 1992.

95. Sateriale, M.; Hart, P. Unexpected death in a black military recruit with sickle cell trait. Case Report. Milit. Med. 150:602-605; 1985.

96. Schoene, R.B.; Escorurou, P.; Robertson, H.T.; Nilson, K.L.; Parsons, J.R.; Smith, N.J. Iron repletion decreases maximal exercise lactate concentrations in female athletes with minimal iron-deficiency anemia. J. Lab. Clin. Med. 102(2):306-312; 1983.

97. Sears, D.A. The morbidity of sickle cell trait; a review of the literature. Am. J. Med. 69:1021-1036; 1978.

98. Seeler, R.A. Deaths in children with sickle cell anemia. A clinical analysis of 19 fatal instances in Chicago. Clin. Pediatr. 11:634-637; 1972.

99. Selby, G.B.; Eichner, E.R. Endurance, swimming, intravascular hemolysis, anemia and iron depletion: new perspective on athlete's anemia. Am. J. Med. 81:791-794; 1986.

100. Shalev, O.; Boylen, A.L.; Levene, C.; Oppenheim, A.; Rachmilewitz, E.A. Sickle cell trait in a white Jewish family presenting as splenic infarction at high altitude. Am. J. Hematol. 27(1):46-48; 1988.

101. Sigler, A.T.; Forman, E.N.; Zinkham, W.H.; Neill, C.A. Severe intravascular hemolysis following surgical repair of endocardial cushion defects. Am. J. Med. 35:467-480; 1963.

102. Smith, D.A.; Perry, P.J. The efficacy of ergogenic agents in athletic competition. Part I: other performance-enhancing agents. Ann. Pharmacother. 26:653-659; 1992.

103. Sproule, B.J.; Halden, E.R.; Miller, W.F. A study of cardiopulmonary alterations in patients with sickle cell disease and its variants. J. Clin. Invest. 37:486-495; 1958.

104. Sproule, B.J.; Mitchell, J.H.; Miller, W.F. Cardiopulmonary physiologic responses to heavy exercise in patients with anemia. J. Clin. Invest. 39:378-388; 1960.

105. Stevens, R.G.; Jones, D.Y.; Micozzi, M.S.; Taylor, P.R. Body iron stores and the risk of cancer. N. Engl. J. Med. 319:1047-1052; 1988.

106. Streeton, J.A. Traumatic haemoglobinuria caused by karate exercises. Lancet 2:191-192; 1967.

107. Thomas, A.N.; Pattison, C.; Serjeant, G.R. Causes of death in sickle cell disease in Jamaica. Br. Med. J. 285(6342):633-635; 1982.

108. Uzsoy, N.K. Cardiovascular findings in patients with sickle cell anemia. Am. J. Cardiol. 13:320-328; 1964.

109. Varat, M.A.; Adolph, R.J.; Fowler, N.O. Cardiovascular effects of anemia. Am. Heart J. 83:415-426; 1972.

110. Viteri, F.E.; Torin, B. Anemia and physical work capacity. Clinics in Hematology 3: 609-626; 1974.

111. Wadler, G.I. Drug use update. Medical Clinics of North America 78:439-455; 1994.

112. Wall, M.A.; Platt, O.S.; Strieder, D.J. Lung function in children with sickle cell anemia. Am. Rev. Respir. Dis. 120(1):210-214;1979.

113. Weiner, M.; Karpatkin, M.; Hart, D.; Seaman, C.; Vora, S.K.; Henry, W.L.; Piomelli, S. Cooley anemia: high transfusion regimen and chelation therapy, results and perspective. J. Pediatr. 92(4):653-658; 1978.

114. Werner, B.; Lindahl, J. Endogenous carbon monoxide production after bicycle exercise in healthy subjects and in patients with hereditary spherocytosis. Scand. J. Clin. Lab. Invest. 40:319-324; 1980.

115. Woodson, R.D. Hemoglobin concentration and exercise capacity. Amer. Rev. Resp. Dis. 129(Suppl):S72-S75; 1984.

116. Woodson, R.D.; Heywood, D.; Lenfont, C. Oxygen transport in hemoglobin Koln. Arch. Intern. Med. 134:711-715; 1974.

CHAPTER 20

Hemophilia

Diana S. Beardsley
Yale University School of Medicine

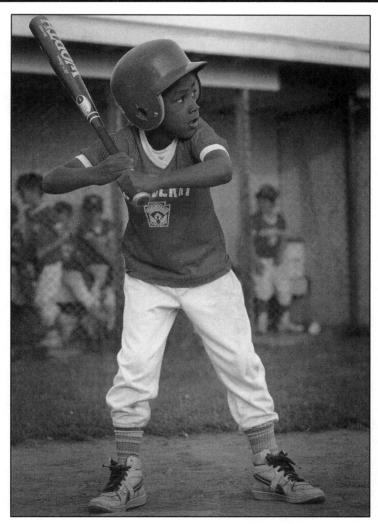

The normal system of hemostasis provides for smooth, fluid flow within normal vascular spaces and for prompt halting of hemorrhage whenever the blood vessels are damaged. There are three major elements of the hemostatic system: blood vessels, platelets (blood clotting cells), and a series of plasma proteins or clotting factors. If a blood vessel is injured, platelets adhere to the site, become activated, and then aggregate together to form a barrier against local blood loss—the platelet plug. This process, called primary hemostasis, provides the initial protection against excessive hemorrhage. After the platelet plug forms, plasma proteins of the clotting cascade become activated and form a strong clot capable of protecting against rebleeding after the platelet bonds are released. This firm clot formation is the process of secondary hemostasis. After clot stabilization and healing, the blood clot is removed by the process of fibrinolysis (see Table 20.1).

Abnormalities of any of the elements of hemostasis can lead to excessive bleeding. Rarely, abnormal blood vessels are more susceptible to hemorrhage because of defective supporting proteins (Marfan's or Ehlers-Danlos' syndromes, steroid effects, or scurvy) or inflammation of the blood vessels (vasculitis). The more common hemostatic defects encountered are those related to abnormalities of platelets or plasma proteins. Abnormalities of platelets that cause defects in primary hemostasis include a low number of platelets (thrombocytopenia) or defective platelet function. Interference with normal platelet

plug formation from any cause predisposes to prolonged bleeding immediately at the time of an injury; this would include epistaxis (nose bleeding) or oral hemorrhage at the time of a facial injury, profuse bleeding from a laceration, or intracranial hemorrhage in the case of a head injury. Abnormalities in primary hemostasis vary considerably in their severity and treatment. Athletic recommendations cannot be generalized for these youngsters, but must be determined on a case-by-case basis. Some children may require no restriction other than avoidance of aspirin and ibuprofen, which interfere with normal platelet function. Others may be so susceptible to excessive bleeding that athletic participation is contraindicated.

Defects of the plasma clotting proteins interfere with the process of secondary coagulation and may result in prolonged hemorrhage after an injury. Abnormalities of plasma clotting proteins may be either congenital or acquired; the acquired defects are variable in severity and etiology. This chapter will focus on the most common of the congenital plasma protein defects, the hemophilias.

PATHOPHYSIOLOGY OF HEMOPHILIA

Hemophilia is caused by an inherited deficiency of one of the important proteins necessary for blood clot formation. Hemophilia A and B (factor VIII and IX deficiencies, respectively) have many similarities in clinical manifestations. Both of these forms of hemophilia have an X-linked recessive inheritance. The genes for factor VIII and factor IX are present on the X chromosome. Females have two X chromosomes; if a woman is a carrier for hemophilia, one of her X chromosomes carries the gene for a defective form of the clotting factor. In general, females who are carriers for hemophilia do not manifest any tendency to bleed excessively, since the normal gene usually causes production of enough clotting factor for normal hemostasis. However, a male has only one X chromosome (from his mother) and one Y chromosome (from the father). If his single X chromosome bears a gene for hemophilia, he will lack sufficient clotting factor to make the firm blood clot necessary to stop hemorrhage at times of injury. The X-linked

Table 20.1   Normal Hemostasis

Primary hemostasis
Blood vessels contract
Platelets adhere to the subendothelium
Platelets are activated and aggregate

Secondary hemostasis
Plasma clotting proteins (clotting factors) are activated in a stepwise cascade of enzymes to activate prothrombin to thrombin
Thrombin catalyzes the polymerization of fibrinogen to fibrin
Fibrin is crosslinked to form a stable clot

Fibrinolysis
After healing, the fibrin clot is lysed by plasmin, the fibrinolytic effector

recessive inheritance pattern for hemophilia means that essentially all individuals affected with hemophilia are male.

LABORATORY ASSESSMENT OF THE SEVERITY OF THE HEMOPHILIAS

The clinical manifestations of hemophilia A and B are identical. Both forms of hemophilia occur in gradations of severity:

- mild,
- moderate, and
- severe.

These clinical gradations correlate directly with the measured deficiency of the clotting factor. In normal individuals, the amount of clotting factors VIII and IX circulating in the blood plasma may range from 50 to 200 units per ml, or 50–200%. Severe hemophilia indicates a factor level less than 1–2% of the average normal level of 100%; moderate hemophilia means that the factor level is up to 5% of normal; mild hemophilia indicates a factor level of 5–40% of normal.

The boy with mild hemophilia usually lives a completely normal life, having excessive bleeding only at times of serious injury or surgery. These individuals are cautioned to avoid contact sports, but usually no other modification of activity is necessary. In order to determine the proper sport program for an individual hemophilic boy, the baseline clotting factor level is very helpful. Actually, exercise may be of direct hemostatic benefit to the youngster with mild hemophilia A, as it has been well documented that strenuous exercise causes an increase in the circulating levels of factor VIII to as much as twice the baseline level (2, 10).

Some boys with mild hemophilia do experience enough bleeding episodes to create a "target joint" (described subsequently). Sport and physical activity recommendations for these youngsters should follow the same guidelines as those for more severe hemophilia (listed subsequently). It must also be recognized that the boy with mild hemophilia can have serious bleeding after significant trauma. Such injuries occasionally occur during sport participation, and it is important that there be a plan for treatment of the athlete with mild hemophilia in case

such an event occurs. The child may downplay the risk if he thinks of himself as "completely normal." Nevertheless, an eye injury caused by a high-speed baseball (for example) could easily lead to blindness if untreated.

It is important to mention that some boys with mild hemophilia are not diagnosed until adolescence or adulthood. In fact, it may be the coach or sport trainer who first notes that the child has experienced a deep hematoma or hemarthrosis of a severity or duration out of proportion to the degree of the trauma sustained. Such observations are extremely important in triggering the initial evaluation for a possible bleeding disorder (3). The comprehensive preparation medical questionnaire and physical exam may not reveal a possibility of a bleeding diathesis unless this has already been diagnosed (21).

NATURAL HISTORY OF SEVERE HEMOPHILIA

The rest of this chapter will discuss boys who have moderate or severe hemophilia. They do not bleed any more easily than anyone else, but they may have more prolonged bleeding from relatively minor traumas. Contrary to a common misconception, boys with hemophilia do not bleed persistently when they suffer a small cut or scratch. These individuals have normal primary hemostasis (platelet plug formation), so such surface hemorrhages usually stop normally. However, a deeper muscle or joint injury may lead to delayed hematoma formation. The excessive hemorrhaging may not become obvious until many hours after the initial injury. It is typical for a hemophilic boy to have many bruises under the skin of the shins and elbow areas. In the toddler years, this excessive bruising may even raise the question of child abuse. Usually, however, the location of these bruises over extensor surfaces is different from those noted in abused children.

The hallmark of hemophilia is the frequent occurrence of hemarthroses—bleeding within the articular joints. In fact, boys with severe hemophilia may experience hemarthrosis after only trivial or even no apparent joint injury. If untreated, recurrent hemarthroses lead to debilitating hemophilic arthropathy and crippling. Frequency and severity of the hemarthroses varies over the years, the middle childhood years being the age of most frequent bleeding episodes. There is considerable individual variability, but in a 1-month period a boy with severe hemophilia typically experiences an average of about 5 significant episodes of joint or muscle bleeding which require replacement therapy.

MANIFESTATIONS OF HEMOPHILIC BLEEDING EPISODES

Bleeding into muscles causes pain and swelling at the site. The bruise may be deep or there may be some overlying purplish discoloration if the hemorrhage includes a superficial component. When bleeding into the closed joint spaces occurs, the initial symptom is a "bubbling" sensation. The boy with hemophilia generally can report this feeling long before the signs of swelling, heat, and decreased range of motion are detectable. It is very important that a hemarthrosis be treated promptly in order to minimize the amount of damage which the affected joint will ultimately sustain. When blood collects in the closed space of a joint, the hemorrhage can be stopped by correction of the clotting factor deficiency. The blood present within the joint is subsequently removed by a natural process involving movement of inflammatory cells into the joint space. After repeated episodes, this normal response to hemorrhage damages the articular cartilages. The end result can be destructive hemophilic arthropathy. As a part of the repair process after recurrent hemarthroses, fragile new blood vessels proliferate in the synovial membranes, which predisposes the joint to bleed more easily in the future, often with no apparent trauma. This vicious cycle creates a particularly vulnerable site for recurrent hemophilic hemorrhage, the "target joint." The individual hemophilic athlete's target joints need to be taken into consideration when advising particular sport activities.

The advent of adequate treatment for each bleeding episode has made it possible to maintain maximum articular health. A number of Queen Victoria's descendants in the royal families of Europe were affected with hemophilia, but during the nineteenth and early twentieth centuries there was no treatment for the condition. Therefore, the affected European princes

and other boys with hemophilia suffered from frequent joint bleeding, and after a more serious injury involving head trauma or damage to internal organs, hemorrhage was often fatal. The average life span for a boy with hemophilia in the 1930s was 7–10 years. More recently, however, the natural history of severe hemophilia has been completely changed by advances which allow effective treatment of the clotting factor deficiency. During the decade from 1971 to 1980, the median life expectancy of a 1-year-old with hemophilia was 68 years (16). Although this has declined recently because of the AIDS epidemic, boys who are now diagnosed with hemophilia are in general expected to enjoy a normal life span, education, and career. In addition to the increase in longevity, quality of life has increased with the advent of effective and now safe treatments for hemophilia (17).

In the 1960s, relatively purified preparations of the clotting factors became available. These were prepared from pooled blood plasma and were dispensed in vials for reconstitution and administration at the time of a bleeding episode. The clotting factor must be given by injection directly into the vein. The factor is stored as a white, lyophilized (freeze-dried) powder in a vial and comes with a separate vial containing sterile water used to reconstitute the factor immediately prior to administration. Most boys with hemophilia receive home treatment, which means that the parents or the child himself will administer the clotting factor without needing to travel to the hemophilia center, emergency room, or pediatrician's office for each dose.

Once the clotting factor is given, there is an immediate increase in the clotting factor level correlated with the dose administered. Minor bleeding episodes such as muscle or joint hemorrhages are treated with a dose calculated to increase the factor level to normal; this means that the child's blood will clot normally until the dose wears off. The half-life of factor VIII is 12–18 hours; that of factor IX is 18–24 hours. The immediate treatment of a bleeding episode is therefore accomplished when the initial dose is administered, and usual first-aid measures are undertaken.

Recently, primary prophylaxis has become a common recommendation for the young child with severe hemophilia (12). This approach to therapy involves infusion of clotting factor every

2 or 3 days as a way to prevent hemorrhage. The aim is to maintain a minimal factor level such that the child with severe hemophilia has at least 1–2% of a normal clotting factor level prior to the next infusion. This has the effect of converting a case of severe hemophilia to one of mild to moderate hemophilia. Sweden has had experience with primary prophylaxis for nearly 20 years, and long-term follow-up studies show that patients treated prophylactically maintain excellent joints while being able to live more normal lives (13). For the young child, primary prophylaxis may require placement of an indwelling vascular access. Special precautions for such vascular devices are discussed in chapter 21.

COMPLICATIONS OF THERAPY

The plasma-derived clotting factor concentrates (often produced from the plasma of more than 20,000 blood donors) which allowed complete correction of clotting factor levels formerly predisposed the hemophilia population to exposure to blood-borne infections including hepatitis and HIV infection. Fortunately, the HIV virus can be completely inactivated by heating or other measures, and clotting factor concentrates available since 1985 have all undergone viral inactivation rendering them free from transmission of the HIV virus. Therefore, most young hemophiliacs are not infected with HIV. Hepatitis C, however, remained a problem until the late 1980s. All patients with hemophilia are immunized against hepatitis B.

Recombinant factor VIII concentrates have been available since December 1992. These synthetic preparations of clotting factor allow the treatment of hemophilia A without the use of clotting factor derived from human blood, thus eliminating the risk of any blood-borne infections. Although universal precautions should be used whenever blood spills occur, no special precautions are necessary when dealing with an individual with hemophilia (1, 8). Universal precautions mean wearing gloves when blood or body secretions are contacted and cleaning up spilled fluids with a bleach solution. The simplest and safest approach is to use full-strength hypochlorite bleach (e.g., "Clorox") from the bottle.

Another complication of therapy for hemophilia is the development of inhibitors. Inhibitors are antibodies formed after exposure to the clotting factor which the patient lacks. Inhibitor antibodies inactivate the therapeutically administered clotting factor, affecting the ability to treat hemorrhagic episodes effectively. Individuals with inhibitors often have more joint damage owing to poor response to therapy. These boys are much more restricted in terms of options for sport.

SPORT, PHYSICAL EDUCATION, AND HEMOPHILIA

Hemophilia does not affect the young athlete's energy level or endurance. Boys with hemophilia are not at an a priori disadvantage for participation in sports which are rated as high or moderate in aerobic intensity. Sports which have varying degrees of neuromuscular skill demands may be appropriate for the child with hemophilia. However, Pietri, Frontera, Pratts, and Suarez found that knees affected by frequent hemarthroses had decreased neuromuscular function as compared to the unaffected knee in the same individual (15). Differences included

- decreased knee extensor strength,
- lower total work, and
- lower average power output (15).

In general, high-top sport footwear will provide the best ankle support for the child with hemophilia. It may be necessary to modify the level and type of exercise, depending upon the recent and cumulative effects of hemophilic arthropathy on a particular joint. It is better to modify a fitness program than to discontinue it completely (6).

The major restriction necessary is to avoid those sports which put the hemophilic athlete at greatest risk for serious internal hemorrhage including intracranial bleeding—i.e., contact sports. Outside of this restriction, it is important that the young man with hemophilia be encouraged to participate in mainstream physical education, recreational, and team sport activities. The benefits to be obtained from such participation are both physical and psychosocial; for example, the boy with hemophilia who has strong, fit muscles and coordinated use of his joints is less likely to suffer from hemarthrosis (10). The types of exercise which are most important in contributing to this protection involve controlled resistance with minimal collision or sudden impact potential. Excellent choices are swimming and Nautilus-type controlled-resistance weight training. Swimming is an outstanding sport for the young man with hemophilia: excellent muscle tone can be achieved, and competition can be experienced with minimal risk of hemorrhage.

In determining whether there is a need to modify the regular school physical education program for the boy with hemophilia, it is often helpful for the hemophilia center's nurse coordinator to visit the school to meet with the physical education instructor, coaches, school nurse, teachers, and aides. Such an educational visit usually results in reassurance that the child can participate in nearly all activities available to his classmates. This is also an excellent opportunity to review the plan for dealing with an injury. Hemophiliacs who perform self-infusion of clotting factor may keep a dose in the school nurse's office for administration at the time of a bleeding episode. If the parent is giving the factor treatments, he or she may need to be contacted to come to school and administer the dose. Some parents carry a pager so that they can be easily contacted at these times. Depending upon the severity of the injury or hemorrhage, the child will either return immediately to the classroom, go home, or need to be evaluated by his physician. Although rarely necessary, it is important to have backup telephone contacts (pediatrician or hemophilia center) so that advice and therapy can be given promptly. The most serious hemorrhages that occur in hemophilia involve the central nervous system, the airway, or vital internal organs. Any change in behavior, unusual headache, or serious trauma demands prompt evaluation and treatment at the hemophilia center or emergency room. If there will be a delay, treatment with a double dose of clotting factor may be given pending full evaluation.

It is advised that all children with hemophilia wear a medical alert bracelet or neck chain. Some boys will discuss their hemophilia openly with classmates, but others wish to keep their bleeding diathesis private. It is important that the wishes of the child and parents be respected in this matter. These boys should be treated as normal group members who do not need special handling from their classmates.

Although a boy with hemophilia can realize a multifaceted and happy life, it should be remembered that he is subject to recurrent, unpredictable hemorrhagic episodes. School absences are more frequent than for nonhemophilic children; in one study they averaged 18 days per year, with a median of 11 days (22).

Team Sports for the Young Man With Hemophilia

A number of benefits result from sport participation by the young man with hemophilia. First is the importance of improved musculoskeletal strength and coordination. In terms of psychosocial development, there is a great reward from cooperating with team members, playing as an important link in a group, and learning to respond to successes and defeats. Furthermore, there is the considerable value of the improved self-esteem to be gained from undertaking a physical challenge and performing well. However, this value depends upon choosing a sport that is unlikely to result in an increased frequency of hemorrhagic episodes. The hemophilic athlete is most likely to persevere in such a sport and reach the level of competence that will contribute to improved self-esteem. It is important to avoid sports in which joint impact is a necessary result. The particular sport for an individual child will depend upon that patient's target joints, the joints most susceptible to hemorrhage. Tables 3.8a and 3.8b in chapter 3 of this text specify motion ratings for the upper and lower body in particular sports. The motions most likely to predispose to frequent bleeding for the hemophilic athlete are those which involve joint compression, especially when sudden stresses are common. A child whose target joint is an elbow will probably find that sports such as mountain climbing, tennis, archery, bowling, or rowing may contribute to elbow hemarthroses. On the other hand, the child with an ankle target joint may be frustrated if he tries to succeed at basketball, skating, or squash. The choice of sports is best made with reference to the child's interests and realistic aspirations, the parents' goals, and the specific recommendations from the hematologist and orthopedist at the hemophilia center (19, 20). It is worth reemphasizing that the best sport for one child with hemophilia may not be wise for another with the same diagnosis, and that recommendations should be taken only as a rough prediction of success for that patient. In many cases, the only way to determine whether a particular sport will be tolerated is by trial participation.

As a general rule, those sports included in the low motion rating group and which are also noncontact sports are likely to be appropriate for most young men with hemophilia. Table 20.2 categorizes the estimated safety of several athletic activities based on recommendations by the Medical and Scientific Advisory Committee of the National Hemophilia Foundation (12). The individual abilities of a particular hemophilic athlete generally guide the recommendations among sports rated to be of intermediate safety.

A recent worldwide questionnaire of hemophilia treatment center medical directors was conducted (9). Sports encouraged by 100% of the physicians included

- swimming,
- table tennis, and
- walking.

The list of banned sports included

- boxing,
- rugby,
- football,
- karate,
- wrestling,
- motorcycling,
- judo,
- hang gliding,
- hockey, and
- skateboarding.

Safe Sport Participation

Proper preparation for sport participation will reduce the risk of injury. Education regarding the rules of the sport and also the types of activity which frequently result in injury will need to come from the coach with expertise in the particular sport. While most organized programs incorporate a full complement of protective gear, the child with hemophilia may benefit from the addition of optional joint supports such as braced knee pads or elbow protection. Specific recommendations are best made in consultation with the orthopedic surgeon or physical therapist who has regularly evaluated that child's joints.

The benefits being obtained from a particular sport should be reevaluated regularly in order to maximize the outcome. If a form of participation becomes a frequent cause of joint hemorrhaging for the athlete, it will be appropriate to modify that sport or choose an alternative to meet the child's needs.

Table 20.2 Sports for Individuals With Hemophilia

Safer ⇒ ⇒	⇒ ⇒ ⇒ ⇒ ⇒	⇒ ⇒ ⇒	⇒ ⇒ ⇒ ⇒	⇒ **More dangerous**
Archery	Baseball	Jogging	Basketball	All-terrain vehicles
Badminton	Bowling	Roller skating	Gymnastics	Boxing
Bicycling	Cross-country skiing	Running	Horseback riding	Diving
Dancing	Weightlifting (controlled resistance)	Tennis	Ice skating	Football
Fishing		Volleyball	Rock climbing	Ice hockey
Golf		Waterskiing	Sailing	Martial arts
Hiking			Soccer	Motorcycling
Swimming				Racquetball
Table tennis				Rugby
Walking				Skateboarding
				Snowmobiling
				Weightlifting (free weights)
				Wrestling

Based on References 9 and 12.

Specific Modifications
for the Child With Hemophilia

Although individual responses to the stresses of a particular sport vary considerably, some recommendations can be made for modifications that may make a sport more tolerable to the athlete with hemophilia. In baseball, pitching and base sliding should be minimized. Joint supports may make basketball less dangerous for the hemophiliac. The gymnast should avoid jumping dismounts. Horseback riding can be a dangerous sport for anyone; for the hemophilic rider, avoiding jumping will decrease the risk of serious hemorrhage. Soccer players should be advised against "heading" the ball as this may lead to intracranial bleeding. Weightlifting with free weights is not recommended because of the risk of joint strain and possible airway hematoma, although controlled-resistance body building is particularly recommended.

Conditioning and
Flexibility Preparation

Most sport training programs include conditioning exercises to prepare the musculoskeletal system for the rigors of competitive participation. This period is extremely important for the athlete with a bleeding disorder. Even for the most frequently recommended low-impact, noncontact sport—swimming—it is advised that participation include warm-up, interval training, and cooldown exercises (4). Specific recommendations for the warm-up exercises include arm swings, leg kicks, neck rotations, wrist extensions, biceps and triceps warm-ups, arm and back stretching, and thigh, leg, and groin stretching against a static resistance. It is important not to bounce in these positions or to overstretch a joint or muscle. A 5-minute cooldown period is advised after the period of training or competition in the water. An added benefit of the isokinetic strengthening program is to be expected in terms of improved joint function outside of the sports program (5).

In some circumstances, prophylactic treatment with clotting factor prior to sport participation is reasonable. This decision should be made by the hemophilia treatment center staff after careful discussion with the parents and child. There are no data available to indicate the actual benefits and risks of prophylactic factor infusion prior to sports participation, as compared to treatment at the time of a bleeding episode. The latter approach is the usual standard in the United States, although prophylaxis has recently been recommended as an option for children with severe hemophilia (12). Prophylactic factor infusion throughout the childhood years is a more common practice in some other countries, however (13, 14).

Camp Experiences for Children
With Hemophilia

In addition to school physical education programs and school- or community-organized sport programs, boys with hemophilia have an opportunity to undertake active, supervised physical activity programs during summer camp. There are at least 44 camps available to youngsters with hemophilia in 17 countries. Many of these facilities provide an on-site hemophilia nurse or physician who is available for the evaluation and prompt treatment of bleeding. A listing of available camps may be obtained from the National Hemophilia Foundation by telephoning 1-800-42-HANDI. Activities at the camps vary widely. One that is frequently deemed to be beneficial is a "ropes" course. The program is safe when carefully supervised, but the challenges undertaken develop problem-solving skills, promote team effort, and build confidence (7, 11, 18).

CONCLUSION

There are a number of conditions that result in an abnormal tendency to bleed excessively. Hemophilia is an inherited deficiency of one of the clotting factors; affected individuals may bleed excessively even after minor traumas. Nevertheless, it is very important to include physical activity and organized team sports in the life of a young man with hemophilia. By careful planning and cooperation between hemophilia center staff members and athletic professionals, a safe and rewarding athletic program can be developed for each child, including those with hemophilia.

REFERENCES

1. American Academy of Pediatrics Committee on Sports Medicine and Fitness. Human Immunodeficiency Virus in the athletic setting. Pediatrics 88:640–641; 1991.
2. Bennet, B.; Ratnoff, O.D. Changes in antihemophilic factor in normal pregnancy, following exercise, and pneumoencephalography. J. Laboratory and Clinical Medicine 80:256–263; 1972.
3. Brown, B.R. Coaches: a missing link in the health care system. Am. J. Dis. Child. 146:211–217; 1992.
4. Goodhew, D.; Buzzard, B.; Jones, P. In the swim: a guide for boys with haemophilia. Paper presented at the World Federation of Hemophilia Meeting. Athens, Greece; 1992.
5. Greene, W.B.; Strickler, E.M. A modified isokinetic strengthening program for patients with severe hemophilia. Developmental Medicine and Child Neurology 25:189–196; 1983.
6. Hede, A.; Hempel-Poulsen, S.; Jensen, J.S. Symptoms and level of sports activity in patients awaiting arthroscopy for meniscal lesions of the knee. J. Bone Joint Surg. (Am.) 72:550–552; 1990.
7. Holtkamp, C. Two hemophilia summer camps in the U.S.A. Paper presented at the World Federation of Hemophilia meeting. Athens, Greece; 1992.
8. Johnson, R.J. HIV infection in athletes. What are the risks? Who can compete? Postgrad. Med. 92:73–75, 79–80; 1992.
9. Jones, P. Unpublished report from the World Federation of Hemophilia Meeting. Athens, Greece; 1992.
10. Koch, B.; Luban, N.L.; Galioto, F.M.; Rick, M.E.; Goldstein, D.; Kelleher, J.F. Changes in coagulation parameters with exercise in patients with classical hemophilia. Am. J. Hematol. 16:227–231; 1984.
11. Mehta, P.; Sandler, E.; Bussing, R.; Cumming, W.; Bendell, W.; Warner, R.; Levine, S.B. Reflections on hemophilia camp (letter). Clin. Pedr. 30:259–260; 1991.
12. National Hemophilia Foundation Medical and Scientific Advisory Committee. (1992). The hemophilia handbook (p. 189). New York: National Hemophilia Foundation.
13. Nilsson, I.M.; Berntorp, E.; Lofqvist, T.; Pettersson, H. Twenty-five years of prophylactic treatment in severe Haemophilia A and B. J. Intern. Med. 232:25–32; 1992.
14. Petrini, P.; Lindvall, N.; Egberg, N.; Blomback, M. Prophylaxis with factor concentrates in preventing hemophilic arthropathy. Am. J. Pediatr. Hematol/Oncol. 13:280–287; 1991.
15. Pietri, M.M.; Frontera, W.R.; Pratts, I.S.; Suarez, E.L. Skeletal muscle function in patients with hemophilia A and unilateral hemarthrosis of the knee. Arch. of Physical Med. and Rehab. 73:22–28; 1992.
16. Ratnoff, O.D.; Jones, P.K. The changing prognosis of classic hemophilia (factor VIII deficiency). Annals of Internal Medicine 114:641–648; 1991.
17. Rosendaal, F.R.; Smit, C.; Varekamp, I.; Brocker-Vriends, A.H.J.T.; van Dijck, H.; Suurmeijer, T.P.B.M.; van den Brouckes, J.P.; Breit, E. Modern haemophilia treatment: medical improvements and quality of life. J. Internal Medicine 228:633–640; 1990.
18. Seeler, R.A.; Ashenhurst, J.B.; Miller, J. A summer camp for boys with hemophilia. J. Pediatr. 87:758–759; 1975.
19. Stern, H.P.; Bradley, R.H.; Prince, M.T.; Stroh, S.E. Young children in recreational sports—participation motivation. Clin. Pediatr. (Phila) 29:89–94; 1990.
20. Stern, P.; Prince, M.T.; Bradley, R.H.; Stroh, S.E. Coaches' goals for young children in a recreational sports program. Clin. Pediatr. (Phila) 28:277–281; 1990.
21. Tanji, J.L. The preparticipation physical examination for sports. Am. Family Physician. 42:397–402; 1990.
22. Woolf, A.; Rappaport, L.; Reardon, P.; Cibarowski, J.; D'Angelo, E.; Bessette, J. School functioning and disease severity in boys with hemophilia. J. Developmental and Behavioral Pediatr. 10:81–85; 1989.

CHAPTER 21

Neoplasms

Clifford Selsky
Walt Disney Memorial Cancer Center at Florida Hospital

Howard A. Pearson
Yale University School of Medicine

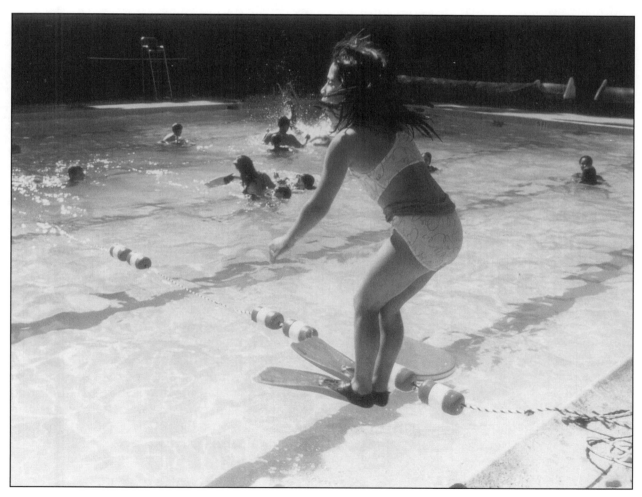

Children with cancer can and should participate in physical activity, both individual and cooperative sports. The kind of activity and intensity of play will be determined with reference to the specific diagnosis and consequences of therapy. Cancer consists of a myriad of diseases, and therapies are no less numerous. Thus, children with a specific diagnosis will represent a spectrum of clinical morbidity. Recommendations cannot be made that apply to all activities and all diagnoses. What follows is a consideration of the factors that need to be kept in mind and evaluated when children with cancer engage in sport.

Childhood cancer is a relatively uncommon pediatric disease. Each year in the United States approximately 6500 children under 15 years of age are diagnosed with malignancy (31). Because almost all childhood cancers are treatable and many are now curable, decisions must be made concerning these patients' lives and activities, both during and after therapy. The diseases as well as their therapies may need to be considered when making recommendations about lifestyles and activities, including participation in sport.

An increased cure rate of many childhood malignancies has resulted from better and especially from more aggressive therapy, including combined chemotherapy, surgery, and radiation therapy for selected kinds of tumors (11). Because it can be anticipated that more than 50% of those children who develop a malignancy will be cured, it is important that their lives be made as normal as possible. Activities such as sport participation should be encouraged to the extent that they are appropriate and safe.

There are general issues that may apply to many kinds of malignancy and others that may apply to only a few specific malignancies. In this presentation, the general issues of chemotherapy, radiation, and surgery will be discussed before specific childhood tumors are considered, with considerations for sport and exercise participation woven throughout.

CHEMOTHERAPY

Much of the therapeutic success leading to the marked improvement in overall survival for pediatric malignancies over the past three de-cades can be attributed to the development of combination chemotherapy (3). Agents of different therapeutic classes are used synergistically to capitalize on their individual therapeutic effects on different biological targets in tumor cells. Because of a narrow therapeutic index for most of these drugs, however, side effects may affect the overall health of persons receiving them.

Except for a few classes, almost all chemotherapeutic agents are toxic to the bone marrow and inhibit the formation of red cells, granulocytes, and platelets. Therapy with myelosuppressive drugs may thus result in single or multiple cytopenias. At times, the depression of circulating blood cells may be so severe that replacement therapy by transfusion or administration of specific growth factor therapy may be required (14).

Close monitoring of the blood cell count is essential during myelosuppressive therapy. Failure to fully anticipate severe marrow depression may result in high-output cardiac failure because of anemia; hemorrhage may be caused by thrombocytopenia and infection secondary to granulocytopenia. During periods of cytopenia, physical activity may need to be restricted because of anemia and its attendant decreased tissue oxygen availability. It is also obvious that because the trauma of sport could result in hemorrhage, physical activity must be restricted in the thrombocytopenic patient (19). Toxicity may also involve rapidly dividing tissues, especially the upper gastrointestinal mucosa, resulting in painful ulcerations (mucositis) (27).

Many chemotherapeutic agents produce partial or total loss of scalp hair. This often produces considerable psychological distress. Head covers of various sorts are used to protect the scalp from direct sunlight and to conserve body heat during winter outdoor activities. The patient should be assured that hair loss is temporary.

Chemotherapeutic agents may also be associated with dose-limiting toxicities that affect different specific organ systems. These effects can impose a limit on the patient's ability to participate in physical activity.

Doxorubicin

Doxorubicin (Adriamycin), an anthracycline tumoricidal antibiotic, is used in the therapy regimens of several pediatric cancers. In addition to myelosuppressive activity, Adriamycin causes hair loss and mucosal ulceration. However, its most significant long-term toxicity is its effect on cardiac muscle. Reversible EKG changes can occur at dosages that are used in standard therapeutic regimens. Cardiomyopathy leading to intractable and irreversible congestive heart failure has also occurred at cumulative doses below 450 mg/m^2 body surface area, a dose generally considered safe. This is especially likely if the heart has been included in an irradiation field (2).

More recently, a disturbing increase in sudden deaths has been described in adolescents and young adults who were treated with Adriamycin during childhood (25). These individuals, usually in their early twenties, did not have previously documented cardiomyopathy or arrhythmias. It has been suggested that deaths may be related to decreased left ventricular wall thickness resulting in high left ventricular enddiastolic pressures and subsequent left ventricular wall stress. It has also been suggested that Adriamycin causes cardiac muscle cell "dropout" that leads to an increased somatic-to-cardiac growth ratio which could result in decreased left ventricular wall thickness (24). It is recommended that patients who have received Adriamycin should be reevaluated on a regular basis with echocardiography and exercise stress tests to identify early signs of increased left ventricular wall stress. Any child or adolescent who has received Adriamycin should have a complete cardiac evaluation done before participation in sport.

Bleomycin

Bleomycin is a tumoricidal, antibiotic mixture of 13 different glycoproteins, and is used for the treatment of Hodgkin's lymphoma, osteosarcoma, and germ cell tumors. Bleomycin does not usually cause significant myelosuppression but can affect pulmonary function. Restrictive changes in ventilation and reduction in diffusion capacity often precede the radiographic abnormality of interstitial pneumonitis (20). These pulmonary changes can lead to progressive limitation of exercise tolerance. Pulmonary function tests should be monitored both during treatment and after therapy is completed.

L-Asparaginase

This enzyme destroys l-asparagine and thus interferes with protein synthesis, including coagulation proteins synthesized in the liver (12).

Vincristine and Vinblastine

Vincristine and Vinblastine are alkaloid chemotherapeutic agents extracted from plants of the vinca family. These drugs inhibit microtubule assembly, thereby disrupting normal cell division (32). Microtubules also play an important role in neural cell function. Because of this, the drugs have neurological side effects. Peripheral neuropathies may result in the loss of deep tendon reflexes, paresthesia, and dysesthesias, as well as foot drop and wrist drop. Eyelid ptosis may also occur (32). These neurological consequences of drug therapy, which may be permanent, can affect participation in sports that involve hand-eye coordination or running.

Taxol

Taxol, a newer chemotherapeutic agent, also affects microtubule function by a different mechanism from that of the vinca alkaloids. Predictably, this drug also causes peripheral neuropathies (7).

Cytosine Arabinoside

Cytosine arabinoside may affect the central nervous system. Toxicity may be manifested as ataxia and other indications of cerebellar dysfunction (33).

6-Mercaptopurine (Purinethol)

This is an oral agent used in maintenance therapy for leukemia. Its major toxicity is dose-related marrow suppression (33).

Methotrexate

This is a folic acid antagonist. Its major toxicities are bone marrow suppression and mucosities. Children receiving methotrexate have actinic sensitivity, and their skin should be protected from direct sunlight (33).

Cisplatinum and Carboplatinum

These platinum coordination complex drugs can cause renal tubular dysfunction leading to the urinary wasting of potassium, calcium, magnesium, and phosphate. Cisplatinum can also affect auditory nerve function leading to selective frequency deafness (26).

Cyclophosphamide (Cytoxan)

This is an alkylating agent of the nitrogen mustard class. It has major myelotoxicities. Excretion of a metabolic derivative can produce severe hemorrhagic cystitis. Alopecia (hair loss) is common (8).

Ifosfamide

Ifosfamide is an alkylating agent requiring hepatic activation. It can cause a profound hypophosphatemia as well as neuromuscular abnormalities. (8).

This discussion of varieties of chemotherapeutic agents is not designed to be exhaustive or complete. A more complete discussion can be found in standard pediatric oncology texts (10, 28). However, it should serve to remind primary care providers and physical activity instructors that children who are currently receiving or who have received chemotherapeutic agents in the past require special evaluation before they engage in sport. Determining the possible sequelae of chemotherapy will permit participation in a specifically designed program of physical activity that will minimize possible risks.

SURGERY

Many children and adolescents with nonhematologic malignancies will undergo some type of surgery as part of diagnosis or therapy (17). Depending upon the procedures employed, there may be functional as well as psychological and physiological consequences that should be recognized when participation in sport by these children is considered.

Children who have one of a pair of organs removed because of unilateral malignancy must minimize risk to the remaining organ. For example, nephrectomy is often performed for Wilms' tumor, and the remaining kidney hypertrophies and could be susceptible to trauma. Thus, contact sports are usually precluded in these children. As another example, retinoblastoma may be treated by enucleation of the affected eye, and sports such as squash which could result in trauma to the remaining eye clearly should not be undertaken without adequate shielding.

Amputation may still be required for optimal local control of some extremity bone malignancies such as osteogenic sarcoma. However, this is not as routinely employed as was the practice in the past. Surgical procedures have been developed over the past 10 years in an attempt to salvage extremities involved by bone tumors such as osteogenic sarcoma (23). Limb salvage procedures result in an extremity that has some degree of limitation in motion and strength. Postoperatively the limb is supported by fixation of bone graft or other internal prosthesis to contiguous uninvolved bone. Aggressive physical therapy programs are initiated to prevent joint contracture and to maintain flexibility. As the graft is gradually replaced by living bone, stress may be put on the affected limb. If this is done too early, however, graft fractures may occur.

Rehabilitation following amputation of an extremity is usually easier and faster than rehabilitation following limb salvage surgery. Most amputees can participate in a wide spectrum of sport activities with the proper conditioning and training. While these activities may be structured for the physically challenged, unique strategies are often devised by the individual patient that permit participation in a surprisingly wide range of sports, including competitive sports.

Procedures on the central nervous system may result in a variety of neurological sequelae (5). The extent of any neurological deficit should be determined prior to establishing a physical activity program. Deficits may include

- intellectual deficits,
- visual field cuts,
- gross motor defects,
- gross or fine defects in position, sense, and balance,
- sensory deficits, and
- others.

It is essential that physicians, therapists, and activity directors design programs of physical activity that are appropriate for the individual patient. These programs should be challenging but feasible. Ideally, the individual program should promote self-esteem as well as providing enjoyment and fun.

RADIATION THERAPY

High-energy radiation delivered as X rays, gamma rays, electrons, or protons are used in the treatment of a variety of malignancies. Radiation can produce significant acute and chronic toxicities. The size and location of the involved radiation field, as well as the radiation dosage, determine the location and degree of these affects. In general, larger involved fields and higher doses delivered are associated with greater effects and consequences (21).

As with chemotherapy, acute effects of radiation primarily affect rapidly dividing tissues, including the gastrointestinal tract mucosa, hair follicles, and bone marrow. If radiation fields involve large areas of active bone marrow such as the pelvis and vertebrae, significant myelosuppression may occur by direct marrow injury.

Desquamation of involved skin of the radiation field can lead to painful radiation burns that must be protected from subsequent mechanical trauma, sun exposure, and infection. When the radiation field includes the gastrointestinal tract, nausea, anorexia, vomiting, diarrhea, and mucosal ulceration result. This may limit a child's desire and ability to participate in sport. Radiation of the head results in alopecia; however, hair regrowth can be expected.

Radiation to the lung parenchyma is often part of the treatment of Hodgkin's disease. Whole lung radiation can cause radiation pneumonitis that may ultimately process to obliteration of air spaces, restrictive lung disease, and decreased diffusion capacity. This complication is usually treated with chronic glucocorticosteroid administration (21). Radiation involving other organs can cause inflammatory responses such as hepatitis or nephritis. Cranial irradiation can cause a syndrome of extreme somnolence. A child or adolescent who has done well during radiation treatment may develop extreme fatigue and somnolence 4 to 8 weeks after therapy is completed, although recovery is usual within a few weeks (18).

Children who receive whole brain irradiation prior to 7 years of age may experience significant intellectual loss. This is believed to be a consequence of radiation-induced failure to myelinization. In such children it has been estimated that there may be an average loss of seven IQ points for each year under the age of 7 when the radiation was given. For example, a child who received whole brain therapy at age 3 years will have a 21-point deficit in the expected final IQ. Many of these children treated in early life are classified as retarded based on low IQ scores. This has lead to experimental protocols for delaying X ray therapy until after myelinization is more complete (13).

A long-term effect of craniospinal radiation therapy is significant reduction in final attained height. This loss is a consequence of inhibition of vertebral body growth as well as growth hormone deficiency secondary to damage to the hypothalamic-pituitary axis (21). Decreased production or secretion of hormones of the hypothalamic-pituitary axis may cause diabetes insipidus and hypothyroidism that require replacement therapy.

It is obvious that there may be long-term consequences of childhood cancer, and some survivors have paid a significant price for their cure. However, this need not exclude them from participating in exercise and sports, even competitive sports.

STEM CELL REPLACEMENT THERAPY

Bone marrow transplantation is an increasingly important modality used for treatment of hematologic malignances and some solid tumors (29). As a prelude to transplantation, the patient receives intensive chemotherapy and/or radiation therapy; theoretically, doses of these are sufficient to destroy all malignant cells throughout the body. Because the patient's bone marrow stem cell compartment and cellular immunity is also destroyed, the patient then requires "rescue" from marrow aplasia by infusion of another source of stem cells. These stem cells then repopulate the marrow and ultimately restore the circulating blood cellular components to normal. Most patients undergoing bone marrow transplant procedure have already received extensive chemotherapy and may also have had surgical procedures and radiation. Thus, increased toxicity may be seen because of an already compromised bone marrow.

Patients undergoing bone marrow transplantation have their immune system significantly impaired by the destruction of T and B lymphocytes and their precursors. Following successful engraftment it may take more than 12 months before adequate humoral immunity is regained, as reflected in low levels of circulating antibody. Full cellular immunity may not be regained for several years. Some transplant programs suggest that patients be isolated at home for as long as 12 months to avoid possible exposure to infectious agents. Other programs do not demand such strict isolation, because most post-transplant infections result from endogenous organisms rather than from contact with other persons. Patients who develop a variety of bacterial, viral, or fungal infections have an increased risk of graft versus host disease (GVHD) (4).

GVHD can be acute or chronic, and accounts for much of the long-term morbidity and mortality associated with bone marrow transplantation (4). Severe GVHD can produce a cutaneous syndrome resembling scleroderma, and may also cause arthritis and decreased joint motion, as well as damaging tear ducts and salivary and sweat glands. GVHD can also result in intractable diarrhea and liver dysfunction. All of these manifestations are debilitating and can limit physical activity and require supportive care.

Preparatory chemotherapy for bone marrow transplantation with Busulfan can produce chronic restrictive lung disease, as can subsequent infectious pneumonitis. High-dose cyclophosphamide may also cause myocarditis or pericarditis, as well as congestive heart failure.

SPECIFIC CHILDHOOD MALIGNANCIES

Leukemia

About 90% of children with leukemia can be classified as acute lymphoblastic (ALL), and 80 percent or more will be cured of their disease using relatively nontoxic therapies, e.g., prednisone, 6-mercaptopurine, Vincristine, Methotrexate, and l-asparaginase. However, some types of agents used for ALL therapy have side effects that could limit physical activity.

Furthermore, during the early months of therapy thrombocytopenia and anemia may necessarily impose limits on sport and physical activity. The neurological toxicity of Vincristine can cause foot drop and loss of deep tendon reflexes, which may affect gross and fine motor activity. Prednisone can cause myopathies, osteoporosis, and aseptic necrosis of the femoral head (3). L-asparaginase inhibits protein synthesis including specific coagulation factors, deficiencies of which can produce a bleeding tendency.

Once complete remission has been attained, children with ALL are hematologically normal and need no special limitations in physical activity; all sport activity can then be encouraged.

About 10% of children with ALL experience relapses of their leukemia and require further cytoxic therapy, which is often more intense than that used initially. Bone marrow transplantation is also employed for relapsed ALL. Children with relapsed ALL require medical surveillance for the associated morbidity of therapy and recurrent disease. Physical activity may need to be limited because of side effects of the therapeutic regimens or consequences of bone marrow transplantation such as GVHD.

A subset of high-risk ALL patients receive Adriamycin as part of their chemotherapy regimen. As emphasized previously, these children must have cardiac function, structure, and stress testing performed prior to strenuous physical activity.

Once remission has been attained, continuous relatively nontoxic maintenance therapy is continued for 18–36 months. After 3 years of continuous and complete remission, relapse is unusual and most children can be considered cured.

Acute Myelogenous Leukemia

Acute myelogenous leukemia often requires several months of intensive myelosuppressive, cytotoxic therapy to attain a complete remission. AML patients may develop bacterial infections because of granulocyte dysfunction associated with the disease. Six weeks or more of hospitalization may be required for initial therapy; during this time, physical activity is neither well tolerated nor usually desired by the patient because of anorexia and nausea, as well as frequent anemia, neutropenia, and thrombocytopenia.

Patients with related HLA-identical donors or donors with one or two antigen mismatches may be considered as candidates for bone marrow transplantation. Other patients may undergo autologous marrow transplants by purging their remission bone marrow with ex vivo alkylating agents, although such therapy is experimental. However, once complete remission is attained full sport participation is possible and desirable.

Hodgkin's Lymphoma

Therapy for Hodgkin's lymphoma is variable and is based upon the extent of involvement (stage) and the histology of the specific tumor (22). Staging depends upon whether disease is present in

- one lymph node (Stage I);
- two lymph node groups on the same side of the diaphragm (Stage II);
- nodes on both sides of the diaphragm (Stage III);
- lymph nodes plus liver, lung, or bone marrow (Stage IV).

The modifier a or b after the stage indicates presence or absence of systemic signs such as fever, night sweats, or weight loss. Stage I–IIa disease is usually treated with radiation therapy. Higher stage patients (IIB–IV) usually receive systemic combined chemotherapy such as MOPD or ABVD and sometimes radiation. Chemotherapy is given in cycles for 6–12 months.

Radiotherapy may also be used for therapy of large mediastinal masses. Radiation of the mediastinum encompasses the heart and, in combination with Adriamycin, chemotherapy can result in decreased cardiac contractibility and reduced ejection fraction. Vincristine therapy may cause neurological dysfunction, and Bleomycin can alter pulmonary function.

The presence and degree of the individual patient's physical impairment needs to be assessed prior to engagement in physical activity. Side effects associated with chemotherapy must be evaluated. Patients whose disease relapses may undergo autologous bone marrow transplantation.

Hodgkin's disease is eminently treatable and often curable: cure rates in lower stages of disease are as high as 80–90%. Even in advanced stages of the disease, 40–50% of patients can be cured. Most patients are able to regain full activity after completion of therapy, and full participation in sport is possible. The much-publicized occurrences of Hodgkin's disease in professional athletes who are able to return to sport after treatment provides encouragement for patients with this disease.

Non-Hodgkin's Lymphoma

Many malignancies fall into the category of non-Hodgkin's lymphoma. The treatment varies depending upon the histological classification and the extent of disease. Adriamycin, Vincristine, Cytoxan, prednisone, and bone marrow transplantation are used as treatments. Initial therapy is usually intensive, and during this aggressive phase of therapy most children cannot engage in any strenuous activity because of anemia.

Cardiac dysfunction, neurological sequelae, and metabolic derangement can all be associated with agents that are used for lymphoma therapy. A complete physical exam and evaluation before beginning exercise or sport is essential. Close collaborative follow-up is necessary between the oncologist, primary care physician, physical education instructors, and other members of the therapeutic team. However, the majority of patients who are cured by chemotherapy are able to participate in all sport activities.

Central Nervous System Tumors

Brain tumors are the second most common type of pediatric malignancy (31). Therapy relies heavily upon initial surgical excision (total or partial), and subsequent cranial or craniospinal radiation therapy. Adjuvant chemotherapy is becoming an increasingly accepted adjunct to therapy.

There are a number of different histological types of intracranial and intraspinal tumors. Because these can involve many neurological structures, therapy can result in a number of neurological deficits. Recent advances in neurosurgery using dissecting microscopic techniques permit more aggressive but definitive operations. Gross total resection has increasingly been the operative goal rather than partial resection or merely excisional biopsy. While these aggressive operations improve the disease-free survival rate, many of the survivors are left with significant neurological impairments.

Radiation continues to be a standard additional therapy for most brain tumors. Chemotherapy has become an accepted adjunctive treatment for many kinds of brain tumors, especially germ cell and primitive blastemal malignancies (13). A number of different chemotherapy regimens are used, but they usually include Vincristine and the alkylating agents (Cytoxan). Recent protocols are investigating the use of high-dose chemotherapy in conjunction with autologous bone marrow rescue.

Children with central nervous system tumors require management by an integrated team approach involving neurologists, neurosurgeons, radiation oncologists, pediatric oncologists, physical therapists, occupational therapists, psychologists, and others. Because of their disease and the potential morbidity of the different treatment modalities, they require extensive and ongoing evaluation before participating in sport or other physical activity. The physical activity instructor should maintain a close working relationship with the rehabilitation specialists involved in the child's care. Despite these caveats many children cured of brain tumors are able to successfully participate even in competitive sports.

Neuroblastoma

Neuroblastomas are malignant tumors that arise from precursors in sympathetic ganglion cells. They can arise anywhere along the sympathetic ganglion chain, as well as in the adrenal medulla from the thorax to the organ of Zuckerkandl at the aortic bifurcation. They may also involve the bone marrow, liver, and subcutaneous tissue by metastatic spread.

Therapy includes surgical excision alone for localized tumors with favorable biological markers. More extensive tumors are usually treated with chemotherapy, with or without radiotherapy. Widely disseminated tumors and those with high-risk biological markers are treated with a combination of chemotherapeutic agents such as doxorubicin, cysplatinum, epidophyllotoxin, and cyclophosphamide given in

alternating cycles (6). While on therapy these patients usually experience myelosuppression with anemia and thrombocytopenia, but can usually resume full activities after therapy is completed. However, cardiac evaluations are indicated because of possible doxorubicin-associated cardiotoxicity. Patients may also require electrolyte supplementation because of cisplatinum-induced renal tubular toxicity.

Wilms' Tumor

Nephroblastoma, more commonly known as Wilms' tumor, arises from renal blastema cells. It occurs throughout childhood: the peak incidence is between 3–6 years of age, but it can occasionally occur in school-age or adolescent children. Hematuria or rapidly increasing abdominal girth are the most common presenting manifestations. Wilms' tumor is usually unilateral but is occasionally seen bilaterally as well. In older patients it can arise in extrarenal tissues. These tumors reach massive size and therefore can easily rupture; they also have a propensity for direct intravenous extension. Metastasis to the lungs and liver may occur.

Surgical staging is important for optimal therapy. Nephrectomy or partial nephrectomy along with adjuvant chemotherapy and/or radiation therapy are the important treatment modalities. Vincristine, actinomycin D plus Adriamycin, and cyclophosphamide are the most widely employed drug combinations (15). Radiation of the tumor bed and abdominal and chest X rays are used for high-stage tumors and for those with metastatic lung lesions.

Children undergoing therapy experience myelosuppression and other acute effects of chemotherapy and radiation. Actinomycin D can cause a condition of "radiation recall" from sensitization of skin areas with radiation fields. This may result in painful erythema and desquamation of previously irradiated areas.

Following completion of therapy, physical activity can be unrestricted except in the event of cardiac dysfunction following Adriamycin administration. In the case of nephrectomy, concern about avoiding trauma to the remaining hypertrophied kidney has been mentioned previously as a rationale for avoiding contact sports; on the other hand, the author knows of several children who have decided to participate in highly competitive contact sports.

Soft Tissue Sarcomas

Rhabdomyosarcoma is the predominant soft tissue sarcoma of childhood. Tumors can occur in the extremities of the axial soma. Rhabdomyosarcoma cells are believed to be primitive skeletal muscle cells—rhabdomyoblasts.

Total surgical excision is indicated unless tumor removal would require a major mutilating procedure. Radiation and adjuvant chemotherapy has been shown to increase the possibility of long-term remission and cure. Vincristine and Adriamycin containing drug regimens usually are used. Actinomycin D and cyclophosphamide are also sometimes included in the chemotherapy regimen. Cisplatinum in combination with the alkylating agent ifosfamide has been used for recurrent tumors (30).

Cyclic myelosuppression can be expected for patients on therapy. Adriamycin-related cardiac toxicity must be addressed before patients engage in extensive physical activity. Extensive surgical procedures may result in physical limitation that should be assessed for designing specific activity programs. Many children with physical limitation do remarkably well, but they should have possible activities clearly delineated.

Bone Tumors

The majority of malignant bone tumors of children and young adults are osteogenic sarcomas. The tumors can affect any bone and can also produce soft-tissue masses. Pulmonary metastases are frequent and often occur early. Many times bone tumors cause pain as their major manifestation; tumors of the extremities may cause pathological fractures (23).

Aggressive surgical resection along with administration of adjuvant combination chemotherapy has increased survival of osteogenic sarcoma to over 70%. Adriamycin, cisplatin, and Methotrexate are used over a 1-year period to treat this tumor. In metastatic disease, ifosfamide is also given. Surgery, including both the amputation and the salvaging of limbs, may be indicated. Metastatic lung nodules can be surgically excised.

Possible Adriamycin cardiotoxicity must be assessed before patients engage in physical activity. Electrolyte abnormalities resulting from renal tubular salt wasting should be monitored, and physical activities should be tailored to the individual because of surgically-induced limitations in limb function.

Ewing's sarcoma is another aggressive bone tumor. Pediatric therapy and adjunctive chemotherapy is effective in curing many children. Most children who have had limb amputation or limb-sparing surgery have adapted themselves to sports such as skiing with great success, despite the very real handicap involved.

Other Tumors

Many other kinds of tumors can occur in children and adolescents. Retinoblastoma occurs either unilaterally or bilaterally and can extend out of the orbit. Chemotherapy containing Adriamycin, surgical extirpation, and radiation therapy are employed (9). Visual impairment, including loss of stereoscopic vision, must be taken into account when designing physical activity programs for these people.

Hepatoblastoma, a malignant tumor of the liver, is treated with Adriamycin-containing chemotherapy regimens (16). Germ cell tumors are often treated with regimens containing Cisplatinum and Vinblastine (1).

CHILDREN WITH CANCER AT CAMP

For the past seven summers the authors have served as resident camp physicians at the Hole In the Wall Gang Camp in Connecticut. This was founded by actor Paul Newman to provide an active and fun-filled camping experience for children with cancer and serious blood diseases. Each summer the camp serves more than 700 children, about two-thirds of whom have a diagnosis of malignancy. The children are in all stages of disease, from recently diagnosed to well beyond completion of therapy. About three-quarters of the campers are still receiving therapy.

As would be expected from the relative frequencies of the various childhood malignancies, most campers have or have had a diagnosis of acute lymphoblastic leukemia. Children who are in the early stages of treatment may be anemic, neutropenic, and thrombocytopenic. These children may have reduced stamina and must be protected from falls. Despite this it is constantly surprising to see how the camp environment energizes these children so that they engage in far more physical activity than their parents or physicians have permitted at home.

It has become almost routine for oncologists to place semipermanent intravenous access catheters ("ports") into new oncology patients in order to facilitate blood drawing and intravenous infusions of chemotherapy and blood products. External ports (Hickman or Broviac catheters) are often used. These entail a plastic catheter which is inserted into an axillary vein and threaded into the superior vena cava. The other end is tunneled out through the skin of the anterior chest.

These implanted devices may become infected. Some physicians prohibit swimming in patients with external catheters because of fear of infections. Over the past 7 years the authors have had more than a hundred campers with external catheters, and with parental and physician consent have permitted these children to swim in the Camp pool. Their external catheters are covered with a sheet of adhesive plastic during swimming, and dressings are changed immediately after swimming. Only one infection has occurred over the past 7 years during or in the 2 weeks following camp. This rate is comparable or less than has been reported as being usual in these patients when they are not swimming.

Another potential sport hazard for children with cancer is the actinic effect of chemotherapeutic agents and X rays. Children receiving Methotrexate and anthrocyclines may develop severe sunburns. Liberal use of sunscreen lotions as well as the wearing of hats and T-shirts while swimming will help to avoid this distressing complication.

The practice at the Hole In The Wall Gang Camp is to encourage children to participate in full in the many activities offered, including softball, horseback riding, swimming, rowing and canoeing, tennis, and others. With appropriate supervision almost all children—even those with significant physical handicaps—can participate in a meaningful and satisfying way. It is the authors' belief that this experience can be widely extrapolated.

SUMMARY

It must be continuously emphasized that the treatment of childhood cancer can be accompanied by both acute and chronic toxicities and sequelae. These may be limiting factors in the design of physical activities for children being actively treated or for those who are off therapy and are long-term survivors. Physical activity instructors need to be aware of present limitations and also to watch for the signs of long-term side effects. They should also be sensitive to acute deterioration in performance that may herald relapse or therapy-induced secondary malignancies. Open communication between physicians, families, and sports counselors is essential for the optimal care of these children. These young lives can be enriched by appropriate physical activity and sport.

Finally, the treatment of many childhood malignancies has improved dramatically over the last two decades, such that most children can now be cured. Although this chapter has pointed out some of the possible long-term consequences of malignancy or its treatment, many such cured children have no significant consequences of their disease or its treatment and can live entirely normal lives.

REFERENCES

1. Ablin, A.; Isaac, H., Jr. Germ cell tumor. In: Pizzo, P.A.; Poplack, D.G., eds. Principles and practices of pediatric oncology. 2d ed. Philadelphia: J.B. Lippincott Company; 1993:881–882.
2. Allen, A. The cardiotoxicity of chemotherapeutic drugs. In: Perry, M.C., ed. The chemotherapy source book. Baltimore: Williams and Wilkins; 1992:582–588.
3. Balis, F.M.; Holcenberg, J.S.; Poplack, D.G. General principles of chemotherapy. In: Pizzo, P.; Poplack, D., eds. Principles and practices of pediatric oncology. 2d ed. Philadelphia: J.B. Lippincott Company; 1993.
4. Barrett, J. Graft-versus-host disease. In: Treleaven, J.; Burrett, J., eds. Bone marrow

transplantation in practice. London: Churchill Livingstone; 1992.

5. Blatt, J.; Copeland, D.R.; Bleyer, W.A. Late effects of childhood cancer and its treatment. In: Pizzo, P.A.; Poplack, D.G., eds. Principles and practice of pediatric oncology. 2d ed. Philadelphia: J.B. Lippincott Company; 1993:291–298.

6. Brodeur, G.M.; Castleberry, R.P. Neuroblastoma. In: Pizzo, P.A.; Poplack, D.G., eds. Principles and practice of pediatric oncology. 2d ed. Philadelphia: J.B. Lippincott Company; 1993.

7. Budman, D.R. Investigational drugs. In: Perry, M.C., ed. The chemotherapy source book. Baltimore: Williams and Wilkins; 1992:462.

8. Clamon, G.H.P. Alkylating agents. In: Perry, M.C., ed. The chemotherapy source book. Baltimore: Williams and Wilkins; 1992: 286–289.

9. Donaldson, S.S.; Egbert, R.P.; Lee, W.H. Retinoblastoma. In: Pizzo, P.A.; Poplack, D.G., eds. Principles and practices of pediatric oncology. 2d ed. Philadelphia: J.B. Lippincott Company; 1993:683–696.

10. Fernbach, D.J.; Vietti, T.J. Clinical pediatric oncology. 4th ed. St. Louis: Mosby Yearbook; 1991a.

11. Fernbach, D.J.; Vietti, T.J. General aspects of childhood cancer. In: Fernbach, D.J.; Vietti, T.J., eds. Clinical pediatric oncology. 4th ed. St. Louis: Mosby Yearbook; 1991b:1–9.

12. Fischer, D.S.; Knobf, M.T. The cancer chemotherapy handbook. Chicago: Year Book Medical Publishers, Inc.; 1989.

13. Friedman, H.S.; Oakes, W.J. New therapeutic options in the management of childhood brain tumors. Oncology 6(5):27–36; 1992.

14. Gabrilove, J.L. Colony-stimulating factor: clinical studies. In: DeVita, V.T., Jr.; Hellman, S.; Rosenberg, S.A., eds. Biologic therapy of cancer. Philadelphia: J.B. Lippincott Company; 1991:445–463.

15. Green, D.M.; D'Angio, G.J.; Beckwith, J.B.; Breslow, N.; Finklestein, J.Z.; Kelalis, P.; Thomas, P.R.M. Wilm's tumor (nephroblastoma, renal embryoma). In: Pizzo, P.A.; Poplack, D.G., eds. Principles and practices of pediatric oncology. 2d ed. Philadelphia: J.B. Lippincott Company; 1993:712–737.

16. Greenberg, M.; Filler, R.M. Hepatic tumors. In: Pizzo, P.A.; Poplack, D.G., eds. Principles

and practices of pediatric oncology. 2d ed. Philadelphia: J.B. Lippincott Company; 1993:705.

17. Hays, D.M.; Atkinson, J.B. General principles of surgery. In: Pizzo, P.A.; Poplack, D.G., eds. Principles and practice of pediatric oncology. 2d ed. Philadelphia: J.B. Lippincott Company; 1993:247–271.

18. Heideman, R.I.; Packer, R.J.; Albright, L.A.; Freeman, C.R.; Rorke, L.B. Tumors of the central nervous system. In: Pizzo, P.A.; Poplack, D.G., eds. Principles and practice of pediatric oncology. 2d ed. Philadelphia: J.B. Lippincott Company; 1993:672–673.

19. Hoagland, H.C. Hematologic complications of cancer chemotherapy. In: Perry, M.C., ed. The chemotherapy source book. Baltimore: Williams and Wilkins; 1992:498–507.

20. Kreisiman, H.; Wolkove, N. Pulmonary toxicity of antineoplastic therapy. In: Perry, M.C., ed. The chemotherapy source book. Baltimore: Williams and Wilkins; 1992: 603–605.

21. Kun, L.E.; Moulder, J.E. General principles of radiation therapy. In: Pizzo, P.A.; Poplack, D.G., eds. Principles and practice of pediatric oncology. 2d ed. Philadelphia: J.B. Lippincott Company; 1993:291–298.

22. Leventhal, B.G.; Donaldson, S.S. Hodgkins disease. In: Pizzo, P.A.; Poplack, D.G., eds. Principles and practice of pediatric oncology. 2d ed. Philadelphia: J.B. Lippincott Company; 1993:579–583.

23. Link, M.P.; Eilber, F. Osteosarcoma. In: Pizzo, P.A.; Poplack, D.G., eds. Principles and practice of pediatric oncology. 2d ed. Philadelphia: J.B. Lippincott Company; 1993:844–866.

24. Lipshultz, S.E.; Colan, S.D.; Gelber, R.D.; Perez-Atayde, A.P.; Sallan, S.E.; Sanders, S.P. Late cardiac effects of doxorubicin therapy for acute lymphoblastic leukemia in childhood. N. Engl. J. Med. 342(12):808–815; 1991.

25. Lipshultz, S.E.; Colan, S.D.; Walsh, E.P.; Sanders, S.P.; Sallan, S.E. Ventricular tachycardia and sudden unexplained death in late survivors of childhood malignancy treated with doxorubicin (abstract). Pediatr. Res. 27(suppl):145A; 1990.

26. Lyss, A.P. Enzymes and random synthetics. In: Perry, M.C., ed. The chemotherapy

source book. Baltimore: Williams and Wilkins; 1992:405–411.

27. Peterson, D.E.; Schibert, M.M. Oral toxicity. In: Perry, M.C., ed. The chemotherapy source book. Baltimore: Williams and Wilkins; 1992:582–588.

28. Pizzo, P.A.; Poplack, D.G., Editors. Principles and practice of pediatric oncology. 2d ed. Philadelphia: J.B. Lippincott Company; 1993.

29. Ramsay, N.K.C. Bone marrow transplantation in pediatric oncology. In: Pizzo, P.A.; Poplack, D.G., eds. Principles and practice of pediatric oncology. 2d ed. Philadelphia: J.B. Lippincott Company; 1993:315–334.

30. Raney, R.B.; Hays, D.M.; Tefft, M.; Triche, T.J. Rhabdomyosarcoma and undifferentiated sarcomas. In: Pizzo, P.A.; Poplack, D.G., eds. Principles and practice of pediatric oncology. 2d ed. Philadelphia: J.B. Lippincott Company; 1993:769–794.

31. Robinson, L.L. General principles of epidemiology of childhood cancer. In: Pizzo, P.A.; Poplack, D.G., eds. Pediatric oncology. 2d ed. Philadelphia: J.B. Lippincott Company; 1993.

32. Rowinsky, E.K.; Donehower, R.C. Vinica alkaloids and epidophyllotoxins. In: Perry, M.C., ed. The chemotherapy source book. Baltimore: Williams and Wilkins; 1992.

33. Schilsky, R.L. Antimetabolites. In: Perry, M.C., ed. The chemotherapy source book. Baltimore: Williams and Wilkins; 1992.

CHAPTER 22

Eating Disorders

Tomas Jose Silber
Children's National Medical Center and
George Washington University School of Medicine and Health Sciences

Nancy S. Mayer
Children's National Medical Center

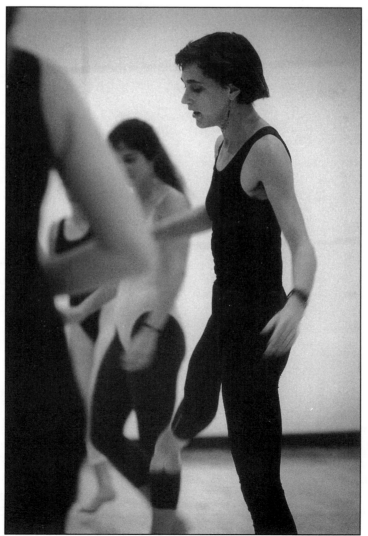

Eating disorders such as anorexia nervosa and bulimia are currently affecting such a significant number of adolescents and young adults that there are few health professionals, trainers, or others involved in sport that have not come across a case, or will not come across a case in their lifetime. Those affected are predominantly female, and there are also special populations at higher risk such as ballet dancers, gymnasts, and runners. Many have an athletic background and become increasingly obsessed with their activity, while others simply discover that intense energy expenditure will contribute to rapid weight loss, and then become compulsive exercisers. Over time, many can become chronically ill, and some will die. It is therefore important that any professional connected with the field of sport and exercise be alert to the clinical manifestations of eating disorders. This chapter will describe eating disorders and their morbidity and mortality, explain the effect of exercise on the condition, and discuss some pertinent management issues.

DESCRIPTION OF EATING DISORDERS

Anorexia nervosa, bulimia, and their variants have more similarities than differences, being united by a constant preoccupation with weight control without regard to the consequences. An eating disorder may be suspected when any of the following warning signs are noted:

- weight loss or failure to recover weight in spite of repeated advice or even admonishment by parents, friends, coaches, or health professionals
- frequent complaint about being fat or having a body area—usually abdomen and thighs—that is "too fat," even when markedly underweight (a body image distortion)
- compulsive exercising
- self-induced vomiting
- use of laxatives, diuretics, or ipecac
- recurrent binge eating
- loss of menstrual periods

Table 22.1 presents the established diagnostic criteria for anorexia nervosa and bulimia (1).

Pathophysiology

The pathophysiology of anorexia nervosa is that of human starvation (2). There is a state of glycogen depletion in the liver, hypoglycemia, ketosis, a hypometabolic state, a virtual shutdown of the endocrine reproductive cycle, diminished cardiovascular contractability, bradycardia, and hypotension. In extreme cases this may eventually lead to loss of consciousness, coma, and death. In bulimia nervosa, on the other hand, the changes are predominantly related to the physiological alterations produced by chronic self-induced vomiting, such as esophagitis and hypokalemic, hyponatremic, hypochloremic, alkalosis. Laxative abuse may lead to abdominal cramps, diarrhea, chronic colonic inflammation, and loss of peristalsis. Abuse of diuretics, intoxication with appetite suppressant stimulants, and ipecac poisoning may result in edema, acidosis, muscle breakdown, and disturbances in cardiac conduction (3).

Physical Symptoms and Clinical Signs

The young adolescent with anorexia nervosa may stand out in her sports gear because of her emaciated appearance; bony extremities; fine, soft (lanugo-like) body hair; dry scaly skin; and brittle head hair. She may also show decreased athletic performance and aerobic capacity, light-headedness, syncope, low heart rate, and low blood pressure. Amenorrhea, delayed gastric emptying, constipation, and insomnia are common. In very severe cases organic brain syndrome can develop. The metabolic effects of starvation are all reversible on refeeding (4).

The person with bulimia may be of normal weight or may also be of very low weight, alternating restrictive eating habits with binges. Initially most are asymptomatic, but over time there can be destruction of dental enamel, esophageal injury leading to bleeding, parotid enlargement ("chipmunk facies"), and menstrual abnormalities. Observation of the hands is important because they may reveal Russell's sign: calluses, sometimes crusted or ulcerated, over the knuckles, caused by pressing them against the upper teeth while inducing vomiting. Electrolyte imbalance may manifest as weakness, muscle cramps, and an irregular pulse. Cardiac

Table 22.1   Diagnostic Criteria for Anorexia Nervosa, Bulimia Nervosa, and Other Eating Disorders

Diagnostic Criteria for 307.1 Anorexia Nervosa

A. Refusal to maintain body weight at or above a minimally normal weight for age and height (e.g., weight loss leading to maintenance of body weight less than 85% of that expected; or failure to make expected weight gain during period of growth, leading to body weight less than 85% of that expected).

B. Intense fear of gaining weight or becoming fat, even though underweight.

C. Disturbance in the way in which one's body weight or shape is experienced, undue influence of body weight or shape on self-evaluation, or denial of the seriousness of the current low body weight.

D. In postmenarcheal females, amenorrhea, i.e., the absence of at least three consecutive menstrual cycles. (A woman is considered to have amenorrhea if her periods occur only following hormone, e.g., estrogen, administration.)

Specify type:
   Restricting type: During the current episode of Anorexia Nervosa, the person has not regularly engaged in binge-eating or purging behavior (i.e., self-induced vomiting or the misuse of laxatives, diuretics, or enemas)
   Binge-eating/purging type: During the current episode of Anorexia Nervosa, the person has regularly engaged in binge-eating or purging behavior (i.e., self-induced vomiting or the misuse of laxatives, diuretics, or enemas)

Diagnostic Criteria for 307.51 Bulimia Nervosa

A. Recurrent episodes of binge eating. An episode of binge eating is characterized by both of the following:
   1. Eating, in a discrete period of time (e.g., within any 2-hour period), an amount of food that is definitely larger than most people would eat during a similar period of time and under similar circumstances
   2. A sense of lack of control over eating during the episode (e.g., a feeling that one cannot stop eating or control what or how much one is eating)

B. Recurrent inappropriate compensatory behavior in order to prevent weight gain, such as self-induced vomiting; misuse of laxatives, diuretics, enemas, or other medications; fasting; or excessive exercise.

C. The binge eating and inappropriate compensatory behaviors both occur, on average, at least twice a week for 3 months.

D. Self-evaluation is unduly influenced by body shape and weight.

E. The disturbance does not occur exclusively during episodes of Anorexia Nervosa.

Specify type:
   Purging type: During the current episode of Bulimia Nervosa, the person has regularly engaged in self-induced vomiting or the misuse of laxatives, diuretics, or enemas
   Nonpurging type: During the current episode of Bulimia Nervosa, the person has used other inappropriate compensatory behaviors, such as fasting or excessive exercise, but has not regularly engaged in self-induced vomiting or the misuse of laxatives, diuretics, or enemas

307.50 Eating Disorder Not Otherwise Specified

The Eating Disorder Not Otherwise Specified category is for disorders of eating that do not meet the criteria for any specific Eating Disorder. Examples include

   1. For females, all of the criteria for Anorexia Nervosa are met except that the individual has regular menses.
   2. All of the criteria for Anorexia Nervosa are met except that, despite significant weight loss, the individual's current weight is in the normal range.
   3. All of the criteria for Bulimia Nervosa are met except that the binge eating and inappropriate compensatory mechanisms occur at a frequency of less than twice a week or for a duration of less than 3 months.
   4. The regular use of inappropriate compensatory behavior by an individual of normal body weight after eating small amounts of food (e.g., self-induced vomiting after the consumption of two cookies).
   5. Repeatedly chewing and spitting out, but not swallowing, large amounts of food.
   6. Binge-eating disorder: recurrent episodes of binge eating in the absence of the regular use of inappropriate compensatory behaviors characteristic of Bulimia Nervosa.

Reprinted from American Psychiatric Association (1994).

dysrhythmia may be fatal (2, 3). Patients who abuse laxatives or diuretics may become dehydrated and/or present with "rebound" edema. Chronic amenorrhea may be followed by osteoporosis (5). Patients with eating disorders who engage in compulsive exercising may be susceptible to overuse injuries (6).

There is also a population of children, adolescents, and young adults who, although they engage in extreme dieting and/or compulsive exercise, do not fulfill the classic criteria and are either asymptomatic or only mildly symptomatic. It is useful to consider them as subclinical and potentially ill, and to apply to their situation the same principles of management as in the full-blown cases, in the hope that early intervention may prevent the onset of the clinical condition.

Clinical and Laboratory Assessment

Nutritional status is determined by anthropometric measurements such as height and weight, best expressed as the body mass index (BMI). This is calculated as weight (in kilograms) divided by height (in meters) squared, or $kg/(m^2)$. A BMI below 16 is highly indicative of very low weight. In addition, triceps skinfold, mid-arm circumference, and body type need to be considered. As noted already, dry hair is typical of poor nutrition, and there is often abundant hair loss after several months of severe dieting, even into the recovery phase. Initially there is marked reduction in body fat, followed by loss of lean muscle mass and, finally, depletion of visceral protein.

Many teenagers and young adults with anorexia nervosa maintain a state of incessant activity and deny their feelings of exhaustion, however objectively one can demonstrate diminished aerobic capacity and loss of fitness and strength (7). The laboratory assessment should include a complete blood count. Leukopenia (decreased white blood cell count) is a marker for progressive malnutrition. The presence of a high hemoglobin and hematocrit, on the other hand, indicates hemoconcentration, as seen in chronic dehydration (2). The urinalysis may show the proteinuria secondary to excessive exercise, a high specific gravity because of fluid depletion, or a low specific gravity caused by excessive water intake. (This practice, known as "water loading," is intended to create a false

impression of weight gain.) Low serum glucose levels are observed in emaciated states, and persistent hypoglycemia has ominous implications. The liver enzymes alanine aminotransferase and aspartate aminotransferase may be elevated and increase further with refeeding, reflecting fatty infiltrates in the liver (7). Bilirubin, total protein, globulin, and albumin are usually normal; in fact, jaundice or hypoalbuminemia are reasons to look for another diagnosis, such as toxic hepatitis or inflammatory bowel disease. Serum amylase is elevated in some patients who self-induce vomiting (3). Blood urea nitrogen (BUN) will vary, reflecting the state of hydration and the protein intake, while creatinine will remain low or normal except in those patients who develop renal complications.

The creatinine height index (CHI) is a laboratory evaluation of somatic protein depletion, in which a daily urinary excretion of creatinine is compared with the ideal urinary creatinine derived from a reference standard. A CHI index of less than 60% is evidence of severe depletion, while an index of 60–80% represents moderate depletion. This is a good method of determining body mass, but is limited by being totally dependent on an accurate urine collection. Serum cholesterol varies but is often paradoxically elevated, reflecting perhaps a diminished cholesterol turnover (2). Minerals need to be assessed because hypophosphatemia and hypomagnesemia can have serious consequences, while low zinc has been associated with loss of taste sensation and worsening anorexia (3). Electrolytes can sometimes be the only clue to the existence of laxative abuse (acidosis) or self-induced vomiting (alkalosis). Hypovolemia often ensues and results in secondary hyperaldosteronism.

Endocrine assessment can demonstrate a host of abnormalities. Clinically the most useful is tri-iodithyronine (T_3), which is low in the presence of normal thyrotropic-stimulating hormone (TSH). This is a reflection of the hypometabolic state of semistarvation and improves with nutritional rehabilitation. While it is seldom clinically necessary to order other endocrine tests, the following abnormalities have been noted in anorexia nervosa: increased growth hormone with impaired growth hormone response to stimulation tests, decreased gonadotropin levels, impaired secretion of antidiuretic hormone, elevation of serum cortisol, loss of diurnal variation of cortisol secretion, and abnormal dexamethasone suppression (3). Other tests known to be abnormal (although of questionable clinical significance) include carotene levels (elevated), electroencephalography (EEG abnormalities are greatest in those who purge), and cranial CT scans (pseudoatrophy) (2). Bone densitometry has been used for the detection of osteopenia (8).

Natural History

In their most severe forms eating disorders may end in death, which may be caused by starvation, electrolyte imbalance leading to cardiac dysrhythmia, prolongation of the QT interval with sudden cardiac arrest, or suicide (2, 3, 7). With treatment 80% of patients recover or have substantial improvement, and the remainder will have a chronic course. Little is known about the natural history of bulimia. Sometimes bulimia is not detected for years because binges and purges occur in complete secrecy.

Therapeutic Intervention

The management of anorexia nervosa and bulimia is difficult because patients—and often their families—tend to deny the illness, and particularly its severity. Often, they avoid or abandon adequate medical and psychiatric follow-up. Treatments are prolonged and may alternate outpatient therapies with periods of hospitalization. Nutritional rehabilitation and regulation of activity are often required. Life-saving intervention may be required at times, because of severe starvation, electrolyte disturbances, seizures, or abuse of laxatives, diuretics, or ipecac. The use of hormonal (estrogen) replacement for amenorrhea has been suggested as a way of preventing osteoporosis, although thus far this has not been proven to be effective. A combination of different treatment approaches may be required, including individual, family, group, and milieu therapies. Approaches may be dynamic, cognitive, behavioral, psychoeducational, or based on self-help; psychotropic medications may also be used. Severely ill or hospitalized patients should be under the care of a multidisciplinary team (9).

Morbidity and Mortality

The short-term mortality ranges from 0 to 5% in a large number of series. The long-term mortality (more than 20 years) from anorexia nervosa has been estimated to be 18% (7). The death rate for bulimia has not been established. As illustrated in Figure 22.1, there is significant morbidity: patients may suffer from amenorrhea; osteoporosis (leading to fractures or vertebral collapse); seizures (caused by water intoxication, hypophosphatemia, or hypomagnesemia); syncope; abdominal distension (caused by delayed gastric emptying or acquired lactose deficiency); constipation (from impaired intestinal motility); diarrhea (from laxative abuse); muscle weakness (caused by hypokalemia or ipecac-induced myositis); hypothermia; or ketosis (2, 3, 7). Thus, many patients are first seen by cardiologists, neurologists, endocrinologists, gynecologists, or other specialists before the true nature of the disease is discovered.

EXERCISE AND EATING DISORDERS

The Effect of Eating Disorders on Exercise Tolerance and Sport Performance

In anorexia nervosa there is usually a component of excessive exercise and/or hyperactivity, constant pacing, and general "fidgetiness," or motor activity not connected with overexercise or physical activity (4). Some patients use exercise to anesthetize themselves by seeking a "high"—a kind of oblivion that blots out the world. As Woodman (10) has put it, "They perform their rituals with food and then exercise until the 'lightness' begins to take over. They go into the Light and then experience themselves lit with an inner radiance" (p. 30). They gravitate to exercise that can obliterate their pain, their anxiety, and their fear, and that can keep them from contacting their real, inner feelings. They choose exhaustive aerobic dance, running, feverishly-paced bicycling, or endless pacing. They exercise and ignore their bodies.

During the acute phase of the illness, the patient will admit to feeling exhausted and lethargic only when her body mass has reached a very

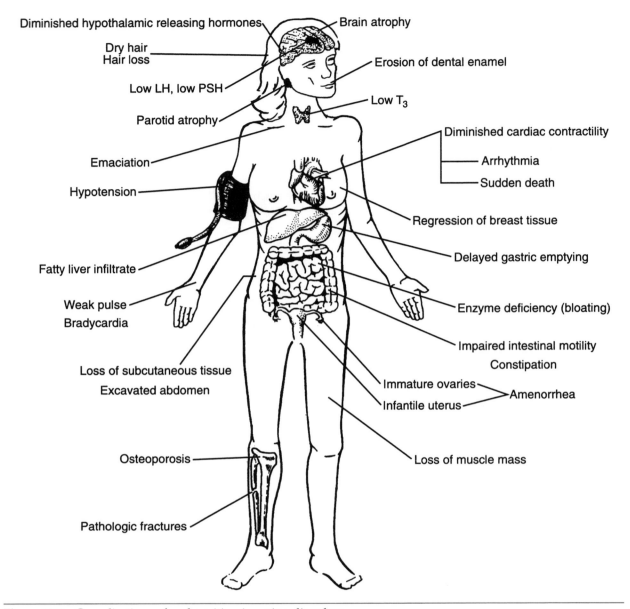

Figure 22.1   Complications of malnutrition in eating disorders.

low level. She may then be pale, cold, and weak. At this point she may not feel like doing much, even if her underlying fidgetiness remains. Before reaching this degree of malnutrition, however, many patients have a very high level of tolerance to exercise, conditioned by habitual exercising and denial of exhaustion. The overexerciser may have strength in certain muscle groups and may exhibit endurance exercises to which she is accustomed, but this specialized endurance is deceptive. There may be a falsely heightened appearance of fitness, an illusion created by the hyperactivity and fidgetiness which seems to suggest an overabundance of energy. When tested objectively, the same patient may show generalized tiredness and fatigue in response to exercise, as well as to manual muscle strength tests graded as low as 3 out of 5. Diminished cardiac aerobic capacity and contractability will also be evident. Marked bradycardia, rhythm irregularities, and low blood pressure are associated with light-headedness and even syncope. Sudden cardiac deaths have resulted from ventricular tachyarrhythmias.

The Special Case of the Competitive Athlete

A special situation is caused by the development of anorexia nervosa in the competitive athlete.

This is not unusual, as dancers, gymnasts, runners, and other athletes may place great emphasis on body weight and perfection. Dieting often occurs in response to criticism or, more often, to unrealistic self-demands and expectations. All problems are reduced to having (or not having) the "ideal weight;" this perceived ideal weight is often redefined each time it is achieved.

Coaches, nurses, and doctors should not be intimidated by the special status of the patient or by pressures from parents, agents, and the like. The same principles that govern the management of the "average" eating-disordered patient need to be applied to the competitive athlete, as well. That is, limits need to be set on training, and activity should be allowed only when the subject is not in danger and should be regulated on the basis of nutritional status and hydration. Putting one professional "in charge," with a clear delineation of authority and responsibility, is crucial to a successful outcome.

Potential Adverse Effects That Can Result From Sport and Exercise

Sport and exercise may become very harmful when athletes with anorexia nervosa are driven by despair and are out of control. This may result in further energy imbalance, weight loss, and malnutrition. Winter sports may lead to severe hypothermia because of defective thermoregulation; similarly, heat stroke, exhaustion, and dehydration are risky in hot environments. Bulimic patients with hypokalemia will be susceptible to muscle cramps and weakness as well as to cardiac rhythm disturbances. In more advanced cases involving persistent hypokalemia and prolonged amenorrhea, contact sports are ill-advised because of muscle weakness and fractures caused by decreased bone mass. Those that are less affected need not be restricted, however.

The primary problem seen in the eating-disordered adolescent's approach to exercise is overindulgence. Exercise is not based on need or on ability; because the patient is out of touch with her body, she has no way of judging when to stop. The compulsive exerciser may experience overuse injuries such as tennis elbow, shoulder tendinitis or bursitis, and running-related injuries (knee pain, tibial stress fracture, or compartment compression syndrome).

Persistent amenorrhea predisposes the patient to osteopenia, probably caused by the associated low estrogen state (8). If osteoporosis has developed there will also be an additional risk of pathological fractures. Vertebral compression fractures may leave a gibus (5). Exercise coupled with severe food restriction may accelerate illness and malnutrition. The fascination with, and addiction to, exercise will continue to compel the person until she has resolved the psychological issues that originally drove her to this behavior.

Precautions to Prevent Adverse Effects

The malnourished athlete needs to be kindly confronted. In cases of persistent weight loss activity needs to be curtailed or even abolished. Target weights (for example, 90% of ideal body weight) may be set to allow for continuation (or resumption) of activity. Since weight can be achieved in fraudulent ways (e.g., by water loading, or by carrying and concealing weights at "weigh-ins"), the weight on the scales should be evaluated in the context of other clinical correlates, such as firmer and higher pulse rate, appropriate increase in blood pressure, and normal body temperature.

In the moderate and severe anorexic patient, restricting activities such as exercise classes, aerobics, and sports helps weight recovery by decreasing caloric expenditures. The desire to be allowed to resume activities can provide the motivation for weight recovery. Typically, the patient will initially protest vehemently about any restrictions; this needs to be explained to coaches and school nurses so that they can reinforce the importance of returning to health and to prevent splitting of the treatment team. As soon as the vital signs improve, a gradual return to activities and sports will enhance social interactions and prevent osteopenia (5).

The goal of treatment is for the affected individual to become more aware of who she really is and what her true needs are. Therefore, exercise must become a conscious process, and mindless, frenetic activity is to be avoided. Whenever exercise is reintroduced it must be at a moderate level. The patient needs to be continually encouraged to breathe correctly with each exercise and not to hold her breath.

Many anorexics display a shallow breathing pattern with decreased inspiration, as noted by minimal lateral costal and diaphragmatic expansion. This pattern, which may be significant enough to require specific attention, is possibly related to the body's attempt to conserve energy in the face of starvation, or it may be associated with psychological stress, or anger. It can be helpful to encourage deeper, less restricted breathing. Emphasis should also be placed on the need to focus, to be aware of proper body alignment, to stay with the pace, and to do only the prescribed number of repetitions. The inclusion of rest periods can enhance the learning of exercise in moderation.

In the case of moderately ill and convalescing patients, the training heart rate level can be set at 60% of the maximum heart rate. Later, the target rate can be at 70% or even 75% of the maximum for short periods of exercise. Some of the medication that anorexics and bulimics may require, such as amitriptyline and impipramine, can increase the resting heart rate, and this too must be taken into consideration. Activities and exercises need to be closely monitored, or patients may quickly exceed their safe level of activity.

Appropriate Response to Adverse Effects

Patients whose eating disorders and exercise compulsion are out of control sometimes require hospitalization. More moderate cases require close observation in the school and recreational environments. Until awareness of body needs is established, balance and moderation have to be enforced by strict guidelines, because the adolescent will not have the ability to stop or slow down until this internal learning is in place. This is often worse with younger anorexics, and when it becomes a problem, the instructor has to intervene. For example, if the anorexic cannot control her impulse to go faster on a stationary bicycle, she has to stop and switch to either resting or gentle stretching. At times it is useful to point out alternatives such as strengthening with small weights (1 to 2 pounds); this can help shift the focus away from speed and calorie burning to the development of form. Another successful alternative is guided movement or dance, where the music and the instructor set the pace and tone.

Conversely, if an eating-disordered patient does not want to move and is in a state of depression, it can be helpful to have her stretch and exercise. Often a sense of isolation and crying can be worked through, and the patient will look and feel much better after an exercise class.

Potential Benefits of Exercise on the Eating Disorder

The planning of appropriate exercise for the anorexic individual may further the development of trust. An exercise session creates an arena for the development of body awareness through the medium of relaxed movement. Exercise can also serve as a support for other processes of internal growth and learning.

Exercise can be an important incentive for eating. Patients who exercise with moderation are often able to eat much more than those who are sedentary, and therefore gain weight more quickly.

Physical Fitness

Severely malnourished individuals are at first very ill and begin a convalescent phase as weight is regained. They are not yet in good physical condition, however. Guided exercise may support the return to a normal and healthy body. The benefits are lean body mass acquisition, osteogenesis, physical endurance, athletic ability, enhanced respiration, and relaxation.

Psychosocial Development

An exercise session allows for interaction with peers and with an instructor. Group structure demands that the anorexics work in conjunction with others, stay with the pace, and, in general, harmonize in some way. They can develop the ability to participate with others, function in a group, and participate in the world. This is more helpful than "prima donna" activities. As changes in body awareness and changes in posture take place there is often an increase in self-esteem and confidence.

Quality of Life

The quality of life is greatly enhanced by the ability to move and to use the body for sport and play. Anorexics and bulimics who are driven to exercise have lost touch with the light quality of fun and play that is present in children. Guided exercise can be the vehicle for relearning how to breathe, to stretch, to move through space, to become more self-content, and to begin to relax and enjoy life. Exercise can indeed then become an emotional outlet and a possibility for a return toward wholeness.

EXERCISE AND SPORT PROGRAMS FOR CHILDREN AND ADOLESCENTS WITH EATING DISORDERS

The exercise prescription both for inpatients and outpatients should be based not only on physical but also on behavioral considerations. Activity recommendations should therefore be made by the coach or physical therapist in coordination with the patient's treatment team (physician, psychotherapist).

It is also necessary to distinguish between different levels of eating disorders. Thus, young people who are becoming obsessed with weight and eating but who do not have anorexia nervosa or bulimia, may have fewer restrictions than those who require more intensive treatment. By contrast, patients who have been recently discharged from the hospital may need the closest monitoring. For example, the following is appropriate for patients who are no longer in the acute phase and are beginning to recover:

- Periods of exercise should be brief, never more than an hour long, including beginning stretches and warm-up, aerobic exercise, and cooldown.
- There should only be one aerobic activity per day.
- Exercises that require relating to others may be particularly encouraged.
- It is very helpful to make conscious breathing and relaxation part of the program.

Specific Exercise and Conditioning Activities to Be Recommended

Aerobic Activities

The full use of the breathing capacity needs to be developed, which can be accomplished with activities such as walking with others, moderate bicycling, and swimming. These provide aerobic activity as well as an opportunity for socialization.

Strength Training

Light weights may be used to begin to develop the upper body. However, if the muscles shake with the effort the weight must be decreased: in some cases, even 1 pound can be too much. Because anorexics tend to focus on abdominal and thigh exercises, usually at the exclusion of other areas of the body, weakness is often seen in the muscles of the arms and upper back. As noted previously, repetitions should be limited.

Movement and Flexibility Training

The hamstrings and heelcords need to be stretched. It is important to maintain proper body alignment and avoid internal hip rotation on hamstring stretches. The whole body can have a sense of tightness and tension to it, yet there is no limitation of motion at any joint. The muscles can be extremely diminished in size and feel almost "stringy" in the severely malnourished girl. Gentle stretching can be particularly helpful. Movements incorporating upper-body or full-body stretches using the arms and trunk are important.

Activities to Be Avoided

These include any that are frenetically paced, or that are highly aerobic in nature. Highly competitive or pressured activities should also be avoided.

Modifications in Activities Due to Changes in the Clinical Stages of Eating Disorders

Severely cachectic individuals admitted to the hospital are not allowed to exercise until the pulse, respiratory rate, and blood pressure come up to a medically safe and stable level. This usually requires a weekly weight gain of 1 to 2 pounds, enforced rest periods, and the like.

As the more severely anorectic patient begins to respond to treatment, she may be evaluated by a physical therapist and started on a modified exercise program. Vital signs are monitored by the therapist for any sign of distress or over-exertion. Sometimes the time allowable for aerobic activities may consist of no more than 5-minute segments, interspersed with rest breaks. If the patient is unable to refrain from frenetically paced exercise she must switch to another form of exercise. The program can be enhanced and modified as the individual starts to regain health and a sense of inner control and connection.

Specific Sports Recommended for the Individual With Eating Disorders

When trying to list specific sports one faces the basic problem that any sport can be abused by the overexerciser. In her blind rush for perfection, the anorexic may overdo any activity; thus, it is not just a matter of which sport to choose.

A good exercise choice would be body movement or dance done within a controlled, workshop setting. Exploratory dance can be extremely therapeutic. Woodman (10) has stated that "what is important to realize is that releasing the body into spontaneous movement or play constellates the unconscious in precisely the same way as does a dream" (p. 78). Ballet is an exercise often favored by anorexics. While ballet can be a medium of self-expression, this aspect of the art usually emerges only after a considerable apprenticeship in technique. Unfortunately, some ballet instructors may place a competitive focus on perfection, to the detriment of the student's balanced development.

In any case patients will choose a variety of sports, and some general guidelines may therefore be considered.

• Moderately ill patients with anorexia nervosa can tolerate only short periods of activities requiring high aerobic output. However, because these patients fervently desire to burn calories and lose weight, they may beg to continue, promising to eat better and so forth. It may be hard to stop this activity, but it is never helpful to allow it to continue.

• More severely afflicted patients are often osteoporotic; hence, collision sports should be excluded in the malnourished with persistent amenorrhea.

• The dominant motions needed in the selected sport should include both the upper and lower extremities, so as to develop the body as a whole. These sports are best kept in the moderate-to-low range of intensity. Sailing and figure skating exemplify sports that tend to elicit balance and variability.

• Sports with high static demands seem somewhat more applicable to the anorexic than do those with high dynamic demands. It must also be taken into consideration that most anorexics do not have the strength for more rugged sports such as speed skating. Tai chi and yoga can also be recommended: the movements are slow and controlled, and promote relaxation and proper breathing techniques.

• Opportunities for success and level of competition should also be considered. Overemphasis on competition presents external demands that can exacerbate rather than alleviate the anorexic's problems. This is not to say that the anorexic must be completely shielded from competition, but the competitive element must be balanced with a sense of play, and the seriousness leavened with fun.

Sports involving low-to-moderate neuromuscular demands would be safer for the anorexic and offer more chances of success. Especially following the acute phase of the illness, the person with anorexia nervosa should be regarded as a convalescent. The physical body has been weakened by malnutrition, and full participation in sports is not desirable. Even when physical health begins to return patients are still not really in tune with their bodies, and remain awkward with obvious muscle weakness.

• The qualities of fun and play should be among the guidelines. For example, if one swims for fun or plays in the water, the result is different from competitive swimming. Dancing, canoeing, equestrian activities, and even some sprinting could be recommended.

• Changes can be made in the program as patients progress or regress. For example, if anorexics begin to lose weight or if the clinical course worsens, they must be guided towards less strenuous and demanding forms of exercise. If weight and health are improving, however, patients can have more freedom and latitude in their choices. Intense, high-collision sports are contraindicated until nutritional rehabilitation has been achieved.

Therapeutic Interventions That Can Enhance Safety and Performance

These include careful monitoring of the intensity of the sport, the time spent each day on the sport, and the relative amount of food required to balance the output of energy. Whenever weight loss takes place it may signal danger of relapse.

Adaptive Changes

Some changes that can be made in sports to permit participation by the person with anorexia include the following:

- Lower the level of competition.
- Increase the sense of play.
- Increase the give-and-take and camaraderie between the players.
- Include periods of rest.
- Include light stretches and full breaths in the warm-up and cooldown periods.
- Include a short "debriefing session" to discuss the game and any subjective responses that emerged during the interaction.

SUMMARY

Eating disorders may become life-threatening illnesses with significant morbidity. Over-exercising and exercise addiction may first call attention to the existence of anorexia nervosa or bulimia nervosa. A very common consequence is loss of menses, which may in turn lead to osteopenia. This may be the most serious long-standing consequence of these conditions.

Osteoporosis occurs in the anorexic as well as in the bulimic with prolonged amenorrhea. Vigorous exercise alone does not protect against osteopenia: a critical factor appears to be the regaining of weight. Only as weight returns to normal, may the menses resume. Normal female levels of estrogen are then gradually reestablished and bone density may sometimes begin to return to normal. Estrogen therapy is a proposed treatment for osteopenia but has not yet been proven to be effective.

While exercise and physical activity may have adverse potential because of caloric expenditure and weight loss, it may also offer some protection from osteoporosis and provide some psychological benefit. The judicious inclusion of exercise in the treatment plan can aid in the development of trust in the instructor, and also provides some monitored physical outlet for anxiety. Exercise can become a backdrop, an arena in which the facets of the activity and the body's response can be discussed, examined, and assimilated.

Until the person with an eating disorder is fully well and has integrated the new learning, exercise must be done in a moderate and balanced way, and it must be complemented with an appropriate intake of food in accordance with the increased demand created by the exercise.

In summary, several recommendations can be made:

1. Young people with established anorexia nervosa and those with low-weight bulimia need to have their physical activity limited. This is important because

   - decreasing caloric expenditure helps maintain and recover weight;
   - it emphasizes the seriousness of the condition;
   - it can act as a motivator to improve nutritional state and to progressively increase and normalize activity.

   Consequently, one would initially encourage sports with low aerobic intensity, low dynamic demands, and low static demands, and contraindicate sports with high or moderate aerobic intensity and high static and dynamic demands. This should be maintained until the patient achieves appropriate weight recovery, e.g., 90% of ideal weight. It should be emphasized that these restrictions are temporary, medically indicated, and not punitive.

2. Prior to participation it is useful to review realistic goals, as well as the importance of hydration, temperature stability (e.g., the danger of hypothermia in winter sports), and training—breathing exercises, warm-up, and relaxation—to avoid extremes.

3. The purpose of restrictions needs to be made clear to school nurses, coaches, and administrators. Although people with

eating disorders may often strenuously object to the controls, most will develop a "healthy side" that will accept and sometimes even welcome the restrictions.

4. When the patient is ready for self-limited activities, as demonstrated by weight recovery, higher and firmer pulse, and normal body temperature, exercise can be increased to the level recommended by the President's Council on Physical Fitness.

REFERENCES

1. American Psychiatric Association. Diagnostic and statistical manual of mental disorders (fourth edition). Washington, DC: Author; 1994.
2. Fisher, M. Medical complications of anorexia and bulimia nervosa. Adol. Med. State of the Art Reviews 3:487–502; 1992.
3. Herzog, D.B.; Copeland, P.M. Eating disorders. N. Engl. J. Med. 313:295–303; 1985.
4. Kaye, W.H.; Gwirtsman, H.E.; Obarzanek, E.; George, D.T. Relative importance of calorie intake needed to gain weight and level of physical activity in anorexia nervosa. Am. J. Clin. Nut. 47:989–994; 1988.
5. Rigotti, N.A.; Nussbaum, S.R.; Herzog, D.B.; Neer, R.M. Osteoporosis in women with anorexia nervosa. N. Engl. J. Med. 291:861–865; 1984.
6. Roy, S. Injuries of exercise. Med. Clin. North Am. 69:197–209; 1989.
7. Silber, T.J. Anorexia nervosa morbidity and mortality. Ped. Ann. 13:851–858; 1984.
8. Silber, T.J.; Cox, J.M. Early detection of osteopenia in anorexia nervosa by radiographic absorptiometry. Adol. Pediatr Gyn. 3:137–140; 1990.
9. Silber, T.J.; D'Angelo, L.J. The role of the primary care physician in the diagnosis and management of anorexia nervosa. Psychosomatics 32:221–225; 1991.
10. Woodman, M. Addiction to perfection. Toronto: Inner City Books; 1982.

RECOMMENDED READING

Bruch, H. The golden cage—the enigma of anorexia nervosa. Cambridge, MA: Harvard University Press; 1978.

Callaway, C.W.; Whitney, C. The Callaway diet—successful permanent weight control for starvers, stuffers and skippers. New York: Bantam Books; 1990.

Prussin, R.; Harvey, P.; DiGeronimo, A. Hooked on exercise: how to understand and manage exercise addiction. New York: Simon & Schuster; 1992.

Rodin, J. Body traps. Breaking the binds that keep you from feeling good about your body. New York: William Morrow and Company, Inc.; 1992.

Siegel, M.; Brisman, J.; Weinshel, M. Surviving an eating disorder: perspectives and strategies for family and friends. New York: Harper and Row; 1988.

Woodman, M. The owl was a baker's daughter: obesity, anorexia nervosa and the repressed feminine. Toronto: Inner City Books; 1980.

Yates, A. Compulsive exercise and the eating disorders. New York: Brunner/Mazel, Inc.; 1991.

CHAPTER 23

Obesity

Oded Bar-Or
Children's Exercise and Nutrition Centre,
McMaster University, Ontario

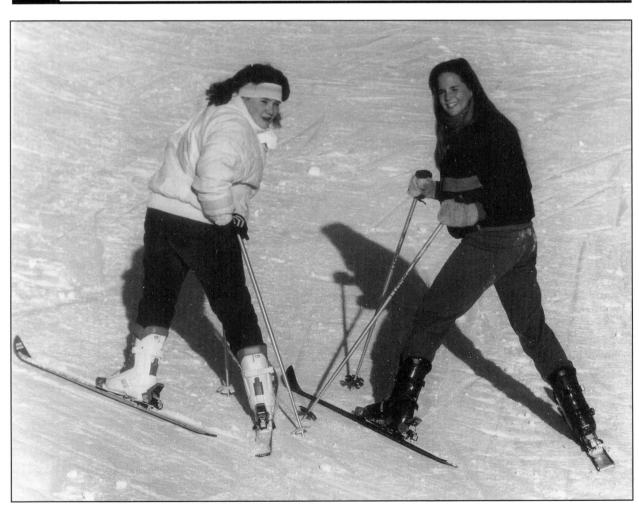

Childhood and adolescent obesity (for brevity's sake referred to here as "juvenile" obesity) is the most common pediatric chronic illness in technologically developed countries. Its prevalence in North America ranges from 10–25% (73, 109), depending on assessment methods and the criteria used to define it. Most importantly, this prevalence has been on the rise in the last decade (73, 132). Overweight and obesity in the USA are particularly prevalent among African-Americans and Hispanics of low socioeconomic status. For example, in a recent survey of Harlem 5- to 11-year-old African-Americans (109), more than a quarter could be considered "obese" and 14% were "superobese" (i.e., above the 95th percentile of weight-for-height national norms). The "tracking" of obesity from childhood to adulthood is only fair, but it is higher from adolescence to adulthood. Still, an obese child has a higher likelihood than a nonobese child of becoming an obese adolescent (140) and adult.

Juvenile obesity is strongly associated with other indices of coronary risk during childhood and youth (17). Furthermore, as shown recently (107), adult females and males who were overweight during adolescence have twice the risk for coronary heart disease and other diseases than those who were not overweight in adolescence. This is true even if they are not obese as adults. Thus, treatment and prevention of obesity at a young age are of a paramount public health importance.

Because enhanced physical activity is one of the cornerstones in the management of obesity, this chapter will focus on five main issues related to physical activity and juvenile obesity:

1. The evidence for a link between juvenile obesity and insufficient physical activity
2. Physiological and medical considerations in the response of the obese child to exertion
3. The role of physical training in the management of juvenile obesity
4. Characteristics of the "optimal" training program and
5. The role of the school in the prevention and management of juvenile obesity.

Information will include a review of the literature, as well as the experience gained at the author's Children's Exercise and Nutrition Centre.

HABITUAL ACTIVITY, ENERGY EXPENDITURE, AND THE OBESE CHILD

It is generally accepted that obesity occurs when energy intake through food exceeds total energy expenditure plus the energy required for growth. Total energy expenditure equals the sum of basal expenditure (often measured as resting metabolic rate), diet-related expenditure (i.e., the energy required for absorption and digestion of food, often referred to as the "thermic effect of food" or "diet-induced thermogenesis"), and expenditure related to physical activity. Basal metabolism accounts for 60–70% of the total energy expenditure. The respective values for dietary and activity expenditures in a sedentary child are 15–20% and 20–25%. However, the activity-related expenditure can rise considerably if the child is physically active. The two questions posed in this section are whether total energy expenditure and physical activity are deficient in children who are already obese, and whether low total energy expenditure and activity are part of the etiology of juvenile obesity. For reviews on the components of energy expenditure in obesity see Matsushima, Kriska, Tajima, and LaPorte (98); Puhl (122); and Schoeller, Bandini, Levitsky, and Dietz (138).

Clinical experience and numerous studies since the 1940s have shown that overweight or obese children are habitually less active than their normal-weight or nonobese peers (30, 35, 40, 41, 49, 52, 80, 104, 117, 144, 154, 162), particularly during nonstructured activities. It has been suggested (e.g., 153) that in the general population, children in the upper adiposity percentiles (even if they are not obese) are less active than those in the lower adiposity percentiles. Other studies, in contrast, have not found the obese or overweight children to be less active (34, 86, 87, 97, 148, 156, 161, 166), to have a lower total daily energy expenditure (9–11, 138), or a lower basal metabolism (11, 95) than their lean peers.

A similar disagreement exists regarding food intake. Several studies have shown that obese children do not have an excessive calorie intake (9, 77, 119). In contrast, Waxman and Stunkard (162) found that the absolute calorie content of food consumed by obese adolescents was higher than that consumed by their nonobese siblings.

One reason for these discrepancies is the low validity and precision of methods often used for the assessment of activity, energy expenditure, and food intake. This is particularly true for recall questionnaires, where obese people seem to underestimate the amount of their food intake and overestimate the amount of activity (92). Another reason for these discrepancies is the way in which energy expenditure has been reported: some of the authors who found the obese to expend as many calories as the lean were calculating energy expenditure in absolute terms, without correction for the larger body mass, or fat-free mass, of the obese. Waxman and Stunkard (162), for example, found a lower degree of activity (as assessed by an observer) among obese boys than among their nonobese siblings, but no intergroup difference in absolute calorie expenditure. However, by correcting for body mass, one would conclude that the obese boys in that study had a lower energy expenditure. Bandini, Schoeller, and Dietz (11) found that when energy expenditure of obese adolescents was related to fat-free mass, it did not differ from that of the nonobese controls. It is thus difficult to reconcile the commonly made clinical observation that obese children are inactive with research findings to the effect that total energy expenditures do not differ.

A major component of North American children's leisure time is spent watching TV. Dietz and Gortmaker (59) have described a dose-response relationship between the prevalence of obesity and the number of hours of TV viewing among US children and adolescents. They have further stated that the likelihood of being obese increases by 2% for each weekly hour spent watching TV, particularly among adolescents. Likewise, The National Children and Youth Fitness Study (117) reported a significant association between adiposity and the extent of TV viewing. In contrast, a recent study (129) found no relationship between the extent of watching TV and body mass index or triceps skinfold thickness among sixth- and seventh-grade females in California. Nor was there any relationship between the level of TV viewing and subsequent changes in body mass index or triceps skinfold thickness over a 2-year period. Similarly, Tucker (155) found no correlation between body mass index and TV watching among adolescent boys, although the "light TV viewers"

scored better than the "heavy TV viewers" on several fitness scores.

If, indeed, TV viewing does increase the likelihood of obesity in children and youth, one possible explanation is that it reduces the leisure time available for activity. However, research so far has shown either a weak relationship (129) or no relationship (152) between the extent of TV watching and the overall activity level of children. An intriguing recent finding, which might suggest a causal relationship between obesity and TV viewing, is that resting metabolic rate dropped significantly among 8- to 12-year-old children while they were watching TV, compared with values obtained while they were resting but not watching TV (88). There is no clear physiological mechanism that explains this finding. Another possible mechanism, as proposed by Dietz and Gortmaker (59), is that TV viewing increases energy intake. Indeed, between-meal snacking increases while watching TV (46), possibly because TV advertising during children's programs often focuses on high-calorie foods (147).

A possible explanation for the reluctance of obese children to exert themselves is that they perceive physical effort to be excessively demanding. As shown by Ward, Blimkie, and Bar-Or (160), the rating of perceived exertion (31) for any given aerobic task is higher among obese adolescents than among nonobese controls. However, when exercise is expressed as a percentage of the person's maximal aerobic power, the effort rating by the obese is not excessive.

These findings are related to children and adolescents who are already obese. The question remains as to whether hypoactivity is actually a cause of juvenile obesity. One approach to this question is to study infants before they are obese and then follow them up longitudinally. The first attempt in this regard was made by Mack and Kleinhenz (94), who studied five newborns, daughters of obese mothers, for the first 8 weeks of life. They found an inverse correlation between activity level and ultimate weight gain. Berkowitz, Agras, Korner, Kraemer, and Zeanah (20) assessed the activity of 1- to 3-day-old babies and then measured their adiposity at ages 4-8 years, but found no correlation between the two values. Ku, Shapiro, Crawford, and Huenemann (89) periodically monitored activity habits of children between age 6 months and 8 years (activity logs were filled in by the parents). An inverse correlation was found between adiposity at age 8 years and activity scores at ages 3 and 4 years in the boys, but not in the girls. The most sophisticated study from a methodological point of view was by Roberts, Savage, Coward, Chew, and Lucas (128). They assessed total energy expenditure of nonobese 3-month-old babies (using the doubly labeled water technique, which is considered a "gold standard" for total energy expenditure), and then measured skinfold thickness at age 1 year. Energy expenditure of those who became overweight at 1 year was only 79% of that of the infants who remained lean. The results did not depend on the adiposity level of the mothers. In animal studies, genetically obese young Zucker rats seem spontaneously less active than their lean controls, even before they become markedly obese (146). These findings do suggest that lower energy expenditure precedes the development of obesity. However, a recent observation (54) found no relationship between total energy expenditure (as measured by doubly labeled water) at age 12 weeks and various indices of body fatness at ages 9 months and 2 years. Unlike in the study by Roberts et al., the mothers of the subjects in this study were not obese. More research, conducted over a longer period and with larger numbers of subjects, is needed to definitively determine the etiological role of low total energy expenditure in juvenile obesity. Such a relationship should be assessed, bearing in mind the strength of the genetic component in becoming obese (149) and in energy expenditure.

PHYSICAL WORKING CAPACITY

Obese children and adolescents, as a group, are less fit than their nonobese peers (see reference 12 for a review). Specific fitness components in which they score low are cardiopulmonary endurance (12, 16, 21, 53, 56, 64, 74, 102, 103, 133) and motor performance (12, 15, 22, 76, 78). They score particularly low in tasks that require carrying or lifting of their own body, such as running, jumping, dips, and chin-ups. Most nonobese 14- to 18-year-old boys in the US, for example, can perform 8 or more chin-ups (131), in contrast to the one or fewer chin-ups achieved by mildly

to moderately obese adolescents (12, p. 205). This low performance, however, does not result from a deficiency in muscle strength, when calculated per cross-sectional area, or from deficient contractile characteristics; these are similar in obese and nonobese children (27, 28). It thus seems that the low score on strength-related fitness tests reflects the excess load that the muscle has to lift, rather than deficient intrinsic contractile characteristics. Obese adolescents have been shown to have a lower rate of motor unit activation during knee extension than their leaner peers (81.5% vs. 95.3%) (28), but the significance of this finding to strength and physical performance is unclear.

Another, often overlooked fitness component that is deficient, particularly in markedly obese people, is economy of movement. Such people require an excessive amount of metabolic energy to perform a given physical task (for a review, see reference 14). This occurs not only during "weight-dependent" tasks such as treadmill running but also in "weight-independent" tasks such as cycling (6, 7). The main reason is the need to carry a large body mass (leg mass, in the case of cycling). Unpublished data from the author's laboratory further seem to indicate that in markedly obese children, energy cost (of treadmill walks) increases because of the wasteful energy expenditure inherent in their "waddle gait." Another reason, as shown for markedly obese adults (164), is the high metabolic cost of ventilation. While Rowland (133) did not find a difference in O_2 cost per kilogram of body mass in obese and nonobese adolescents during treadmill walking, for the same walking speed, the obese consumed 89% of their maximal O_2 uptake, compared with only 82% in the nonobese. This difference can explain the earlier fatigability displayed by the obese. Confirming this assumption is the low ventilatory threshold among obese adolescents (51, 127, 133).

It is important to emphasize that low aerobic fitness does not, in itself, constitute an abnormal cardiorespiratory response to exercise. As shown by Cooper, Poage, Barstow, and Springer (51), when corrections were made for body size, cardiorespiratory functions during maximal cycling exercise were normal in most of 18 obese children and adolescents. A similar conclusion was reached by Rowland (133), whose subjects were tested on a treadmill. The deficiency in performance is therefore a reflection of the excess weight carried by the obese, rather than of a malfunctioning cardiorespiratory system. A practical implication is that weight loss per se, even without aerobic training, can improve the aerobic performance of the obese child. It should be realized, however, that extreme obesity may be accompanied by a right ventricular (2) or left ventricular (3) cardiac dysfunction.

EFFECTS OF ENHANCED PHYSICAL ACTIVITY ("TRAINING")

It is now quite clear that the most effective and long-lasting approach to managing juvenile obesity is by a combination of training (to increase the total daily energy expenditure), changes in food intake, and behavior modification (4, 38, 39, 66, 70, 96). To understand the specific role of training one should study its effects in isolation from the other two therapeutic modalities; however from clinical and practical points of view it is extremely important to understand how training affects obesity when prescribed in combination with nutritional education and behavior modification.

Training as a Single Intervention

Table 23.1 is a summary of anthropometric, physiological, and biochemical changes that training induces in obese children and adolescents. While it is beyond the scope of this chapter to analyze these in detail, the following is an overview of such changes, with emphasis on those most relevant to weight control and health. For detailed reviews, see Björntorp (24) and Pacy, Webster, and Garrow (110).

Based on a review of 55 studies of adolescents and adults (both obese and nonobese), Wilmore (167) reported a training-induced reduction in body mass and percent fat and an increase in lean body mass. These effects were quite mild, however: the average loss of body fat following 6 to 104 weeks of training was only 1.6%, although the effect appeared greater in obese (e.g., 105) than in nonobese subjects. Similarly, modest training-induced increases in fat-free mass and decreases in percent fat have been found in children (26, 112, 115, 137, 143). Training can

Table 23.1 Anthropometric, Physiological, Biochemical, and Appetite Changes Induced by Training, or by Training Plus Low-Calorie Diets, in Obese Children and Adolescents

Variable	Increase	Decrease	No change
Height increase			x
Weight increase		x	x
% body fat		x	
Fat-free mass	x		x
Fat patterning			x
Heart rate, rest and submax.		x	
Arterial blood pressure, rest and submax.		x	
Basal and resting energy expenditure			x
Thermic effect of food			x
O₂ uptake, submax.		x	
O₂ uptake, max.	x		
Ventilation, submax.		x	
Ventilation, max.	x		
Plasma insulin		x	
Sensitivity to insulin	x		
Glucose tolerance	x		
Free fatty acid mobilization	x		
Low-density lipoprotein		x	x
High-density lipoprotein	x		x
Total cholesterol		x	x
Triglycerides		x	x
Appetite		x	x

Note. More than one effect reflects disagreement in the literature regarding some variables.

From "Juvenile Obesity: The Importance of Exercise—and Getting Children to Do It" by D.F. Parker and O. Bar-Or, 1991, *The Physician and Sportsmedicine,* **19**(6), pp. 113-125. Copyright 1991. Reprinted with permission of McGraw-Hill, Inc.

effect changes in the distribution of body fat in male adults (58), but there are no similar data for children.

Even though training by itself is efficacious in weight control, the effect is slower than that of a low-calorie diet. The main reason is that the negative calorie balance that can be induced by training seldom exceeds 300 calories per day in obese children and youth (as will be discussed subsequently). This contrasts with the reduction of 1000 or more calories per day that can be achieved through low-calorie diets. As shown for healthy children, aerobic training causes an increase in aerobic fitness and a reduction in resting and submaximal exercise heart rate.

Because training-induced changes in body mass and percent fat often do not tally with the caloric value of the added activities (e.g., 105), it has been suggested (65) that obese children, when given a regimented program, may compensate by reducing other activities, such that the actual daily energy expenditure is lower than the expected. This possibility was tested recently (26) in mildly obese Dutch boys who underwent a 4-week, laboratory-based aerobic program. Results showed that total daily energy expenditures increased even more than was expected from the program, suggesting that there was no decrease in spontaneous activities. It has yet to be shown whether the same holds true for children with more severe obesity or those living in other societies.

Finally, one should note that anthropometric, physiological, and biochemical changes in response to training may differ markedly among individuals, most probably because of genetic predisposition (33). This may explain the clinically observed differences in the effectiveness of intervention programs among patients.

Training as Part of a Multidisciplinary Management

Even though low-calorie diets, particularly if extreme, can induce fast weight loss, it is important to assess the combined effects of low-calorie diets and training. The general pattern in most studies is a reduction in body mass (or in the rate of mass increase) and percent body fat—more so than by training alone—and other physiological changes, as outlined in Table 23.1 (4, 63, 83, 101, 108, 113, 115, 118, 121, 126, 130, 143, 165). Some studies (e.g., 17, 67, 70), although not all (82), have shown that when training is added to a low-calorie diet along with behavior modification, the physiological effects are greater than for diet plus behavior modification without training.

Some of these changes are relevant to the child's present and future cardiovascular health. Among these, one should highlight the reduction in resting arterial blood pressure (39, 101, 130). Even though this is a mild reduction (7–12 mmHg), it is particularly relevant to adolescents with mild hypertension; for them, such a reduction may make the difference between needing or not needing hypotensive medication. Furthermore, if sustained, even a mild reduction in blood pressure may be important for reducing coronary risk.

Another health-related effect is on lipid profile. Some cross-sectional studies have shown that physically active or physically fit healthy children have lower total cholesterol, triglycerides, and low-density lipoprotein concentrations and a greater high-density lipoprotein concentration than do their less active or less fit peers. Nevertheless, the few controlled longitudinal studies that exist show no evidence that enhanced physical activity is the cause of an improved lipid profile in healthy children and adolescents (for reviews see 13, 57). Among the obese, interventions by training or, more often, by low-calorie diets plus training have yielded more encouraging results. Most authors (17, 63, 101, 121, 137, 165) have found an improved profile, while others (170) have found equivocal effects. The design of these studies does not make it possible to determine whether the beneficial effects resulted directly from the intervention or from the weight loss that accompanied the intervention. One practical implication, however, is that improvement in lipid profile is more likely to occur in children who had an abnormal profile, than in those who had a normal one.

Juvenile obesity is often accompanied by above-normal plasma insulin concentrations and/or a low sensitivity to insulin (55, 108, 170). However, training or training-plus-diet studies have yielded a decrease in plasma insulin levels and/or an increase in sensitivity to insulin (108, 145, 170).

A concern often expressed by parents is that children's appetite might increase as a result of training, which would prevent weight loss. Results in the literature do not confirm this concern. Young athletes do indeed eat more than less active children (18); however, as originally pointed out by Mayer (99, 100), at low levels of activity people eat more than when they are more active. A similar pattern was shown for obese children whose appetite decreased following a 4-month program of an extra physical activity (29). More recent studies with obese women (168, 169) also found no increase in appetite as a result of training.

An important benefit of adding training to a low-calorie diet is that the latter may induce, at least for several weeks, a loss of fat-free mass and a negative nitrogen balance (particularly in very low calorie regimens involving 750 calories per day or less). Indeed, as shown in obese adults (123) and children (25, 36), the body mass lost by a low-calorie diet includes nearly 30% fat-free mass. It has also been shown that low-calorie diets may be accompanied by a reduction in height velocity (i.e., the rate at which body height increases) (60). Such responses, if sustained for a long period, are particularly undesirable during the years of growth, when a positive nitrogen balance is needed. The question then remains whether this catabolic effect of diet can be slowed down or reversed by the anabolic effect of training. Some (139, 172), although not all (44) studies with adults have shown that this is indeed the case. While training in obese children can increase their fat-free mass (26), there are no studies in which the addition of exercise to diet, as a means of preserving fat-free mass, has been studied. An additional safeguard might be provided by a resistance training regimen; this has been suggested both for adults (8) and for children (150).

Even when a program is successful in reducing percent body fat, its long-term effects are usually disappointing. While very few scientists have followed up their subjects beyond the duration of an intervention program, it has been a common clinical experience that the effectiveness of diet-plus-training programs is short-lived once the intervention has been concluded. This frustrating phenomenon may in part have biological roots: most people with a propensity for obesity will remain so no matter what the short-term changes are. Other reasons, however, are behavioral: unless a person changes his or her daily eating and activity habits during the program, it is unlikely that the effects of the program will be sustained beyond its duration. Indeed, several studies have shown that behavior modification is extremely important for achieving sustained, long-term effects (37, 39, 68–70). It has further been shown that programs in which the parents—whether obese or not—also undergo behavior modification promise a long-term carryover (39, 48, 71, 96), particularly when the parents are counselled separately from their children (39).

Safety Considerations

Clinical experience, and the lack of reports about detrimental side-effects, strongly suggest that training programs are safe for obese children and adolescents. However, very few studies have addressed this issue directly. Hayashi, Fujino, Shindo, Hiroki, and Arakawa (75), in a controlled study, monitored obese 10- to 11-year-old children before and after a 1-year, 5-days-per-week jogging program. The mild increase in left ventricular end-diastolic volume was similar to that found in nonobese children and adults. There was also a transitory decrease in the combined ECG voltage of SV_1 plus RV_5. Obese adolescents have a higher than average risk for arterial hypertension. However, the author's experience as well as that of others (130) suggests that the increase in blood pressure during exercise is similar in obese and nonobese individuals. Therefore, an elevated blood pressure in an obese child is no contraindication for intense activity. Another issue to recognize is the association between obesity and asthma. In our clinic approximately 10–15% of obese patients also have asthma, and some of these have exercise-induced bronchoconstriction. According to Kaplan, Campbell-Shaw, and Moccia (81), there are young obese patients who respond to exertion with bronchoconstriction, even in the absence of asthma or atopic disease. Such patients benefit from beta-sympathomimetic drugs. A practical implication is that when an obese child complains of shortness of breath with exertion, one should entertain the possibility of bronchoconstriction rather than assume that this is merely a reflection of low fitness. Finally, when obesity is marked, some patients may complain of back, knee, or ankle pain during exertion. In the absence of clear musculoskeletal abnormality, it seems that such pain results from the excessive mechanical load imposed on the back and lower limbs during exercise. Indeed, these complaints usually disappear when the child switches to non-weight-bearing activities such as swimming and cycling. In conclusion, it seems that training programs for obese children and youth do not carry excessive risk.

THE OPTIMAL EXERCISE PROGRAM

The main considerations in planning an exercise program for obese children and youth are physiological and motivational. Ideally, one would like the program to induce an increase in energy expenditure that is sufficient to cause a negative calorie balance. However, the specific activities must take into account the child's likes and dislikes. In addition, the program should be feasible for the family, taking into account its financial means and the availability of exercise facilities around home. Table 23.2 summarizes the main characteristics of an optimal program that takes the physiological and motivational aspects into account.

Physiological Considerations

An exercise program should be constructed so that the child will burn off as many calories as possible. To achieve this, the activities should include large muscle groups (e.g., thigh, shoulder, and trunk) and move the whole body over distances. Examples include walking, jogging, cycling, swimming, dancing, cross-country skiing, snowshoeing, and skating. Even though physical fitness of the obese child is often low (as has been discussed), an increase in fitness should not be regarded as the main objective of an exercise program, but as a by-product of the

Table 23.2 Characteristics of an Optimal Training Program for the Management of Juvenile Obesity

Emphasizes use of large muscle groups

Moves the whole body over distance

Deemphasizes intensity, emphasizes duration

Raises daily total energy expenditure by 10-15%

Includes muscle strength elements

Daily, or near-daily exercise

Gradual increase in frequency and daily volume

Activities must be liked by the child

Token remuneration to be provided

Parental participation to be encouraged

Group activities to include other obese children

Fun, fun, fun!!

decrease in excess body mass and body fat. Therefore, the intensity of each activity can be kept quite low, at least during the first few months. One should remember that the caloric value of walking a mile is practically identical to that of jogging a mile; the advantage of walking is that the child will not become as fatigued and will, therefore, be able and willing to pursue the exercise over longer distances.

Based on research (e.g., 26) and on experience accumulated at the author's Children's Exercise and Nutrition Centre, a 10–15% increase in daily caloric expenditure is feasible for obese children and youth (e.g., from 2,000 to 2,200–2,300 calories per day). This can be achieved by 30 to 45 minutes of mild- to moderate-intensity exercise. When calculating calories one must take into account the weight of the child; for example, a 30-kilogram child expends approximately 20 calories during a 10-minute walk at 2.5 miles per hour, compared with 30 calories per 10 minutes for a 50-kilogram adolescent. Table 23.3 provides a sample of calorie equivalents for various activities, in children who vary in their body mass. For a more detailed list, see Bar-Or (12, pp. 349–350).

Some patients, adolescent boys in particular, show interest in resistance training, to

Table 23.3 Calorie Equivalents of Activities Performed by Children and Adolescents of Various Body Masses

Activity	Body mass in kg			
	20	40	60	80
Basketball (game)	34	68	102	130
Cross-country skiing (leisure pace)	24	48	72	96
Cycling, 6 mph	15	26	39	52
Ice hockey (on-ice)	52	104	156	208
Running, 5 mph	37	66	90	110
8 mph	—	93	126	156
Swimming 35 yards per min				
breast	20	40	60	80
front crawl	27	51	77	90
back	19	36	54	78
Walking 2.5 mph	17	26	34	41

Note. Values are for 10 min of exercise. These are approximate values. Actual calorie equivalents will vary with the intensity of the game and with the child's proficiency. Adapted from Bar-Or (1983).

strengthen and build up their muscles. It has been shown (163) that girls and boys, even before puberty, can increase their strength through such a program. In addition to increasing the child's strength and self-confidence, resistance training may help to preserve fat-free mass. As already suggested, this may be particularly important when training is prescribed in combination with a very low-calorie diet. Resistance training in children is safe provided they are supervised by an adult—at least at the start of their program—and adhere to safety guidelines (43). Also worthy of consideration are weight-bearing activities. (An example would be jumping and landing, in which compression forces are exerted on the spinal column and lower limbs. Likewise, pushing with the hands will exert compression forces on the upper limbs.) Even though there is as yet no scientific evidence about its benefit to the obese child, weight-bearing exercise may increase the peak mineral content of the bone during the years of growth. This is particularly important for an individual who is undergoing dietary restriction and weight loss.

Ideally, some activity or another should be performed each day. However, it is not likely that an obese child who has been inactive prior to the program will be able to start it at such a high frequency. One therefore should devise a program that starts with 1–2 brief sessions (10–15 minutes each) per week, gradually increasing in frequency and time per session, until the child can be active for 30–45 minutes daily.

An exercise prescription should specify the frequency, intensity, type, and time ("FITT") of the activities. It is usually easy for children and parents to understand the concept of type, time, and frequency, but much harder to grasp the notion of intensity. This has been an ongoing challenge in exercise prescription for children. Adults are often advised to measure their own pulse rate as a way of gauging exercise intensity. This technique was also attempted with children at the author's laboratory at the Wingate Institute, Israel, but the results were disappointing: the children, even when successfully palpating their radial or carotid pulse, reported heart rates that were much different from those monitored by ECG.

An alternative approach to prescribing exercise intensity is the use of Rating of Perceived Exertion (RPE). Ward and Bar-Or (159) taught a group of mildly obese girls and boys how to rate their perceived efforts using the Borg RPE scale (31), while riding a cycle ergometer. In subsequent visits, when the children were asked to perform cycling, walking, and running intensities prescribed to them as numbers on the Borg scale, they were indeed successful in discriminating among the various prescribed intensities, as judged from their heart rates, power outputs, and walking/running velocities. However, they did seem to choose intensities higher than expected, based on each child's predetermined HR-over-RPE regression line. A practical implication is that RPE can be used as a means for prescribing exercise intensity, but that one should reduce the prescribed number on the scale if the child seems to exert at an excessive level.

While the RPE approach can yield prescriptions at various intensities, it requires the services of an exercise laboratory. This makes it impractical for most physicians' office situations. A simpler way of prescribing moderate intensity is to instruct the child to work out at levels that cause an increase in breathing effort and frequency, but not to the extent that the child cannot talk during the exercise (the "walk and talk" principle).

Motivational Considerations

Most obese patients are quite reluctant to become more physically active. When obese children or adolescents start an exercise program, they may feel inadequate in their ability to participate in sport. Indeed, such individuals will often not be welcome by their peers. An activity that is perceived as too hard, too boring, or too embarrassing may therefore not be engaged in consistently, and it is thus important to make it as attractive as possible to the child. One should first identify the activities that the child likes the most. These should be the first ones attempted, even if their caloric equivalent may be less than optimal. For example, a baseball match has a low caloric value because the participants stand or sit most of the time. However, if an obese child expresses interest in this sport, he or she should be encouraged to join in. Then, when additional confidence has been gained, activities with a higher energy cost should be phased in.

For the same reason, activity goals set for the child should be attainable. Increments in volume and intensity, made every 1–2 weeks, should be small.

Unlike adults, children do not join a weight control program because of concern for their future health. It is unrealistic to expect a 10-year-old girl, for example, to join a program because it may help prevent hypertension 30 years later. Typically, children are motivated by gratifications that are extrinsic to the program itself. Token rewards should be given once the child has reached a certain goal or milestone. Whenever possible, such goals should not be based on changes in body mass, but rather on changes in behavior (e.g., logging a certain mileage per week, or sustaining activities for a certain period of time). A contract can be signed between the parent (or therapist) and the child, which specifies the activities and the rewards. However, the emphasis on tokens and extrinsic rewards may become counterproductive if it is used for prolonged periods, and the therapist should switch gradually to intrinsic rewards that reinforce the desirable behavior.

As stated earlier, behavior modification of activity and eating patterns is most important, particularly with patients who seem refractory to making lifestyle changes through an educational program alone. Behavioral strategies regarding modifications of activity patterns include

- self-monitoring of activities;
- collecting points for minutes of daily exercise (or miles covered) which, in analogy to a "frequent flyer" program, are subsequently traded for rewards;
- modeling, which is the teaching of the child and the parent to set examples for each other; and
- contingency contracting, in which the parent deposits money at the start of the program and the money is returned to the parent in proportion to the number of sessions attended.

The latter may not be effective for the child, but is geared primarily to the parent to enhance clinic attendance. A modification of the contingency approach is that the child rather than the parent will receive the balance.

Similar approaches can be taken regarding modification of eating habits. Additional measures include

- identifying and subsequently eliminating specific cues that trigger uncontrolled eating;
- reducing the size of the child's plate at the dinner table if the child insists on having "a full plate," similar to other family members;
- forbidding any eating in front of the TV (where one often does not notice what and how much one is consuming, and is influenced by food-related commercials); and
- attempting to eat at a slow pace.

For further discussion of behavior modifications, see references 37, 38, 66, 67, and 96.

A main reason that obese children may be reluctant to participate in sport is that they are embarrassed about displaying their bodies. Adolescent boys, for example, often have fat accumulation that enlarge their breasts. Such boys are reluctant to wear T-shirts, let alone take them off. Likewise, obese girls are often reluctant to wear shorts. Such individuals should be prescribed activities that do not require them to display their bodies.

For physiological and motivational reasons, swimming and water-based games are among the best activities for the obese child. Because of their low body density, people with a high fat content float well in the water. This gives them an advantage over lean people. In addition, subcutaneous fat is a very effective thermal insulator, which reduces heat loss from the body. As a result, children and adolescents with thick skinfolds tolerate cool water better than do their leaner peers (84). Most important, obese children like swimming because their bodies are submerged under water and cannot be seen by others.

Our experience at the Children's Exercise and Nutrition Centre has been that while obese children and, in particular, adolescents are often inhibited when expected to exercise with nonobese persons, they feel quite at ease when exercising with other obese individuals. Whenever possible, activity groups should be limited to obese people, ideally of a similar age and gender group.

Finally, one cannot overestimate the value of fun, recreation, and variety in any exercise program. Activities should include games and other playful situations, with a minor element of competition. It is unlikely that any child, obese or nonobese, will adhere to a program that is regimented and monotonous. For example, a prescription that includes intermittent running as part of a game is much preferred to prolonged jogging or to riding a stationary bike. This principle must be explained and reinforced to parents, therapists, and educators. Another principle is that some activities should also be encouraged outside a regimented program. These include "lifestyle" elements such as free play, walking to and from school, helping in household chores, and taking the dog out for a walk. Such activities have been proven to be efficacious and to have long-lasting effects on weight control (66, 68).

ROLE OF THE SCHOOL IN THE MANAGEMENT OF JUVENILE OBESITY

Most research on the effects of training on juvenile obesity has been done under laboratory or clinic conditions, and much valuable practical experience in management of this illness has been generated in clinics and hospitals. Nevertheless, such programs can attend to only a small segment of the young obese population, usually at the higher ranges of adiposity. In addition, medical programs require expensive resources, which makes them impractical for large-scale interventions. Thus, even if most successful, it is unlikely that clinic-based programs will ever be able to resolve, on a nationwide basis, this major public health challenge. Alternative sites for delivery of obesity-related health care should therefore be sought.

One suggested alternative is to institute home-based programs. The idea is that parental involvement and role-playing can strongly influence a child's lifestyle habits, including physical activity (e.g., 106), and eating and smoking (136). While this notion seems plausible, such an approach requires a certain level of knowledge, skill, and commitment on the parents' part. In one study (23), 11 families were tutored, and subsequently supervised, by 10 consultants (physical education students) on how to implement a home-based activity program for their obese children. The program lasted 10–11 weeks, requiring weekly visits by the consultants, and yielded an increase in the activity of most of the

children but no change in adiposity. This highly labor-intensive program did not address eating habits. Obviously, much more research is needed to optimize and evaluate the efficacy and cost-effectiveness of home-based programs.

Another approach to managing juvenile obesity is with the use of summer camps (101, 114, 118, 120). Such programs seem efficacious in reducing body fat and other coronary risk factors, but the effects are short-lived. A case in point is a study by Parizková, Vanecková, Sprynarová, and Vamberová (114), in which obese boys attended a summer camp for 4 consecutive summers. Each time, the program yielded a reduction in body mass and adiposity and an improved aerobic fitness. However, each year the effect disappeared during the subsequent months and the children resumed their precamp characteristics. One can therefore assume that, once obese children return home from a camp, they revert to their previous lifestyle habits and cannot sustain the changes made during camp.

The most promising alternative to the clinic approach is through the school system. As summarized in Table 23.4, the school environment has several characteristics that are conducive to successful prevention and management of juvenile obesity. The vast majority of North American children and youth who are obese or at risk of becoming obese attend schools daily, 8–9 months of the year. Many schools have professionals such as nurses (or nurse's aides), counselors, physical educators, and health educators who can assess the eating and activity habits of their pupils and administer related programs. Food service personnel can help in providing

Table 23.4 Characteristics of Schools That Are Conducive to Effective Prevention and Management of Juvenile Obesity

Pooling of experts (nurse, counselor, physical and health educator)

Pooling of at-risk children and adolescents

Available volunteer role models among the students

Available indoor and outdoor sports facilities

Daily, almost year-round contact with children

Effective lines of communication with parents

No "medical" stigma

proper lunches. Sport facilities are available in schools, and they are often occupied only partially, if at all, after school hours. These facilities, and the related equipment, are specifically geared for children and adolescents. Schools have built-in lines of communication with parents. These can help to keep the parents involved in the program and maintain its continuity. Involving the parents in a school program can improve its success (38). An important and often overlooked reason for the reluctance of children and, in particular, adolescents to join obesity-management programs is the medical stigma attached to them. School-based programs have the advantage of not having this stigma. Another potential advantage of school-based programs is that students who have successfully controlled their body adiposity can assist those who start the program the following year. The use of peers as role models may be particularly useful in junior and senior high schools, although less so in primary schools.

Among teachers, the physical education expert is in a unique position. Many physical education teachers are skilled in performing basic anthropometric measurements and assessing body composition. They are thus in an excellent position to identify those pupils who already are obese and others who gain weight excessively. Furthermore, these teachers are proficient in measuring physical fitness and administering exercise programs. Physical education teachers would therefore be the most logical coordinators of such school-based intervention programs. In one survey (142), more than 90% of pediatricians and family physicians acknowledged the desirability of collaborating with physical educators for the assessment of obesity at school. A similar percentage acknowledged the potential benefit of including a nutrition education program within physical education.

Numerous studies have been conducted since the 1960s, but mostly in the last decade, to assess the feasibility and effectiveness of school-based, weight control programs in the US and Canada (19, 32, 38, 42, 45, 47, 50, 72, 79, 85, 90, 91, 105, 125, 134, 141, 157, 171). Similar studies have been conducted outside North America (1, 5, 61, 62, 93, 151). For reviews of the rationale for, and success of, school-based programs, see Parcel,

Green, and Bettes (111), Resnicow (124), Sallis and McKenzie (135), and Ward and Bar-Or (158). Most of these programs, particularly those that combined exercise with nutrition education (with or without behavior modification), have induced a reduction in overweight and/or adiposity. However, in only one out of two studies that included a follow-up was the benefit sustained for up to 10 months following the intervention (171). As reviewed by Parcel et al. (111), school-based interventions seem more successful among younger than among older schoolchildren.

In conclusion, while schools differ in size, sport facilities, and availability and proficiency of professionals, the school environment seems to represent the best potential medium, on a nationwide basis, for shaping health-related attitudes and behaviors of children and adolescents. As stated by Parcel, Green, and Bettes (111), "School-based programs can contribute to shifting social norms for exercise behaviors (increasing energy expenditure) and for the eating behaviors" (p. 143). Obviously, however, much more research is need to refine and optimize such programs. If found efficacious, school-based interventions will require the allocation of major resources currently unavailable to most school systems. Clinics and hospitals will then be able to concentrate on those children and adolescents with morbid obesity, who often need aggressive therapeutic approaches, as well as on those whose obesity is accompanied by other medical or psychiatric conditions.

REFERENCES

1. Alexandrov, A.; Isakova, G.; Maslennikova, G.; et al. Prevention of atherosclerosis among 11-year-old schoolchildren in two Moscow administrative districts. Health Psych. 7(Suppl.):247–252; 1988.
2. Alpert, M.A.; Singh, A.; Terry, B.E.; Kelly, D.L.; El-Deane, S.; Mukerji, V.; Villareal, D.; Artis, A.K. Effect of exercise and cavity size on right ventricular function in morbid obesity. Am. J. Cardiol. 61:1361–1365; 1989.
3. Alpert, M.A.; Singh, A.; Terry, B.E.; Kelly, D.L.; Villareal, D.; Mukerji, V. Effect of

The author is indebted to Tom Baranowski, PhD, for his most constructive critique of the manuscript.

exercise on left ventricular systolic function and reserve in morbid obesity. Am. J. Cardiol. 63:1478–1482; 1989.

4. Amador, M.; Flores, P.; Pena, M. Normocaloric diet and exercise: a good choice for treating obese adolescents. Acta Paediatr. Hung. 30:123–138; 1990.

5. Angelico, F.B.; Fabiani, L.; et al. Management of childhood obesity through a school-based programme of general health and nutrition education. Public Health 105:393–398; 1991.

6. Anton-Kuchly, B.; Roger, P.; Varene, P. Determinants of increased energy cost of submaximal exercise in obese subjects. J. Appl. Physiol. Respir. Environ. Exerc. Physiol. 56:18–23; 1984.

7. Åstrand, I.; Åstrand, P.-O.; Stunkard, A. Oxygen intake of obese individuals during work on a bicycle ergometer. Acta Physiol. Scand. 50:294–299; 1960.

8. Ballor, D.L.; Katch, V.L.; Becque, M.D.; Mark, C.R. Resistance weight training during caloric restriction enhances lean body weight maintenance. Am. J. Clin. Nutr. 47:19–25; 1988.

9. Bandini, L.G. Energy expenditure in obese and nonobese adolescents. Cambridge, MA: Massachusetts Institute of Technology; 1987.

10. Bandini, L.G.; Schoeller, D.A.; Cyr, H.; Young, V.R.; Dietz, W.H. A validation of energy intake and energy expenditure in obese and nonobese adolescents. Int. J. Obesity 11:437A; 1987.

11. Bandini, L.G.; Schoeller, D.A.; Dietz, W.H. Energy expenditure in obese and nonobese adolescents. Pediatr. Res. 27:198–203; 1990.

12. Bar-Or, O. Pediatric sports medicine for the practitioner: from physiological principles to clinical applications. New York: Springer Verlag; 1983.

13. Bar-Or, O. Response to physical conditioning in children with cardiopulmonary disease. Exerc. Sport Sci. Rev. 13:305–334; 1985.

14. Bar-Or, O. Pathophysiologic factors which limit the exercise capacity of the sick child. Med. Sci. Sports Exerc. 18:276–282; 1986.

15. Barry, A.J.; Cureton, T.K. Factorial analysis of physique and performance in prepubescent boys. Res. Quart. 32:283–300; 1961.

16. Barta, L.; Szöke, L.; Vándor-Szobotka, V. Working capacity for obese children. Acta Paediatr. Acad. Scient. Hung. 9:17–21; 1968.

17. Becque, M.D.; Katch, V.L.; Socchini, A.P.; Charles, R.M.; Moorhead, C. Coronary risk incidence of obese adolescents: reduction by exercise plus diet intervention. Pediatrics 81:605–612; 1988.

18. Berg, K. Body composition and nutrition of adolescent boys training for bicycle racing. Nutr. Metab. 14:172–180; 1972.

19. Berg, K.; Sady, S.P.; Savage, M.; Smith, J. Developing an elementary school CHD prevention program. Physician Sportsmed. 11(10):99–105; 1983.

20. Berkowitz, R.I.; Agras, W.S.; Korner, A.F.; Kraemer, H.C.; Zeanah, C.H. Physical activity and adiposity: a longitudinal study from birth to childhood. Pediatrics 106:734–738; 1985.

21. Berndt, I.; Rehs, H.J.; Rutenfranz, J. Sportpädagogische Gesichtpunkte zur Prophylaxe Adipositas im Kindesalter. Öff. Gesundh.-Wesen 37:1–9; 1975.

22. Beunen, G.; Malina, R.M.; Ostyn, M.; Rensen, R.; Simons, J.; Van-Gerven, D. Fatness, growth and motor fitness of Belgian boys 12 through 20 years of age. Human Biol. 55:599–613; 1983.

23. Bishop, P.; Donnelly, J.E. Home based activity program for obese children. Am. Corr. Ther. J. 41:12–19; 1987.

24. Björntorp, P. Exercise in the treatment of obesity. Clin. Endocr. Metab. 5:431–453; 1976.

25. Blaak, E.E.; Bar-Or, O.; Westerterp, K.R.; Saris, W.H.M. Effect of VLCD on daily energy expenditure and body composition in obese boys. Int. J. Obesity 14(Suppl. 2):86; 1990.

26. Blaak, E.E.; Westerterp, K.R.; Bar-Or, O.; Wouters, L.J.M.; Saris, W.H.M. Total energy expenditure and spontaneous activity in relation to training in obese boys. Am. J. Clin. Nutr. 55:777–782; 1992.

27. Blimkie, C.J.R.; Ebbesen, B.; MacDougall, D.; Bar-Or, O.; Sale, D. Voluntary and electrically evoked strength characteristics of obese and nonobese preadolescent boys. Human Biol. 61:515–532; 1989.

28. Blimkie, C.J.R.; Sale, D.G.; Bar-Or, O. Voluntary strength, evoked twitch contractile

properties and motor unit activation of knee extensors in obese and non-obese adolescent males. Euro. J. Appl. Physiol. 61:313–318; 1990.

29. Blomquist, B.; Börjeson, M.; Larsson, Y.; et al. The effect of physical activity on the body measurements and work capacity of overweight boys. Acta Paediatr. Scand. 54:566–572; 1965.

30. Bloom, W.L.; Eidex, M.F. Inactivity as a major factor in adult obesity. Metabolism 8:679–684; 1967.

31. Borg, G. Perceived exertion as an indicator of somatic stress. Scand. J. Rehab. Med. 2–3:92–98; 1970.

32. Botvin, G.J.; Cantlon, A.; Carter, B.J.; Williams, C.L. Reducing adolescent obesity through a school health program. J. Pediatr. 95:1060–1062; 1979.

33. Bouchard, C.; Tremblay, A.; Nadeau, A.; Dussault, J.; Després, J.-P.; Theriault, J.; Lupien, O.J.; Serresse, O.; Boulay, M.R.; Fournier, G. Long-term exercise training with constant energy intake. 1: effect on body composition and selected metabolic variables. Int. J. Obesity 14:57–73; 1990.

34. Bradfield, R.B.; Paulos, J.; Grossman, L. Energy expenditure and heart rate of obese high school girls. Am. J. Clin. Nutr. 24:1482–1488; 1971.

35. Bronstein, I.P.; et al. Obesity in childhood: childhood studies. Am. J. Dis. Child. 63:130; 1953.

36. Brown, M.R.; Klish, W.J.; Hollander, J.; Campbell, M.A.; Forbes, G.B. A high protein, low calorie liquid diet in the treatment of very obese adolescents: long-term effect on lean body mass. Am. J. Clin. Nutr. 38:20–31; 1983.

37. Brownell, K.D. Obesity: understanding and treating a serious, prevalent, and refractory disorder. J. Consult. Clin. Psychol. 50:820–840; 1982.

38. Brownell, K.D.; Kaye, F.S. A school-based behavior modification, nutrition education, and physical activity program for obese children. Am. J. Clin. Nutr. 35:277–283; 1982.

39. Brownell, K.D.; Kelman, S.H.; Stunkard, A.J. Treatment of obese children with and without their mothers. Changes in weight and blood pressure. Pediatrics 71:515–523; 1983.

40. Bruch, H. Obesity in childhood. Am. J. Dis. Child. 60:1082–1109; 1940.

41. Bullen, B.A.; Reed, R.B.; Mayer, J. Physical activity of obese and nonobese adolescent girls appraised by motion picture sampling. Am. J. Clin. Nutr. 14:211–223; 1964.

42. Bush, P.J.; Zuckerman, A.E.; Taggart, V.S. Cardiovascular risk factor prevention in black school children: the "Know Your Body" evaluation project. Health Education Quarterly 16:215–227; 1989.

43. Cahill, B.R., Editor. Proceedings of the conference on strength training and the prepubescent. Chicago: American Orthopedic Society for Sports Medicine; 1988.

44. Calles-Escandón, J.; Horton, E.S. The thermogenic role of exercise in the treatment of morbid obesity: a critical evaluation. Am. J. Clin. Nutr. 55:533S–537S; 1992.

45. Christakis, G.; Sajecki, S.; Hillman, R.W.; Miller, E.; Blumanthal, S.; Archer, M. Effect of a combined nutrition education and physical fitness program on the weight status of obese high school boys. Fed. Am. Soc. Exper. Biol. 25:15–19; 1966.

46. Clancey-Hepburn, K.; Hickey, A.A.; Nevill, G. Children's behavior responses to TV food advertisements. J. Nutr. Ed. 6:93–96; 1974.

47. Coates, T.J.; Jeffery, R.W.; Slinkard, L.A. Heart healthy eating and exercise: introducing and maintaining changes in health behaviors. Am. J. Publ. Health 71:15–23; 1981.

48. Coates, T.J.; Killen, J.D.; Slinkard, L.A. Parent participation in a treatment program for overweight adolescents. Int. J. Eating Disord. 1:37–48; 1982.

49. Cohen, C.J. Physical activity and dietary patterns of lean versus obese middle-school children. Pediatr. Exerc. Sci. 4:187–188; 1992.

50. Collip, P.J. An obesity program in the public schools. Pediatr. Ann. 4:276–282; 1975.

51. Cooper, D.M.; Poage, J.; Barstow, T.J.; Springer, C. Are obese children truly unfit? Minimizing the confounding effect of body size on the exercise response. J. Pediatr. 116:223–230; 1990.

52. Corbin, C.B.; Pletcher, P. Diet and physical activity patterns of obese and nonobese elementary school children. Res. Quart. 39:922–928; 1968.

53. Davies, C.T.M.; Godfrey, S.; Light, M.; Sargeant, A. J.; Zeidifard, E. Cardiopulmonary responses to exercise in obese girls and young women. J. Appl. Physiol. 38: 373–376; 1975.

54. Davies, P.S.W.; Day, J.M.E.; Lucas, A. Energy expenditure in early infancy and later body fatness. Int. J. Obesity 15:727–731; 1991.

55. Dechamps, I.; Giron, B.J.; Lestradet, H. Blood glucose, insulin, and free fatty acid levels during oral glucose tolerance tests in 158 obese children. Diabetes 26:89–93; 1977.

56. DeMeersman, R.E.; Stone, S.; Schaefer, D.C.; Miller, W.W. Maximal work capacity in prepubescent obese and nonobese females. Clin. Pediatr. 24:199–200; 1985.

57. Després, J.P.; Bouchard, C.; Malina, R.M. Physical activity and coronary risk factors during childhood and adolescence. Exerc. Sport Sci. Rev. 18:243–261; 1990.

58. Després, J.P.; Bouchard, C.; Tremblay, A.; Savard, R.; Marcotte, M. Effects of aerobic training on fat distribution in male subjects. Med. Sci. Sports Exerc. 17:113–118; 1985.

59. Dietz, W.H.; Gortmaker, S.L. Do we fatten our children at the television set? Obesity and television viewing in children and adolescents. Peds. 75:807–812; 1985.

60. Dietz, W.H.; Hartung, R. Changes in height velocity of obese preadolescents during weight reduction. Am. J. Dis. Child. 139: 705–707; 1985.

61. Dwyer, T.; Coonan, W.E.; Leitch, D.R.; Hetzel, B.S.; Baghurst, R.A. An investigation of the effects of daily physical activity on the health of primary school students in South Australia. Int. J. Epidemiol. 12: 308–313; 1983.

62. Dwyer, T.; Coonan, W.E.; Worsley, A.; Leitch, D.R. An assessment of the effects of two physical activity programs on coronary heart disease risk factors in primary school children. Comm. Health Stud. 3: 196–202; 1979.

63. Endo, H.; Takagi, Y.; Nazue, T.; Kuwahata, K.; Uemasu, F.; Kobayashi, A. Beneficial effects of dietary intervention on serum lipid and apolipoprotein levels in obese children. Am. J. Dis. Child. 146:303–305; 1992.

64. Epstein, L.H.; Koeske, R.; Zidansek, J.; Wing, R.R. Effects of weight loss on fitness in obese children. Am. J. Dis. Child 137:654–657; 1983.

65. Epstein, L.H.; Wing, R.R. Aerobic exercise and weight. Addict. Behav. 5:371–388; 1980.

66. Epstein, L.H.; Wing, R.R.; Koeske, R.; Ossip, D.; Beck, S. A comparison of lifestyle changes and programmed aerobic exercise on weight and fitness changes in obese children. Behav. Ther. 13:651–665; 1982.

67. Epstein, L.H.; Wing, R.R.; Koeske, R.; Valoski, A. Effects of diet plus exercise on weight changes in parents and children. J. Consult. Clin. Psychol. 52:429–437; 1984.

68. Epstein, L.H.; Wing, R.R.; Koeske, R.; Valoski, A. A comparison of lifestyle exercise, aerobic exercise, and calisthenics on weight loss in obese children. Behav. Ther. 16:345–356; 1985.

69. Epstein, L.H.; Wing, R.R.; Koeske, R.; Valoski, A. Long-term effect of family-based treatment of childhood obesity. J. Consult. Clin. Psychol. 55:91–95; 1987.

70. Epstein, L.H.; Wing, R.R.; Penner, B.C.; Kress, M.J. Effect of diet and controlled exercise on weight loss in obese children. Pediatrics 107:358–361; 1985.

71. Epstein, L.H.; Wing, R.R.; Woodall, K.; Penner, B.C.; Kress, M.J.; Koeske, R. Effects of family-based behavioral treatment on obese 5–8-year-old children. Behav. Ther. 16:205–212; 1985.

72. Foster, G.D.; Wadden, T.A.; Brownell, K.D. Peer-led program for the treatment and prevention of obesity in the schools. J. Consult. Clin. Psychol. 53:538–540; 1985.

73. Gortmaker, S.L.; Dietz, W.H.; Sobol, A.M.; Wehler, C.A. Increasing pediatric obesity in the United States. Am. J. Dis. Child. 141:535–540; 1987.

74. Gracey, M.; Hitchcock, N.E.; Wearne, K.L.; Garcia-Webb, P.; Lewis, R. The 1977 Busselton children's survey. Med. J. Austr. 2:265–267; 1979.

75. Hayashi, T.; Fujino, M.; Shindo, M.; Hiroki, T.; Arakawa, K. Echocardiographic and electrocardiographic measures in obese children after an exercise program. Int. J. Obesity 11:465–472; 1987.

76. Hensley, L.D.; East, W.B.; Stillwell, J.L. Body fatness and motor performance during preadolescence. Res. Q. Exer. Sport 53:133–140; 1982.

77. Huenemann, R.L.; Shapiro, L.R.; Hampton, M.C.; Mitchell, B.W. Teen-agers' activities and attitudes toward activity. J. Am. Diet. Ass. 51:433–440; 1967.

78. Ismail, A.H.; Christian, J.E.; Kessler, W.V. Body composition relative to motor aptitude in prepubescent boys. Res. Quart. 34:462–470; 1963.

79. Jetté, M.; Barry, W.; Pearlman, L. The effects of an extracurricular physical activity program on obese adolescents. Canad. J. Publ. Health 68:39–42; 1977.

80. Johnson, M.L.; Burke, B.S.; Mayer, J. Relative importance of inactivity and overeating in the energy balance of obese high school girls. Am. J. Clin. Nutr. 4:37–44; 1956.

81. Kaplan, T.A.; Campbell-Shaw, M.H.; Moccia, G. Association of exercise-induced bronchospasm with obesity. Pediatr. Exerc. Sci. 4:351–359; 1992.

82. Katch, V.; Becque, M.D.; Marks, C.; Moorehead, C.; Rocchini, A. Oxygen uptake and energy output during walking of obese male and female adolescents. Am. J. Clin. Nutr. 47:26–32; 1988a.

83. Katch, V.; Becque, M.D.; Marks, C.; Moorehead, C.; Rocchini, A. Basal metabolism of obese adolescents: inconsistent diet and exercise effects. Am. J. Clin. Nutr. 48:565–569; 1988b.

84. Keatinge, W.R. Body fat and cooling rates in relation to age. In: Folinsbee, L.J. et al., ed. Environmental stress. Individual human adaptation. New York: Academic Press; 1978.

85. Killen, J.D.; Telch, M.J.; Robinson, T.N.; Maccoby, N.; Taylor, C.B.; Farquhar, J.W. Cardiovascular disease risk reduction for tenth graders. A multiple-factor school-based approach. JAMA 260:1728–1733; 1988.

86. Klesges, R.C.; Eck, L.H.; Hanson, C.L.; Haddock, C.K.; Klesges, L.M. Effects of obesity, social interactions, and physical environment on physical activity in preschoolers. Health Psychol. 9:435–449; 1990.

87. Klesges, R.C.; Haddock, C.K.; Eck, L.H. A multimethod approach to the measurement of childhood physical activity and its relationship to blood pressure and body weight. J. Pediatr. 116:888–893; 1990.

88. Klesges, R.C.; Shelton, M.L.; Klesges, L.M. Effects of television on metabolic rate: potential implications for childhood obesity. Pediatrics 91:281–286; 1993.

89. Ku, L.C.; Shapiro, L.R.; Crawford, P.B.; Huenemann, R.L. Body composition and physical activity in 8-year-old children. Am. J. Clin. Nutr. 34:2770–2775; 1981.

90. Lansky, D.; Brownell, K.D. Comparison of school-based treatment for adolescent obesity. J. School Health 5:384–387; 1982.

91. Lansky, D.; Vance, M.A. School-based intervention for adolescent obesity: analysis of treatment, randomly selected control, and self-control subjects. J. Consult. Clin. Psychol. 51:147–148; 1983.

92. Lichtman, S.W.; Pisarska, K.; Berman, E.R.; Pestone, M.; Dowling, H.; Offenbacher, E.; Weisel, H.; Heshka, S.; Matthews, D.E.; Heymsfield, S.B. Discrepancy between self-reported and actual caloric intake and exercise in obese subjects. New Engl. J. Med. 327:1893–1898; 1992.

93. Lionis, C.; Kafatos, A.; Vlachonikolis, J. The effects of a health education intervention program among Cretan adolescents. Prev. Med. 20:685–699; 1991.

94. Mack, R.W.; Kleinhenz, M.E. Growth, caloric intake, and activity levels in early infancy: a preliminary report. Human Biol. 46:345–354; 1974.

95. Maffeis, C.; Micciolo, R.; Zoccante, L.; Zaffanello, M.; Pinelli, L. Basal energy expenditure in obese and normal weight schoolchildren. Acta Paediatr. Scand. 80:1145–1149; 1991.

96. Mahan, L.K. Family-focused behavior approach to weight control in children. Pediatr. Adolesc. Endocr. 34:983–996; 1987.

97. Marti, B.; Vartianen, E. Relations between leisure time exercise and cardiovascular risk factors among 15 year olds in Finland. J. Epidem. Comm. Health 43:228; 1989.

98. Matsushima, M.; Kriska, A.; Tajima, N.; LaPorte, R. The epidemiology of physical activity and childhood obesity. Diabetes Research and Clinical Practice 10:S95–S102; 1990.

99. Mayer, J. The best diet is exercise. In: Collipp, P.J., ed. Childhood obesity. Littleton, MA: PSG Publishing Co.; 1980: 207–222.

100. Mayer, J.; Roy, P.; Mitra, K.P. Relations between caloric intake, body weight and physical work: studies in industrial male population in West Bengal. Am. J. Clin. Nutr. 4:169–175; 1956.

101. McKenzie, T.L.; Buono, M.; Nelson, J. Modification of coronary heart disease (CHD) risk factors in obese boys through diet and exercise. Am. Corr. Ther. J. 38:35–37; 1984.

102. Mocellin, R.; Rutenfranz, J. Investigations on the physical working capacity of healthy and sick adolescents. III. The physical working capacity of obese children and adolescents [in German]. Zeitsch. Kinder. 104:179–196; 1968.

103. Mocellin, R.; Rutenfranz, J. Investigations of the physical working capacity of obese children. Acta Paediatr. Scand. 217 (suppl.): 77–79; 1971.

104. Montoye, H.J. Risk indicators for cardiovascular disease in relation to physical activity in youth. In: Binkhorst, R.A.; Kemper, H.C.G.; Saris, W.A., eds. Children and exercise XI. Champaign, IL: Human Kinetics; 1985:3–25.

105. Moody, D.L.; Wilmore, J.H.; Girandola, R.N.; Royce, J.P. The effects of a jogging program on the body composition of normal and obese high school girls. Med. Sci. Sports 4:210–213; 1972.

106. Moore, L.L.; Lombardi, D.A.; White, M.J.; Campbell, J.L.; Oliveria, S.A.; Ellison, R.C. Influence of parents' physical activity levels on activity levels of young children. J. Pediatr. 118:215–219; 1991.

107. Must, A.; Jacques, P.; Dallali, G.E.; Bajema, C.J.; Dietz, W.H. Long-term morbidity and mortality of overweight adolescents. New Engl. J. Med. 327:1350–1355; 1992.

108. Nichols, J.F.; Bigelow, D.M.; Canine, K.M. Short-term weight loss and exercise training effects on glucose-induced thermogenesis in obese adolescent males during hypocaloric feeding. Int. J. Obesity 13: 683–690; 1989.

109. Okamoto, E.; Davidson, L.L.; Conner, D.R. High prevalence of overweight in inner-city schoolchildren. Am. J. Dis. Child. 147: 155–159; 1993.

110. Pacy, P.J.; Webster, J.; Garrow, J.S. Exercise and obesity. Sports Med. 3:89–113; 1986.

111. Parcel, G.S.; Green, L.W.; Bettes, B.A. School-based programs to prevent or reduce obesity. In: Krasengor, G.D.; Grave, G.D.; Kretchmer, N., eds. Childhood obesity: biobehavioral perspective. Caldwell, NJ: Telford Press; 1988:143–157.

112. Parizková, J. Physical training in weight reduction of obese adolescents. Ann. Clin. Res. 14(suppl. 34):63–68; 1982.

113. Parizková, J.; Vamberová, M. Body composition as a criterion of suitability of reducing regimens in obese children. Develop. Med. Child Neurol. 9:202–211; 1967.

114. Parizková, J.; Vaneckova, M.; Sprynarová, S.; Vamberová, M. Body composition and fitness in obese children before and after special treatment. Acta Paediatr. Scand. 217 (suppl.):80–85; 1971.

115. Parizková, J.; Vaneckova, M.; Vamberová, M. A study of the changes in some functional indicators following reduction of excessive fat in obese children. Physiol. Bohemoslov. 11:351–357; 1962.

116. Parker, D.F.; Bar-Or, O. Juvenile obesity: the importance of exercise—and getting children to do it. Physician Sportsmed. 19(6):113–125; 1991.

117. Pate, R.; Ross, J.G. The National Children and Youth Fitness Study II: factors associated with health-related fitness. J. Phys. Ed. Rec. Dance. 58:93–95; 1987.

118. Pazourek, M. Vigorous exercise and reduced food intake in obese children. Obes. Bariatr. Med. 2:50–53; 1973.

119. Peckos, P.S. Caloric intake in relation to physique in children. Science 117:631–633; 1953.

120. Peckos, P.S.; Spargo, J.A.; Heald, F.P. Program and results of a camp for obese adolescent girls. Postgrad. Med. 27:527–533; 1960.

121. Peja, M.; Velkey, L. The joint influence of diet and increased physical activity in obese children. Acta Paediatr. Hung. 29: 373–381; 1989.

122. Puhl, J.L. Energy expenditure among children: implications for childhood obesity. I. Resting and dietary energy expenditure. Ped. Exerc. Sci. 1:212–229; 1989.

123. Ravussin, E.; Burnard, B.; Schutz, Y.; Jéquier, E. Energy expenditure before and during energy restriction in obese patients. Am. J. Clin. Nutr. 41:753–759; 1985.

124. Resnicow, K. School-based interventions: populations vs. high-risk approach. Presented at the New York Academy of

Sciences conference on prevention and treatment of childhood obesity. Bethesda, MD; 1993.

125. Resnicow, K.; Cohn, L.; Reinhardt, J.; et al. A three-year evaluation of the Know Your Body program in minority schoolchildren. Health Educ. Quarter. 19:463–480; 1992.

126. Reybrouck, T.; Vinckx, J.; Van Den Berge, G.; Vanderschueren-Lodeweyckx, M. Exercise therapy and hypocaloric diet in the treatment of obese children and adolescents. Acta Paediatr. Scand. 79:84–89; 1990.

127. Reybrouck, T.; Weymans, M.; Vinckx, J.; Stijns, H.; Vanderschueren-Lodeweyckx, M. Cardiorespiratory function during exercise in obese children. Acta Paediatr. Scand. 76:342–348; 1987.

128. Roberts, S.B.; Savage, J.; Coward, W.A.; Chew, B.; Lucas, A. Energy expenditure and intake in infants born to lean and overweight mothers. New Engl. J. Med. 318: 461–466; 1988.

129. Robinson, T.N.; Hammer, L.D.; Killen, J.D.; Kraemer, H.C.; Wilson, D.M.; Hayward, C.; Taylor, C.B. Does television viewing increase obesity and reduce physical activity? Cross-sectional and longitudinal analyses among adolescent girls. Pediatrics 91:273–280; 1993.

130. Rocchini, A.P.; Katch, V.; Anderson, J.; Hinderliter, J.; Becque, D.; Martin, M.; Marks, C. Blood pressure in obese adolescents: effect of weight loss. Pediatrics 82: 16–23; 1988.

131. Ross, J.G.; Dotson, C.O.; Gilbert, G.G.; Katz, S.J. New standards for fitness measurement. J. Phys. Ed. Rec. Dance. 56:62–66; 1985.

132. Ross, J.G.; Pate, R.R.; Lohman, T.G.; Christenson, G.M. Changes in body composition of children. J. Phys. Ed. Rec. Dance 58: 74–77; 1987.

133. Rowland, T.W. Effects of obesity on aerobic fitness in adolescent females. Am. J. Dis. Child 145:764–768; 1991.

134. Ruppenthal, B.; Gibbs, E. Treating childhood obesity in a public school setting. J. School Health 49:569–571; 1979.

135. Sallis, J.F.; McKenzie, T.L. Physical education's role in public health. Res. Q. Exer. Sport 62:124–137; 1991.

136. Sallis, J.F.; Nader, P.R. Family determinants of health behaviors. In: Gochman, D.S., ed. Health behaviors: emerging research perspectives. New York: Plenum; 1988: 107–124.

137. Sasaki, J.; Shindo, M.; Tanaka, H.; Ando, M.; Arakawa, K. A long-term aerobic exercise program decreases the obesity index and increases the high density lipoprotein cholesterol concentration in obese children. Int. J. Obesity 11:339–345; 1987.

138. Schoeller, D.A.; Bandini, L.G.; Levitsky, L.L.; Dietz, W.H. Energy requirements of obese children and young adults. Proc. Nutr. Soc. 47:241–246; 1988.

139. Schrub, J.-C.; Wolf, L.-M.; Courtois, H. Fasting with muscular exercise, changes in weight and nitrogen balance [in French]. Nouv. Press. Med. 4:875–878; 1975.

140. Seidman, D.S.; Laor, A.; Gale, R.; Stevenson, D.K.; Danon, Y.L. A longitudinal study of birth weight and being overweight in late adolescence. Am. J. Dis. Child. 145: 782–785; 1991.

141. Seltzer, C.C.; Mayer, J. An effective weight control program in a public school system. Am. J. Publ. Health 60:679–689; 1970.

142. Sintek, S.; Bishop, P. Physicians' perceptions of using physical education for managing childhood obesity. Physician Sportsmed. 13(5):119–124; 1985.

143. Sprynarová, S.; Parizková, J. Changes in aerobic capacity and body composition in obese boys after reduction. J. Appl. Physiol. 20:934–937; 1965.

144. Stefanik, P.A.; Heald, F.P.; Mayer, J. Caloric intake in relation to energy output of obese and non-obese adolescent boys. Am. J. Clin. Nutr. 7:55–62; 1959.

145. Sterky, G. Clinical and metabolic aspects of obesity in childhood. In: Pernow, B.; Saltin, B., eds. Muscle metabolism during exercise. New York: Plenum Press; 1971: 521–527.

146. Stern, J.S.; Johnson, P.R. Spontaneous activity and adipose cellularity in the genetically obese Zucker rat (fafa). Metabolism 26:371–379; 1977.

147. Story, M.; Faulkner, P. The prime-time diet: a content analysis of eating behavior in television program content and commercials. Am. J. Publ. Health 80:738–740; 1990.

148. Stunkard, A.; Pestka, Y. The physical activity of obese girls. Am. J. Dis. Child 103:116–121; 1962.

149. Stunkard, A.J.; Sorensen, T.I.A.; Hanis, C.; Teasdale, T.; Chakraborty, R.; Schull, W.J.; Schulsinger, F. An adoption study of human obesity. New Engl. J. Med. 314:193–198; 1986.

150. Suskind, R.M.; Sothern, M.; Farros, R.P.; von Almen, T.; Schumacher, H.; Vargas, A.; Escobar, O.; Loftin, M.; Brown, R.; Udall, J.N., Jr. Recent advances in the treatment of childhood obesity. Presented at the New York Academy of Sciences Conference on Prevention and Treatment of Childhood Obesity. Bethesda, MD; 1993.

151. Tamir, D.; Feurstein, A.; Brunner, S. Primary prevention of cardiovascular disease in childhood: changes in serum total cholesterol, high density lipoprotein, and body mass index after 2 years of intervention in Jerusalem schoolchildren age 7–9 years. Prev. Med. 19:22–30; 1990.

152. Taras, H.F.; Sallis, J.F.; Patterson, T.L.; Nader, P.R.; Nelson, J.A. Television's influence on children's diet and physical activity. J. Behav. Devel. Pediatr. 10:176–180; 1989.

153. Taylor, W.; Baranowski, T. Physical activity, cardiovascular fitness, and adiposity in children. Res. Q. Exer. Sport 62:157–163; 1991.

154. Thomson, M.E.; Cruickshank, F.M. Survey into the eating and exercise habits of New Zealand pre-adolescents in relation to overweight and obesity. N.Z. Med. J. 89:7–9; 1979.

155. Tucker, L.A. The relationship of television viewing to physical fitness and obesity. Adolescence 21:797–806; 1986.

156. Vara, L.; Argas, S. Caloric intake and activity levels are related in young children. Int. J. Obesity 13:613–617; 1989.

157. Walter, H.J.; Hofman, A.; Vaughan, R.D.; Wynder, E.L. Modification of risk factors for coronary heart disease: five-year results of a school-based intervention trial. New Engl. J. Med. 318:1093–1100; 1988.

158. Ward, D.S.; Bar-Or, O. Role of the physician and physical education teacher in the treatment of obesity at school. Pediatrician 13:44–51; 1986.

159. Ward, D.S.; Bar-Or, O. Use of the Borg scale in exercise prescription for overweight youth. Canad. J. Sports Sci. 15:120–125; 1990.

160. Ward, D.S.; Blimkie, C.J.R.; Bar-Or, O. Rating of perceived exertion in obese adolescents. Med. Sci. Sports Exerc. 18:S72; 1986.

161. Watson, A.W.S.; O'Donovan, D.J. The relationship of level of habitual activity to measures of leanness-fatness, physical working capacity, strength and motor ability in 17 and 18 year-old males. Euro. J. Appl. Physiol. 37:93–100; 1977.

162. Waxman, M.; Stunkard, A.J. Caloric intake and expenditure of obese boys. J. Pediatr. 96:187–193; 1980.

163. Weltman, A. Weight training in prepubertal children. Physiological benefits and potential damage. In: Bar-Or, O., ed. Advances in pediatric exercise sciences. Volume 3. Champaign, IL: Human Kinetics; 1989:101–129.

164. Whipp, B.J.; Davis, J.A. The ventilatory stress of exercise in obesity. Am. Rev. Respir. Dis. 129(suppl.):S90–S92; 1984.

165. Widhalm, K.; Maxa, E.; Zyman, H. Effect of diet and exercise upon the cholesterol and triglyceride content of plasma lipoproteins in overweight children. Eur. J. Pediatr. 127:121–126; 1978.

166. Wilkinson, P.W.; Parkin, J.M.; Pearlson, G.; Strong, H.; Sykes, P. Energy intake and physical activity in obese boys. Brit. Med. J. 1:756; 1977.

167. Wilmore, J.H. The 1983 C.H. McCloy research lecture. Appetite and body composition consequent to physical activity. Res. Q. Exer. Sport 54:415–425; 1983.

168. Woo, R.; Garrow, J.S.; Pi-Sunyer, F.X. Effect of exercise on spontaneous calorie intake in obesity. Am. J. Clin. Nutr. 36:470–477; 1982a.

169. Woo, R.; Garrow, J.S.; Pi-Sunyer, F.X. Voluntary food intake during prolonged exercise in obese women. Am. J. Clin. Nutr. 36:478–484; 1982b.

170. Ylitalo, V. Treatment of childhood obesity, with special reference to the mode of therapy, cardiorespiratory performance and the carbohydrate and lipid metabolism. Acta Paediatr. Scand. 290 (suppl.):1–108; 1981.

171. Zakus, G.; Chin, M.L.; Cooper, H.; et al. Treating adolescent obesity: a pilot project in school. J. School Health 51:663–666; 1981.

172. Zuti, W.B.; Golding, L.A. Comparing diet and exercise as weight reduction tools. Physician Sportsmed. 4(1):49–53; 1976.

CHAPTER 24

Diabetes Mellitus

Edward S. Horton
Joslin Diabetes Center, Boston, MA

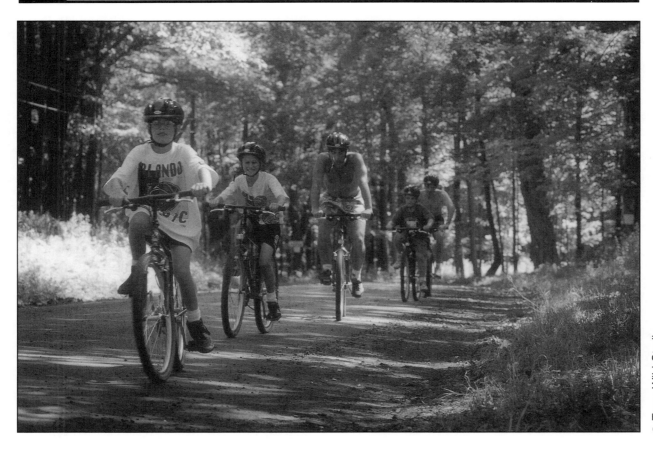

Today the outlook for children with diabetes mellitus is much more optimistic than it was a generation ago, both in terms of day-to-day management of the disease and the prevention of long-term complications. With the advent of self–blood glucose monitoring and training in self-management, people with diabetes are empowered to make adjustments in their own daily regimen and thus participate successfully in a wide range of activities, including participation in sports and exercise, often at the level of world-class athletes. This chapter will present information on both the physiological and practical aspects of diabetes and exercise in children.

BRIEF DESCRIPTION OF DIABETES MELLITUS

Pathophysiology

Diabetes mellitus is not a single disease, but a group of disorders of varying etiology and pathogenesis that are characterized by increased fasting and postprandial blood glucose concentrations, insulin deficiency and/or decreased insulin action, abnormalities of glucose, lipid, and protein metabolism, and the development of both acute and long-term complications.

Diabetes is currently classified into four clinically different types. They are

- insulin-dependent (IDDM or Type I) diabetes,
- non-insulin-dependent (NIDDM or Type II) diabetes,
- gestational diabetes (GDM), and
- other types of diabetes secondary to or associated with other diseases that damage the pancreas or produce severe resistance.

A diagnosis of diabetes can be made when a random plasma glucose value exceeds 200 mg/dl and the patient has the classic signs and symptoms. Alternatively, the diagnosis can be established by a fasting plasma glucose value that equals or exceeds 140 mg/dl on at least two occasions, or a fasting plasma level of less than 140 mg/dl accompanied by a sustained, elevated plasma glucose of over 200 mg/dl during at least two oral glucose tolerance tests.

IDDM or Type I

The most common form of diabetes in children is IDDM or Type I diabetes. It is currently estimated that there are approximately 600,000 cases in the United States. Patients with IDDM have severe insulinopenia and, by definition, are absolutely dependent on exogenous insulin to prevent ketoacidosis and death. These patients are often lean and frequently have experienced recent weight loss at the time of diagnosis. IDDM is more common in Caucasians than in nonwhite populations and is estimated to account for only 5 to 10 percent of all known cases of diabetes mellitus. Onset is most frequently during childhood, although IDDM may occur at any age.

The primary defect in IDDM is inadequate insulin secretion caused by an autoimmune process that destroys the pancreatic B-cells. Clinical onset of symptoms is usually preceded by an asymptomatic period of months or years during which the B-cells are progressively destroyed by a T-lymphocyte-mediated process in genetically susceptible individuals. The evolving process of B-cell destruction with progressive insulin loss gives rise to a broadly predictable pattern of glucose homeostasis both before and for some time after diagnosis of diabetes. Anti-islet cell and anti-insulin antibodies can be detected in the plasma before clinical diabetes develops, and defective insulin secretion in response to a glucose load is also present. Overt glucose intolerance emerges when insulin secretory reserves are decreased to less than 20% of normal. At this point all phases of the insulin secretory response are reduced so that glucose uptake by peripheral tissues is impaired and hepatic glucose production becomes excessive, resulting in fasting hyperglycemia and abnormal glucose tolerance. Once metabolic derangements are corrected by treatment with insulin, significant residual endogenous insulin secretion can often be demonstrated, indicating that some B-cell function remains. This period is called the honeymoon period, and some individuals may temporarily cease to require exogenous insulin. It is unusual for the honeymoon period to last for more than several months to one year, when the need for insulin treatment becomes inevitable. Current research is directed towards identification of genetically susceptible individuals who have evidence of autoimmune B-cell destruction but who have not yet developed clinical diabetes. Various treatments are being developed and tested to suppress the immune response and thus prevent diabetes from developing, or to prolong the honeymoon phase in those who do develop diabetes.

NIDDM or Type II

Although relatively uncommon in children, NIDDM or Type II diabetes is by far the most common form of diabetes, accounting for over 90% of cases worldwide. It is usually diagnosed after age 30, and the incidence increases significantly with increasing age. A form of NIDDM called maturity onset diabetes of the young (MODY) may occur in children of families affected by this autosomal dominant disorder.

NIDDM is a heterogeneous disorder characterized by a genetic predisposition and interaction between insulin resistance and decreased B-cell function. Patients with NIDDM may have few or none of the classic symptoms of diabetes mellitus when first discovered. They are not absolutely dependent on exogenous insulin for survival and are not prone to the development of ketoacidosis except during conditions of severe stress such as those caused by infections, trauma, or surgery. There is a strong association between the presence of obesity and low levels of physical exercise, and the development of NIDDM. However, NIDDM may also develop in lean individuals.

GDM

The term *gestational diabetes mellitus* (GDM) is used to describe glucose intolerance that has its onset or is first detected during pregnancy. GDM occurs in about 2% of pregnant women, usually during the second or third trimester when levels of insulin-antagonist hormones increase and insulin resistance normally occurs. In most cases, glucose tolerance returns to normal following parturition, although over time a significant percentage of women with a history of GDM will develop overt NIDDM.

Other Types of Diabetes

Finally, a variety of conditions that damage the pancreatic islets or produce severe insulin resistance may result in the development of diabetes mellitus. These include pancreatitis, subtotal or total pancreatectomy, hemochromatosis, exposure to pancreatic toxins, and in rare cases the presence of anti-insulin receptor or anti-insulin antibodies. Depending on the severity of the defect, patients with these disorders may require treatment with diet, oral hypoglycemic agents, or insulin.

Since the majority of children with diabetes have Type I or IDDM and require insulin treatment, this chapter will focus on the benefits and risks associated with exercise and sport in this group and discuss precautions and strategies that can be used to make it possible to participate safely and successfully in a wide variety of individual and team sports.

Physical Symptoms and Clinical Signs

Although the autoimmune process of pancreatic B-cell destruction may proceed undetected for months or years prior to the development of clinical diabetes, the onset of signs and symptoms of diabetes is often quite rapid. Insulin deficiency results in a catabolic state characterized by hyperglycemia, increased lipid and protein metabolism, weight loss, and, if insulin deficiency is severe, the development of ketoacidosis and ultimately death. Symptoms associated with hyperglycemia include polyuria, polyphagia, increased thirst, dehydration, blurred vision, and fatigue. If ketoacidosis develops, patients become progressively lethargic, stuporous, and eventually comatose; breathing is deep and rapid (Kussmaul respirations), and there is the odor of acetone on the breath. Laboratory tests reveal a severe metabolic acidosis with increased plasma ketone bodies and electrolyte disturbance. Fortunately, diabetic ketoacidosis in children is rarely fatal if diagnosed promptly and treated appropriately with insulin, rehydration, and correction of acidosis and electrolyte abnormalities. However, children with inadequate treatment or poorly controlled glycemia may have symptoms of hyperglycemia including increased thirst, increased urination, weight loss, blurred vision, and fatigue. Chronic hyperglycemia is also associated with an increased risk for infections and decreased wound healing. Insulin treatment may result in hypoglycemic reactions which are characterized by

- low blood glucose concentrations (less than 50 mg/dl),
- activation of the sympathetic nervous system leading to tachycardia, increased perspiration, tremulousness, and a sense of anxiety or fright, or
- altered central nervous system function leading to mental confusion, loss of consciousness, or even death in the presence of prolonged, untreated hypoglycemia.

When blood glucose concentrations are maintained in the normal or nearly normal range by appropriate balancing of insulin administration, food intake, and exercise, children with diabetes function normally. While even brief periods of hypoglycemia may result in symptoms, children usually respond promptly to treatment with oral glucose or carbohydrate-containing foods or beverages. More severe or prolonged hypoglycemia may require treatment by subcutaneous or intramuscular injection of glucagon or administration of glucose intravenously. In contrast, recurrent or sustained periods of hyperglycemia may be associated with less acute symptoms or even no symptoms, and may be tolerated for long periods of time.

Most children with IDDM do not manifest any of the long-term complications of diabetes because of the relatively short duration of their disease and the 5- to 15-year time span required for them to become clinically evident. However, if diabetes is present for more than 5 years a careful evaluation for the presence and/or progression of long-term complications is mandatory, since exercise performance may be affected and the risks of exercise increased. Long-term complications include

- the development of microvascular abnormalities leading to retinopathy and nephropathy,
- the development of peripheral neuropathy and other neuropathic disorders,
- premature cataract formation,
- premature coronary artery disease,
- cerebrovascular disease, and
- peripheral vascular disease.

Clinical and Laboratory Assessment

Children with IDDM should have ready access to comprehensive health care including the services of physicians, diabetes educators, nutritionists, exercise physiologists, and mental health professionals. A minimum of three to four visits per year to the health care team is recommended for evaluation and management of diabetes. This should include a complete physical examination at least once a year and, at each visit, an assessment of overall glycemic regulation, problems with hypo- or hyperglycemia, and a review of the patient's insulin regimen, diet and exercise habits, growth and development, intercurrent illnesses, and self-management skills. Depending on age, children should be taught how to assume appropriate responsibility for their own care and be trained in techniques of self glucose monitoring; adjustment of diet, exercise and insulin regimens; and management of acute complications of diabetes and intercurrent illness.

If diabetes has been present for 5 years or longer, an annual examination by a trained ophthalmologist is indicated to evaluate and treat diabetic retinopathy. Patients should also be screened for the presence of microalbuminuria (defined as a 24-hour albumin excretion of at least 40 milligrams), an early sign of renal damage. Also indicated is a careful neurological examination for detection of early peripheral neuropathy and, in some cases, an evaluation for autonomic neuropathy.

Routine laboratory evaluation should include measurement of glycated hemoglobin as an indication of average glycemic control during the preceding 2 to 3 months, as well as periodic evaluation of lipid profiles, urinalysis, hemograms, and chemistry profiles consistent with current standards of pediatric care.

Other than careful evaluation of glycemic control, the patient's self-management skills, and screening and evaluation of long-term diabetic complications, no special testing is required for children who wish to participate in sport. The major problems for most children with diabetes are appropriate management of blood glucose prior to, during, and following exercise, and the long-term adjustments in diabetic management imposed by rigorous programs of training and competition.

Natural History, Morbidity, and Mortality

When insulin was discovered in 1921 and the first children with IDDM were treated successfully, it was thought that a cure for this once fatal disease had been found. Only after several years did it become evident that numerous long-term complications were occurring and contributing significantly to the morbidity and mortality of diabetes. Microvascular disease in the retina leading to proliferative retinopathy, macular edema, retinal hemorrhage, retinitis proliferans, and impaired vision or blindness occurs in many, although not all, patients with diabetes. The incidence and severity of retinopathy increases with the duration of the diabetes and is related to the level of glycemic control. Likewise, the development of diabetic nephropathy occurs in some but not all patients with diabetes, affecting approximately 35% after a period of 10 to 15 years. Diabetic end-stage renal disease is currently the leading cause of chronic renal failure in the United States, accounting for approximately one third of patients on dialysis therapy. Peripheral sensory neuropathy, motor neuropathies, and autonomic neuropathy develop in a high percentage of patients with diabetes, and there is an increased incidence of macrovascular disease which is associated with a two- to threefold increased risk for myocardial infarction, as well as an increased risk for cerebrovascular accidents and peripheral vascular disease. Thus, diabetes mellitus is associated with significantly increased morbidity and mortality due to long-term complications of the disease.

There is now compelling evidence that the development and/or progression of long-term complications may be significantly reduced by improved glycemic control in patients with IDDM. The Diabetes Control and Complications Trial (10), a large multicenter study carried out in 29 diabetes centers in the United States and Canada, examined whether intensive treatment of patients with IDDM could decrease the long-term complications of diabetes. The goal was to maintain blood glucose concentrations as close to the normal range as possible. A total of 1441 patients with IDDM were followed for up to 9 years and monitored closely for the development or worsening of diabetic retinopathy, nephropathy, neuropathy, hyperlipidemia, and macrovascular disease. The primary prevention cohort consisted of 726 patients with no retinopathy at baseline, and the secondary intervention cohort consisted of 715 patients with mild retinopathy. Patients in both groups were randomly assigned to intensive therapy either with an external insulin pump or by three or more daily insulin injections, plus frequent blood glucose monitoring and diabetic team support or to conventional therapy with one or two daily insulin injections and less stringent monitoring.

In the primary prevention cohort, intensive therapy reduced the adjusted mean risk for the development of retinopathy by 76% compared to conventional therapy. In the secondary intervention cohort, intensive therapy slowed the progression of retinopathy by 54% and reduced the development of proliferative or severe nonproliferative retinopathy by 47%. In the two cohorts combined, intensive therapy reduced the occurrence of microalbuminuria by 39%, that of clinical albuminuria by 54%, and that of clinical neuropathy by 60%. (As noted previously, microalbuminuria is defined as a urinary albumin excretion of at least 40 milligrams over a 24-hour period; clinical albuminuria is defined as an excretion of at least 300 milligrams.) Modest improvements in hypercholesterolemia and hypertriglyceridemia were also observed in the intensively treated groups, but these changes were not statistically significant. The chief adverse event associated with intensive therapy was a two- to threefold increase in severe hypoglycemia reactions. A lesser problem associated with intensive therapy was a somewhat greater gain in weight compared to those patients receiving conventional therapy. Throughout the study the intensively treated group maintained an average glycated hemoglobin (HbA1C) and an average daily blood glucose profile that was significantly lower than in the conventionally treated group. The mean (± SD) value for all glucose profiles in the intensive therapy group was 155 ± 30 mg/dl, as compared with 231 ± 55 mg/dl in the conventional therapy group; HbA1C levels were approximately 2% lower, with a mean of 7.2% vs. 9.1%.

This study has demonstrated conclusively that intensified therapy and improved glycemic control in patients with IDDM has a major impact on the development of long-term complications of diabetes, decreasing significantly the development and progression of retinopathy, nephropathy, and neuropathy, and improving lipid profiles associated with increased risk of macrovascular disease.

Therapeutic Interventions

There are four major goals of therapy in the treatment of IDDM:

- to achieve normal metabolic and biochemical control through appropriate use of insulin, diet and exercise;
- to avoid severe hypo- or hyperglycemic reactions and other acute complications of diabetes;
- to avoid or delay the development of long-term complications; and
- to make it possible for people with diabetes to live a full and satisfying life with their disease.

Numerous insulin preparations are available including human, pork, beef, or beef-pork types. Most patients are now treated with human insulin, which is available in short- (regular and semi-lente), intermediate- (NPH and lente), or long-acting (ultralente) forms. Although some patients are well controlled on one or two injections daily of a combination of short- and intermediate-acting insulin, most require three or four injections to achieve good glycemic control. In some cases, insulin pumps that infuse regular insulin subcutaneously are preferable to multiple injection treatment. Numerous regimens exist and treatment should be individualized to provide the best possible glycemic control and the flexibility to accommodate changes in diet and exercise, and to avoid episodes of hypoglycemia and severe hyperglycemia.

Self blood glucose monitoring before meals, at bedtime, and at other times such as before, during, or after exercise is extremely important so that the patient can make adjustments in insulin dosage and food intake and learn how different types, intensities, and durations of exercise affect blood glucose. Education is an integral part of diabetes care, and should address the effects of diabetes on metabolism; the interactions among insulin, food intake, and exercise; and the skills needed to make management decisions. Members of the health care team must be available to educate and assist patients with management of their disease.

EXERCISE AND DIABETES MELLITUS

Effects of IDDM on Exercise Tolerance and Sport Performance

Shortly after the discovery of insulin, it was observed (19) that exercise potentiates the hypo-glycemic effect of injected insulin and that the combination of insulin and exercise may lead to acute or delayed symptomatic hypoglycemia and decreased insulin requirements in patients with IDDM. More recently, it has also been recognized that exercise may result in a further rise in blood glucose and the rapid development of ketosis in insulin-deficient diabetics in poor metabolic control (3), and that even in well-controlled individuals exercise of high intensity may produce sustained hyperglycemia (27). Because of these problems with the regulation of blood glucose and ketone metabolism during or after exercise, many children with IDDM have found it difficult to participate in sport or other recreational activities in which physical exercise may be intermittent and of varied intensity and duration. In fact, in the past it has not been uncommon that young, physically active, and otherwise healthy people with Type I diabetes have not been allowed to participate in organized athletics and have been discouraged from participating in potentially dangerous recreational sports because of these risks. As more is learned about the multiple neural and endocrine factors that regulate blood glucose and other metabolic fuels during and after exercise, this information can be used to develop strategies to make it both possible and safe for children with IDDM to participate in sport or other forms of vigorous physical activity. Today, with the use of multiple dose insulin (MDI) or insulin pump therapy and self blood glucose monitoring (SBGM), many children and young adults are achieving the same level of athletic training and success in competition as their nondiabetic peers. In cross sectional studies, however, children with IDDM tend to be less physically fit and have lower aerobic capacity than children without diabetes. It is not clear whether this results from a lower average level of physical training in diabetic children (because of inherent problems in blood glucose regulation with exercise), or from subclinical autonomic neuropathy with impaired cardiovascular response to exercise. Most patients with Type I diabetes show normal cardiovascular and peripheral adaptations to physical training, with the possible exception of deficient proliferation of capillaries in skeletal muscle (23), and many have achieved the status of world-class athletes.

Potential Adverse Effects That Can Result From Sports and Exercise

Exercise presents several risks for people with diabetes, and these risks must be weighed against the potential benefits when advising children with diabetes about participation in vigorous physical activity. As already noted, hypoglycemia may occur during or after exercise in insulin-treated individuals, and when exercise is superimposed on the insulin-deficient state rapid increases in blood glucose and the development of ketosis may occur. Even in well-controlled individuals brief periods of high-intensity exercise may cause hyperglycemia.

In adults, exercise may precipitate angina pectoris, myocardial infarction, cardiac arrhythmias, or sudden death if there is underlying coronary artery disease. In addition, several of the long-term complications of diabetes may be worsened by exercise. Individuals who have proliferative retinopathy are at increased risk for developing retinal or vitreous hemorrhages during vigorous exercise, and retinal detachment may occur. Vigorous exercise also increases proteinuria (35), although this is probably a transient hemodynamic response; it is not yet known whether there is any deleterious effect of exercise on the progression of renal disease. In patients with peripheral neuropathy, soft tissue and joint injuries are more likely to occur and may go unrecognized. In those with autonomic neuropathy, physical working capacity may be significantly decreased (32). This is associated with an increased resting pulse rate and a decreased cardiovascular response to exercise (24), lower maximum aerobic capacity ($\dot{V}O_2$max), and an impaired response to dehydration. However, recent epidemiological data from long-term follow-up of children with Type I diabetes suggest that regular physical activity early in life is not associated with an adverse effect on health and may, in fact, be beneficial (18). This had led many diabetologists to recommend that physical exercise be encouraged in people with diabetes if they enjoy it and if there are no specific contraindications, but that exercise not be regarded as part of the therapeutic prescription for every diabetic. Instead, the goal should be to develop educational programs for those with diabetes who want to participate in sport or other forms of physical exercise; in this way, they will be able to maintain good metabolic control before, during, and after exercise and avoid or minimize the various complications.

Precautions to Prevent Adverse Effects

During the past 15 years much new information has been acquired about the hormonal and metabolic adaptations that occur during physical exercise and several excellent reviews have been written on exercise and diabetes (15, 41). As more is learned about the physiology of exercise in normal subjects and the alterations that occur in diabetes mellitus, it is clear that much can be done to make it possible for insulin-treated diabetic patients who wish to exercise to do so with minimal risk. In this section, current concepts regarding the regulation of glucose and other metabolic fuels during and after exercise will be summarized and comparisons made between the normal condition and the abnormalities observed in Type I diabetes mellitus. This information may be used to develop strategies for the management of exercise in children with diabetes who wish to participate in sport or other vigorous recreational activities.

During exercise, numerous cardiovascular, hormonal, and neural responses occur in a highly integrated fashion to ensure the delivery of oxygen and metabolic fuels to working muscle groups, and to remove metabolic end products. Increased oxygen delivery and carbon dioxide removal from tissues are accomplished by increased respiration and cardiac output, redistribution of blood flow, and increased capillary perfusion of working muscles. Metabolic fuels are made available by a more complex system that involves breakdown of glycogen and triglyceride stores within muscle itself and increased delivery of substrates via the blood. Glucose and fatty acids, the major metabolic fuels for muscle, are released into the circulation from the liver and adipose tissue, respectively, and amino acids are made available by increased release from muscle.

In the resting, postabsorptive state, the blood glucose concentration is maintained at a constant level by a closely matched balance between glucose utilization and hepatic glucose production. Approximately 50% of glucose turnover is accounted for by uptake in the brain, where glucose is the major (usually the only) metabolic substrate utilized. Between 30 and 35% is taken up by other tissues including blood cells, kidneys, and the splanchnic bed, while only 15-20% is used by muscles. Hepatic glucose production is maintained by a combination of breakdown of hepatic glycogen stores through glycogenolysis, and the formation of new glucose by gluconeogenesis. In normal subjects in the postprandial state, hepatic glucose production stems predominantly from glycogenolysis, whereas in diabetes gluconeogenesis is much higher and may account for as much as 40% of hepatic glucose production. The major gluconeogenic precursors (lactate, pyruvate, alanine, and glycerol) are derived from glycolysis and oxidation of amino acids in muscle and other peripheral tissues, and from lipolysis in adipose tissue. Free fatty acids are also released by lipolysis and provide a major substrate for energy production.

At rest, approximately 10% of the energy generated in skeletal muscle comes from glucose oxidation; 85-90% comes from the oxidation of fatty acids; and only 1-2% is from amino acids (1). With the onset of exercise, carbohydrate utilization in muscle increases abruptly and is associated with the rapid breakdown of muscle glycogen stores. The marked increase in glycolysis results in lactate formation which accumulates in muscle and is released into the circulation. Within the first few minutes of exercise, blood flow to the muscles is increased, glucose uptake from the circulation occurs, and lactate release declines as aerobic metabolism is established. The increase in glucose uptake by exercising muscles is closely matched by increased hepatic glucose production; blood glucose concentrations stay relatively constant for up to several hours during sustained, moderate-intensity exercise.

The onset of exercise is also associated with the activation of lipolysis in adipose tissue and the release of free fatty acids (FFA) and glycerol into the circulation. FFA concentrations rise and are taken up and utilized by exercising muscle in proportion to their concentration in plasma. Lactate, pyruvate, alanine, and other gluconeogenic amino acids released from both exercising and non-exercising muscle are extracted by the liver and utilized for gluconeogenesis, as is glycerol released from adipose tissue. Several factors influence the relative amounts of carbohydrate and FFA utilized during exercise. These include

- the intensity and duration of exercise,
- the level of physical training,
- the antecedent diet, and
- the effects of meals taken shortly before or during exercise.

As the intensity of exercise is increased, carbohydrate becomes a progressively more important substrate for energy production. During exercise of moderate intensity, i.e., at 50% of $\dot{V}O_2$max, muscle derives approximately 50% of its energy from carbohydrate oxidation. At intensities of 70-75% $\dot{V}O_2$max carbohydrate becomes the predominant metabolic fuel, and when exercise is at or near 100% of $\dot{V}O_2$max nearly all of the energy is derived from carbohydrate oxidation. Amino acids contribute only 1-2% of the energy required for muscular contraction at all intensities of exercise; oxidation of lipids makes up the difference (11). Thus, during very high-intensity exercise, carbohydrate oxidation rates are markedly increased, muscle glycogen stores are depleted rapidly, and glucose uptake from the circulation is high. If hepatic glycogen stores are adequate, hepatic glucose production is able to match or exceed peripheral utilization, and blood glucose concentration remains constant or may actually increase.

With increasing duration of low- to moderate-intensity exercise, muscle and hepatic glycogen stores decline and plasma FFA concentrations increase in conjunction with increased lipolysis in adipose tissue. Fatty acid oxidation by exercising muscle increases gradually and carbohydrate oxidation decreases, so that after 2 or 3 hours of continuous exercise, FFA becomes the major substrate for energy production. With increasing duration of exercise, hepatic glucose production decreases and becomes progressively more dependent on gluconeogenesis, but is usually sufficient to maintain normal blood glucose concentrations. Hypoglycemia rarely develops, although it may occur during prolonged, exhaustive exercise such as long-distance running or cycling. This is usually associated with depletion of muscle and hepatic glycogen stores and the inability of hepatic glucose production to keep up with the high rates of peripheral glucose utilization.

Physical training has a major effect on the pattern of metabolic fuel utilization during exercise. Compared to untrained individuals, trained subjects perform the same amount of work at a lower percentage of $\dot{V}O_2$max and thus utilize less carbohydrate and more FFA. Even when exercising at the same relative intensity, i.e., the same percent $\dot{V}O_2$max, trained subjects utilize less carbohydrate and more FFA than untrained subjects. This results in a slower rate of decline of muscle and liver glycogen stores and is associated with greater endurance.

The antecedent diet is also an important factor in determining substrate utilization during exercise and endurance. A carbohydrate-rich diet is associated with increased rates of carbohydrate oxidation during exercise, and endurance is greater after feeding a high carbohydrate diet than after a high fat diet. The dietary effects on endurance during prolonged exercise are correlated with the pre-exercise muscle glycogen content, an observation that has led to the practice of "carbohydrate loading" by some participating in endurance sports.

Following exercise, glucose uptake by muscle continues to increase, and is utilized to rebuild muscle glycogen stores. Without feeding, muscle glycogen stores are replenished rather slowly, depending on continued hepatic glucose production and maintenance of normal plasma glucose concentrations. With feeding, particularly during the first 2 hours after exercise, muscle glycogen stores are replenished more rapidly, reaching normal levels within 12-14 hours. Ingested glucose is taken up preferentially in previously exercised muscle groups, whereas hepatic glycogen stores recover at a slower rate.

The hormonal response to exercise is a complex, highly integrated system that involves activation of the sympathetic nervous system and the hypothalamic pituitary axis, as well as the suppression or release of a large number of hormones that regulate the mobilization and/or metabolism of glucose, FFA, and amino acids, as well as fluid and electrolyte balance. The magnitude and pattern of the hormonal adaptation to physical activity depends on multiple factors such as the intensity and duration of the exercise performed, and the level of physical training and the physiological state under which exercise is being performed. The latter includes such variables as body and environmental temperature, hydration, the supply of oxygen, and the availability of glucose and other metabolic substrates to working muscles. These responses have been reviewed extensively by Galbo (14) and Sutton and Farrell (34).

The major physiological effects of sympathetic nervous system activation during exercise are to increase heart rate and cause vasoconstriction in the vascular beds supplying the splanchnic circulation, kidneys, and nonexercising muscles. This results in a redistribution of blood flow away from these areas and increases flow to exercising muscle groups. Norepinephrine and epinephrine also play major roles in the regulation of metabolic fuel mobilization and utilization, both by direct and indirect mechanisms (7). Insulin secretion is suppressed by alpha-adrenergic stimulation; lipolysis is stimulated by beta-adrenergic stimulation; and catecholamines stimulate glycogenolysis in both liver and muscle tissue, making glucose available to provide energy for muscular contraction.

Insulin plays a key role in the regulation of metabolic fuel delivery and utilization during exercise. Its secretion is suppressed during physical activity in response to alpha-adrenergic inhibitory effects on the pancreatic beta cells. In addition, increased blood flow to working muscles results in increased insulin delivery to these tissues. The falling insulin concentration in plasma has major effects on glucose, lipid, and amino acid metabolism, making these fuels more readily available for energy production. Insulin is the major inhibitor of hepatic glucose production; the fall in plasma insulin during exercise, coupled with no change or a rise in plasma glucagon, results in increased hepatic glucose output. This is closely correlated with peripheral glucose utilization and maintenance of blood glucose concentration within a normal range. In addition, the falling insulin concentrations decrease the inhibitory effects on lipolysis in adipose tissue and the release of amino acids from muscle. Since little or no insulin is needed for glucose uptake in exercising muscle (29), the fall in plasma insulin concentrations does not impair glucose utilization during exercise.

Glucagon secretion increases during exercise, primarily in response to falling glucose concentration. Glucagon responses are minimal during mild- to moderate-intensity exercise; however, with very high-intensity or prolonged exercise, glucagon concentration increases and plays a role in maintaining glucose homeostasis. Glucagon responses are greater in untrained than in trained individuals. The major role of glucagon is to increase uptake of amino acids in the liver and to stimulate gluconeogenesis. Glucagon also has glycogenolytic activity in the liver and, along with epinephrine, is the major glucose counter-regulatory hormone during exercise (38).

During physical activity, growth hormone and cortisol concentrations also increase and are important in maintaining glucose levels during prolonged exercise. Cortisol and growth hormone antagonize insulin action in peripheral tissues and may serve to limit glucose utilization in nonexercising, insulin-sensitive tissues, making more glucose available to working muscle. Several other hormones also increase during physical activity, although much less is known about their physiological roles or their relevance to metabolic homeostasis during exercise in diabetes mellitus.

Exercise-Induced Hypoglycemia

Whereas changes in blood glucose are very small in normal subjects during exercise, several factors may complicate glucose regulation during and following exercise in patients with insulin-treated diabetes. Exercise potentiates the hypoglycemic effect of injected insulin, and regular physical activity leads to decreased insulin requirements but an increased risk of hypoglycemic reactions in insulin-treated diabetics. Several studies have confirmed that physical training increases sensitivity to insulin. Athletes have normal or increased tolerance to oral glucose in conjunction with low basal and glucose-stimulated insulin responses (21), and physical inactivity rapidly results in decreased glucose tolerance (20). Both normal control subjects and patients with NIDDM have been shown to have a 30-35% increase in insulin-stimulated glucose disposal after physical training when studied by the hyperinsulinemic-euglycemic clamp technique (9). This increase in insulin sensitivity correlates well with the training induced increase in $\dot{V}O_2$max and is thought to be caused primarily by increased glucose uptake by muscle, since no changes have been observed in hepatic glucose production rates.

Acute exercise in untrained subjects is also associated with increased insulin sensitivity and glucose metabolism, which persists for several hours following the exercise (4). This is related both to the need for replenishment of decreased muscle and liver glycogen stores, and to increased glucose metabolism in muscle.

The blood glucose lowering effects of exercise led Joslin (16) and others to advocate physical exercise as a major method of improving blood glucose control in insulin-treated diabetics, and for many years regular physical exercise has been considered, along with diet and insulin, to be a key part of the triad of good diabetic management. Some studies, however, have failed to show a beneficial effect of exercise on long-term metabolic control in Type I diabetes (37, 41), whereas others have shown that a program of regular exercise does result in improved glucose control (25, 33). The questionable effects of physical training in improving long-term glucose control, along with the increased acute risks and complications of exercise, have cast doubts on the concept that exercise should be advocated for all diabetics. Most diabetologists, as already noted, now believe that the best advice is to encourage exercise for those who do not have any significant contraindications and who wish to participate, but not to recommend it for everyone. The youth who wants to exercise and is free of complications should be instructed in the effects of exercise on blood glucose regulation, and strategies should be developed to avoid hypoglycemia during or after exercise and to prevent exercise-induced hyperglycemia. These individuals should also be taught to postpone exercise and take corrective steps when it is contraindicated by poor metabolic control. With proper instruction, careful monitoring, appropriate adjustments in insulin and food intake, and individual experience, many youths with insulin-treated diabetes can learn to exercise safely (see Figure 24.1).

One of the major problems for children with IDDM is that plasma insulin concentrations do not respond to exercise in a normal manner, thus upsetting the balance between peripheral glucose utilization and hepatic glucose production. In normals, plasma insulin concentrations decrease to low levels during exercise. This, in conjunction with constant or increasing plasma concentrations of glucagon, promotes increased hepatic glucose production to match the increased rate of peripheral glucose utilization.

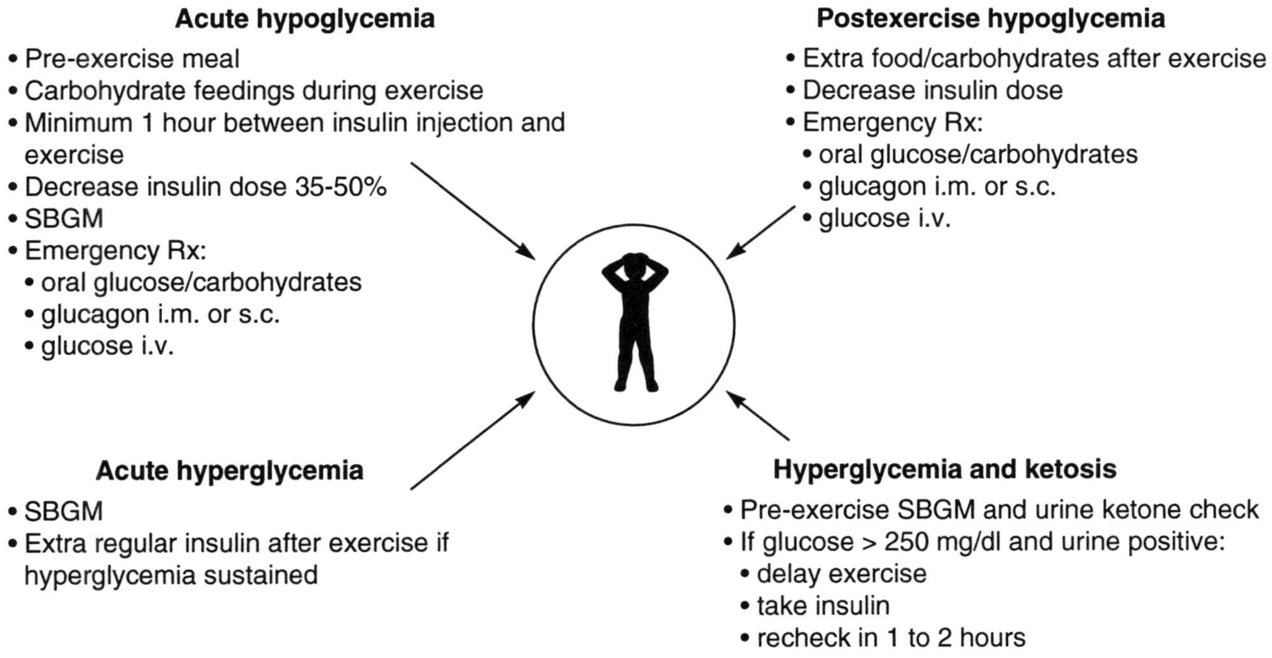

Acute hypoglycemia

- Pre-exercise meal
- Carbohydrate feedings during exercise
- Minimum 1 hour between insulin injection and exercise
- Decrease insulin dose 35-50%
- SBGM
- Emergency Rx:
  - oral glucose/carbohydrates
  - glucagon i.m. or s.c.
  - glucose i.v.

Postexercise hypoglycemia

- Extra food/carbohydrates after exercise
- Decrease insulin dose
- Emergency Rx:
  - oral glucose/carbohydrates
  - glucagon i.m. or s.c.
  - glucose i.v.

Acute hyperglycemia

- SBGM
- Extra regular insulin after exercise if hyperglycemia sustained

Hyperglycemia and ketosis

- Pre-exercise SBGM and urine ketone check
- If glucose > 250 mg/dl and urine positive:
  - delay exercise
  - take insulin
  - recheck in 1 to 2 hours

Figure 24.1 Diabetes-related exercise complications, and strategies for their prevention and treatment.

The low insulin concentration during exercise also increases the lipolytic response to catecholamines, making FFA available for oxidation by exercising muscle, and glycerol available to the liver for gluconeogenesis. In insulin-treated diabetes, plasma insulin concentrations do not decrease during exercise and may even increase substantially if exercise is undertaken within an hour or so of an insulin injection. This results from increased absorption of insulin from the subcutaneous tissue. This effect of exercise on insulin absorption is most marked if regular insulin is used and the injection site is in an exercising part of the body (17). At rest, soluble human insulin is absorbed more rapidly than is porcine insulin, but during exercise this difference disappears, both being absorbed more rapidly than in the resting condition. The increased absorption rate during exercise is not associated with increased cutaneous blood flow, but may be due to mechanical stimulation of the injection site (12).

Enhanced insulin absorption during exercise is most likely to occur when the insulin injection is given immediately before or within a few minutes of the onset of exercise. The longer the interval between injection and onset of exercise, the less significant this effect will be and the less important it is to choose the site of injection to avoid an exercising area. Since there is considerable variation in insulin absorption rates from different injection sites such as the thigh, abdomen, or arm, this may have more of an effect on the rate of insulin absorption than the exercise itself. To avoid this problem, a good plan is to postpone vigorous exercise for at least 60-90 minutes after an insulin injection. However, even with this precaution, plasma insulin concentrations do not fall normally during exercise in insulin-treated patients, and glucose homeostasis may be impaired.

The sustained insulin levels during exercise may enhance peripheral glucose uptake and stimulate glucose oxidation by exercising muscle. However, the major effect is to inhibit hepatic glucose production (40). Both glycogenolysis and gluconeogenesis are inhibited by the high insulin levels and, even though counterregulatory hormone responses may be normal or even enhanced, the hepatic glucose production rate cannot match the rate of peripheral glucose utilization, and blood glucose concentration falls. During mild to moderate exercise of short duration, this may be considered to be a beneficial effect of exercise, but during more prolonged exercise hypoglycemia may result. This is particularly true in some diabetics in whom glucagon deficiency coexists, since the combination of high insulin and low glucagon concentrations may result in decreased gluconeogenesis and impaired hepatic glucose production.

Several factors may affect the epinephrine response to hypoglycemia in youths with diabetes. It is now well recognized that one of the trade-offs for tight metabolic control is an increased incidence of severe hypoglycemic reactions, many of which are associated with exercise. One possible mechanism for the increased incidence of exercise-induced hypoglycemia in patients on intensive insulin therapy is a subnormal response of epinephrine, growth hormone, and cortisol when blood glucose is lowered to 50 mg/dl (31). This observation, coupled with the finding that, in diabetics, epinephrine secretion is stimulated when blood glucose is decreased rapidly from 200 to 100 mg/dl, is consistent with the hypothesis that the preceding plasma glucose concentration has a major effect on the magnitude of the counterregulatory hormone response to a falling blood glucose level. Furthermore, it has been clearly demonstrated that strict control of blood glucose by insulin pump therapy results in a significant decrease in the threshold glucose concentration for epinephrine and growth hormone release, as well as an increase in the sensitivity of the liver to insulin for inhibition of glucose production (2). Thus, intensively treated patients achieve much lower blood glucose concentrations before counterregulatory mechanisms become activated and hepatic glucose production increases.

Another factor which may contribute to exercise-induced hypoglycemia is autonomic neuropathy. Defective autonomic nervous system function has been associated with decreased catecholamine responses and inadequate glucose counterregulation to insulin-induced hypoglycemia in a group of patients who experienced frequent hypoglycemic reactions during intensive insulin therapy (39). In addition, patients with autonomic neuropathy often do not develop the classic warning signs of hypoglycemia before developing severe neuroglucopenia, which further compounds the problem of exercise-induced hypoglycemia.

Strategies to avoid hypoglycemia during prolonged, vigorous exercise include decreasing insulin dosage prior to exercise and taking supplemental carbohydrate feedings before and during exercise. For example, in exhaustive, competitive events such as marathon running, insulin-dependent diabetics may omit their usual insulin dose altogether and start with an elevated blood glucose concentration which gradually falls to a normal range during the first 60 to 90 minutes of the run. As long as insulin deficiency is not severe enough to result in ketosis prior to exercise, metabolic fuel regulation during exercise is fairly normal, although lactate and pyruvate concentrations are greater and several of the glucose counterregulatory hormones (glucagon, catecholamines, growth hormone, and cortisol) increase more in diabetics than in normals (26). This counterregulatory response is probably a key factor in preventing hypoglycemia from occurring.

Since the vast majority of young people with IDDM do not participate in marathon running or similar exhausting events, it is important to develop strategies for managing more moderate forms of exercise. The metabolic responses to moderate-intensity exercise performed 30 minutes after breakfast have been studied in insulin-dependent diabetics and compared to normals (6). In normal subjects the expected postprandial rise in blood glucose and insulin concentrations is rapidly reversed by exercise, returning to fasting levels within 45 minutes. When exercise is stopped, there is a moderate rebound increase in glucose and insulin concentrations which do not exceed those occurring after breakfast alone. Thus, 45 minutes of cycle exercise started 30 minutes after a meal has a significant but transient effect of lowering blood glucose concentrations.

In subjects with IDDM treated with a closed-loop "artificial endocrine pancreas," blood glucose responses following breakfast and in response to exercise are similar to those in normal control subjects, and there is an appropriate 30% decrease in insulin requirement during exercise. When insulin is infused at a constant rate, i.e., not decreased during exercise, symptomatic hypoglycemia occurs, further demonstrating the interaction between insulin and exercise in lowering blood glucose concentrations in insulin-treated subjects (28).

In patients treated with subcutaneous insulin, responses to exercise started 30 minutes after breakfast have been found to be variable, with the majority having improved blood glucose concentrations which persist even through lunch. Some subjects, however, show improved glucose levels only during lunch, and a few show no significant improvement at all (6).

Thus, the effect of postprandial exercise on blood glucose concentrations and the appropriate adjustments in insulin dosage may vary considerably, and individual responses should be determined to achieve improved glucose control and avoid symptomatic hypoglycemia.

Postexercise Hypoglycemia

Another major problem for the youth with insulin-treated diabetes is the occurrence of post-exercise hypoglycemia. Many diabetics experience increased insulin sensitivity and have hypoglycemic reactions several hours following exercise, in some cases even the following day. In one study (22), 16% of 300 young patients with IDDM who were followed prospectively for 2 years experienced postexercise, late-onset hypoglycemia, usually occurring at night 6 to 15 hours after the completion of unusually strenuous exercise or play. Although the mechanism of postexercise hypoglycemia is not well understood, it most likely results from increased glucose uptake and glycogen synthesis in the previously exercised muscle groups, associated with increased insulin sensitivity and activation of glycogen synthase in skeletal muscle (4). Hepatic glycogen stores also recover following exercise but at a slower rate than occurs in muscle, so that increased requirements for dietary carbohydrate may persist for up to 24 hours following prolonged, glycogen-depleting exercise. Various strategies have been used to prevent postexercise hypoglycemia, including decreasing preexercise doses of intermediate- or short-acting insulin and taking supplemental feedings after exercise; however, no universal guidelines are totally effective and treatment regimens must be individualized.

Exercise-Induced Hyperglycemia

In contrast to moderate-intensity, sustained exercise during which blood glucose concentrations remain constant or decrease slightly, short term, high-intensity exercise at 80% of $\dot{V}O_2$max or greater is normally associated with a transient increase in blood glucose levels (27). The rise in blood glucose during exercise reaches a peak 5 to 15 minutes after exercise is stopped, and then gradually returns to the preexercise level within 40 to 60 minutes. This glycemic response to intense exercise results from a marked stimulation of hepatic glucose production, which exceeds the rate of glucose uptake in muscle and is associated with activation of the sympathetic nervous system, a sharp rise in glucose counterregulatory hormones (particularly epinephrine), and a suppression of insulin secretion. The energy for muscular contraction is provided predominantly from glycolysis and from oxidation of glucose derived from breakdown of muscle glycogen stores; glucose uptake from the circulation increases only gradually. Hepatic glucose production, on the other hand, is stimulated rapidly by the decrease in portal vein insulin concentration, an increase in the glucagon to insulin ratio, and the rapid rise in plasma epinephrine. When exercise is stopped there is a rapid, two- to three-fold increase in plasma insulin, which has an inhibitory effect on hepatic glucose production and may enhance postexercise glucose uptake in muscle. As a result, the transiently elevated blood glucose concentration returns rapidly to normal (5).

In the youth with insulin-dependent diabetes this highly integrated response to brief, high-intensity exercise is abnormal, and sustained hyperglycemia may occur. Mitchell, Abraham, Shiffrin, Leiter, and Marliss (27) have studied the effects of exercise to exhaustion at 80% $\dot{V}O_2$max on glucose substrate and hormone responses in Type I diabetics treated with insulin pumps and in normal controls. In contrast to the normals, blood glucose rose to much higher levels during postexercise recovery in the diabetic subjects, and remained elevated for the entire 2-hour postexercise observation period. The pattern of postexercise hyperglycemia was influenced by the initial, preexercise glucose concentration, being considerably greater when the preexercise level was elevated. The most likely mechanism of the sustained hyperglycemic response to the high-intensity exhausting exercise is the absence of any increase in plasma insulin during postexercise recovery in the diabetic subjects.

Since many sports and recreational activities require relatively short periods of very high-intensity exercise, the sustained hyperglycemic response to this type of exercise may present a problem for children with diabetes. At present there are no clear-cut guidelines for prevention or management of this response, although it is possible that the administration of small doses of insulin following exercise might shorten the period of hyperglycemia. Careful self-monitoring of blood glucose levels before, during, and following exercise of different intensities and duration may provide the individual patient with useful information that will allow him or her to develop strategies to minimize the risks of either hyper- or hypoglycemia.

Exercise-Induced Ketosis

Another problem encountered by insulin-treated diabetics occurs when exercise is undertaken in the presence of severe insulin deficiency. In this situation, plasma insulin concentrations are very low or absent, and hyperglycemia and ketosis are present. With the onset of exercise, peripheral glucose utilization is impaired, lipolysis is enhanced, and hepatic glucose production and ketogenesis are stimulated. This results in a rapid rise in the already elevated blood glucose concentration and the rapid development of ketosis (3). In this situation, the already poor metabolic control rapidly becomes worse, and instead of lowering blood glucose the exercise causes a rapid deterioration of the metabolic state. The mechanism for the rapid development of ketosis is not altogether clear, but recent studies suggest that in insulin-deprived individuals there is a defect in peripheral clearance of ketones rather than a marked increase in ketogenesis during exercise (13). To avoid this, the youth with insulin-dependent diabetes should check his or her blood glucose concentration and urine ketones prior to undertaking vigorous physical activity. If blood glucose is greater than 250 mg/dl and ketones are present in urine or blood, the exercise should be postponed and supplemental insulin taken to reestablish good metabolic control. Likewise, if blood glucose is less than 100 mg/dl and the individual has taken insulin within the past 60-90 minutes, supplemental feedings should be taken prior to and during exercise to avoid hypoglycemia.

Strategies for Management of Exercise in Children With IDDM

A list of factors to consider prior to the onset of exercise is provided in Table 24.1. It is obviously impossible to predict all situations since physical

Table 24.1 Checklist for Children With Diabetes Before Starting Exercise

1. The exercise plan
   a. Will the exercise be habitual or unusual?
   b. What is the anticipated intensity of exercise?
   c. How does it relate to the level of physical training?
   d. How long will it last?
   e. Will it be continuous or intermittent?
   f. How many calories will be expended?

2. The plan for meals and supplemental feedings
   a. When was the last meal eaten?
   b. Should a high-carbohydrate snack be eaten before starting?
   c. Should supplemental carbohydrate feedings be taken during exercise? If so, how much and how often?
   d. Will extra food be required after exercise to avoid post-exercise hypoglycemia?

3. The insulin regimen
   a. What is the usual insulin mixture and dosage? Should it be decreased prior to or after exercise?
   b. When was the last insulin injection?
   c. Should the injection site be changed to avoid exercising areas?

4. The preexercise blood glucose concentration
   a. Is the blood glucose concentration in a safe range to exercise (100 to 250 mg/dl)?
   b. If blood glucose is less than 100 mg/dl a preexercise carbohydrate snack should be taken to decrease the risk of exercise-induced hypoglycemia.
   c. If blood glucose is greater than 250 mg/dl, urine ketones should be checked. If they are negative and the high glucose is due to recent food intake it is generally safe to exercise. If they are positive, supplemental insulin should be taken and exercise delayed until ketones are negative and blood glucose is less than 250 mg/dl.

exercise is often spontaneous, intermittent, and varies greatly in intensity and duration from one time to the next. However, a number of strategies which may be useful to avoid either hypo- or hyperglycemia are outlined in Table 24.2. If exercise can be anticipated, ideally it should occur 1-3 hours following a meal when the starting blood glucose is above 100 mg/dl. If exercise is prolonged and vigorous, frequent carbohydrate feedings should be taken during exercise, as well as extra food following exercise, to avoid postexercise hypoglycemia. If exercise is intermittent and of high intensity and short duration, hyperglycemia may be a problem, and small supplemental doses of insulin may be needed during postexercise recovery.

Table 24.2 Suggested Strategies to Avoid Hypo- or Hyperglycemia During and After Physical Exercise

1. Adjustments to the insulin regimen
   a. Take insulin at least one hour before exercise. If less than one hour before exercise, inject in a non-exercising area of the body.
   b. Decrease the dose of both short and intermediate acting insulin before exercise.
   c. Alter daily insulin schedule.
2. Meals and supplemental feedings
   a. Eat a meal one to three hours before exercise and check to see that blood glucose is in a safe range (100 to 250 mg/dl) before starting exercise.
   b. Take supplemental carbohydrate feedings during exercise, at least every 30 minutes if exercise is vigorous and of long duration. Monitor blood glucose during exercise if necessary to determine size and frequency of feedings needed to maintain safe glucose levels.
   c. Increase food intake for up to 24 hours after exercise, depending on intensity and duration of exercise to avoid late-onset postexercise hypoglycemia.
3. Self-monitoring blood glucose and urine ketones
   a. Monitor blood glucose before, during, and after exercise to determine the need and effect of changes in insulin dosage and feeding schedule.
   b. Delay exercise if blood glucose is <100 mg/dl or >250 mg/dl and ketones are present. Use supplemental feedings or insulin to correct glucose and metabolic control before starting exercise.
   c. Learn individual glucose responses to different types, intensities, and conditions of exercise. Determine effects of exercise at different times of the day (e.g., morning, afternoon or evening) and effects of training versus competition on blood glucose responses.

There are no precise guidelines regarding how much carbohydrate should be eaten during prolonged exercise to avoid hypoglycemia. However, one can make some estimate of energy requirements based on the intensity and duration of the physical exercise to be performed. For example, if one is planning to go jogging, cycling, backpacking, or swimming, it might be estimated that the activity will require 600 calories per hour, or 10 calories per minute. This might represent 50% of the patient's maximum aerobic capacity, an exercise intensity at which about 50% of the energy would be derived from carbohydrate oxidation. Thus, the energy requirement from carbohydrate would be approximately 5 calories per minute, equivalent to 1.25

grams of glucose per minute. A 30-minute period of exercise at this intensity would utilize 37.5 grams of carbohydrate, some from glycogen breakdown in muscle and some from circulating glucose. Since glucose uptake by muscle can range from 0.2 to 0.8 grams per minute in a 70-kilogram person during cycling for up to 40 minutes (36), and up to 1.1 grams per minute after 3 hours of cycling at 70% $\dot{V}O_2$max (8), the precise amount of exogenous carbohydrate needed to maintain a normal blood glucose concentration is difficult to determine. Youths, because of their smaller muscle mass, will generally require less exogenous carbohydrate during exercise than adults. However, based on an estimated glucose uptake of 0.5 to 0.8 grams per minute in the example given, the patient might be instructed to eat a carbohydrate snack containing 15 to 25 grams of carbohydrate every 30 minutes to maintain a normal blood glucose concentration during exercise.

This kind of calculation is obviously only approximate, and actual carbohydrate requirements will depend on multiple factors such as the intensity and duration of exercise, the level of physical conditioning, the antecedent diet, the circulating insulin levels, and the relative need for exogenous carbohydrate to maintain blood glucose concentration in a normal range. For example, lower-intensity exercise would decrease the requirements initially, but if exercise is continued for several hours muscle and liver glycogen levels will become depleted and more exogenous carbohydrate will be required to prevent hypoglycemia. It is often very helpful to monitor blood glucose at frequent intervals during exercise of different types and duration to determine individual responses and learn from experience.

If the exercise is planned in advance, the insulin dosage and schedule may be altered to decrease the likelihood of hypoglycemia during or following exercise. Individuals who take a single dose of intermediate-acting insulin may decrease the dose by 30-35% on the morning prior to exercise. Alternatively, they may change to a split dose regimen, taking two-thirds of the usual dose in the morning and one third before the evening meal, if supplemental insulin is needed following the exercise. Those who are taking a combination of intermediate- and short-acting insulin may decrease the latter by 50% or omit it altogether prior to exercise. They may also decrease the intermediate-acting insulin before exercise and take supplemental doses of short-acting insulin later if needed.

For those on MDI therapy with short-acting insulin, the dose before exercise may be decreased by 30-50%, and postexercise doses adjusted based on glucose monitoring and experience with postexercise hypoglycemia. If an insulin pump is used, the basal infusion rate may be decreased during exercise, and premeal boluses decreased or omitted. If this is not done hypoglycemia may occur during exercise (30), although this has not been a universal finding in studies of the effects of moderate-intensity exercise on glucose homeostasis in patients treated with insulin pumps. In practice, both the intra- and postexercise basal infusion rates and the premeal boluses can be adjusted based on glucose monitoring and personal experience. In advising a patient regarding these strategies, it is important to stress the individual nature of the problem and the need for careful glucose monitoring and experience. If exercise patterns are relatively consistent with respect to time of day and the intensity and duration of exercise, a routine program can often be developed to avoid either hypo- or hyperglycemia during the following exercise. If exercise is unusual, then frequent glucose monitoring will be helpful to make adjustments in insulin dosage and the frequency and size of supplemental feedings.

Although children with diabetes are frequently free of any long-term complications of the disease, a final comment should be made about the necessity for a thorough medical evaluation prior to undertaking unusual or particularly vigorous exercise programs. Diabetic children should be screened carefully for the presence of proliferative retinopathy, nephropathy, and both peripheral and autonomic neuropathy, all of which present increased risks for exercise. Some types of exercise should be avoided if specific risks are present. For example, those with proliferative retinopathy should not do heavy lifting or straining, and should avoid positions with the head low or excessive jarring of the head, all of which may precipitate a vitreous hemorrhage. Those with peripheral neuropathy should be particularly careful to avoid cuts, blisters, and pounding exercises of the lower extremities (e.g., jogging

or running sports), and those with autonomic neuropathy should be careful to maintain appropriate fluid and electrolyte balance during prolonged exercise in a warm climate.

Appropriate Response to Adverse Effects in the School and Recreational Environment

In supervising, coaching, or advising children with IDDM who are participating in sport or recreational activities involving exercise, the most important thing is to be aware of the inherent risks of hypoglycemia during or after exercise, to be alert to the signs and symptoms that may occur, and to be prepared to provide assistance if needed. It is also important to recognize the risks of exercise-induced hyperglycemia and ketosis that may occur in children who are insulin-deficient. Knowledge of the normal metabolic responses to exercise and the abnormalities in metabolic fuel homeostasis that occur in IDDM is critical for instructing diabetic children in the skills needed to manage exercise successfully. An appropriate environment and support system must be provided to make it possible for children to coordinate meals and exercise; to perform SBGM before, during, and after exercise if indicated; to test urine for ketones and, if needed, to take food, carbohydrate-containing drinks, or oral glucose to prevent or treat hypoglycemia.

If symptomatic hypoglycemia occurs, supervising individuals should recognize the signs and symptoms and be prepared to assist the child in taking carbohydrate-containing foods, beverages, or glucose tablets. Severe hypoglycemic reactions associated with stupor or loss of consciousness are medical emergencies. If the child is unable to take oral food or fluids, intramuscular or subcutaneous injection of glucagon (1 milligram) and/or intravenous administration of glucose (5-10 grams) by appropriately trained individuals is indicated as an emergency measure. Following oral carbohydrates or treatment with glucagon or intravenous glucose administration the signs and symptoms of hypoglycemia should clear rapidly, usually within 5 to 15 minutes. If the child is unconscious or there is evidence of seizures, appropriate measures must be taken to establish and maintain a clear airway and prevent aspiration. Attempts to provide oral carbohydrates should be avoided because of the danger of aspiration. In this circumstance, glucagon or glucose administration is indicated.

For participation in recreational exercise, physical training, or competition, the guidelines outlined in Tables 24.1 and 24.2 should be followed, making appropriate allowances for individual circumstances and experience. The goal is to ascertain that the preexercise blood glucose level is in an appropriate range and that overall metabolic control is adequate for exercise to be safe. Adjustments in insulin dosage and plans for supplemental feeding before, during, and after exercise are the responsibility of the child and the supervising medical team. However, the coach, teacher, or other supervisory personnel should be aware of the plans and assist in implementing them.

Potential Benefits of Exercise in Diabetes

Regular physical exercise is now recognized as having several benefits to health, not only for those with diabetes but for everyone. In addition to lowering blood glucose and increasing insulin sensitivity, regular exercise improves several of the recognized risk factors for cardiovascular disease. Serum cholesterol and triglyceride concentrations decrease with physical training (an effect attributable to decreases in low-density and very low-density lipoproteins), and high-density lipoprotein cholesterol increases. Also, mild to moderate hypertension improves, resting pulse rate and cardiac work decrease, and physical working capacity increases with physical training. Since young people with diabetes are at increased risk for developing long-term complications of their disease, including premature cardiovascular disease, retinopathy, nephropathy, and neuropathy, all of these effects of regular exercise may have long-term benefits to health and provide the rationale for encouraging exercise as part of daily life. Psychological benefits of exercise such as an increased sense of well-being, improved self-esteem, and an enhanced quality of life are also important for children with diabetes, who have to cope with the anxieties and limitations of living with a chronic disease.

EXERCISE AND SPORT PROGRAMS FOR CHILDREN WITH DIABETES

If a child with diabetes is well educated in the skills of self-management, understands the principles and strategies for regulation for blood glucose before, during, and after exercise, and is well motivated to put them into practice, there are no major limitations to participation in any type of exercise or sport program. Exercise of short duration and moderate intensity is usually well tolerated without major changes in blood glucose concentrations. Hypoglycemia is most likely to occur during prolonged, aerobic exercises such as

- running,
- cycling,
- swimming,
- cross-country skiing, or
- team sports lasting an hour or more.

Intermittent, high-intensity exercise such as occurs in ice hockey, basketball, or soccer may result in hyperglycemia or in hypoglycemia, depending on individual reactions. The use of SBGM and individual experience will allow the child to determine his or her characteristic reaction and to make the appropriate adjustments. While transient or sustained hyperglycemia during exercise is not associated with symptoms or impaired performance, hypoglycemia is, and should be guarded against and treated promptly.

The occurrence of hypoglycemia may be dangerous to the individual in situations requiring mental alertness, neuromuscular coordination, or sustained effort. These dangers should be recognized and minimized by adequate precautions to maintain blood glucose concentrations in a normal range and appropriate supervision and support from others. For example, participation in activities such as scuba diving, long-distance swimming or running, technical mountaineering, and similar activities should be undertaken only with appropriate training and support systems to assist the individual should severe hypoglycemia develop. Each situation should be evaluated on an individual basis, taking into consideration the child's knowledge and skills in self-management, prior experience with blood glucose regulation during exercise, and the support systems available to recognize and treat hypoglycemia if it occurs.

REFERENCES

1. Ahlborg, G.; Felig, P.; Hagenfeldt, L.; Hendler, R.; Wahren, J. Substrate turnover during prolonged exercise. J. Clin. Invest. 53:1080-1090; 1974.

2. Amiel, S.A.; Tamborlane, W.V.; Simonson, D.C.; Sherwin, R.S. Defective glucose counterregulation after strict control of insulin-dependent diabetes mellitus. N. Engl. J. Med. 316:1376-1383; 1987.

3. Berger, M.; Berchtold, P.; Cuppers, H.-J.; Drost, H.; Kley, H.K.; Muller, W.A.; Wiegelmann, W.; Zimmerman-Telschow, H.; Gries, F.A.; Kruskemper, H.L.; and Zimmerman, H. Metabolic and hormonal effects of muscular exercise in juvenile type diabetics. Diabetologia 13:355-365; 1977.

4. Bogardus, C.; Thuillez, P.; Ravussin, E.; Vasquez, B.; Narimiga, M.; Azhar, S. Effect of muscle glycogen depletion on in vivo insulin action in man. J. Clin. Invest. 72:1605-1610; 1983.

5. Calles, J.; Cunningham, J.J.; Nelson, L.; Brown, N.; Nadel, E.; Sherwin, R.S.; Felig, P. Glucose turnover during recovery from intensive exercise. Diabetes 32:734-738; 1983.

6. Caron, D.; Poussier, P.; Marliss, E.B.; Zinman, B. The effect of postprandial exercise on meal-related glucose tolerance in insulin-dependent diabetic individuals. Diabetes Care 5:364-369; 1982.

7. Clutter, W.E.; Rizza, R.A.; Gerich, J.E.; Cryer, P.E. Regulation of glucose metabolism by sympathochromaffin catecholamines. Diabetes/Metabolism Reviews 4(1):1-15; 1988.

8. Coggan, A.R.; Coyle, E.F. Reversal of fatigue during prolonged exercise by carbohydrate infusion or ingestion. J. Appl. Physiol. 63:2388-2395; 1987.

9. DeFronzo, R.A.; Ferrannini, E.; Koivisto, V. New concepts in the pathogenesis and treatment of non-insulin dependent diabetes mellitus. Am. J. Med. 74:52-81; 1983.

10. Diabetes Control and Complications Trial Research Group. The effect of intensive treatment of diabetes on the development and progression of long term complications of insulin dependent diabetes mellitus. New Engl. J. Med. 329:977-986; 1993.

11. Felig, P.; Wahren, J. Fuel homeostasis in exercise. New Engl. J. Med. 293:1078-1084; 1975.

12. Fernqvist, E.; Linde, B.; Ostman, J.; Gunnarsson, R. Effects of physical exercise on insulin absorption in insulin-dependent diabetics. A comparison between human and porcine insulin. Clin. Physiology 6:489-498; 1986.

13. Fery, F.; deMaertelaer, V.; Balasse, E.O. Mechanism of the hyperketonaemic effect of prolonged exercise in insulin-deprived type 1 (insulin-dependent) diabetic patients. Diabetologia 30:298-304; 1987.

14. Galbo, H. Hormonal and metabolic adaptation to exercise. New York: Thieme-Stratton Inc.; 1983.

15. Horton, E.S. Role and management of exercise in diabetes mellitus. Diabetes Care 11:201-211; 1988.

16. Joslin, E.P. The treatment of diabetes mellitus. In: Joslin, E.P.; Root, H.F.; White, P.; Marble, A., ed. Treatment of diabetes mellitus. Philadelphia: Lea & Febiger; 1959:243-300.

17. Koivisto, V.; Felig, P. Effects of leg exercise on insulin absorption in diabetic patients. N. Engl. J. Med. 298:77-83; 1978.

18. LaPorte, E.E.; Dorman, J.S.; Tajima, N.; Cruickshanks, K.J.; Orchard, T.J.; Cavender, D.E.; Becker, D.J.; Drash, A.L. Pittsburgh insulin-dependent diabetes morbidity and mortality study: physical activity and diabetic complications. Pediatrics 78:1027-1033.

19. Lawrence, R.D. The effects of exercise on insulin action in diabetes. Br. Med. J. 1:648-652; 1926.

20. Lipman, R.L.; Raskin, P.; Love, T.; Triebwasser, J.; LeCocq, F.R.; Schnure, J.J. Glucose intolerance during decreased physical activity in man. Diabetes 21:101-107; 1972.

21. Lohmann, D.; Liebold, F.; Heilmann, W.; Senger, H.; Pohl, A. Diminished insulin response in highly trained athletes. Metabolism 27:521-542; 1978.

22. MacDonald, M.J. Postexercise late-onset hypoglycemia in insulin-dependent diabetic patients. Diabetes Care 10:584-588; 1987.

23. Mandroukas, K.; Krotkiewski, M.; Holm, G.; Stromblad, G.; Grimby, G.; Lithell, H.; Wroblewski, Z.; Bjorntrop, P. Muscle adaptations and glucose control after physical training in insulin-dependent diabetes mellitus. Clinical Physiology 6:39-52; 1986.

24. Margonato, A.; Gerundini, P.; Vicedomini, G.; Gilardi, M.C.; Pozza, G.; Fazio, F. Abnormal cardiovascular response to exercise in young asymptomatic diabetic patients with retinopathy. Am. Heart J. 112:554;1986.

25. Marrero, D.G.; Fremion, A.S.; Golden, M.P. Improving compliance with exercise in adolescents with insulin-dependent diabetes mellitus: results of a self-motivated home exercise program. Pediatrics 81:519-525; 1988.

26. Meinders, A.E.; Willekens, F.L.A.; Heere, L.P. Metabolic and hormonal changes in IDDM during long-distance run. Diabetes Care 11:1-7; 1988.

27. Mitchell, T.H.; Abraham, G.; Shiffrin, A.; Leiter, L.A.; Marliss, E.B. Hyperglycemia after intense exercise in IDDM subjects during continuous subcutaneous insulin infusion. Diabetes Care 11:311-317; 1988.

28. Nelson, J.D.; Poussier, P.; Marliss, E.B.; Albisser, A.M.; Zinman, B. Metabolic response of normal man and insulin-infused diabetics to postprandial exercise. Am. J. Physiol. 242:E309-E316; 1982.

29. Richter, E.A.; Ploug, T.; Galbo, H. Increased muscle glucose uptake following exercise: no need for insulin during exercise. Diabetes 34:1041-1048; 1985.

30. Schiffrin, A.; Parikh, S.; Marliss, E.B.; Desrosier, M.M. Metabolic response to fasting exercise in adolescent insulin-dependent diabetic subjects treated with continuous subcutaneous insulin infusion and intensive conventional therapy. Diabetes Care 7:255-260; 1984.

31. Simonson, D.C.; Tamborlane, W.V.; DeFronzo, R.A.; Sherwin, R.S. Intensive insulin therapy reduces the counterregulatory hormone responses to hypoglycemia in patients with type 1 diabetes. Ann. Int. Med. 103:184-190; 1985.

32. Storstein, L.; Jervell, J. Response to bicycle exercise testing of long standing juvenile diabetics. Acta. Med. Scan. 205:227-230; 1979.

33. Stratton, R.; Wilson, D.P.; Endres, R.K.; Goldstein, D.E. Improved glycemic control after supervised 8-wk exercise program in insulin-dependent diabetic adolescents. Diabetes Care 10:589-593; 1987.

34. Sutton, J.R.; Farrell, P.A. Endocrine responses to prolonged exercise. In: Lamb, D.R.; Murray, R., eds. Perspectives in exercise science and sports medicine. vol. 1: Prolonged exercise. Indianapolis: Benchmark Press; 1988:153-212.

35. Viberti, G.C.; Jarrett, R.J.; McCartney, M.; Keen, H. Increased glomerular permeability to albumin induced by exercise in diabetic subjects. Diabetologia 14:293-300; 1978.

36. Wahren, J.; Felig, P.; Ahlborg, G.; Jorfeldt, L. Glucose metabolism during leg exercise in man. J. Clin. Invest. 50:2715-2725; 1971.

37. Wallberg-Henriksson, H.; Gunnarsson, R.; Rossner, S.; Wahren, J. Long-term physical training in female type I (insulin-dependent) diabetic patients: absence of significant effect on glycemic control and lipoprotein levels. Diabetologia 29:53-57; 1986.

38. Wasserman, D.H.; Lickley, H.L.A.; Vranic, M. Interactions between glucagon and other counterregulatory hormones during normoglycemic and hypoglycemic exercise in dogs. J. Clin. Invest. 74:1404-1413; 1984.

39. White, N.H.; Skor, D.; Cryer, P.E.; Bier, D.M.; Levandoski, L.; Santiago, J.V. Identification of type I diabetic patients at increased risk for hyperglycemia during intensive therapy. N. Engl. J. Med. 308:485-491; 1983.

40. Zinman, B.; Murray, F.T.; Vranic, M.; Albisser, A.M.; Leibel, B.S.; McClean, P.A.; Marliss, E.B. Glucoregulation during moderate exercise in insulin treated diabetics. J. Clin. Endocrinol. Metab. 45:641-652; 1977.

41. Zinman, B.; Vranic, M. Diabetes and exercise. Medical Clinics of North America 69:145-157; 1985.

Credits

Borg's RPE Scale on p. 36 from *An Introduction to Borg's RPE Scale* (Table 7.5) by G. Borg, 1985, Ithaca, NY: Mouvement Publications. Copyright © 1985 by Gunnar Borg. Reprinted with permission.

Table 6.1: From "Proposal for Revised Clinical and Electronencephalographic Classification of Epileptic Seizures" by the Commission on Classification and Terminology of the International League Against Epilepsy, 1981, *Epilepsia*, **22**, pp. 489-501. Copyright 1981 by the International League Against Epilepsy. Reprinted with permission.

Tables 6.2 and 6.3: From "Clinical Pharmacology of Antiepileptic Drugs." In *Epilepsy: Diagnosis, Management, Quality of Life* (pp. 22-27) by J.K. Penry (Ed.), 1986, New York: Raven Press. Copyright 1986 by Raven Press. Reprinted with permission.

Figures 9.1 and 9.3: From "Exercises in Patients With Inflammatory Arthritis" by J.E. Hicks, 1990, *Rheumatic Disease Clinics of North America*, **16**, pp. 846, 857. Copyright 1990 by WB Saunders. Reprinted with permission of WB Saunders and J.E. Hicks.

Figure 10.1: Reprinted with permission of HealthScan Products Inc., Cedar Grove, NJ 07009.

Figure 10.3: From "An Evaluation of Pharmacotherapy for Exercise-Induced Asthma" by S. Anderson, J.P. Seale, L. Ferris, R. Schoeffel, and D.A. Lindsay, 1979, *Journal of Allergy and Clinical Immunology*, **64**, pp. 612-624. Adapted with permission of Mosby-Year Book, Inc.

Figure 11.1: From "Cystic Fibrosis" by D. Orenstein, 1991, *Respiratory Care*, **36**(7), p. 748. Adapted with permission of American Association for Respiratory Care, Daedalus Enterprises, Inc.

Figure 11.2: From "Patients With Cystic Fibrosis" by D.M. Orenstein and P.A. Nixon. In *Exercise in Modern Medicine* by B.A. Franklin, S. Gordon, and G.C. Timmis (Eds.), 1989, Baltimore: Williams and Wilkins. Copyright 1989. Reprinted with permission of Williams and Wilkins.

Figure 11.5: From "Hospital Therapy Improves Exercise Tolerance and Lung Function in Cystic Fibrosis" by F.J. Cerny, G.J. Cropp, and M.R. Bye, 1984, *American Journal of Diseases of Children*, **138**(3), p. 262. Copyright 1984 by the American Medical Association. Reprinted with permission.

Table 12.1: From "Human Immunodeficiency Virus in the Athletic Setting" by the American Academy of Pediatrics Committee on Sports Medicine and Fitness, 1991, *Pediatrics*, **88**, pp. 640-641. Copyright 1991 by the American Academy of Pediatrics. Adapted with permission.

Figures 14.1 and 14.2: From *If Your Child Has a Congenital Heart Defect* (#50-1109) (pp. 24, 34) by the American Heart Association, 1991, Dallas, TX: American Heart Association. Copyright 1991 by the American Heart Association. Reprinted with permission.

Table 22.1: From *Diagnostic and Statistical Manual of Mental Disorders* (4th ed.) (pp. 544 and 548-550) by the American Psychiatric Association, 1994, Washington, DC: Author. Copyright 1994 by the American Psychiatric Association. Reprinted with permission.

Table 23.3: From *Pediatric Sports Medicine for the Practitioner: From Physiologic Principles to Clinical Applications*, by O. Bar-Or, 1983, New York: Springer-Verlag. Reprinted with permission.

Index

About the Editor and Contributors

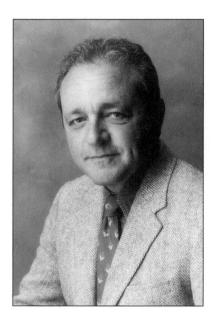

Dr. Barry Goldberg, MD, has spent his career studying sports and exercise activities for children with chronic health conditions and working to enrich their quality of life. In 1964 he received a bachelor's degree in biology/chemistry from Queens College in New York; he earned his medical degree from the Downstate Medical Center in New York City in 1968.

Director of Sports Medicine at Yale University Health Services, Dr. Goldberg is also clinical professor of pediatrics at the Yale University School of Medicine and codirector of the Pediatric Cardiopulmonary Stress-Testing Facility at Yale New Haven Hospital.

As a researcher, Goldberg has published more than 30 scholarly articles in the field, contributing one of the first studies of children with corrected congenital heart disease and their responses to rehabilitation programs that included exercise and physical training. He served as past editor of *Pediatrics in Review* and is the editor of

an ongoing pediatric series for *The Physician and Sportsmedicine*.

Goldberg has been actively involved in establishing guidelines for children's activity. He is chair of the Medical Advisory Committee for U.S.A. Baseball, which establishes policy for all amateur baseball in the U.S. He is also a member of the Executive Committee of the American Academy of Pediatrics section on Sports Medicine and Physical Fitness. From 1986 to 1992 as a member of the American Academy of Pediatrics Sports Medicine Committee, Goldberg was involved in establishing Academy policies for youth sports. He is also a member of the Youth Sports Committee of the American College of Sports Medicine and the Connecticut Sports Medicine Committee, and he serves on the board of directors of the Volvo Grassroots Tennis program.

Goldberg lives with his wife, Betty, and their three children in Orange, CT.

Carol Adams Mushett, MEd
Georgia State University

Bruce S. Alpert, MD
University of Tennessee, Memphis

Balu H. Athreya, MD
Children's Seashore House, Philadelphia, PA

Oded Bar-Or, MD
Children's Exercise and Nutrition Centre
McMaster University, Ontario

Diana S. Beardsley, MD, PhD
Yale University School of Medicine

Donald R. Bennett, MD
University of Nebraska College of Medicine

David S. Braden, MD
University of Mississippi Medical Center

Sarah D. Cohn, JD
Yale-New Haven Hospital

Nancy M. Cummings, MD
University of Massachusetts Medical Center

David Cypcar, MD
Regional Allergy and Asthma Consultants
Asheville, NC

Lawrence J. D'Angelo, MD, MPH
Children's National Medical Center
and George Washington University

Charles C. Duncan, MD
Yale University School of Medicine

John T. Fahey, MD
Yale University School of Medicine

Mary E. Fox, MS
University of Tennessee, Memphis

Sally S. Harris, MD, MPH
Palo Alto Medical Clinic

Edward S. Horton, MD
Joslin Diabetes Center, Boston, MA

Thomas L. Kennedy III, MD
Bridgeport Hospital, Bridgeport, CT

David D. Kilmer, MD
University of California, Davis,
School of Medicine

Nancy E. Lanphear, MD
Genesee Developmental Unit, Rochester, NY

Robert F. Lemanske, Jr., MD
University of Wisconsin Medical School

Gregory S. Liptak, MD
University of Rochester School of Medicine

Nancy S. Mayer, RPT
Children's National Medical Center

Craig M. McDonald, MD
University of California, Davis,
School of Medicine

Michael A. Nelson, MD
University of New Mexico School of Medicine

Eileen M. Ogle, PA-C
Yale University School of Medicine

David M. Orenstein, MD
University of Pittsburgh
and Children's Hospital of Pittsburgh

Arthur M. Pappas, MD
University of Massachusetts Medical Center

Howard A. Pearson, MD
Yale University School of Medicine

Kenneth J. Richter, DO
Michigan State University

Leonard Rieser, JD
Education Law Center, Philadelphia, PA

Thomas W. Rowland, MD
Baystate Medical Center, Springfield, MA

Shirley A. Scull, MS, PT
Children's Seashore House, Philadelphia, PA

Clifford Selsky, MD
Walt Disney Memorial Cancer Center
at Florida Hospital

Norman J. Siegel, MD
Yale University School of Medicine

Arnold T. Sigler, MD
Johns Hopkins University School of Medicine

Tomas Jose Silber, MD, MASS
Children's National Medical Center
and George Washington University School
of Medicine and Health Sciences

William B. Strong, MD
Medical College of Georgia Hospital and Clinics

Reginald Louis Washington, MD
Rocky Mountain Pediatric Cardiology
Denver, CO

Michael Weitzman, MD
University of Rochester School of Medicine
and Dentistry

Duncan O. Wyeth, MA
Michigan Jobs Commission, Lansing, MI

William H. Zinkham, MD
Johns Hopkins University School of Medicine

Important resources on children's physical activity

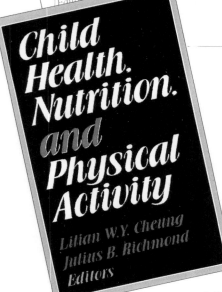

An international forum on current and emerging topics

New Horizons in Pediatric Exercise Science

Cameron J.R. Blimkie, PhD, and
Oded Bar-Or, MD, Editors

1995 • Cloth • 272 pp • Item BBLI0528
ISBN 0-87322-528-7 • $39.00 ($58.50 Canadian)

An important review of current research and practice

Child Health, Nutrition, and Physical Activity

Lilian W.Y. Cheung, DSc, RD, and
Julius B. Richmond, MD, Editors

1995 • Cloth • 392 pp • Item BCHE0774
ISBN 0-87322-774-3 • $35.00 ($48.95 Canadian)

The only comprehensive reference on laboratory and field assessment of children's physical activity

Measurement in Pediatric Exercise Science

David Docherty, PhD, Editor

1996 • Cloth • Approx 376 pp • Item BDOC0960
ISBN 0-87322-960-6 • Call for price

Prices are subject to change.

Human Kinetics
The Information Leader in Physical Activity

2335